Pediatric Endocrinology

CONTEMPORARY ENDOCRINOLOGY

P. Michael Conn, SERIES EDITOR

Pediatric Endocrinology: **A Practical Clinical Guide,** edited by SALLY RADOVICK AND MARGARET H. MACGILLIVRAY, 2003

Androgens in Health and Disease, edited by CARRIE BAGATELL AND WILLIAM J. BREMNER, 2003

Endocrine Replacement Therapy in Clinical Practice, edited by A. WAYNE MEIKLE, 2003

Early Diagnosis of Endocrine Diseases, edited by ROBERT S. BAR, 2003

Type I Diabetes: **Etiology and Treatment,** edited by MARK A. SPERLING, 2003

Handbook of Diagnostic Endocrinology, edited by JANET E. HALL AND LYNNETTE K. NIEMAN, 2003

Diseases of the Thyroid, 2nd ed., edited by LEWIS E. BRAVERMAN, 2003

Developmental Endocrinology: **From Research to Clinical Practice,** edited by ERICA A. EUGSTER AND ORA HIRSCH PESCOVITZ, 2002

Osteoporosis: **Pathophysiology and Clinical Management,** edited by ERIC S. ORWOLL AND MICHAEL BLIZIOTES, 2002

Challenging Cases in Endocrinology, edited by MARK E. MOLITCH, 2002

Selective Estrogen Receptor Modulators: **Research and Clinical Applications,** edited by ANDREA MANNI AND MICHAEL F. VERDERAME, 2002

Transgenics in Endocrinology, edited by MARTIN MATZUK, CHESTER W. BROWN, AND T. RAJENDRA KUMAR, 2001

Assisted Fertilization and Nuclear Transfer in Mammals, edited by DON P. WOLF AND MARY ZELINSKI-WOOTEN, 2001

Adrenal Disorders, edited by ANDREW N. MARGIORIS AND GEORGE P. CHROUSOS, 2001

Endocrine Oncology, edited by STEPHEN P. ETHIER, 2000

Endocrinology of the Lung: **Development and Surfactant Synthesis,** edited by CAROLE R. MENDELSON, 2000

Sports Endocrinology, edited by MICHELLE P. WARREN AND NAAMA W. CONSTANTINI, 2000

Gene Engineering in Endocrinology, edited by MARGARET A. SHUPNIK, 2000

Endocrinology of Aging, edited by JOHN E. MORLEY AND LUCRETIA VAN DEN BERG, 2000

Human Growth Hormone: **Research and Clinical Practice,** edited by ROY G. SMITH AND MICHAEL O. THORNER, 2000

Hormones and the Heart in Health and Disease, edited by LEONARD SHARE, 1999

Menopause: **Endocrinology and Management,** edited by DAVID B. SEIFER AND ELIZABETH A. KENNARD, 1999

The IGF System: **Molecular Biology, Physiology, and Clinical Applications,** edited by RON G. ROSENFELD AND CHARLES T. ROBERTS, JR., 1999

Neurosteroids: **A New Regulatory Function in the Nervous System,** edited by ETIENNE-EMILE BAULIEU, MICHAEL SCHUMACHER, AND PAUL ROBEL, 1999

Autoimmune Endocrinopathies, edited by ROBERT VOLPÉ, 1999

Hormone Resistance Syndromes, edited by J. LARRY JAMESON, 1999

Hormone Replacement Therapy, edited by A. WAYNE MEIKLE, 1999

Insulin Resistance: **The Metabolic Syndrome X,** edited by GERALD M. REAVEN AND AMI LAWS, 1999

Endocrinology of Breast Cancer, edited by ANDREA MANNI, 1999

Molecular and Cellular Pediatric Endocrinology, edited by STUART HANDWERGER, 1999

Gastrointestinal Endocrinology, edited by GEORGE H. GREELEY, JR., 1999

The Endocrinology of Pregnancy, edited by FULLER W. BAZER, 1998

Clinical Management of Diabetic Neuropathy, edited by ARISTIDIS VEVES, 1998

G Proteins, Receptors, and Disease, edited by ALLEN M. SPIEGEL, 1998

Natriuretic Peptides in Health and Disease, edited by WILLIS K. SAMSON AND ELLIS R. LEVIN, 1997

Endocrinology of Critical Disease, edited by K. PATRICK OBER, 1997

Diseases of the Pituitary: **Diagnosis and Treatment,** edited by MARGARET E. WIERMAN, 1997

Diseases of the Thyroid, edited by LEWIS E. BRAVERMAN, 1997

Endocrinology of the Vasculature, edited by JAMES R. SOWERS, 1996

PEDIATRIC ENDOCRINOLOGY

A Practical Clinical Guide

Edited by

Sally Radovick, MD
*University of Chicago Medical Center,
Chicago, IL*

Margaret H. MacGillivray, MD
*Children's Hospital of Buffalo,
Buffalo, NY*

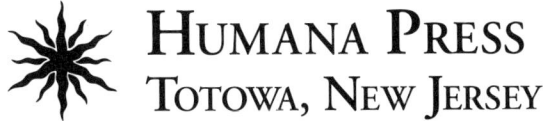

© 2003 Humana Press Inc.
999 Riverview Drive, Suite 208
Totowa, New Jersey 07512
www.humanapress.com

For additional copies, pricing for bulk purchases, and/or information about other Humana titles, contact Humana at the above address or at any of the following numbers: Tel: 973-256-1699; Fax: 973-256-8341; E-mail: humana@humanapr.com or visit our website at humanapress.com

All rights reserved. No part of this book may be reproduced, stored in a retrieval system, or transmitted in any form or by any means, electronic, mechanical, photocopying, microfilming, recording, or otherwise without written permission from the Publisher.

Due diligence has been taken by the publishers, editors, and authors of this book to assure the accuracy of the information published and to describe generally accepted practices. The contributors herein have carefully checked to ensure that the drug selections and dosages set forth in this text are accurate and in accord with the standards accepted at the time of publication. Notwithstanding, as new research, changes in government regulations, and knowledge from clinical experience relating to drug therapy and drug reactions constantly occurs, the reader is advised to check the product information provided by the manufacturer of each drug for any change in dosages or for additional warnings and contraindications. This is of utmost importance when the recommended drug herein is a new or infrequently used drug. It is the responsibility of the treating physician to determine dosages and treatment strategies for individual patients. Further it is the responsibility of the health care provider to ascertain the Food and Drug Administration status of each drug or device used in their clinical practice. The publisher, editors, and authors are not responsible for errors or omissions or for any consequences from the application of the information presented in this book and make no warranty, express or implied, with respect to the contents in this publication.

All articles, comments, opinions, conclusions, or recommendations are those of the author(s), and do not necessarily reflect the views of the publisher.

This publication is printed on acid-free paper. ∞
ANSI Z39.48-1984 (American National Standards Institute)
Permanence of Paper for Printed Library Materials.

Production Editor: Mark J. Breaugh.

Cover Design by Patricia F. Cleary.

Photocopy Authorization Policy:
Authorization to photocopy items for internal or personal use, or the internal or personal use of specific clients, is granted by Humana Press Inc., provided that the base fee of US $10.00 per copy, plus US $00.25 per page, is paid directly to the Copyright Clearance Center at 222 Rosewood Drive, Danvers, MA 01923. For those organizations that have been granted a photocopy license from the CCC, a separate system of payment has been arranged and is acceptable to Humana Press Inc. The fee code for users of the Transactional Reporting Service is: [0-89603-946-3/03 $10.00 + $00.25].

Printed in the United States of America.   10   9   8   7   6   5   4   3   2

Library of Congress Cataloging-in-Publication Data:

Pediatric endocrinology : a practical clinical guide / edited by Sally Radovick, Margaret H. MacGillivray
    p. ; cm. -- (Contemporary endocrinology)
    Includes bibliographical references and index.
    ISBN 0-89603-946-3 (alk. paper)   1-59259-336-4 (e-ISBN)
    1. Pediatric endocrinology. I. Radovick, Sally. II. MacGillivray, Margaret H., 1930–
III. Contemporary endocrinology (Totowa, N. J.)
    [DNLM: 1. Endocrine Diseases--Child. WS 330 P3715 2003]
RJ418 .P435 2003
618.92'4--dc21

                                                  2002032813

PREFACE

The aim of *Pediatric Endocrinology: A Practical Clinical Guide* is to provide practical detailed and concise guidelines for the clinical management of pediatric endocrine diseases and disorders. The audience is thus all those pediatric endocrinologists, pediatricians, and primary care physicians who provide medical care for children and adolescents. The scope of the text includes the most common and the most challenging diseases and disorders seen by both primary care physicians and pediatric endocrinologists. We have encouraged the involvement of a junior coauthor for many articles to give recognition to our young investigators in the field. We believe we have assembled a state-of-the-art book on the "how to's" of pediatric endocrinology.

Although the main focus is on diagnosis and treatment, each author has included a brief discussion on pathophysiology and molecular mechanisms. The chapters are prepared in such a way that there is a consistency of organization. After the introductory discussion of the problem with background information, there is a brief overview of recent progress on the mechanism involved. The clinical features that characterize each condition are discussed. Criteria used to establish a diagnosis are delineated. The therapy section is the most comprehensive and reviews the options available and the risks and benefits of each approach. Outcome data are included as well as information on the long-term safety and efficacy of the treatment modality. Where relevant, psychosocial and quality-of-life issues are discussed.

Sally Radovick, MD
Margaret H. MacGillivray, MD

Contents

Preface v
Contributors xi

Part I   GROWTH DISORDERS

   1   Hypopituitarism 3
       Diego Botero, Olcay Evliyaoglu, and Laurie E. Cohen

   2   Growth Hormone Insensitivity Syndrome 37
       Arlan L. Rosenbloom

   3   Growth Hormone Treatment of Children with Idiopathic Short
       Stature or Growth Hormone Sufficient Growth Failure 67
       *Jean-Claude Desmangles, John Buchlis,
       and Margaret H. MacGillivray*

   4   Growth Hormone Treatment of Children
       Following Intrauterine Growth Failure 79
       Steven D. Chernausek

   5   Growth Suppression by Glucocorticoids:
       Mechanisms, Clinical Significance, and Treatment Options 93
       David B. Allen

   6   Growth Hormone Therapy in Prader-Willi Syndrome 105
       Aaron L. Carrel and David B. Allen

   7   Turner Syndrome 117
       Marsha L. Davenport and Ron G. Rosenfeld

   8   Management of Adults
       with Childhood Growth Hormone Deficiency 139
       David M. Cook

Part II   HYPOTHALAMIC AND PITUITARY DISORDERS

   9   Diabetes Insipidus 155
       Frederick D. Grant

  10   Management of Endocrine Dysfunction
       Following Brain Tumor Treatment 173
       Stuart Alan Weinzimer and Thomas Moshang, Jr.

  11   Endocrinologic Sequelae of Anorexia Nervosa 189
       Catherine M. Gordon and Estherann Grace

Part III	ADRENAL DISORDERS
12	Adrenal Insufficiency 203
	Kathleen E. Bethin and Louis J. Muglia
13	Congenital Adrenal Hyperplasia 227
	Lenore S. Levine and Sharon E. Oberfield
14	Cushing Syndrome in Childhood 249
	Sandra Bonat and Constantine A. Stratakis
15	Mineralocorticoid Disorders 261
	Christina E. Luedke

Part IV	THYROID DISORDERS
16	Congenital Hypothyroidism 275
	Cecilia A. Larson
17	Autoimmune Thyroid Disease 291
	Stephen A. Huang and P. Reed Larsen
18	Resistance to Thyroid Hormone and TSH Receptor Mutations 309
	Ronald N. Cohen
19	Thyroid Cancer in Children and Adolescents 327
	Charles A. Sklar and Michael P. La Quaglia

Part V	CALCIUM AND BONE DISORDERS
20	Abnormalities in Calcium Homeostasis 343
	Ruben Diaz
21	Rickets: *The Skeletal Disorders of Impaired Calcium or Phosphate Availability* 365
	Bat-Sheva Levine and Thomas O. Carpenter

Part VI	REPRODUCTIVE DISORDERS AND CONTRACEPTION
22	Delayed Puberty 383
	Diane E. J. Stafford
23	Precocious Puberty: *Clinical Management* 399
	Henry Rodriguez and Ora H. Pescovitz
24	Management of Infants Born with Ambiguous Genitalia 429
	Margaret H. MacGillivray and Tom Mazur
25	Menstrual Disorders and Hyperandrogenism in Adolescence 451
	Robert L. Rosenfield
26	Contraception 479
	Helen H. Kim

Part VII	METABOLIC DISORDERS
27	Hypoglycemia 511
	Charles A. Stanley

	28	Diabetes Mellitus in Children and Adolescents .... 523 *William V. Tamborlane and JoAnn Ahern*
Part VIII	MEN	
	29	Multiple Endocrine Neoplasia Syndromes .... 535 *Michael S. Racine and Pamela Thomas*
Part IX	ENDOCRINE AND CRITICAL ILLNESS	
	30	The Endocrine Response to Critical Illness .... 551 *Michael S. D. Agus*
	Index 565	

CONTRIBUTORS

MICHAEL S. D. AGUS, MD, *Division of Pediatric Critical Care, Boston Medical Center, Boston, MA*
JOANN AHERN, MSN, APRN, CDE, *Department of Pediatrics and The Yale Children's Clinical Research Center, New Haven, CT*
DAVID B. ALLEN, MD, *Department of Pediatrics, University of Wisconsin Children's Hospital, Madison, WI*
KATHLEEN E. BETHIN, MD, PhD, *Department of Pediatrics, Washington University School of Medicine, St. Louis, MO*
SANDRA BONAT, MD, *National Institute of Child Health and Human Development, National Institutes of Health, Bethesda, MD*
DIEGO BOTERO, MD, *Division of Pediatric Endocrinology, Children's Hospital, Boston, MA*
JOHN BUCHLIS, MD, *Division of Endocrinology, Children's Hospital of Buffalo, Buffalo, NY*
THOMAS O. CARPENTER, MD, *Department of Pediatrics, Yale University School of Medicine, New Haven, CT*
AARON L. CARREL, MD, *Department of Pediatrics, University of Wisconsin Children's Hospital, Madison, WI*
STEVEN D. CHERNAUSEK, MD, *Division of Endocrinology, Children's Hospital Medical Center, Cincinnati, OH*
LAURIE E. COHEN, MD, *Division of Pediatric Endocrinology, Children's Hospital, Boston, MA*
RONALD N. COHEN, MD, *Section of Endocrinology, Department of Medicine, The University of Chicago, Chicago, IL*
DAVID M. COOK, MD, *Division of Endocrinology, Oregon Health Sciences University, Portland, OR*
MARSHA L. DAVENPORT, MD, *Division of Pediatric Endocrinology, University of North Carolina School of Medicine, Chapel Hill, NC*
JEAN-CLAUDE DESMANGLES, MD, *Division of Endocrinology, Children's Hospital of Buffalo, Buffalo, NY*
RUBEN DIAZ, MD, PhD, *Division of Endocrinology, Children's Hospital, Boston, MA*
OLCAY EVLIYAOGLU, MD, *Division of Pediatric Endocrinology, Children's Hospital, Boston, MA*
CATHERINE M. GORDON, MD, MSC, *Divisions of Endocrinology and Adolescent Medicine, Children's Hospital, Boston, MA*
ESTHERANN GRACE, MD, *Division of Adolescent Medicine, Children's Hospital, Boston, MA*
FREDERICK D. GRANT, MD, *Endocrine-Hypertension Division, Brigham and Women's Hospital, Boston, MA*
STEPHEN A. HUANG, MD, *Division of Endocrinology, Children's Hospital, Boston, MA*
HELEN H. KIM, MD, *Department of Obstetrics and Gynecology and Section of Pediatric Endocrinology, The University of Chicago, Chicago, IL*
MICHAEL P. LA QUAGLIA, MD, *Department of Surgery, Memorial Sloan-Kettering Cancer Center, New York, NY*

P. Reed Larsen, MD, *Thyroid Diagnostic Center, Brigham and Women's Hospital, Boston, MA*
Cecilia A. Larson, MD, *New England Newborn Screening Program, Jamaica Plain, MA*
Bat-Sheva Levine, MD, MPH, *Division of Endocrinology, Children's Hospital, Boston, MA*
Lenore S. Levine, MD, *Division of Pediatric Endocrinology, Diabetes and Metabolism, Columbia University College of Physicians and Surgeons, New York, NY*
Christina E. Luedke, MD, PhD, *Division of Endocrinology, Children's Hospital, Boston, MA*
Margaret H. MacGillivray, MD, *Division of Endocrinology, Children's Hospital of Buffalo, Buffalo, NY*
Tom Mazur, PsyD, *Division of Endocrinology, Children's Hospital of Buffalo, Buffalo, NY*
Thomas Moshang, Jr., MD, *Division of Endocrinology and Diabetes, The Children's Hospital of Philadelphia, Philadelphia, PA*
Louis J. Muglia, MD, PhD, *Department of Pediatrics, Washington University School of Medicine, St. Louis, MO*
Sharon E. Oberfield, MD, *Division of Pediatric Endocrinology, Diabetes and Metabolism, Columbia University College of Physicians and Surgeons, New York, NY*
Ora H. Pescovitz, MD, *Section of Pediatric Endocrinology and Diabetology, James Whitcomb Riley Hospital for Children, Indiana University School of Medicine, Indianapolis, IN*
Michael S. Racine, MD, *Division of Pediatric Endocrinology, University of Michigan Medical Center, Ann Arbor, MI*
Sally Radovick, MD, *Section of Pediatric Endocrinology, University of Chicago Medical Center, Chicago, IL*
Henry Rodriguez, MD, *Section of Pediatric Endocrinology and Diabetology, James Whitcomb Riley Hospital for Children, Indiana University School of Medicine, Indianapolis, IN*
Arlan L. Rosenbloom, MD, *Division of Endocrinology, Department of Pediatrics, University of Florida College of Medicine; Florida Department of Health, Children's Medical Services, Gainesville, FL*
Ron G. Rosenfeld, MD, *Department of Pediatrics, Oregon Health & Science University, Portland, OR*
Robert L. Rosenfield, MD, *Department of Pediatrics, The University of Chicago Children's Hospital, Chicago, IL*
Charles A. Sklar, MD, *Department of Pediatrics, Memorial Sloan-Kettering Cancer Center, New York, NY*
Diane E. J. Stafford, MD, *Division of Endocrinology, Children's Hospital, Boston, MA*
Charles A. Stanley, MD, *Division of Endocrinology/Diabetes, The Children's Hospital of Philadelphia, Philadelphia, PA*
Constantine A. Stratakis, MD,D(MED)SC, *National Institute of Child Health and Human Development, National Institutes of Health, Bethesda, MD*
William V. Tamborlane, MD, *Department of Pediatrics, Pediatric Pharmacology Research Unit and Children's Clinical Research Center, Yale University School of Medicine, New Haven, CT*
Pamela Thomas, MD, *Division of Pediatric Endocrinology, University of Michigan Medical Center, Ann Arbor, MI*
Stuart Alan Weinzimer, MD, *Department of Pediatrics, Yale University School of Medicine, New Haven, CT*

I GROWTH DISORDERS

1 Hypopituitarism

Diego Botero, MD, Olcay Evliyaoglu, MD, and Laurie E. Cohen, MD

CONTENTS

INTRODUCTION
GH PHYSIOLOGY
GROWTH HORMONE DEFICIENCY
DIAGNOSIS OF GROWTH HORMONE DEFICIENCY
GH THERAPY
GH REPLACEMENT IN ADULTS
CONCLUSIONS
REFERENCES

INTRODUCTION

The pituitary gland is formed of anterior (adenohypophysis) and posterior (neurohypophysis) parts, which are embryologically derived from two different sources *(1)*. The primordium of the anterior pituitary, Rathke's pouch, forms by the upward invagination of the stomodeal ectoderm in the region of contact with the neuroectoderm of the primordium of the ventral hypothalamus *(2)*. Rathke's pouch can be identified by the third week of pregnancy *(3)*. The posterior pituitary arises from the neural ectoderm of the forebrain.

The anterior pituitary is formed of three parts; the pars distalis (pars anterior or anterior lobe), the pars intermedia (intermediate lobe), and the pars tuberalis (pars infundibularis or pars proximalis), and forms 80% of the pituitary gland. In humans, the pars distalis is the largest part of the anterior pituitary and is where most of the anterior pituitary hormones are produced *(3)*. The intermediate lobe is poorly developed in humans and although it is only a rudimentary vestige in adults, it is relatively obvious in pregnant women and in the fetus *(4)*. The upward extension of the pars distalis onto the pituitary stalk forms the pars tuberalis, which may contain a small number of gonadotropin-producing cells *(3)*.

Peptides produced in neurons of the hypothalamus are transported via a capillary plexus in the pituitary stalk to the anterior pituitary, where they regulate the release of several hormones that are synthesized there *(5)*. These hormones are somatotropin (growth hormone, GH), prolactin (PRL), thyrotropin (thyroid-stimulating hormone, TSH), fol-

From: *Contemporary Endocrinology: Pediatric Endocrinology: A Practical Clinical Guide*
Edited by: S. Radovick and M. H. MacGillivray © Humana Press Inc., Totowa, NJ

licle-stimulating hormone (FSH), luteinizing hormone (LH), and adrenocorticotropin (ACTH). Posterior pituitary hormones are synthesized in cell bodies of neurons in the hypothalamus and transported along their axons through the neurohypophyseal tract of the pituitary stalk. These hormones, arginine vasopressin (antidiuretic hormone, DDAVP) and oxytocin, are stored in and secreted from the posterior pituitary *(6)*.

Hypopituitarism is the deficiency in varying degrees of any or multiple pituitary hormones. In this chapter, GH deficiency will be discussed, while other hormonal deficiencies are presented elsewhere in this book. To understand GH deficiency, an understanding of the growth hormone axis is important.

GH PHYSIOLOGY
GH Gene

GH is the most abundant hormone in the pituitary. It is a single-chain α-helical non-glycosylated polypeptide with 191 amino acids and two intramolecular disulfide bonds, with a molecular weight of 22 kDa. This mature hormone accounts for 75% of the GH produced in the pituitary gland *(3)*. The 20 kDa variant arises from alternative splicing of one of the intervening sequences during the processing of hGH pre-mRNA and differs from the 22 kDa form by deletion of amino acids 32–46. The 20 kDa form constitutes 10–25% of the total pituitary human(h) GH *(7,8)*. The remainder of the GH produced by the pituitary is in the N-acetylated and desaminated forms and oligomers *(3)*. Secreted GH circulates both unbound and attached to binding proteins of several sizes, which are portions of the extracellular domain of the GH receptor (GH-R) *(9)*.

GH is encoded by the *GH-1* gene. It is part of a 50-kb cluster of five genes located on human chromosome 17q22-24 that evolved from a series of three sequential gene duplications followed by sequence divergence: 5' to 3', they are *GH-1, chorionic somatomammotropin-like (CS-L), CS-A, GH-2,* and *CS-B (10)*. The *CS-L* gene is translated and undergoes alternative splicing, but the resultant protein products appear nonfunctional *(11)*. The *CS-A* and *CS-B* genes are placentally expressed and encode human chorionic somatomammotropin (hCS), also known as human placental lactogen. hCS is produced in massive amounts by syncytiotrophoblastic cells. hCS has 85% homology to GH-N and also contains two disulfide bonds that occur at the same positions as in GH-N, but it only has 0.5% the affinity for the GH-R. hCS production is shared by both genes, and deletion of both genes is necessary to have hCS deficiency. hCS is present in very high concentrations in maternal serum. Complete deficiency of hCS during pregnancy is associated with the presence of a normal growth pattern during fetal life and infancy, suggesting that hCS is not required for fetal or extrauterine growth. It also does not appear essential for maintenance of pregnancy or lactation *(12)*. The *GH-2* gene product is known as GH variant (GH-V) and differs from GH-N by 13 amino acids that are distributed along its peptide chain. It is expressed as at least four alternatively-spliced mRNAs in the placenta and is continuously secreted during the second half of pregnancy, suppressing maternal pituitary *GH-1* gene function *(13,14)*.

GH Secretion (Fig. 1)

GH secretion is under the control of two hypothalamic hormones: growth hormone releasing hormone (GHRH) and somatotropin release-inhibiting factor (SRIF), also known as somatostatin (sst).

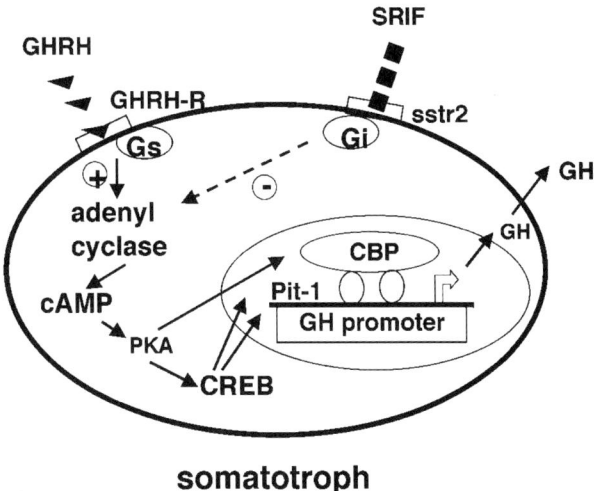

Fig. 1. Simplified model of GH gene activation. GH synthesis and release from somatotrophs is regulated by GHRH stimulation and SRIF inhibition. GHRH activation of its Gs-protein coupled receptor leads to an increase in cAMP and intracellular calcium resulting in activation of PKA. PKA phosphorylates and activates CREB, which binds to cAMP response elements in the *GH* promoter to enhance *GH-1* gene transcription. There is also a PKA-dependent, CREB-independent mechanism of human *GH* gene activation by Pit-1 and CBP. SRIF activation of its Gi-coupled protein leads to a decrease in cAMP and a reduction in calcium influx.

GHRH is a 44 amino acid protein with high homology to members of the vasoactive intestinal polypeptide/glucagon family of peptides *(15)*. GHRH binds to the GHRH receptor (GHRH-R), a G-protein-coupled receptor with seven transmembrane spanning domains with three extracellular and three cytoplasmic loops *(16)*. On binding GHRH, the GHRH-R activates a Gs-coupled protein with a resultant increase in cAMP and intracellular calcium, leading to activation of protein kinase A (PKA) *(17,18)*. PKA phosphorylates and activates cyclic AMP-response element binding protein (CREB), which binds to cAMP response elements in the *GH* promoter to enhance *GH-1* gene transcription *(19,20)*. There is also a PKA-dependent, CREB-independent mechanism of *hGH* gene activation by Pit-1 and CREB binding protein (CBP) *(21)*.

SRIF is a 14 amino acid neuropeptide that regulates GH-mediated negative feedback. Via the SRIF receptor (sstr) subtype 2 *(22)*, SRIF activates a Gi-coupled protein *(23, 24)*, which decreases cyclic (cAMP) *(25)* and reduces calcium influx *(25)* resulting in inhibition of GH secretion. SRIF controls the pulse frequency of GH *(26,27)*.

Infants have nonpulsatile GH secretion. GH pulse frequency and amplitude decrease and tonic secretion diminishes *(28)* until a pulsatile pattern of GH secretion is seen in prepubertal children *(29)*. There is a gradual increase in 24-h integrated GH secretion during childhood, and the amplitudes of GH pulses are increased during puberty, probably secondary to the effect of gonadal steroids on GHRH *(30–32)*. hGH production continues throughout life, but declines with age *(33,34)*.

GH-releasing peptides (GHRP) or GH-secretagogues (GHS) are man-made ligands that stimulate GH release but do not act through the GHRH or SRIF receptors. GHS receptor (GHS-R) ligands regulate GHRH release by initiating and amplifying pulsatile

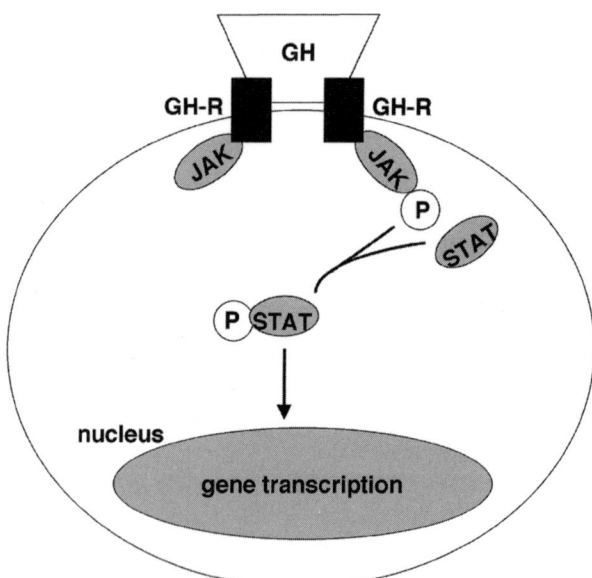

Fig. 2. Schematic model of GH-R binding and signaling. A single GH molecule binds asymmetrically to the extracellular domain of two receptor molecules, causing the receptor to dimerize. Dimerization triggers interaction of the GH-R with Jak 2 and tyrosine phosphorylation of both Jak2 and the GH-R, followed by phosphorylation of cytoplasmic transcription factors known as STATS. After phosphorylation, STATs dimerize and move to the nucleus, where they activate gene transcription.

GH release *(35)*. Their receptor, GHS-R, was identified after their invention. The GHS-R is a seven transmembrane G-protein-coupled receptor that acts via protein kinase C activation and is expressed in the hypothalamus, including the arcuate nucleus, and in pituitary somatotrophs *(36)*.

Recently, an endogenous ligand for GHS-R was purified and identified from the rat stomach. It was named ghrelin, which is the Proto-Indo-European root of "grow" *(37)*. Ghrelin stimulates GH secretion from rat pituitary cells through an increase in intracellular calcium. Ghrelin-producing neurons have been identified in the hypothalamic arcuate nucleus, and ghrelin appears to be a physiological mediator of feeding *(38)*.

GH Action (Fig. 2)

At least 50% of circulating GH is bound to GH-binding protein (GHBP). GHBP is the extracellular domain of the GH receptor (GH-R) found circulating in the serum as a soluble form *(9)*. The source or mechanism of generation of GHBP is not entirely known. It may be shed from membrane-bound receptors by proteolytic cleavage or synthesized *de novo* from an alternatively spliced receptor mRNA.

The GH-R belongs to the cytokine family of receptors *(39)*. It is a 620 amino acid protein localized on the plasma membrane of GH-responsive cells. It has a large extracellular domain, a single transmembrane helix, and an intracellular domain *(40)*. A single GH molecule binds asymmetrically to the extracellular domain of two receptor molecules, causing the receptor to dimerize. Dimerization triggers interaction of the GH-R with Janus kinase (Jak 2) and tyrosine phosphorylation of both Jak2 and the GH-R *(41–44)*, followed by phosphorylation of cytoplasmic transcription factors known as signal transducers and activators of transcription (STATS). After phosphorylation, STATs dimerize, move to the nucleus, and activate gene transcription *(45,46)*.

Many of the actions of GH are mediated by insulin-like growth factors (IGFs) or somatomedins, which were first identified by their ability to incorporate sulfate into rat cartilage *(47)*. Because of their resemblance to proinsulin, these peptides were named insulin-like growth factors *(48)*. The actions of GH on extrauterine growth are primarily through stimulation of production of IGF-1, a basic 70 amino acid peptide *(49)*.

Human fetal serum IGF-1 level is relatively low and is positively correlated with gestational age *(50,51)*. In newborns, serum IGF-1 levels are 30%–50% of adult levels. During childhood, serum IGF-1 levels gradually increase, reaching adult values at the onset of puberty. Gonadal steroids increase IGF-1 production, contributing to the pubertal growth spurt. During puberty, serum IGF-1 levels peak achieving two to three times adult values *(52,53)*. After adolescence, serum IGF-1 concentrations decline gradually with age *(54,55)*. Both systemic IGF-1 *(56)*, predominantly produced by the liver, and local IGF-1 *(57–60)* stimulate longitudinal bone growth by increased osteoblast activity and increased collagen synthesis in bone *(61)*.

In serum, IGFs are complexed to high-affinity binding proteins (IGFBPs). IGFBPs serve to extend an IGFs serum half-life, to transport IGFs to target cells *(62)*, and to modulate the IGFs interaction with their receptors by competing with IGF receptors for IGF peptides *(63)*. Six distinct human and rat IGFBPs have been cloned and sequenced *(64,65)*. The concentrations of the different types of IGFBPs are variable in different biological fluids. IGFBP-3 is the major IGFBP in human serum and transports over 90% of the circulating IGF-1 *(3)*. IGFBP-3 is GH-dependent *(3)*.

The IGF-1 receptor is structurally related to the insulin receptor with two alpha subunits and two beta subunits *(66, 67)*. The alpha subunits are linked by disulfide bonds and contain binding sites for IGF-1. The beta subunits are composed of a transmembrane domain, an ATP binding site, and a tyrosine kinase domain. The tyrosine kinase domain is responsible for transduction of the presumed signal *(3,68)*.

GROWTH HORMONE DEFICIENCY

Hypopituitarism can be caused by anything that damages the hypothalamus, pituitary stalk, or pituitary gland. The incidence of congenital GH deficiency has been reported as between 1:4000 and 1:10,000 live births *(69,70)*. Growth failure is the most common sign of GH deficiency presenting in infancy and childhood. Children with mild GH deficiency usually present after 6 mo of age, when the influences of maternal hormones wane *(71)*. They generally have normal birth weights, with slightly below average lengths *(72)*. The growth rate of a child with GH deficiency will progressively decline, and typically the bone age will be delayed. They develop increased peri-abdominal fat *(73)* and decreased muscle mass, and may also have delayed dentition, thin hair, poor nail growth, and a high-pitched voice *(71)*. Severe GH deficiency in the newborn period may be characterized by hypoglycemia and conjugated hyperbilirubinemia, as well as a small phallus in boys, consistent with multiple anterior pituitary hormone deficiencies *(71)*.

Acquired Forms of Hypopituitarism (Table 1)

Head trauma can damage the pituitary stalk and infundibulum and can lead to the development of transient and permanent diabetes insipidus, as well as other hormonal deficiencies *(74,75)*. There are a number of reports suggesting an association between hypopituitarism and complicated perinatal course, especially breech delivery *(69,76,*

Table 1
Etiologies of GH Deficiency

Trauma	Cranial and central nervous system abnormalities
head injury	septo-optic dysplasia
perinatal events	cleft lip +/– palate
Infiltrative and autoimmune diseases	empty sella syndrome
Langerhans histiocytosis	holoprosencephaly, anencephaly
sarcoidosis	pituitary aplasia or hypoplasia
lymphocytic hypophysitis	thin or absent pituitary stalk
	hydrocephalus
Infections	
meningitis	Genetic (mutations, deletions)
granulomatous diseases	GRHR receptor
	pituitary transcription factors
Metabolic	Rpx/Hesx1
hemachromatosis	Ptx2/Rieg
cerebral edema	Lhx3/Lim-3/P-LIM
	Prop-1
Neoplasms	Pit-1/GHF-1
craniopharyngioma	GH-1 gene
germinoma	types Ia, Ib, II, and III
hypothalamic astrocytoma/optic glioma	multiple GH family gene deletions
	bioinactive GH
Cranial Irradiation	GH receptor
	IGF-1
Idiopathic	IGF-1 receptor

77). It is not clear if a complicated perinatal course causes hypopituitarism, or if a brain anomaly leads to both complicated delivery and hypopituitarism. The finding that some of these patients have a microphallus at birth suggests pituitary dysfunction may precede the birth trauma *(6)*.

Infiltrative conditions can also disrupt the pituitary stalk. Diabetes insipidus can be the first manifestation of Langerhans cell histiocytosis *(78–80)* or sarcoidosis *(81)*. Lymphocytic hypophysitis, usually in adult women in late pregnancy or the postpartum period, can result in hypopituitarism *(82)*.

Metabolic disorders can cause hypopituitarism through destruction of the hypothalamus, pituitary stalk, or pituitary. Hemochromatosis is characterized by iron deposition in various tissues, including the pituitary. It may be idiopathic or secondary to multiple transfusions (e.g., for thalassemia major). Gonadotropin deficiency is the most common hormonal deficiency, but GH deficiency has also been described *(83,84)*.

Hypothalamic or pituitary tissue can also be destroyed by the mass of suprasellar tumors or by their surgical resection. These tumors include craniopharyngiomas, low-grade gliomas/hypothalamic astrocytomas, germ-cell tumors, and pituitary adenomas *(85)*. Treatment of brain tumors or acute lymphoblastic leukemia (ALL) with cranial irradiation may also result in GH deficiency. Lower doses preserve pharmacologic response of GH to stimulation, but spontaneous GH secretion may be lost *(86)*. The higher the radiation dose, the more likely and the earlier GH deficiency will occur after treatment *(87,88)*. Clayton et al. reported that 84% of children who received greater than 3000 cGy to the hypothalamopituitary area had evidence of GH deficiency more than five years after irradiation *(87)*. The higher the dose, the more likely the development of other anterior pituitary hormone deficiencies as well *(88)*. Cranial radiation can also be associated with precocious puberty leading to premature epiphyseal fusion *(86)*, and spinal irradiation can lead to skeletal impaired spinal growth *(89)*, both of which will further compromise adult height.

Congenital Forms of Hypopituitarism (Table 1)

Cranial malformations, such as holoprosencephaly, septo-optic dysplasia (SOD), and midline craniocerebral or midfacial abnormalities can be associated with anomalies of the pituitary gland. Embryonic defects such as pituitary hypoplasia, pituitary aplasia, and congenital absence of the pituitary gland can also occur *(6)*. Although the etiology of these conditions is often unknown, it has recently been recognized that some have a genetic basis.

Multiple molecular abnormalities have been found in many of the factors involved in the GH axis. To date, no mutations in GHRH, SRIF, or the sstr have been identified.

GHRH Receptor Mutations

There is a mouse strain, the *little* dwarf mouse, that has an autosomal recessive missense mutation at codon 60 (aspartic acid to glycine) preventing hypothalamic GHRH binding *(90,91)*. These mice exhibit postnatal growth failure and delayed pubertal maturation. There is biochemical evidence of GH deficiency with high levels of GHRH *(91)*.

A consanguineous Indian Moslem kindred has a nonsense mutation at codon 72 (glutamic acid to a stop codon) yielding a truncated GHRH-R that lacks the membrane spanning regions and a G-protein site *(92)*. A similar mutation is found in codon 50 in "Dwarfism of Sindh" *(93)*.

Pituitary Transcription Factor Mutations

Several pituitary-specific transcription factors play a role in the determination of the pituitary cell lineages (Fig. 3), and patients with hypopituitarism have been found to have mutations in them.

Rpx, also known as *Hesx1*, is a member of the paired-like class of homeobox genes originally described in *Drosophila melanogaster (94)*. It is the earliest known specific marker for the pituitary primordium, suggesting that it has a role in early determination or differentiation of the pituitary *(95)*, although no target genes for *Rpx* have yet been identified *(96)*. Mice lacking Rpx have abnormalities in the corpus callosum, anterior and hippocampal commisures, and septum pellucidum similar to the defects seen in SOD in man *(94)*. Two siblings with agenesis of the corpus callosum, optic nerve hypoplasia, and panhypopituitarism were found to have a homozygous mutation at codon 53 (arginine to cysteine) in the homeodomain (DNA binding domain) of *Hesx1* resulting in a drastic reduction in DNA binding *(94)*.

Thomas et al. scanned 228 patients with a wide spectrum of congenital hypopituitarism phenotypes: 85 with isolated pituitary hypoplasia (including isolated GH deficiency and combined pituitary hormone deficiency [CPHD]), 105 with SOD, and 38 with holoprosencephaly or related phenotypes. They identified three missense mutations: 1)

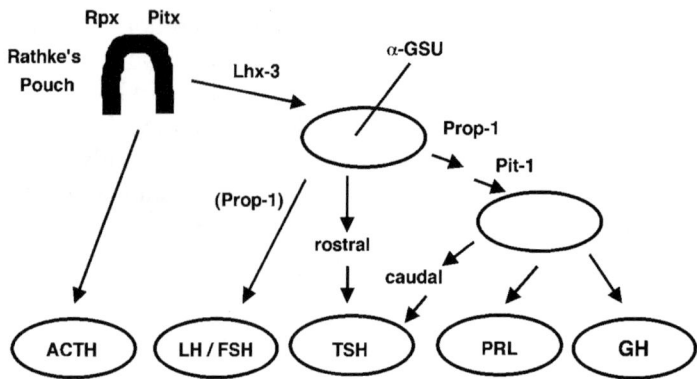

Fig. 3. Anterior pituitary development. Several pituitary-specific transcription factors play a role in the determination of the pituitary cell lineages. Rpx (also known as Hesx1) is the earliest known specific marker for the pituitary primordium, suggesting that it has a role in early determination or differentiation of the pituitary. Ptx (also known as Pitx and P-OTX) has two subtypes, Ptx1 and Ptx2, both present in the fetal and adult pituitary. Ptx2 is expressed in the thyrotrophs, gonadotrophs, somatotrophs, and lactotrophs. Lhx3 (also known as LIM-3 and P-Lim) appears to have a maintenance function in the gonadotrophs, thyrotrophs, somatotrophs, and lactotrophs. Prop-1 is required for somatotroph, lactotroph, and thyrotroph determination and appears to have a role in gonadotroph differentiation. Pit-1 (also known as GHF-1, POU1F1) has been shown to be essential for the development of somatotrophs, lactotrophs, and thyrotrophs, as well as for their cell specific gene expression and regulation.

a serine to leucine at codon 170, located immediately C-terminal to the homeodomain, was identified in two affected brothers, both with GH deficiency and one with optic nerve hypoplasia; 2) a threonine to alanine at codon 181 (T181A) was identified in one patient with isolated GH deficiency; and 3) a glutamine to histidine at codon 6 causing a non-conservative substitution in exon 1 was identified in an individual with multiple pituitary hormone deficiencies. All affected individuals had inherited the mutation from one of their parents, who were not affected, and the T181A mutation was identified in a non-affected sibling *(97)*. These sequence changes may represent polymorphisms that do not compromise Hesx1 function. However, 100 control sequences were identical to previously published wild type data. Incomplete penetrance would not be surprising, given that heterozygous Rpx+/– mice display low penetrance of a mild phenotype *(97)*.

Ptx2 (Pitx2, P-OTX2) is a paired-like homeodomain transcription factor closely related to the mammalian *Otx* genes that are expressed in the rostral brain during development and are homologous to the *Drosophila orthodenticle (otd)* gene essential for the development of the head in *Drosophila melanogaster (98)*. Ptx2 is present in the fetal pituitary and is expressed in the adult pituitary gland in the thyrotrophs, gonadotrophs, somatotrophs, and lactotrophs, but not in the corticotrophs *(99)*, as well as in the adult kidney, lung, testis, and tongue *(100)*.

RIEG is the human homolog of Ptx2. In individuals with Rieger syndrome, an autosomal dominant condition with variable manifestations including anomalies of the anterior chamber of the eye, dental hypoplasia, a protuberant umbilicus, mental retardation, and pituitary alterations, six mutations in one allele of RIEG have been found *(101)*. Five mutations were found to affect the homeobox region: three were missense mutations causing nonconsensus amino acid changes in the homeodomain, and two were splicing mutations in the intron dividing the homeobox sequence *(102)*. Two of the missense mutations have been studied: the first, a leucine to histidine at codon 54 in helix 1 of the homeodomain, leads to an unstable protein; the other, a threonine to proline at codon 68 in helix 2 of the homeodomain only mildly diminishes DNA binding but impairs transactivation of the *PRL* promoter. GH promoter activity was not evaluated, but since there is GH insufficiency in a subset of affected individuals with Rieger syndrome, Ptx2 may also have a role in activation of the *GH* gene *(101)*.

Lhx3, also known as LIM-3 and P-Lim, is a LIM-type homeodomain protein *(103–105)*. The LIM proteins contain two tandomly repeated unique cysteine/histidine LIM domains located between the N-terminus and the homeodomain that may be involved in transcriptional regulation *(103)*. During development, there is Lhx3 expression in the anterior and intermediate lobes of the pituitary gland, the ventral hindbrain, and the spinal cord. *Lhx3* expression persists in the adult pituitary, suggesting a maintenance function in one or more of the anterior pituitary cell types *(103)*. Lhx3 is expressed in GH_1 cells, which secrete GH, GH_3 cells which secrete GH and PRL, and α-TSH cells which express the α-glycoprotein subunit (α-GSU) *(103)*, suggesting a common cell precursor for gonadotrophs, thyrotrophs, somatotrophs, and lactotrophs *(106)*.

Patients with complete deficits of GH, PRL, TSH, and gonadotropins and a rigid cervical spine leading to limited head rotation have been found to have mutations in the *Lhx3* gene. A tyrosine to cysteine at codon 116 (Y116C) in the LIM2 domain is associated with a hypoplastic anterior pituitary. An intragenic 23 amino acid deletion predicting a severely truncated protein lacking the entire homeodomain is associated with an enlarged pituitary (107). Whereas the intragenic gene deletion mutant protein does not bind DNA, the Y116C mutant does. Both mutant Lhx3 proteins have a reduced gene activation capacity *(108)*.

Prop-1 is a paired-like homeodomain transcription factor *(109)*. Prop-1 expression is restricted to the anterior pituitary during development *(2)*. Several human mutations of Prop-1 resulting in CPHD of GH, PRL, and TSH have also been described. Some subjects do not produce LH and FSH at a sufficient level to enter puberty spontaneously *(110)*, while others have a loss of gonadotropin secretion with age but enter puberty spontaneously (albeit delayed), suggesting that Prop-1 is not needed for gonadotroph determination, but may have a role in gonadotroph differentiation *(109)*.

Multiple nonconsanguineous patients from at least eight different countries have a documented recurring homozygous autosomal recessive mutation of Prop-1, delA301,G302 (also known as 296delGA) in exon 2, which changes a serine to a stop codon at codon 109 resulting in a truncated gene product with only the N-terminus and first helix of the homeodomain *(111–113)*. This mutant lacks promoter binding and transcriptional activation *(110)*. Interestingly, one family was noted to have progressive ACTH deficiency with age *(114)*. Likewise, several patients in a large consanguineous Indian pedigree, bearing a 112–124del mutation resulting in a premature stop codon at position 480, had an impaired pituitary-adrenal axis *(115)*. These clinical findings suggest that signals from the other pituitary cell lineages may be important in maintaining corticotroph function *(114)*. Several other mutations in Prop-1 have been described *(109, 110,112,116,117)*.

Pit-1 or GHF-1 (official nomenclature now POU1F1) is a member of a family of transcription factors, POU, responsible for mammalian development. Pit-1 expression is restricted to the anterior pituitary lobe *(118)*. Pit-1 has been shown to be essential for

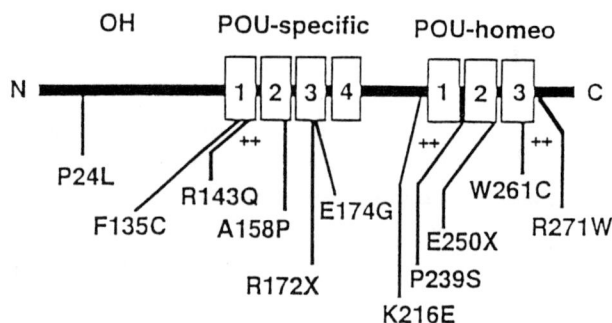

Fig. 4. Pit-1 Gene Mutations. Point mutations of the *Pit-1* gene in patients with CPHD. OH indicates the transactivation domain, which is rich in serine and threonine amino acid residues. The four α-helices of the POU-specific and the three α-helices of the POU-homeodomain (the DNA binding domains) are shown as boxes.

the development of somatotrophs, lactotrophs, and thyrotrophs, as well as for their cell specific gene expression and regulation *(119)*.

A number of humans with CPHD of GH, PRL, and TSH have been found to have *Pit-1* gene mutations (Fig. 4). The inheritance pattern and phenotypic presentation are quite different among these patients, reflecting the location of the mutation in Pit-1. The arginine to tryptophan mutation at codon 271 (R271W) in one allele of the *Pit-1* gene is the most common mutation and has been described in several unrelated patients of different ethnic backgrounds *(120–128)*. The mutant Pit-1 binds normally to DNA, but the mutant protein acts as a dominant inhibitor of transcription *(120)* and may act by impairing dimerization *(129)*. Thus, the mutation need only be present in one allele to cause CPHD.

A patient with GH deficiency, but dysregulation of PRL and TSH, bears a lysine to glutamic acid mutation at codon 216 (K216E) in one allele. The mutant Pit-1 binds to DNA and does not inhibit basal activation of the *GH* and *PRL* genes. However, the mutant Pit-1 is unable to support retinoic acid induction of the *Pit-1* gene distal enhancer either alone or in combination with wild type Pit-1. Thus, the ability to selectively impair interaction with the superfamily of nuclear hormone receptors is another mechanism responsible for CPHD *(130)*.

Several other point mutations in the Pit-1 gene resulting in CPHD have been described. Some alter residues important for DNA-binding and/or alter the predicted α-helical nature of the Pit-1 protein (phenylalanine to cysteine at codon 135 [F135C]) *(131)*, arginine to glutamine at codon 143 [R143Q]) *(122)*, lysine to a stop codon at codon 145 [K145X] (unpublished data), alanine to proline at codon 158 [A158P] *(132)*, arginine to a stop codon at codon 172 [R172X] *(133–135)*, glutamic acid to glycine at codon 174 [E174G] *(133)*, glutamic acid to a stop codon at codon 250 [E250X] *(136)*, and tryptophan to cysteine at codon 261 [W261C] *[137]*). The A158P mutant Pit-1, however, has a minimal decrease in DNA binding. Others have been shown to or postulated to impair transactivation of target genes (proline to leucine at codon 24 [P24L] *(122)*, A158P *(132)*, and proline to serine at codon 239 [P239S] *[138]*).

GH Gene Mutations

Type IA GH deficiency is associated with growth retardation in infancy with subsequent severe dwarfism. There is autosomal recessive inheritance with absent endogenous GH due to complete *GH-1* gene deletion. Heterogeneous deletions of both alleles ranging 6.7-45 kb have been described *(139–142)*. The *GH-1* gene is predisposed to such mutations, because it is flanked by long stretches of highly homologous DNA *(143)*. These patients frequently develop antibodies to exogenous GH owing to lack of immune tolerance because of prenatal GH deficiency *(144,145)*. These antibodies may block the response to GH, but some patients do not develop a decline in growth velocity. In some cases, no antibodies develop.

Type IB is a partial GH deficiency. Patients are less severely affected than those with deletions. There is autosomal recessive inheritance with decreased endogenous GH on provocative stimulation due to point mutations in the *GH-1* gene *(146,147)* (Fig. 5A). Several families have been studied. One has a homozygous splice site G to C transversion in intron 4 of the *GH-1* gene causing a splice deletion of half of exon 4, as well as a frameshift within exon 5. These changes affect the stability and biological activity of the mutant GH protein and may also derange targeting of the GH peptide into secretory granules *(148)*. There has also been a G to T transversion described at the same site *(146)*, as well as a deletion/frameshift mutation in exon 3 *(149)*. Other homozygous nonsense, splicing, and frameshift mutations have been described *(150,151)*.

Type II is a partial GH deficiency similar to type IB, but with autosomal dominant inheritance. Several patients have been found to have intronic transitions in intron 3 *(147,148,152–154)* inactivating the donor splice site of intron 3 and deleting exon 3 (Fig. 5B). Autosomal dominant mutations act in a dominant-negative manner, but the mechanism is not known.

Type III is a partial GH deficiency with X-linked inheritance due to interstitial Xq13.3-Xq21.1 deletions or microduplications of certain X regions. Patients may also have hypogammaglobulinemia, suggesting a contiguous Xq21.2-Xq22 deletion *(155,156)*.

Multiple GH family gene deletions have been described. One family has a homozygous 40 kb deletion that eliminates the *GH-1, GH-2, CS-A,* and *CS-B* genes *(157)*. Another family has a 45 kb deletion that eliminates the *GH-1, CS-L, CS-A,* and *GH-2* genes *(158)*. These patients have normal birth weights, subsequent severe growth retardation, and hypoglycemia. The mothers have normal postpartum lactation. It appears that placental expression of *CS-L* or *CS-B* alone may be sufficient to sustain a normal pregnancy and prenatal growth, supporting the concept of significant duplication in the function of these genes.

Bioinactive GH has also been reported. A child was described with severe growth retardation and high serum GH levels, elevated GHBP, low IGF-1 levels, and increased GH levels after provocative testing. He had an autosomal arginine to cysteine mutation at codon 77 inherited from his unaffected father, who only produced wild type GH. The child expressed both mutant and wild type GH. The mutant GH has a higher affinity for GHBP, less phosphorylating activity, and an inhibitory or dominant-negative effect on wild type GH activity. The cysteine may change the molecular configuration by forming a new disulfide bond, resulting in lower bioactivity *(159)*. An aspartic acid to lysine mutation at codon 112 has also been identified, which is believed to prevent GH-R dimerization *(160)*.

GH-R MUTATIONS

Laron dwarfism is an autosomal recessive disorder characterized by clinical features of severe GH deficiency but with normal to high levels of hGH after provocative testing

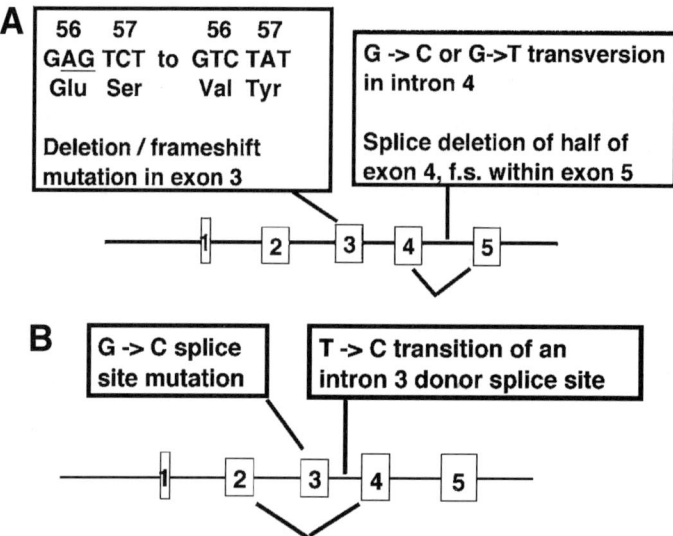

Fig. 5. GH-1 gene point mutations. (A) GH deficiency type IB. Partial GH deficiency with autosomal recessive inheritance. A deletion/frameshift mutation in exon 3; and homozygous splice site G to C and G to T transversions in intron 4 causing a splice deletion of half of exon 4, as well as a frameshift (f.s.) within exon 5. Other homozygous nonsense, splicing, and frameshift mutations have been described. (B) GH deficiency type II. Partial GH deficiency with autosomal dominant inheritance. Several patients have been found to have intronic transitions in intron 3 inactivating the donor splice site of intron 3 and deleting exon 3.

(161). Plasma IGF-1 levels are low and do not respond to exogenous hGH. Several deletions and point mutations of several GH-R exons have been described *(162–171)*. There is a lack of GH binding activity. Many of these mutations affect the extracellular domain and therefore present with absent or decreased levels of GHBP *(172)*. Other mutations that do not affect the extracellular domain region manifest with normal or elevated GHBP levels. Recombinant IGF-1 can be used for treatment *(173,174)*. It has also been hypothesized that some patients with idiopathic short stature, normal GH secretion, and low serum concentrations of GHBP may have partial insensitivity to GH due to mutations in the *GH-R* gene. Four of 14 children, but none of 24 normal subjects, had mutations in the region of the *GH-R* gene that codes for the extracellular domain of the receptor *(166)*.

IGF-1 MUTATIONS

A boy with severe prenatal and postnatal growth failure was found to have a homozygous partial IGF-1 gene deletion with undetectable levels of IGF-1. He also had bilateral sensorineural deafness, mental retardation, moderately delayed motor development, and behavioral difficulties with hyperactivity and a short attention span. He did not have a significant delay in his bone age, and his IGFBP-3 level was normal *(175)*.

African pygmies have normal levels of hGH, peripheral unresponsiveness to exogenous hGH, and decreased IGF-1 levels. An isolated deficiency of IGF-1 has been hypothesized, but Bowcock et al. found no differences in restriction fragment length polymorphisms in the IGF-1 gene in Pygmies vs non-Pygmie black Africans *(176)*. Pygmie T-cell lines show IGF-1 resistance at the receptor level with secondary GH resistance *(177,178)*. However, more recent data suggest that in growing and adult

African pygmies showing no clinical or biochemical signs of nutritional deficiency, serum IGF-1 and IGFBP-3 are essential normal *(179)*.

Other patients are suspected to have IGF-1 resistance, as they have elevated GH levels and elevated IGF-1 levels *(180–182)*. In one patient, cultured fibroblasts had a 50% reduction in IGF-1 binding capacity *(181)*. Another patient had marked diminished ability of IGF-1 to stimulate fibroblast α-aminoisobutyric acid uptake compared to control subjects *(182)*. Their birth lengths less than 5th percentile suggest the importance of IGF-1 in fetal growth.

Post-signal transduction defects and mutations in IGF-binding proteins may occur but have not yet been demonstrated.

DIAGNOSIS OF GROWTH HORMONE DEFICIENCY

The diagnosis of growth hormone GH deficiency in childhood must be based on auxological criteria. Evaluation of the GH-IGF axis is indicated in children with a height below 2 standard deviation scores (SDS) and a growth velocity (over at least 6 mo) below the 10–25th percentile, in whom other causes of growth retardation have been ruled out. Several pharmacological tests have been implemented to assess the GH status *(183)*. Conventionally, the criteria for diagnosis of GH deficiency is peak serum GH <10 ng/mL after two different GH stimulation tests. The sensitivity and specificity of these tests is limited owing to their dependence on physiological parameters such as age, gender, and body weight, the implementation of different pharmacological stimuli, arbitrary cut-off values, poorly reproducible results, and the use of different laboratory techniques for the measurement of GH. Assessment of serum levels of IGF-I and its binding protein IGFBP-3 is a major advance in the diagnosis of GH deficiency.

Growth Hormone Stimulation Tests

GH is secreted episodically, mostly during rapid eye movement sleep. Between the pulses of pituitary GH secretion, serum concentrations are typically below the sensitivity of most conventional assays (<1–2 ng/mL), which limits the usefulness of random samples. Radioimmunoassays (RIAs) and immunometric assays are the most commonly used laboratory-techniques for determination of GH levels. Estimations performed by RIA use polyclonal antibodies, which render low specificity and higher GH levels when compared with the more specific immunoradiometric assays using two highly specific monoclonal antibodies. Discrepancies up to two- to four-fold have been reported among different assays.

A variety of pharmacological tests have been implemented to assess the GH secretory capacity of the pituitary gland *(183)*. They are expensive, not free of side effects, and require fasting conditions as high glucose levels inhibit GH secretion. GH provocative tests have been divided into two groups: screening tests (including exercise, levodopa, and clonidine), and definitive tests (including arginine, insulin, and glucagon). Due to their low specificity and sensitivity, and to exclude normal children who might fail a single stimulation test, the performance of two different provocative tests, sequentially or in combination, has been implemented *(184,185)*. An inappropriate low secretory response in the second test is supposedly confirmatory of GH deficiency. As these tests are not physiologic, they may not always identify children with growth failure who will respond to GH treatment.

CLONIDINE

Clonidine is an α2 adrenergic agonist that increases GHRH secretion and inhibits SRIF. Blood pressure monitoring is necessary as hypotension may occur. Dosage and sampling: 5 µg/kg (max 250 µg). Samples for GH are drawn at 0, 30, 60, and 90 min *(186)*.

LEVODOPA

Due to its α-adrenergic stimulatory effect, levodopa increases the secretion of GHRH. The addition of a β-adrenergic receptor antagonist, such as propranolol, increases its stimulatory effect. Dosage and sampling: It is administered orally, giving 125 mg for children less than 13.5 kg body weight, 250 mg for those between 13.5 and 31.5 kg, and 500 mg for children over 31.5 kg. Serum samples should be obtained at 0, 30, 60, and 90 min *(187)*.

INSULIN TOLERANCE TEST (ITT)

It was the first established pharmacological stimulus for assessment of GH status and is considered the gold standard of GH provocative tests. Induced hypoglycemia is a strong stimulus to elicit maximal GH response. In addition, the reserve of the adrenal cortex can be evaluated, as hypoglycemia induces the release of cortisol as well. Insulin-induced hypoglycemia may result in seizures and neurological sequelae. It is usually not recommended in children under 5 yr of age. Children with severe GH deficiency may be particularly prone to hypoglycemia and for this reason, half of the usual insulin dose is recommended when severe hypopituitarism is suspected. Serum glucose levels must be evaluated at the bedside at each time point during the protocol. For the test to be valid, serum glucose levels must decrease to 50% of the initial value, or less than 40 mg/dL. The patient must be monitored until serum glucose levels return to normal. Symptomatic hypoglycemia should be treated with a bolus of 2 cc/kg of 10% dextrose. If hypopituitarism is suspected, a bolus of 100 mg of hydrocortisone may be administered as well. Fatalities have been described during the performance of this test. Dosage and sampling: 0.1 units/kg body weight of regular insulin iv bolus. Serum samples should be obtained at 0, 15, 30, 45, and 60 min *(188)*.

ARGININE

Arginine inhibits the secretion of SRIF and induces the secretion of glucagon. Dosage and sampling: 0.5 g/kg (max 30 g) of arginine hydrochloride 10% iv over 30 min. Sampling: 0, 30, 45, 60, 90, and 120 min *(189)*.

GLUCAGON

By inducing hyperglycemia with subsequent release of insulin, GH is secreted in response to a moderate fall in blood glucose. In addition, glucagon inhibits the secretion of SRIF. Normal reserves of glycogen are necessary to produce hyperglycemia and subsequently to induce the release of insulin. The test is considered safe in small children and infants *(190)*. False positive results have been reported in up to 20% *(191)*. Dosage and sampling: 0.03 mg/kg to a maximum of 1 mg im. Samples are obtained at 0, 60, 120, and 180 min *(190)*.

GHRH

Although the use of GHRH allows direct assessment of the secretory capacity of the somatotrophs, there is great variability in the GH response, very likely owing to fluctuations in endogenous SRIF tone *(192)*. Up to 15% of normal children will show a peak response lower than 10 ng/mL *(193)*, and normal stimulated levels of GH cannot rule out GH deficiency of hypothalamic origin, the most common cause of GH deficiency.

Inhibitors of endogenous SRIF such as pyridostigmine and arginine have been used in combination with GHRH (194) to enhance the GH response and to reduce the inter-individual and the intra-individual variability. Priming with arginine appears to enhance the GH response to an acute bolus of GHRH in normal children, which might discriminate between children with GH deficiency and normal short children *(194)*. Dosage and sampling: 1 µg/kg/iv of GHRH over 1 min. Samples are obtained at 0, 15, 30, 45, and 60 min. The GH peak secretion occurs in the first hour after administration.

Sex Steroid Priming

In normal children, serum levels of GH are age and sex dependent and show a sharp pubertal increase. Immediately before puberty, GH secretion may normally be very low, making the discrimination between GH deficiency and constitutional delay of growth and puberty difficult *(195)*. Sex steroid priming with estrogen *(196)* or androgen *(197)*, administered for Tanner Stage I or II children, has been recommended to distinguish between GH deficiency and constitutional delay in growth and puberty *(198)*. In girls, 50–100-mg ethinyl estradiol po once a day or Premarin 5-mg p.o. twice a day for two or three days has been used. As an alternative in boys, 100 mg testosterone enanthate im may be given one week prior to the test. While children with GH deficiency might have an attenuated response, those with constitutional growth delay will have a normal secretory pattern. In a study by Marin et al. *(198)*, 61% of normal stature prepubertal children who were not primed with sex steroids failed to raise their peak serum GH concentration above 7 ng/L following a provocative test.

Summary

In summary, the threshold to define GH deficiency to various provocative stimuli is arbitrary and based on no physiological data. Pharmacological tests involve the use of potent GH secretagogues, which may not reflect GH secretion under physiological circumstances, masking the child with partial GH deficiency. GH stimulation tests are reliable only in the diagnosis of severe or complete GH deficiency. In addition to their low reproducibility *(199)*, a "normal" secretory response does not exclude the possibility of various forms of GH insensitivity or partial GH deficiency. Caution must be taken in obese children who undergo provocative testing for GH secretion, owing to a negative impact of adipose tissue on GH secretion *(200)*. Table 2 shows the protocols most commonly used in the assessment of GH secretion.

Physiologic Assessment of Growth Hormone Secretion

Exercise Test

It has been implemented as a screening test. Three to four hours of fasting should precede the test. Twenty minutes of mild-to-moderate exercise should be performed with the final heart rate exceeding 120 beats/min for the test to be valid. Although it is simple, safe, and inexpensive, up to one-third of normal children have an absent GH response. Samples are obtained at 20 and 40 min *(201)*.

Overnight Test for Spontaneous Growth Hormone Secretion

Sleep-induced GH release appears to be the result of an increment in the secretion of GHRH. Most consistent surges occur during slow-wave electroencephalographic rhythms in phases 3 and 4 of sleep. The term "GH neurosecretory dysfunction" refers to

Table 2
Growth Hormone Stimulation Tests

Test	Administration	Time of peak GH	Side effects
Insulin-induced hypoglycemia (ITT)	0.05–0.1 IU/kg, iv bolus	30–60 min	severe hypoglycemia
Clonidine	0.125 mg/m2, oral	60–120 min	drowsiness, hypotension
L-dopa / propanolol			
L-dopa	125 mg body weight <13.5 kg 250 mg >13.5, <31.5 kg 500 mg >31.5 kg, oral	60–120 min	headache, nausea, emesis
Propranolol	0.75 g/kg/oral		induced asthma
Glucagon	0.03 mg/kg (max 1 mg), sc or im	120–180 min	late hypoglycemia
Arginine hydrochloride	0.5g/kg, iv over 20 min	40–70 min	late hypoglycemia
GHRH	1 or 2 µg/kg, i.v. bolus	30–60 min	flushing
Exercise	20 min of moderate exercise	20–40 min	exhaustion, post-exercise induced asthma

patients with an abnormally slow growth rate and low integrated GH concentration (mean serum 24-h GH concentration) but appropriate GH response to provocative tests *(202,203)*. The pathophysiology and the incidence of this condition remain unknown. Although the integrated GH concentration has better reproducibility compared to the standard provocative tests, there is still significant intra-individual variation and overlapping with the values found in normal short children *(204)*. Lanes et al. reported decreased overnight GH concentrations in 25% of normally growing children *(205)*. Sampling is required every 20 min for a minimum of 12–24 h. For the 12 h test, samples are obtained every 20 min from 8 PM to 8 AM. Most reports suggest that the mean level of GH has a normal lower limit of 3 ng/L. In addition, the number and height of surges of GH secretion must be assessed. Six to ten surges, with at least four of them with a GH concentration over 10 ng/L, must be present in a normal subject. The test is difficult to perform, expensive, and unspecific. No normative data for comparison purposes are available. This method uncovers GH deficiency in children who have had a normal GH response to provocative tests after cranial irradiation.

URINARY GROWTH HORMONE

GH is excreted in urine in small amounts, which correspond to approx 0.05% of the total daily circulating GH. Although the measurement of GH in urine is more reliable because of the use of ultrasensitive enzyme-linked immunosorbent assays and immunoradiometric assays *(206)*, the interpretation of the results is difficult due to large inter- and intra-individual variation and the effect of renal function. The test might be useful in the diagnosis of severe GH deficiency. Adequate age- and sex-related standards have to be developed.

IGFs

The IGFs are related GH-dependent peptide factors that mediate many of the anabolic and mitogenic actions of GH. GH induces the expression of IGF-I in liver and cartilage. IGF-II is highly expressed in multiple fetal tissues and is less regulated by GH. Because of little diurnal variation, their quantification in random samples is useful. The use of age- and puberty-corrected IGF-I has become a major tool in the diagnosis of GH deficiency *(207)*. However, sensitivity is still limited due to a significant overlap with normal values. Low levels of IGF-I may be found in normal children, especially in those less than five years of age. Low levels are also reported in children with malnutrition, hypothyroidism, renal failure, hepatic disease, and diabetes mellitus. Serum levels of IGF-I do not correlate perfectly with GH status as determined by provocative GH testing *(208, 209)*. Simultaneous measurement of IGF-I and IGF-II, although recommended by some *(210)*, is not commonly used in the clinical practice.

IGFBPs

IGFBP-3 is the major carrier of IGF-1 *(211)*. It is GH-dependent but has less age variation and is less affected by the nutritional status compared to IGF-I, and it seems to correlate more accurately with GH status *(212)*. Although low levels of IGFBP-3 are suggestive of GH deficiency, up to 43% of normal short children have been reported to have low concentrations *(213)*. Similarly, normal values have been reported in children with partial GH deficiency *(208,214)*. Although determinations of IGFBP-2 have been recommended, normal levels may be found in patients with GH deficiency *(215)*.

In summary, determinations of IGF-I and IGFBP-3 are reliable tests in the diagnosis of severe GH deficiency and have better reproducibility when compared with GH provocative tests. However, their sensitivity and specificity are still sub-optimal.

Bone Age Evaluation

The evaluation of skeletal maturation is crucial in the assessment of growth disorders, as osseous growth and maturation is influenced by nutritional, genetic, environmental and endocrine factors. Skeletal maturation is significantly delayed in patients with GH deficiency, hypothyroidism, hypercortisolism, and chronic diseases. Children with constitutional growth delay will show a delayed bone age, which corresponds with the height age.

In children over one year of age, the radiograph of the left hand is commonly used to evaluate the skeletal maturation. The bone age is determined by comparing the epiphyseal ossification centers with chronological standards from normal children. Comparison of the distal phalanges renders better accuracy. Several methods to determine the skeletal age are available, with the Greulich and Pyle *(216)* and Tanner-Whitehouse 2 (TW2) *(217)* methods the most widely used. For the Greulich and Pyle method, a radiograph of the left hand and wrist is compared with the standards of the Brush Foundation Study of skeletal maturation in normal boys and girls *(216)*, and is based on current height and chronological age. The standards correspond to a cohort of white children, so applicability to other racial groups may be less accurate. The TW2 method assigns a score to each one of the epiphyses. This more accurate method is also based on current height and chronological age, but is also more time consuming. Neither of the methods is accurate, as bone age estimation has technical difficulties owing to inter- and intra-observer variations, as well as ethnic and gender differences among children.

Prediction of Adult Height

Ultimate adult height can be predicted from the bone age, as there is a direct correlation in a normal individual between the degree of skeletal maturation and the time of epiphyseal closure, the event that ends skeletal growth. Predictions of ultimate height are based on the fact that the more delayed the bone age is for the chronological age, the longer the time before epiphyseal fusion ends further growth.

The growth potential of an individual must be evaluated according to the parents' and siblings' heights, as genetic influences play a crucial role in determining the final height. An approximation of the ultimate adult height is obtained by calculating the mid-parental height. For girls, mid-parental height is (mother's height + father's height – 13 cm) / 2; for boys, (mother's height + father's height + 13 cm) / 2. The child's target height is the mid-parental height +/– 2 SD (10 cm or 4 in) *(218)*. When the growth pattern deviates from the parental target height, an underlying pathology must be ruled out. Three methods to estimate the final adult height are available: 1) Bayley-Pinneau (B-P) which is based on current stature, chronological age (CA), and bone age (BA) obtained by the Greulich and Pyle method *(219)*. This method probably under predicts growth potential *(220)*; 2) The TW2 method considers current height, chronologic age, TW2 assessment of bone age, mid-parental stature, and pubertal status *(217)*; and 3) The Roche-Wainer-Thissen (R-W-T) method requires recumbent length, weight, chronological age, mid-parental stature, and Greulich and Pyle bone age assessment. Predictions of the ultimate adult height are not totally accurate and are of limited value in children with growth disorders.

Magnetic Resonance Imaging

Brain anomalies are common in patients with GH deficiency. Magnetic resonance imaging (MRI) of the brain is a sensitive and specific indicator of hypopituitarism. A triad of radiological findings has been described in GH deficient subjects: small or absent anterior pituitary gland, truncated/absent pituitary stalk, and ectopic posterior pituitary gland. Mass lesions such as suprasellar tumors, or thickening of the pituitary stalk due to infiltrative disorders such as histiocytosis may be found. Structural abnormalities are more common in patients with CPHD or panhypopituitarism (93%) and in those with severe GH deficiency *(221)* compared to those with isolated GH deficiency (80%). Patients with SOD present with hypoplasia of the optic chiasm, optic nerves, and infundibular region of the hypothalamus. The absence of the septum pellucidum is not a constant finding.

Conclusions on Evaluation

Clinical assessment of height and growth velocity is the single most useful parameter in the evaluation of a growth-retarded child. When hormonal evaluation is warranted, determinations of skeletal age, thyroid function, and IGF axis provide an effective way to assess the GH status. A single measurement of IGF-I and IGFBP-3 allows the evaluation of the GH-IGF axis, contributing not only to the evaluation of GH deficiency but to GH sensitivity as well. The response of IGF-I and IGFBP-3 to GH stimulation will probably be an important diagnostic tool once normal reference values are determined. The reliability of GH measurements after provocative tests has been questioned because of poor sensitivity, specificity and reproducibility. Confirmation of a severe defect of

GH secretion should lead to appropriate imaging studies of the hypothalamus and the pituitary gland.

GH THERAPY

The use of GH from human cadaver pituitary glands dates from the late 1950s. In 1985, the distribution of this type of GH was banned in the US due to a possible causal relationship with Creutzfeld-Jakob disease. More than 20 young adults who had received human cadaveric pituitary GH developed this entity. Future cases can still emerge due to the potential long incubation period of prion diseases *(222)*. In the same year as the ban, DNA-derived human recombinant GH became available and replaced the pituitary-derived GH.

The use of recombinant human GH targets the normalization of height and the attainment of a normal adult stature. In the United States, human recombinant GH has been approved for administration in several clinical entities: GH deficiency, Turner syndrome, chronic renal failure prior to transplantation, Prader-Willi syndrome, small for gestation age, AIDS wasting, and adult GH deficiency. However, the spectrum of conditions where GH might be of benefit is expanding, considering its metabolic effects.

The use of GH in short non-GH deficient children has been proposed as a therapeutic intervention to reduce the physiological and psychological risks associated with short stature. A recent study, involving 109 children with GH deficiency and 86 children with idiopathic short stature, found that GH therapy can ameliorate some previous behavioral problems, especially in the group of children with GH deficiency *(223)*. However, at present, there are not conclusive data to prove that GH therapy in children with normal short stature improves social, physiological or educational functions.

Several studies on the use of GH in normal short children or children with idiopathic short stature have rendered controversial results. The administration of GH may produce a short-term increase in height velocity, but the ultimate adult height is not necessarily augmented. Similarly, there is some concern that treatment of normal short children with GH may induce an earlier fusion of the epiphyses and acceleration of the tempo of pubertal development *(224)*. Long-term data are still unavailable. Clinical trials of non-GH deficient children carried out until adulthood are mandatory.

A study involving 187 short children with appropriate GH response to provocative testing and normal growth rate showed a moderate increase in the growth rate during the first year (7.7–9.2 cm/yr), but this effect declined rapidly after, returning to the pretreatment growth velocity *(225,226)*. Other studies have shown a more sustained effect, but the final height did not increase for the genetic height potential. Another study involving Japanese children without GH deficiency who received GH until reaching final height did not show a significant improvement in the height SDS for bone age during the prepubertal period. From this study, it was concluded that GH administration during puberty might be detrimental, as it shortened the height SDS for bone age, resulting in a shorter final height that might have been obtained *(227)*. A recent study by Hintz et al. *(228)*, which included 80 children with idiopathic short stature and slow growth but normal GH response to provocative stimuli, documented an average height gain of 5 cm for boys and 5.4 cm for girls. They received GH therapy until complete bone maturation was reached. Regardless of height gain, all remained shorter than mid-parental target height. This was a heterogeneous group of patients, and some of them had growth retardation which might be indicative of GH deficiency regardless of a normal response to provocative tests. Thus, GH may be of benefit to some patients with idiopathic short stature.

Alternative modes of therapy including GHRH and GH secretagogues have been developed, but their clinical utility is still being assessed *(229)*.

Growth Hormone Dosage

The dose of GH is calculated per kg body weight or body surface area and is expressed in terms of international units (IU) or milligrams (3 IU = 1 mg). It ranges from 0.18–0.30 mg/kg/wk and is administered subcutaneously six to seven times per week (manufacturers' instructions). The lower dose mimics the physiologic production rate in prepubertal children and should not induce an early onset of puberty nor abnormally accelerate the skeletal maturation *(230)*. Recently, a depot preparation has been placed on the market.

No correlation has been found between the indices of spontaneous GH secretion and the results of provocative testing with the therapeutic response *(231)*. A successful response is obtained when the pretreatment growth rate increases more than 2.5 cm/yr after six months of GH administration. The greatest response is observed during the first year of treatment, when growth velocity can double or triple. The response later attenuates, but still remains higher than the pretreatment growth rate.

Two factors have the greatest influence on final height during GH therapy in subjects with idiopathic GH deficiency: the genetic potential (expressed as the mid-parental height) *(232)* and the age at onset of therapy. The longer the replacement therapy, the better the ultimate height. To optimize prepubertal growth, there is a strong argument for early diagnosis and treatment in children with GH deficiency. As shown by the National Collaborative Growth Study (NCGS), there is a significant negative correlation between age at the onset of Tanner stage 2 of pubertal development on the total height gained during puberty and the percentage of adult final height gained *(233)*. Thus, subjects who are diagnosed with GH deficiency during puberty have less growth potential. For this group of patients, two strategies have been recommended. In the first approach, the GH dose is increased to the upper therapeutic range to support pubertal growth and to match the normal physiological increase in GH that occurs at this age. However, significant improvement in final height has not been documented *(234)*. In the second approach, a combination of GH and gonadotropin releasing hormone (GnRH) is administered to arrest pubertal development and prolong peripubertal growth. Preliminary results seem more encouraging with this kind of therapy. Only selected patients, especially those with an unfavorable height SDS for bone age in terms of final height prognosis, would be candidates for this regimen *(234)*.

Follow-up

To evaluate the GH response, the most important parameter is determination of height velocity (expressed as change in height Z score). Suboptimal response may be indicative of an incorrect diagnosis of GH deficiency, lack of compliance, improper preparation and/or administration of GH, associated hypothyroidism, concurrent chronic disease, complete osseous maturation, and rarely, anti-GH antibodies. Development of antibodies to exogenous GH has been reported in 10–30% of recipients of human recombinant GH. This finding is more common in children lacking the *GH* gene. However, the presence of GH antibodies does not usually attenuate the hormonal effect, as growth failure has been reported in less than 0.1% *(235)*.

Monitoring of the IGF-I and IGFBP-3 levels has gained wide acceptance for assessment of safety and compliance; however, serum levels do not always correlate with the obtained increment in growth velocity. Although recommended by some *(236)*, regular monitoring of the bone age in children under GH therapy is questionable. Interobserver differences in bone age interpretation and erratic changes over time in skeletal maturation make the estimation of final adult height inaccurate. Similarly, predictions of final height may be artificially overestimated, as GH may accelerate the bone maturation in advance to any radiographic evidence *(237)*.

Side Effects

DIABETES AND INSULIN RESISTANCE

The development of diabetes mellitus in patients under GH therapy has been a concern, considering the anti-insulinic effect of GH. However, no higher incidence of type I insulin dependent diabetes mellitus (IDDM) in children and adults on GH therapy has been reported. A retrospective study of more than 23,000 GH recipients found 11 cases of type I IDDM, an incidence not different from expected values. However, 18 patients developed type II DM for an incidence of 3.4/100,000, six-fold higher than in children not receiving GH. The higher incidence for type II DM indicates that the use of GH in predisposed individuals might accelerate the onset of diabetes *(238)*.

LEUKEMIA

Concern was raised about the development of *de novo* leukemia after a cluster of leukemia in patients under GH therapy was reported in Japan in 1988 *(239)*. However, recent data from Japan obtained from more than 32,000 GH-recipients reported the development of leukemia in 14 cases for an incidence of 3/100,000 patient years, not higher than in the general population *(240)*. In the United States, three cases of leukemia occurred in 59,736 patient-yr of follow-up, not significantly higher than the 1.66 cases expected in the US age-, race- and gender-matched general population ($p = 0.23$). Three additional cases, found in an extended follow-up that provided 83,917 person-years of risk, yielded a minimum rate of leukemia that was statistically increased (2.26 cases expected, $p = 0.028$). However, five of the six subjects had antecedent cranial tumors as the cause of GH deficiency, and four had received radiotherapy. There was no increase in leukemia in patients with idiopathic growth hormone deficiency *(241)*. From these data and other data registry information, it has been concluded that the incidence of leukemia in GH-recipient individuals without risk factors is not higher than in the general population.

RECURRENCE OF CENTRAL NERVOUS SYSTEM TUMORS

Considering the mitogenic effect of GH, the possibility of an induced carcinogenic effect has been investigated. Several possible mechanisms that could account for the association of GH/IGF-I and the development of cancer have been proposed *(242)*. However, data from the Kabi International Growth Study (KIGS) *(243)* and the National Cooperative Growth Study (NCGS) *(244)* do not support an increase in the risk of brain tumor recurrence. A similar study in 170 children with GH deficiency secondary to treatment for medulloblastoma did not reveal an increase in tumor relapse *(245)*.

Skin Cancer

The statistics of the NCGS have not shown a higher incidence of melanocyte nevi or skin cancer in individuals treated with GH *(246)*.

Benign Intra-Cranial Hypertension

This neurological complication has been described in patients receiving GH, but the incidence is very low. A prospective study collecting data on 3332 children in Australia and New Zealand found a low incidence of 1.2 cases per 1000 patients. However, ophthalmologic evaluation is mandatory in GH recipients in the event of persistent headaches, nausea, visual symptoms, and dizziness *(247)*.

Slipped Capital Femoral Epiphysis (SCFE)

NCGS reported that children with GH deficiency were significantly more likely to develop SCFE while on GH (91.0/100,000 patient yr) than the general population. Typically, these children were older, heavier, and grew more slowly during the first year of GH treatment than those who did not. Children with idiopathic short stature on GH treatment did not show an increased incidence (9.5/100,000 patient-yr). It is possible that the increased incidence seen in patients with GH deficiency could be due to osteopenia associated with delayed exposure to gonadal steroids contributing to instability of the growth plate. Untreated hypothyroidism may also have been a contributing factor in one patient *(248)*.

Summary

In summary, significant side effects of GH therapy are unusual. Although still in investigation, it appears that in the absence of additional risk factors, there is no evidence that long-term GH therapy increases the risk of developing diabetes, brain tumor recurrence, and leukemia. The possibility of a casual relationship of GH therapy with slipped femoral epiphysis, as well as Perthes disease, scoliosis, kyphosis, and sleep apnea, has not been established.

GH REPLACEMENT IN ADULTS

GH deficiency in adults is recognized as a clinical syndrome characterized by several metabolic disturbances, which ameliorate with GH supplementation. Adults with GH deficiency present with an abnormal body composition including increased subcutaneous and visceral fat mass, reduced extracellular fluid volume, and subnormal muscle mass. In addition, low bone density, reduced cardiac performance, lipid abnormalities, reduced physical performance, impaired cognitive function, and reduced quality of life have been described *(249,250)*. Changes in body composition have been reported in adolescents with childhood-onset GH deficiency after discontinuing GH for one year *(251)*. These changes are characterized by an increment in the total body fat and by a reduction of the resting metabolic rate.

There is clear evidence that GH improves body composition, exercise capacity and bone mineral density in adults with GH deficiency *(252,253)*. GH therapy in adults has shown significant reduction of body fat *(252)*, normalization of the lipid profile *(253)*, increase in muscle mass *(254)*, and improvements in bone density *(255,256)*, cardiac structure and function *(257)*, physical performance and exercise capacity, and cognitive function. The effects appear to be sustained after long-term treatment *(255)*. Considering these findings, it seems advisable not to stop GH therapy in recipients who have reached their final height.

Diagnosis of Adult GH Deficiency

Diagnosis of GH deficiency in childhood does not always indicate a similar diagnosis in adulthood. Although children with panhypopituitarism, severe isolated GH deficiency, or growth hormone deficiency associated with brain anomalies very likely will require lifelong therapy, a high number of children with GH deficiency have no persistency of this hormonal defect in adult life and do not require treatment. Thus, reassessment of the GH status after discontinuing GH administration is recommended. Normalization of the GH response to provocative testing has been reported in more than 20% of children with diagnosis of severe GH deficiency *(258)* and up to 71% of those with partial GH deficiency *(259)*. Likewise, many adults with history of childhood-onset GH deficiency will have a normal GH response to provocative stimuli. Longobardi et al. showed that 40% of adult patients with prior diagnosis of isolated GH deficiency in childhood had a normal GH response to a standard ITT *(260)*.

Both the pediatric and the adult endocrinologist play an important role during the transition of children with GH deficiency into adulthood *(261)*. Currently, the diagnosis of GH deficiency in adults is based on the GH peak-response to a provocative stimulus, with the ITT being the stimulus of choice *(262)*. A GH response less than 3 ng/L supports the diagnosis. Serum IGF-I and IGFBP-3 have limited diagnostic accuracy. Normal levels of IGF-I are frequently found in adults with GH deficiency, even in those with a GH peak-response less than 3 ng/L *(263)*. The sensitivity of this test seems to be better in adults with childhood-onset GH deficiency. In this group of patients, concentrations of IGF-I below 2 SD are frequently found *(263,264)*.

CONCLUSIONS

Congenital anomalies or anything that damages the hypothalamus, pituitary stalk, or pituitary gland can result in GH deficiency. It is now recognized that there are molecular defects at multiple levels of the GH axis that can also result in growth hormone deficiency. Diagnosis of GH deficiency, however, remains problematic. Once it is diagnosed, recombinant human growth hormone is a safe and effective treatment.

REFERENCES

1. Asa SI, Kovacs K. Functional morphology of the human fetal pituitary. Pathol Annu 1984. 19: 275–315.
2. Dutour A. A new step understood in the cascade of tissue-specific regulators orchestrating pituitary lineage determination: the Prophet of Pit-1 (Prop-1). Eur J Endocrinol 1997;137(6):616–617.
3. Rosenfeld RG. Disorders of growth hormone and insulin-like growth factor secretion and action, in Pediatric Endocrinology Sperling MA, ed. 1996, W.B. Saunders, PA. Philadelphia. 117–169.
4. Reichlin S. Neuroendocrinology, in: Williams Textbook of Endocrinology Wilson JD and Foster DW, eds. 1991, W.B. Saunders: Philadelphia. 1079–1138.
5. Gorcyzca W, Hardy J. Arterial supply of human pituitary gland. Neurosurgery 1987;20:360.
6. Blethen SL. Hypopituitarism, in: Pediatric Endocrinology, Lifshitz F, ed. 1996, Marcel Dekker Inc. New York. 19–31.
7. DeNoto FM, Moore DD, Goodman HM. Human growth hormone DNA sequence and mRNA structure: possible alternative splicing. Nucl Acids Res 1981;9(15):3719–3730.
8. Cooke NE, Ray J, Watson MA, et al. Human growth hormone gene and the highly homologous growth hormone variant gene display different splicing patterns. J Clin Invest 1988;82(1):270–275.
9. Baumann G, Stolar WM, Ambarn K, et al. A specific growth hormone-binding protein in human plasma: initial characterization. J Clin Endocrinol Metab 1986;62:134–141.
10. Chen EY, Lino Y-C, Smith DH, et al. The human growth hormone locus: nucleotide sequence, biology, and evolution. Genomics 1989;4:479–497.

11. Misra-Press A, Cooke NE, Liebhaber SA. Complex alternative splicing partially inactivates the human chorionic somatomammotropin-like (hCS-L) gene. J Biol Chem 1994;269:23,220–23,229.
12. Nielsen PV, Pedersen H, Kampmann EM. Absence of human placental lactogen in an otherwise uneventful pregnancy. Am J Obstetr Gynecol 1979;135:322–326.
13. Frankenne F, Scippo, ML, van Beeumen J, et al. Identification of placental human growth hormone as the growth hormone-V gene expression product. J Clin Endocrinol Metab 1990;71:15–18.
14. de Zegher F, Vanderschueren-Lodeweyckx M, Spitz B, et al. Perinatal growth hormone (GH) physiology: Effect of GH-releasing factor on maternal and fetal secretion of pituitary and placental GH. J Clin Endocrinol Metab 1990;71:520–522.
15. Campbell RM, Scanes CG. Evolution of the growth hormone-releasing factor (GHRF) family of peptides. Growth Reg 1992;2:175–191.
16. Mayo KE. Molecular cloning and expression of a pituitary-specific receptor for growth hormone-releasing hormone. Mol Endocrinol 1992;6(10):1734–1744.
17. Chen C, Clarke IJ. Modulation of Ca^{2+} influx in the ovine somatotroph by growth hormone-releasing factor. Am J Physiol , 1995;268:E204–E212.
18. Mayo KE, Godfrey PA, Suhr ST, et al. Growth hormone-releasing hormone: synthesis and signaling. Recent Prog Horm Res 1995;50:35–73.
19. Barinaga M, Yamonoto, G, Rivier C, et al., Transcriptional regulation of growth hormone gene expression by growth hormone-releasing factor. Nature 1983;306:84–85.
20. Bilezikjian LM, Vale MM. Stimulation of adenosine 3',5'-monophosphate production by growth hormone-releasing factor and its inhibition by somatostatin in anterior pituitary cells in vitro. Endocrinology 1983;113:1726–1731.
21. Cohen LE, et al. CREB-independent regulation by CBP is a novel mechanism of human growth hormone gene expression. J Clin Invest 1999;104(1123–1128).
22. Raynor K, Murphy W, Coy D, et al. Cloned SRIF receptors: identification of subtype selective peptides and demonstration of high affinity binding of linear peptides. Mol Pharmacol 1993;43:838–844.
23. Law S, Manning D, Reisine T. Identification of the subunits of GTP binding proteins couples to SRIF receptors. J Biol Chem 1991;266:17,885–17,897.
24. Law S, Yasuda, K, Bell GI, et al. Gias and Goa selectively associate with the cloned SRIF receptor subtype STR2. J Biol Chem 1993;268;10,721–10,727.
25. Fujii Y, Gonoi T, Yamada Y, et al. Somatostatin receptor subtype SSTR2 mediates the inhibition of high voltage activated calcium channels by somatostatin and its analogue SMS. FEBS Letters 1996;355:117–120.
26. Tannenbaum GS, Ling N. Evidence for autoregulation of growth hormone secretion via the central nervous system. Endocrinology 1980;115:1952–1957.
27. Turner P, Tannenbaum GS. In vivo evidence of a positive role for somatostatin to optimize pulsatile growth hormone secretion. Am J Physiol 1995;269:E683–E690.
28. Miller JD, Esparaza, A, Wright NM, et al. Spontaneous growth hormone release in term infants: Changes during the first four days of life. J Clin Endocrinol Metab 1993;76:1058–1062.
29. Costin G, Ratman-Kaufman F, Brasel J. Growth hormone secretory dynamics in subjects with normal stature. J Pediatr 1989;115:537–544.
30. Mauras N, Blizzard RM, Link K, et al. Augmentation of growth hormone secretion during puberty: Evidence for a pulse amplitude-modulated phenomenon. J Clin Endocrinol Metab 1987;64:596–601.
31. Rose SR, Municchi, G, Barnes KM, et al. Spontaneous growth hormone secretion increases during puberty in normal girls and boys. J Clin Endocrinol Metab 1991;73:428–435.
32. Martha PM, Gorman KM, Blizzard RM, et al. Endogenous growth hormone secretion and clearance rates in normal boys as determined by deconvolution analysis: Relationship to age, pubertal status and body mass. J Clin Endocrinol Metab 1992;74:336–344.
33. Dudl RJ, Ensinck JW, Palmer HE, et al. Effect of age on growth hormone secretion in man. J Clin Endocrinol Metab 1973;37(1):11–16.
34. Rudman D, Kutner MH, Rogers CM, et al. Impaired growth hormone secretion in the adult population: relation to age and adiposity. J Clin Invest 1981;67(5):1361–1369.
35. Smith RG, Van der Ploeg LHT, Cheng K, et al. Peptidomimetic regulation of growth hormone (GH) secretion. Endo Rev 1997;18:621–645.
36. Howard AD, Feighner SD, Cully DF, et al. A receptor in pituitary and hypothalamus that functions in growth hormone release. Science 1996;273:972–977.
37. Kojima M, Hosoda, H, Date Y, et al. Ghrelin is a growth-hormone-releasing acylated peptide from stomach. Nature 1999;402(1999):656–660.

38. Nakazato M, Murakami M, Date Y, et al. A role for ghrelin in the central regulation of feeding. Nature 200;1409:194–198.
39. Bazan JF. Structural design and molecular evolution of a cytokine receptor superfamily. Proc Natl Acad Sci USA, 1990;87:6934–6938.
40. Godowski PJ, Leung DW, Meacham LR, et al. Characterization of the human growth hormone receptor gene with demonstration of a partial gene deletion in two patients with Laron-type dwarfism. Proc Natl Acad Sci USA 1989;86:8083–8087.
41. Campbell GS, Christian LJ, Carter-Su C. Evidence for involvement of the growth hormone receptor-associated tyrosine kinase in actions of growth hormone. J Biol Chem 1993;268:7427–7434.
42. Argetsinger LS, Cambell GS, Yang X, et al. Identification of JAK2 as a growth hormone receptor-associated tyrosine kinase. Cell 1993;74:237–244.
43. Finbloom DS, Petricoin EF, Hackett RH, et al. Growth hormone and erythropoietin differentially activate DNA-binding proteins by tyrosine phosphorylation. Mol Cell Biol 1994;14:2113–2118.
44. Silva CM, Weber MJ, Thorner MO. Stimulation of tyrosine phosphorylation in human cells by activation of the human growth hormone receptor. Endocrinology 1995;132:101–108.
45. Silva CM, Lu H, Day RN. Characterization and cloning of STAT5 from IM-9 cells and its activation by growth hormone. Mol Endocrinol 1996;10:508–518.
46. Smit LS, Meyer DJ, Billestrup N, et al. The role of the growth hormone receptor and Jak1 and Jak2 kinases in the activation of STATs 1, 3, and 5 by growth hormone. Mol Endocrinol. 1996;10:519–533.
47. Salmon WDJ, Daughaday WH. A hormonally controlled serum factor which stimulates sulfate incorporation by cartilage in vivo. J Lab Clin Med 1957; 49:825.
48. Rinderknecht E, Humbel RE. The amino acid sequence of human insulin-like growth factor I and its structural homology with proinsulin. J Biol Chem 1978;253(8):2769–2776.
49. Daughaday WH, Rotwein, IP. Insulin-like growth factors I and II. Peptide, messenger ribonucleic acid and gene structures, serum, and tissue concentrations. Endo Rev 1989;10(1):68–91.
50. Gluckman PD, Barrett-Johnson JJ, Butler JH, et al. Studies of insulin-like growth factor I and II by specific radioligand assays in umbilical cord blood. Clin Endocrinol 1983;19:405.
51. Bennet A, Wilson DM, Wibbelsman CJ, et al. Levels of insulin-like growth factor-I and -II in human cord blood. J Clin Endocrinol Metab 1983;57:609.
52. Luna AM, Wilson DM, Wibbelsman CJ, et al. Somatomedins in adolescence: A cross sectional study of the effect of puberty on plasma insulin-like growth factor I and II levels. J Clin Endocrinol Metab 1983;57:258.
53. Cara FJ, Rosenfield RL, Furlanetto RW. A longitudinal study of the relationship of plasma somatomedin-C concentrations to the pubertal growth spurt. Am J Dis Child 1987;141:562.
54. Johanson AJ, Blizzard RM. Low somatomedin-C levels in older men rise in response to growth hormone administration. John Hopkins Med J 1981;149:115.
55. Rudman D, Feller AG, Nagraj HS, et al. Effects of human gorwth hormone in men over 60 years old. N Engl J Med 1990;312:1.
56. Ohlsson C, Bengtsson, B-A, Isaksson OGP, et al. Growth hormone and bone. Endocr Rev 1998;19(1);55–79.
57. Isaksson O, Jansson G, Gause IA. Growth hormone stimulates longitudinal bone growth directly. Science, 1982;216(4551):1237–1239.
58. Maor G, Hochberg Z, Silbermann M. Growth hormone stimulates the growth of mouse neonatal condylar cartilage in vitro. Acta Endocrinol 1989;120(4):526–532.
59. Maor G, Hochberg Z, von der Mark K, et al. Human growth hormone enhances chondrogenesis and osteogenesis in a tissue culture system of chondroprogenitor cells. Endocrinology 1989;125(3):1239–1245.
60. Isgaard J, Moller COG, Nilsson A, et al. Regulation of insulin-like growth factor messenger ribonucleic acid in rat growth plate by growth hormone. Endocrinology 1988;122(4):1515–1520.
61. Zamboni G, Antoniazzi F, Radetti G, et al. Effects of two different regimens of recombinant human growth hormone therapy on the bone mineral density of patients with growth hormone deficiency. J Pediatr 1991;119:483–485.
62. Elgin RG, Busby WHJ, Clemmons DR. An insulin-like growth factor (IGF) binding protein enhances the biologic response to IGF-I. Proc Natl Acad Sci USA 1987;84(10):3254–3258.
63. Ritvos O, Ranta T, Jalkanen J, et al. Insulin-like growth factor (IGF) binding protein from human decidua inhibits the binding and biological action of IGF-I in cultured choriocarcinoma cells. Endocrinology 1988;122(5):2150–2157.

64. Lamson G, Giudice LD, Rosenfeld RG. Insulin-like growth factor binding proteins (IGFBPs): Structural and molecular relationships. Growth Factors 1991;5:19–28.
65. Kelley KM, Oh Y, Gargosky SE, et al. Insulin-like growth factor binding proteins (IGFBPs) and their regulatory dynamics. Intl J Biochem Cell Biol 1996;28:619–637.
66. Chernausek S, Jacobs S, van Wyk, JJ. Structural similarities between receptors for somatomedin C and insulin: analysis by affinity labeling. Biochem 1981;20:7345.
67. Massague J, Czech MP. The subunit structures of two distinct receptors for insulin-like growth factors I and II and their relationship to the insulin receptor. J Biol Chem 1982;257:5038.
68. Oh Y, Muller HL, Neely EK, et al. New concepts in insulin-like growth factor receptor physiology. Growth Reg 1993;3:113.
69. Rona RJ, Tanner JM. Aetiology of idiopathic growth hormone deficiency in England and Wales. Arch Dis Child 1977;52:197–208.
70. Vimpani GV, Vampani AF, Lidgard GP, et al. Prevalence of severe growth hormone deficiency. Br Med J 1977;2:427–430.
71. Shulman DI. Growth hormone therapy: An update. Contemporary Pediatrics, 1998;15(8):95–100.
72. Gluckman PD, Gunn AJ, Wray A, et al. Congenital idiopathic growth hormone deficiency associated with prenatal and early postnatal growth failure. J Pediatr 1992;121:920–923.
73. Wabitsch M, Heinze E. Body fat in GH deficient children and the effect of treatment. Horm Res 1993;5:43–52.
74. Barreca T, Perrie C, Sannia A, et al. Evaluation of anterior pituitary function in patients with post-traumatic diabetes insipidus. J Clin Endocrinol Metab 1980;51:1279–1282.
75. Yamanaka C, Momoi T, Fuisawa I, et al. Acquired growth hormone deficiency due to pituitary stalk transection after head trauma in childhood. Eur J Pediatr 1993;152(2):99–101.
76. Craft WH, Underwood JJ, van Wyk LE. High incidence of perinatal insult in children with idiopathic hypopituitarism. J Pediatr 1980;96:397–402.
77. Cruikshank DP. Breech presentation. Clin Obstet Gynecol 1986;29:255–263.
78. Dunger DB, Broadbent V, Yoeman E. The frequency and natural history of diabetes insipidus in children with Langerhans-cell histiocytosis. N Engl J Med 1989;321:1157–1162.
79. Tien RD, Newton TH, McDermott MW, et al. Thickened pituitary stalk on MR images in patients with diabetes insipidus and Langerhans-cell histiocytosis. Am J Neuro Radiol 1990;11:703–708.
80. O'Sullivan RM, Sheehan M, Poskitt KJ, et al. Langerhans cell histiocytosis of hypothalamus and optic chiasm: CT and MR studies. J Comput Assist Tomogr 1991;15:52–55.
81. Freda PU, Silverberg SJ, Kalmon KD, et al. Hypothalamic-pituitary sarcoidosis. Trends Endo-crinol Metab 1992;2:321–325.
82. Bevan JS, Othman S, Lazarus JH, et al. Reversible adrenocorticotropin deficiency due to probably autoimmune hypophysitis in a woman with postpartum thyroiditis. J Clin Endocrinol Metab 1992;74:548–552.
83. Duranteau L, Chanson P, Bumberg-Tick J, et al. Non-responsiveness of serum gonadotropins and testosterone to pulsatile GnRH in hemochromatosis suggesting a pituitary defect. Acta Endocrinol 1993;128(4):351–354.
84. Oerter KE, Kamp GA, Munson PJ, et al. Multiple hormone deficiencies in children with hemochromatosis. J Clin Endocrinol Metab 1993;76:357–361.
85. Pollack IF. Brain tumors in children. New Engl J Med 1994;331(22):1500–1507.
86. Rappaport R, Brauner R. Growth and endocrine disorders secondary to cranial irradiation. Pediatr Res 1989;25:561–567.
87. Clayton PE, Shalet, SM. Dose dependency of time on onset of radiation-induced growth hormone deficiency. J Pediatr 1991;118:226–228.
88. Shalet SM. Growth and endocrine sequelae following the treatment of childhood cancer, in Clinical Paediatric Endocrinology, B. C.G.D., ed. 1995; Blackwell Science Ltd.: Oxford. 383–396.
89. Shalet SM, Gibson B, Swindell R, et al. Effect of spinal irradiation on growth. Arch Dis Child 1987;62:461–464.
90. Godfrey P, Rahal JO, Beamer WG, et al. GHRH receptor of little mice contains a missense mutation in the extracellular domain that disrupts receptor function. Nat Genet 1993; 4(3):227–232.
91. Lin SC, Lin CR, Gukovsky I, et al. Molecular basis of the little mouse phenotype and implications for cell type-specific growth (see comments). Nature 1993;364(6434):208–213.
92. Wajnrajch MP, Gertner JM, harbison MD, et al. Nonsense mutation in the human growth hormone-releasing hormone receptor causes growth failure analogous to the little (lit) mouse. Nat Genet 1996;12:88–90.

93. Maheshwari HG, Silverman BL, Dupuis J, et al. Phenotype and genetic analysis of a syndrome caused by an inactivating mutation in the growth hormone-releasing hormone receptor: Dwarfism of Sindh. J Clin Endocrinol Metab 1998;83(11):4065–4074.
94. Dattani M, Martinez-Barbera J-P, Thomas PQ, et al. Mutations in the homeobox gene HESX1/Hesx1 associated with septo-optic dysplasia in human and mouse. Nat Genet 1998;19:125–133.
95. Hermesz E, Mackem S. Mahon, Rpx: a novel anterior-restricted homeobox gene progressively activated in the prechordal plate, anterior neural plate and Rathke's pouch of the mouse embryo. Development 1996;122(1):41–52.
96. Tremblay JJ, C. Lanctot, Drouin J. The pan-pituitary activator of transcription, Ptx1 (pituitary homeobox 1), acts in synergy with SF-1 and Pit1 and is an upstream regulator of the Lim-homeodomain gene Lim3/Lhx3. Mol Endocrinol 1998. 12(3):428–441.
97. Thomas PQ, Dattani MT, Brickman JM, et al. Heterozygous HESX1 mutations associated wtih isolated congenital pituitary hypoplasia and septo-optic dysplasia. Hum Mol Genet 2001;10(1):39–45.
98. Lamonerie T, Tremblay JJ, Lanctot C, et al. Ptx1, a bicoid-related homeo box transcription factor involved in transcription of the pro-opiomelanocortin gene. Genes Dev 1996;10(10):1284–1295.
99. Drouin J, Lamolet B, Lamonerie T, et al. The PTX family of homeodomain transcription factors during pituitary development. Mol and Cell Endocrinol 1998;140:31–36.
100. Gage PJ, Camper SA. Pituitary homeobox 2, a novel member of the bicoid-related family of homeobox genes, is a potential regulator of anterior structure formation. Hum Mol Genet 1997; 6(3):457–464.
101. Semina EV, Reiter R, Leysens NJ, et al. Cloning and characterization of a novel bicoid-related homeobox transcription factor gene, RIEG, involved in Rieger Syndrome. Nat Genet 1996;14(4):392–399.
102. Amendt BA, Sutherland LB, Semina EV, et al. The molecular basis of Rieger syndrome. J Biol Chem 1998;273(32):20,066–20,072.
103. Zhadanov AB, Bertuzzi S, Taira M, et al. Expression pattern of the murine LIM class homeobox gene Lhx3 in subsets of neural and neuroendocrine tissues. Dev Dyn 1995; 202(4):354–364.
104. Mbikay M, Tadros H, Seidah NG, et al. Linkage mapping of the gene for the LIM-homeoprotein LIM3 (locus Lhx3) to mouse chromosome 2. Mamm Genome 1995; 6(11):818–819.
105. Bach I, Rhodes SJ, Pearse RV, et al. P-Lim, a LIM homeodomain factor, is expressed during pituitary organ and cell commitment and synergizes with Pit-1. Proc Natl Acad Sci USA, 1995;92(7):2720–2724.
106. Sheng HZ, Zhadanov AB, Mosinger B, Jr., et al., Specification of pituitary cell lineages by the LIM homeobox gene Lhx3. Science 1996;272(5264):1004–1007.
107. Netchine I, Sobrier M-L, Krude H, et al. Mutations in LHX3 result in a new syndrome revealed by combined pituitary hormone deficiency. Nat Genet 2000;25:182–186.
108. Sloop KW, Parker GE, Hanna KR, et al. LHX3 transcription factor mutations associated with combined pituitary hormone deficiency impair the activation of pituitary target genes. Gene 2001;265:61–69.
109. Fluck C, Deladoey J, Rutishauser K, et al. Phenotypic variability in familial combined pituitary hormone deficiency caused by a PROP1 gene mutation resulting in the substitution of Arg –> Cys at codon 120 (R120C). J Clin Endocrinol Metab 1998;83(10):3727–3734.
110. Wu W, Cogan JD, Pfaffle RW, et al. Mutations in PROP1 cause familial combined pituitary hormone deficiency. Nat Genet 1998;18(2):147–149.
111. Fofanova OV, Takamura N, Kinoshita E-J, set al. A mutational hot spot in the Prop-1 gene in Russian children with combined pituitary hormone deficiency. Pituitary 1998;45–49.
112. Fofanova O, Takmura N, Kinoshita E, et al. Compound heterozygous deletion of the Prop-1 gene in children with combined pituitary hormone deficiency. J Clin Endocrinol Metab 1998;83(7):2601–2604.
113. Cogan JD, Wu W, Phillips III JA, et al. The PROP1 2-base pair deletion is a common cause of combined pituitary hormone deficiency. J Clin Endocrinol Metab 1998;83(9):3346–3349.
114. Pernasetti F, Toledo SPA, Vasilyev VV, et al. Impaired adrenocorticotropin-adrenal axis in combined pituitary hormone deficiency caused by a two-base pair deletion (301-302delAG) in the Prophet of Pit-1 Gene. J Clin Endocrinol Metab 2000;85:390–397.
115. Agarwal G, Bhatia V, Cook S, et al. Adrenocorticotropin deficiency in combined pituitary hormone deficiency patients homozygous for a novel PROP1 mutation. J Clin Endocrinol Metab., 2000;85(12):4556–4561.
116. Osorio MGF, Kopp P, Marui S, et al. Combined pituitary hormone deficiency caused by a novel mutation of a highly conserved residue (F88S) in the homeodomain of PROP-1. J Clin Endocrinol Metab 2000; 85(8):2779–2785.

117. Duquesnoy P, Roy A, Dastot F, et al. Human Prop-1: cloning, mapping, genomic structure. Mutations in familial combined pituitary hormone deficiency. FEBS Letters, 1998;437(3):216–220.
118. Bodner M, Castrillo JL, Theill LE, et al. The pituitary-specific transcription factor GHF-1 is a homeobox-containing protein. Cell 1988;55(3):505–518.
119. Simmons DM, Voss JW, Ingraham HA, et al. Pituitary cell phenotypes involve cell-specific Pit-1 mRNA translation and synergistic interactions with other classes of transcription factors. Genes Dev 1990;4(5): 695–711.
120. Radovick S, Nations M, Du Y, et al. A mutation in the POU-homeodomain of Pit-1 responsible for combined pituitary hormone deficiency. Science 1992;257(5073):1115–1118.
121. Cohen LE, Wondisford FE, Salvatoni A, et al. A "hot spot" in the Pit-1 gene responsible for combined pituitary hormone deficiency: clinical and molecular correlates. J Clin Endocrinol Metab 1995;80(2):679–684.
122. Ohta K, Nobukuni Y, Mitsubuchi H, et al. Mutations in the Pit-1 gene in children with combined pituitary hormone deficiency. Biochem Biophys Res Commun 1992;189(2):851–855.
123. Okamoto N, Wada Y, Ida S, et al. Monoallelic expression of normal mRNA in the PIT1 mutation heterozygotes with normal phenotype and biallelic expression in the abnormal phenotype. Human Mol Genet 1994;3:1565–1568.
124. de Zegher F, Pernasetti F, Vanhole C, et al. The prenatal role of thyroid hormone evidenced by fetomaternal Pit-1 deficiency. J Clin Endocrinol Metab 1995;80(11):3127–3130.
125. Holl RW, Pfaffle R, Kim C, et al. Combined pituitary deficiencies of growth hormone, thyroid stimulating hormone and prolactin due to Pit-1 gene mutation: a case report. Eur J Pediatr 1997;156(11):835–837.
126. Aarskog D, Eiken HG, Bjerknes R, et al. Pituitary dwarfism in the R271W Pit-1 gene mutation. Eur J Pediatr 1997;156(11):829–34.
127. Arnhold IJ, Nery M, Brown, MR, et al. Clinical and molecular characterization of a Brazilian patient with Pit-1 deficiency. J Ped Endocrinol Metab 1998;11(5):623–630.
128. Ward L, Chavez M, Huot C, et al. Severe congenital hypopituitarism with low prolactin levels and age-dependent anterior pituitary hypoplasia: A clue to a PIT-1 mutation. J Pediatr 1998;132:1036–1038.
129. Jacobson EM, Li P, Leon-del-Rio A. et al. Structure of Pit-1 POU domain bound to DNA as a dimer: unexpected arrangement and flexibility. Genes Dev 1997;11(2):198–212.
130. Cohen LE, Zanger K, Brue T, et al. Defective retinoic acid regulation of the pit-1 gene enhancer: A novel mechanism of combined pituitary hormone deficiency. Mol Endocrinol 1999;13:476–484.
131. Pellegrini-Bouiller I, Belicar P, Barlier A, et al. A new mutation of the gene encoding the transcription factor Pit-1 is responsible for combined pituitary hormone deficiency. J Clin Endocrinol Metab 1996;81(8):2790–2796.
132. Pfaffle RW, DiMattia GE, Parks JS, et al. Mutation of the POU-specific domain of Pit-1 and hypopituitarism without pituitary hypoplasia. Science 1992;257(5073):1118–1121.
133. Brown MR, Parks JS, Adess ME, et al. Central hypothyroidism reveals compound heterozygous mutations in the Pit-1 gene. Horm Res 1998;49(2):98–102.
134. Tatsumi K, Miyai K, Notomi T, et al. Cretinism with combined hormone deficiency caused by a mutation in the PIT1 gene. Nat Genet 1992;1(1):56–58.
135. Frisch H, Kim, C, Hausler G, et al. Combined pituitary hormone deficiency and pituitary hypoplasia due to a mutation of the Pit-1 gene. Clin Endocrinol 2000;52(5):661–665.
136. Irie Y, Tatsumi K, Ogawa M, et al. A novel E250X mutation of the PIT1 gene in a patient with combined pituitary hormone deficiency. Endocr J 1995;42(3):351–354.
137. Li S, Crenshaw EB, Rawson EJ, et al. Dwarf locus mutants lacking three pituitary cell types result from mutations in the POU-domain gene pit-1. Nature 1990;347(6293):528–533.
138. Pernasetti F, Milner RDG, Al Ashwal AAZ, et al. Pro239Ser: A novel recessive mutation of the Pit-1 gene in seven Middle Eastern children with growth hormone, prolactin, and thyrotropin deficiency. J Clin Endocrinol Metab 1998;83:2079–2083.
139. Illig R, Prader A, Ferrandez A, et al. Hereditary prenatal growth hormone deficiency with increased tendency to growth hormone antibody formation (A-type) of isolated growth hormone deficiency. Acta Paed Scand 1971;60:607.
140. Phillips JA, Hjelle BL, Seeburg PH, et al. Molecular basis of familial isolated growth hormone deficiency. Proc Natl Acad Sci USA, 1981;78:6372–6375.
141. Braga S, Phillips JA, Joss E, et al. Familial growth hormone deficiency resulting from a 7.6 kb deletion within the growth hormone gene cluster. Am J Med Genet 1986;25:443–452.
142. Perez Jurado LA, Argente J. Molecular basis of familial growth hormone deficiency. Horm Res 1994;42(4-5):189–197.

143. Vnencak-Jones CL, Phillips JA. Hot spots for growth hormone gene deletions in homologous regions outside of Alu repeats. Science 1990;250:1745–1748.
144. Prader A, Zachmann M, Poley JR, et al. Long-term treatment with human growth hormone (Raben) in small doses: evaluation of 18 hypopituitary patients. Helv Paediatr Acta 1967;22:423–440.
145. Phillips JA. Inherited defects in growth hormone synthesis and action, in Metabolic Basis of Inherited Disease CR, Scriver, et al., eds. 1995, McGraw Hill: St. Louis, MO. p. 3023–3044.
146. Phillips JA, Cogan JD. Molecular basis of familial human growth hormone deficiency. J Clin Endocrinol Metab 1994;78:11–16.
147. Binder G, Ranke MB. Screening for growth hormone (GH) gene splice-site mutaitons in sporadic cases with severe isolated GH deficiency using ectopic transcript analysis. J Clin Endocrinol Metab 1995;80:1247–1252.
148. Cogan JD, Phillips, JA, Schenkman SS, et al. Familial growth hormone deficiency: A model of dominant and recessive mutations affecting a monomeric protein. J Clin Endocrinol Metab 1994;79:1261–1265.
149. Igarashi Y, Kamijo T, Ogawa M, et al. A new type of inherited growth hormone deficiency: A compound heterozygote of a 6.7 kb deletion, including the GH-1 gene, and two base deletion deletion in the third exon of the GH-1 gene. Pediatr Res 1993;33:S35.
150. Duquesnoy P, Amselem S, Gourmelen M, et al. A frameshift mutaiton causing isolated growth hormone deficiency type IA. Am J Hum Genet 1990;47:A110.
151. Cogan JD, Phillips JA, Sakati N, et al. Heterogeneous growth hormone (GH) gene mutations in familial GH deficiency. J Clin Endocrinol Metab 1993;76:1224–1228.
152. Cogan, JD, Ramel B, Lehto M, et al. A recurring dominant negative mutation causes autosomal dominant growth hormone gene deficiency - A clinical research center study. J Clin Endocrinol Metab 1995;80:3591–3595.
153. Kamijo T, Kinoshita E, Yoshimoto M, et al. An identical mutation in GH 1 gene associated with IGHD in two sporadic Japanese patients. Horm Res 1997;48(suppl 2):92.
154. Saitoh H, Fukushima T, Kamoda T, et al. A Japanese family with autosomal dominant growth hormone deficiency. Eur J Pediatr 1999;158:624–627.
155. Fleisher TA, White RM, Broder S, et al. X-linked hypogammaglobulinemia and isolated growth hormone deficiency. N Engl J Med 1980;302:1429–1434.
156. Conley ME, Burk W, Herrod HG, et al. Molecular analysis of X-linked agammaglobulinemia with growth hormone deficiency. J Pediatr 1991;119:392–397.
157. Goossens M, Brauner R, Czernichow P, et al. Isolatd growth hormone (GH) deficiency type Ia associated with a double deletion in the human GH gene cluster. J Clin Endocrinol Metab 1986;62:712–716.
158. Akinci A, Kanaka C, Eble A, et al. Isolated growth hormone (GH) deficiency type IA associated with a 45-kilobase gene deletion within the human GH gene cluster. J Clin Endocrinol Metab 1992;75:437–441.
159. Takahashi Y, Kaji, H, Okimura Y, et al. Brief report: Short stature caused by a mutant growth hormone. N Engl J Med 1996;334:432–436.
160. Takahashi Y, Shirono H, Arisaka O, et al. Biologically inactive growth hormone caused by an amino acid substitution. J Clin Invest 1997;100:1159–1165.
161. Laron A, Pertzelan A, Mannheimer S. Genetic pituitary dwarfism with high serum concentration of growth hormone. A new inborn error of metabolism? Israel J Med Science 1966;2:152–155.
162. Amselem S, Duquesnoy P, Attree O, et al. Laron dwarfism and mutations of the growth hormone-receptor gene. N Engl J Med 1989;321:989–995.
163. Amselem S, Sobrier ML, Duquesnoy P, et al. Recurrent nonsense mutations in the growth hormone receptor from patients with Laron dwarfism. J Clin Invest 1991;87:1098–1102.
164. Berg MA, Guevara-Agurre J, Rosenbloom AL, et al. Mutation creating a new splice site in the growth hormone receptor genes of 37 Ecuadorean patients with Laron syndrome. Human Mutation 1992;1:24–34.
165. Berg MA, Argente J, Chernausek S, et al. Diverse growth hormone receptor gene mutations in Laron Syndrome. Am J Hum Genet 1993;52:998–1005.
166. Goddard AD, Covello R, Luoh SM, et al. Mutations of the growth hormone receptor in children with idiopathic short stature. N Engl J Med 1995;333:1094–1098.

167. Woods KA, Fraser NC, Postel-Vinay MC, et al. A homozygous splice site mutation affecting the intracellular domain of the growth hormone (GH) receptor resulting in Laron syndrome with elevated GH-binding protein. J Clin Endocrinol Metab 1996;81:1686–1690.
168. Ayling RM, Ross R, Towner P, et al. A dominant-negative mutation of the growth hormone receptor causes familial short stature. Nat Genet 1997;16:13–14.
169. Kaji H, Nose O, Tajiri H, et al. Novel compound heterozygous mutations of growth hormone (GH) receptor gene in a patient with GH insensitivity syndrome. J Clin Endocrinol Metab 1997;82:3705–3709.
170. Iida K, Takahashi Y, Kaji H, et al. Growth hormone (GH) insensitivity syndrome with high serum GH-binding protein levels caused by a heterozygous splice site mutation of the GH receptor gene producing a lack of intracellular domain. J Clin Endocrinol Metab 1998;83:531–537.
171. Walker JL, Crock PA, Behncken SN, et al. A novel mutation affecting the interdomain link region of the growth hormone receptor in a Vietnamese girl, and response to long-term treatment with recombinant human insulin-like growth factor-I and luteinizing hormone-releasing hormone analogue. J Clin Endocrinol Metab 1998;83:2554–2561.
172. Baumann G, Shaw MA, Winter RJ. Absence of the plasma growth hormone binding-protein in Laron-type dwarfism. J Clin Endocrinol Metab 1987;65: 814–816.
173. Backeljauw PF, Underwood LE, a.t.G.C. Group. Prolonged treatment with recombinant insulin-like growth factor-I in children with growth hormone insensitivity syndrome: A clinical research center study. J Clin Endocrinol Metab 1996;81:3312–3317.
174. Laron Z, Anin S, Klinger B. Long-term IGF-1 treatment of children with Laron syndrome. Lessons from Laron syndrome 1966–1992. Pediatr Adolesc Endocrinol 1993;24:226–236.
175. Woods KA, Camacho-Hubner, C, Savage MO, et al. Intrauterine growth retardation and postnatal growth failure associated with deletion of the insulin-like growth factor I gene. N Engl J Med 1996;335(18):1363–1367.
176. Bowcock A, Sartorelli V. Polymorphism and mapping of the IGF1 gene, and absence of association with stature among African Pygmies. Human Genetics, 1990;85(3):349–354.
177. Geffner ME, Bailey RC, Bersch N, et al. Insulin-like growth factor-I unresponsiveness in an Efe Pygmy. Biochem Biophys Res Commun1993;193(3):1216–1223.
178. Geffner ME, Bersch N, Bailey RC, et al. Insulin-like growth factor I resistance in immortalized T cell lines from African Efe Pygmies. J Clin Endocrinol Metab 1995;80(12):3732–3738.
179. Dulloo AG, Shahkhalili Y, Atchou G, et al. Dissociation of systemic GH-IGF-1 axis from a genetic basis for short stature in African Pygmies. Eur J of ClinNutr 1996;50(6):371–380.
180. Lanes R, Plotnick LP, Spencer EM, et al. Dwarfism associated with normal serum growth hormone and increased bioassayable, receptorassayable, and immunoassayable somatomedin. J Clin Endocrinol Metab 1980;50:85–488.
181. Bierich Jr, Moeller H, Ranke MB, et al. Pseudopituitary dwarfism due to resistance to somatomedin: A new syndrome. Eur J Pediatr 1984;142:186–188.
182. Heith–Monnig E, Wohltmann HJ, Mills-Dunlap B, et al. Measurement of insulin-like growth factor I (IGF-1) responsiveness of fibroblasts of children with short stature: Identification of a patient with IGF-1 resistance. J Clin Endocrinol Metab 1987;64:501–507.
183. Shalet SM, Toogood A, Rahim A, et al. The diagnosis of growth hormone deficiency in children and adults. Endocr Rev 1998;19(2):203–223.
184. Penny R. Sequential arginine and insulin tolerance test on the same day. J Clin Endocrinol Metab 1969;29:1499–1501.
185. Fass B. Relative usefulness of three growth hormone screening tests. Amer J Dis Child 1974;133:931–933.
186. Gil-Ad I. Oral clonidine as a growth hormone stimulation test. Lancet, 1979;2:278–279.
187. Weldom VV, Gupta SK, Klingensmith G, et al. Evaluation of growth hormone release in children using arginine and L-dopa in combination. J Pediatr 1975;87:540–544.
188. Gale EA, Bennett T, MacDonald IA, et al. The physiological effects of insulin-induced hypoglycemia in man: responses at different levels of blood glucose. Clin Sci 1983;65:263–271.
189. Merimee TJ, Rabinowitz D, Fineberg SE. Arginine-initiated release of human growth hormone. N Engl J Med 1969;(280):1434–1438.
190. Mitchell ML, Byrne MJ, Sanchez Y, et al. Detection of growth hormone deficiency: the glucagon stimulation test. N Engl J Med 1979;282:539–541.

191. Chanoine JP, Rebuffat E, Kahn A, et al. Glucose, growth hormone, cortisol, and insulin responses to glucagon injection in normal infants, aged 0.5–12 months. J Clin Endocrinol Metab 1995;80:3032–3035.
192. Gelato MC, Malozowski S, Caruso-Nicoletti M, et al. Growth hormone responses to GH-releasing hormone during pubertal development in normal boys and girls: comparison to idiopathic short stature and GH deficiency. J Clin Endocrinol Metab 1986;63:174–179.
193. Ghigo E, Bellone J, Aimaretti G, et al. Reliability of provocative tests to assess growth hormone secretory status. Study in 472 normally growing children. J Clin Endocrinol Metab 1996;81:3323–3327.
194. Ghigo E. Neutransmitter control of growth hormone secretion. Excerpta Medica 1992;103–106.
195. Rosenfeld RG. Evaluation of growth and maturation in adolescence. Pediatr Rev 1982;4:175.
196. Deller JJ, Bolulis MW, Harris WE, et al. Growth hormone response patterns to sex hormone administration in growth retardation. Am J Med Sci 1979;259:292–296.
197. Martin LG, Clark JW, Connor TB. Growth hormone secretion enhanced by androgens. J Clin Endocrinol Metab 1968;28:425–428.
198. Marin G, Domene HM, Barnes KM, et al. The effects of estrogen priming and puberty on the growth hormone response to standardized treadmill exercise and arginine-insulin in normal girls and boys. J Clin Endocrinol Metab 1994;79(2):537–541.
199. Zadik Z, Chalew SA, Gilula Z, et al. Reproducibility of growth hormone testing procedures: a comparison between 24-hour integrated concentration and pharmacological stimulation. J Clin Endocrinol Metab 1990;71:1127–1130.
200. Carel JC, Tresca JP, Letrait M, et al. Growth hormone testing for the diagnosis of growth hormone deficiency in childhood: a population register-based study. J Clin Endocrinol Metab 1997;82(7):2117–2121.
201. Greene SA, Torresani T, Prader A. Growth hormone response to a standardized exercise test in relation to puberty and stature. Arch Dis Child 1987;62: 53–56.
202. Spiliotis BE, August GP, Hung W, et al. Growth hormone neurosecretory dysfunction: a treatable cause of short stature. JAMA 1984;251:2223–2230.
203. Bercu BB, Shulman DJ, Root AW, et al. Growth hormone provocative testing frequently does not reflect endogenous GH secretion. J Clin Endocrinol Metab 1986;63:709–716.
204. Rose SR, Ross JL, Uriarte M, et al. The advantage of measuring stimulated as compared with spontaneous growth hormone levels in the diagnosis of growth hormone deficiency. N Engl J Med 1988;319:201–207.
205. Lanes R. Diagnostic limitations of spontaneous growth hormone measurements in normally growing prepubertal children. Amer J Dis Child 1989;143:1284.
206. Pirazzoli P, Mandini M, Zucchini S, et al. Urinary growth hormone estimation in diagnosing severe growth hormone deficiency. Arch Dis Child 1996;75:228–231.
207. Juul A, Skakkebaek NE. Prediction of the outcome of growth hormone provocative testing in short children by measurement of serum levels of insulin-like growth factor 1 and insulin-like growth factor binding protein 3. J Pediatr 1997;130:197–204.
208. Tillmann V, Buckler JMH, Kibirige MS, et al. Biochemical test in the diagnosis of childhood growth hormone deficiency. J Clin Endocrinol Metab 1997;82: 531–535.
209. Reiter EO, Lovinger R. The use of commercially available somatomedin-C radioimmunoassay in patients with disorders of growth. J Pediatr 1981; 99:720–724.
210. Rosenfeld RG, Wilson DM, Lee PDK, et al. Insulin-like growth factors I and II in the evaluation of growth retardation. J Pediatr 1986;109(3):428–433.
211. Martin JL, Baxter RC. Insulin–like growth factor-binding protein from human plasma. Purification and characterization. J Biol Chem 1986;261(19):8754–8760.
212. Blum WF, Ranke MB, Kietzmann K, et al. A specific radioimmunoassay for the growth hormone-dependent somatomedin-binding protein: its use for diagnosis of GH deficiency. J Clin Endocrinol Metabol 1990;70:1292–1298.
213. Hasegawa Y, Hasegawa T, Aso T, et al. Usefulness and limitiation of measurement of insulin-like growth factor binding protein-3 (IGFBP-3) for diagnosis of growth hormone deficiency. Endocrinol Jpn 1992;1992:585–591.
214. Sklar C, Sarafoglou K, Whittam E. Efficacy of insulin-like growth factor-I and IGF-binding protein-3 in predicting the growth hormone response to provocative testing in children treated with cranial irradiation. Acta Endocrinol 1993;129: 511–515.

215. Smith WJ, Nam TJ, Underwood LE, et al. Use of insulin-like growth factor binding protein-2 (IGFBP-2), IGFBP-3, and IGF-I for assessing growth hormone status in short children. J Clin Endocrinol Metab 1993;77:1294–1299.
216. Greulich WW, Pyle SI. Radiographic atlas of skeletal development of the hand and wrist. Vol. 2. 1959, Stanford, CA: Stanford University Press.
217. Tanner JM. Assessment of skeletal maturity and prediction of adult height (TW2 method). 1975, New York, Academic Press.
218. Vogiatzi MG, Copeland, KC. The short child. Pediatr Rev 1998;19(3):92–99.
219. Bayley N, Pinneau SR. Tables for predicting adult height from skeletal age: Revised for use with the Greulich-Pyle hand standards. J Pediatr 1952;40:432.
220. Shulman DI, Bercu, BB. Abstract 1079: Predicted heights in children with growth retardation and bone age delay following 1 to 3 years of growth hormone therapy. in 72nd Annual Meeting of the Endocrine Society. 1990.
221. Hamilton J, Blaser S, Daneman D. MR imaging in idiopathic growth hormone deficiency. Am J Neuroradiol 1998;19(9):1609–16015.
222. Fradkin JE. Creutzfeldt-Jakob disease in pituitary growth hormone recipients. Endocrinologist, 1993;3:108.
223. Stable B, Siegel PT, Clopper RR, et al., Behavior change after growth hormone treatment of children with short stature. J Pediatr 1998;1998(3):366–373.
224. Attie KM, Hintz RL, Hopwood NJ, et al. Genenthech Collaborative Study Group. Growth hormone treatment of idiopathic short stature and its effect on the onset and tempo of puberty (abstract). Pediatr Res 1992;31:72A.
225. Hopwood NJ, Hintz RL, Gertner JM, et al. Growth response of children with non-growth hormone deficiency and marked short stature during three year of growth hormone therapy. J Pediatr 1993;123:215–227.
226. Moore WV, Moore KC, Gifford R, et al. Long-term treatment with growth hormone of children with short stature and normal growth hormone secretion. J Pediatr 1992;120:702–708.
227. Kawai M, Momoi T, Yorifuji T, et al. Unfavorable effects of growth hormone therapy on the final height of boys with short stature not caused by growth hormone deficiency. J Pediatr 1997;130(2):205–209.
228. Hintz RL, Attie KM, Baptista J, et al. Effect of growth hormone treatment on adult height of children with idiopathic short stature. N Engl J Med 1999;340:502–507.
229. Duck SC, Rappaport R. Long-term treatment with GHRH (1-44) amide in prepubertal children with classical growth hormone deficiency. J Pediatr Endocrinol Metab 1999;12(4):531–536.
230. MacGillivray MH, Blithe SL, Bushels JG, et al. Current dosing of growth hormone in children with growth hormone deficiency: how physiologic? Pediatrics 1998;102(2 pt 3):527–530.
231. Bell JJ, Dana K. Lack of correlation between growth hormone provocative test results and subsequent growth rate during growth hormone therapy. Pediatrics 1998;102(2 pt 3):518–520.
232. Cutfield W, Lindberg A, Albertsson Wikland K, et al. Final height in idiopathic growth hormone deficiency: The KIGS experience. KIGS international board. Acta Paediatrica 1999;88(428):72–75.
233. August GP, Julius JR, Blethen SL. Adult height in children with growth hormone deficiency who are treated with biosynthetic growth hormone: The National Cooperative Growth Study experience. Pediatrics 2001;102(2 pt 3):512–516.
234. Saggese G, Federico G, Barsanti S. Management of puberty in growth hormone deficient children. J Pediatr Endocrinol Metab 1999;12:329–334.
235. Blethen SL, Allen DB, Graves D, et al. Safety of recombinant deoxyribonucleic acid-derived growth hormone: The National Cooperative Growth Study experience. J Clin Endocrinol Metab 1996;81(5):1704–1710.
236. Kaufman FR, Sy JP. Regular monitoring of bone age is useful in children treated with growth hormone. Pediatrics 1999;104(4 pt 2):1039–1042.
237. Wilson DM. Regular monitoring of bone age is not useful in children treated with growth hormone. Pediatrics 1999;104(4 pt 2):1036–1039.
238. Cutfield WS, Wilton P, Bennmarker H, et al. Incidence of diabetes mellitus and impaired glucose tolerance in children and adolescents receiving growth-hormone treatment. Lancet 2000. 355(9204):610–13.
239. Watanabe S, Yamaguchi N, Tsunematsu Y, et al. Risk factors for leukemia occurring among growth hormone users. Jpn J Cancer 1989;80:822.

240. Nishi Y, Tanaka T, Kakano K, et al. Recent status in the occurrence of leukemia in growth-hormone-treated patients in Japan. GH Treatment Study Committee of the Foundation for Growth Science, Japan. J Clin Endocrinol Metab 1999;84(6):1961–1965.
241. Fradkin JE, Millis JL, Schonberger LB, et al. Risk of leukemia after treatment with pituitary growth hormone. JAMA 1993;270(23):2829–2832.
242. Holly JM, Gunnell DJ, Davey Smith G. Growth hormone, IGF-I and cancer. Less intervention to avoid cancer? More intervention to prevent cancer? J Endocrinol 1999;162(3):321–330.
243. Wilton P. Adverse events during GH treatment: 10 years' experience in KIGS, a pharmaco-epidemiological survey, in Growth Hormone Therapy in KIGS – 10 Years' Experience. Ranke, MB and Wilton P, eds. 1999, Johann Ambrosius Barth Verlag: Heidelberg. p. 349–364.
244. Moshang T, Rundle AC, Graves DA, et al. Brain tumor recurrence in children treated with growth hormone: The National Cooperative Growth Study experience. J Pediatr 1996;128:S4–7.
245. Packer RJ, Boyett JM, Janss AJ, et al. Growth hormone replacement therapy (GH Rx) for children with GH deficiency secondary to treatment for medulloblastoma is not associated with increased likelihood of disease relapse. J Clin Oncol 2001;18:480.
246. Wyatt D. Melanocytic nevi in children treated with growth hormone. Pediatrics 1999;104(4 pt 2): 1045–1050.
247. Crock PA, McKenzie JD, Nicoll AM, et al. Benign intracranial hypertension and recombinant growth hormone therapy in Australia and New Zealand. Acta Paediatrica 1998;87(4): 381–386.
248. Blethen SL, Rundle AC, o.b.o.t.G.N.C.G.S. (NCGS), Slipped capital femoral epiphysis in children treated with growth hormone. Horm Res 1996;46:113–116.
249. Cuneo RC, Salomon F, McGauley GA, et al. The growth hormone deficiency syndrome in adults. Clin Endocrinol 1992; 37:387–397.
250. de Boer H, Blok GJ, van der Veen EA. Clinical aspects of growth hormone deficiency in adults. Endocr Rev 1995;16:63–86.
251. Cowan FJ, Evans WD, Gregory JW. Metabolic effects of discontinuing growth hormone treatment. Arch Dis Child 1999;80(6):517–523.
252. Ter Maaten JC, de Boer H, Kamp O, et al. Long-term effects of growth hormone (GH) replacement in men with childhood-onset GH deficiency. J Clin Endocrinol Metab 1999;84(7):2373–2380.
253. Binnerts A, Swart GR, Wilson JHP, et al. The effect of growth hormone administration in growth hormone deficient adults on bone, protein, carbohydrate and lipid homeostasis, as well as on body composition. Clin Endocrinol 1992;37:79–87.
254. Jorensen JOL, Thuesen L, Muller J, et al. Three years of growth hormone treatment in growth hormone deficient adults: near normalization of body composition and physical performance. Eur J Endocrinol 1994;130: 224–228.
255. Gomez JM, Gomez N, Fiter J, et al. Effects of long-term treatment with GH in the bone mineral density of adults with hypopituitarism and GH deficiency after discontinuation of GH replacement. Horm Metab Res 2000;32(2):66–70.
256. Amato G, Izzo G, la Montagna G, et al. Low-dose recombinant human growth hormone normalizes bone metabolism and cortical bone density and improves trabecular bone density in growth hormone deficient adults without causing adverse effects. Clin Endocrinol 1996;45A:27–32.
257. Amato G, Carella C, Fazio S, et al. Body composition, bone metabolism, and heart structure and function before and after GH replacement therapy at low doses. J Clin Endocrinol Metab 1993 1993:1671–1676.
258. Cacciari E, Tassoni P, Cicognani A, et al. Value and limits of pharmacological and physiological tests to diagnose growth hormone (GH) deficiency and predict therapy response: first and second retesting during replacement therapy of patients defined as GH deficient. J Clin Endocrinol Metab 1994;79:1663–1669.
259. Tauber M, Moulin P, Pienkowski C,et al. Growth hormone (GH) retesting and auxological data in 131 GH-deficient patients after completion of treatment. J Clin Endocrinol Metab 1997;82:352–356.
260. Longobardi S, Merola B, Pivonello R, et al. Reevaluation of growth hormone (GH) secretion in 69 adults diagnosed as GH-deficient patients during childhood. J Clin Endocrinol Metab 1996;81:1244–1247.
261. Allen DB. Issues in the transition from childhood to adult growth hormone therapy. Pediatrics 1999;104(4 pt 2):1004–1010.
262. Hoffman DM, O'Sullivan AJ, Baxter RC, et al. Diagnosis of growth hormone deficiency in adults. Lancet 1994;343: 1064–1068.
263. Gills MS, Toogood AA, O'Neill PA, et al. Urinary growth hormone (GH), insulin-like growth factor I (IGF-I), and IGF-binding protein-3 measurements in the diagnosis of adult GH deficiency. J Clin Endocrinol Metab 1998;83(7):2562–2565.

264. Hilding A, Hall K, Wivall-Helleryd IL, et al. Serum levels of insulin-like growth factor I in 152 patients with growth hormone deficiency, aged 19–82 years, in relation to those in healthy subjects. J Clin Endocrinol Metab 1999;84(6):2013–2019.

2 Growth Hormone Insensitivity Syndrome

Arlan L. Rosenbloom, MD

CONTENTS

> DEFINITION AND CLASSIFICATION
> THE GH–IGF-I AXIS
> DISCOVERY OF LARON SYNDROME AND PRE-MOLECULAR STUDY
> THE MOLECULAR BASIS OF GHI
> EPIDEMIOLOGY
> CLINICAL FINDINGS
> BIOCHEMICAL FEATURES
> DIAGNOSTIC ISSUES IN GH RESISTANCE
> TREATMENT
> CONCLUSION
> REFERENCES

DEFINITION AND CLASSIFICATION

Growth hormone insensitivity (GHI) is defined as the absence of an appropriate growth and metabolic response to endogenous GH or to GH administered at physiologic replacement dosage *(1)*. Table 1 lists the known conditions associated with GH resistance and their clinical and biochemical features. Only GH receptor (GH-R) deficiency (GHRD) and GH-GHR signal transduction defects are appropriately described as primary GH resistance or insensitivity. Inability to generate insulin-like growth factor-I (IGF-I) resulting from mutation of the IGF-I gene *(2)* and resistance to IGF-I due to mutation of the IGF-I receptor *(3)* are properly considered primary IGF-I deficiency and IGF-I resistance.

The conditions that have been associated with secondary or acquired GHI do not consistently demonstrate elevated serum GH concentrations, low levels of IGF-I, or even growth failure. Acquired GH resistance occurs in some patients with GH gene deletion for whom injections of recombinant human GH stimulate the production of GH inhibiting antibodies; such patients have extremely low or unmeasurable serum concentrations of GH *(4)*. Growth failure associated with chronic renal disease is thought to be

From: *Contemporary Endocrinology: Pediatric Endocrinology: A Practical Clinical Guide*
Edited by: S. Radovick and M. H. MacGillivray © Humana Press Inc., Totowa, NJ

Table 1
Conditions Characterized by Unresponsiveness
to Endogenous or Exogenous Growth Hormone: Clinical and Biochemical Features

	Clinical			Biochemical			
Condition	Growth Failure	GH deficiency phenotype	GH	GHBP	IGF-I	IGFBP-3
IGF-I gene deletion	severe (with IUGR)	no	increased	normal	absent	normal
IGF-I receptor deficiency	severe (with IUGR)	no	increased	normal	increased	increased
Primary GH insensitivity						
GHR deficiency/autosomal recessive forms	severe	yes	increased (child) normal/elevated (adult)	absent/low/ normal	markedly decrease	decreased
GHR deficiency/dominant negative forms	moderate	no or mild	increased elevated	2 × normal	marked decrease	low normal
GH–GHR signal transduction defect	severe (Arab) moderate (Pakistani)	yes (Arab) no (Pakistani)	elevated	normal	marked decrease	normal (Arab) low (Pakistani)
Acquired GH insensitivity						
GH inhibiting antibodies	severe	yes	absent	normal decrease	marked decreased	decreased
Malnutrition	none to mild	no	increased	decreased	variable decreased	normal or
Diabetes mellitus	none to mild	no	increased	decreased	decreased	increased
Renal disease	mild to severe	no	normal	decreased	normal	increased

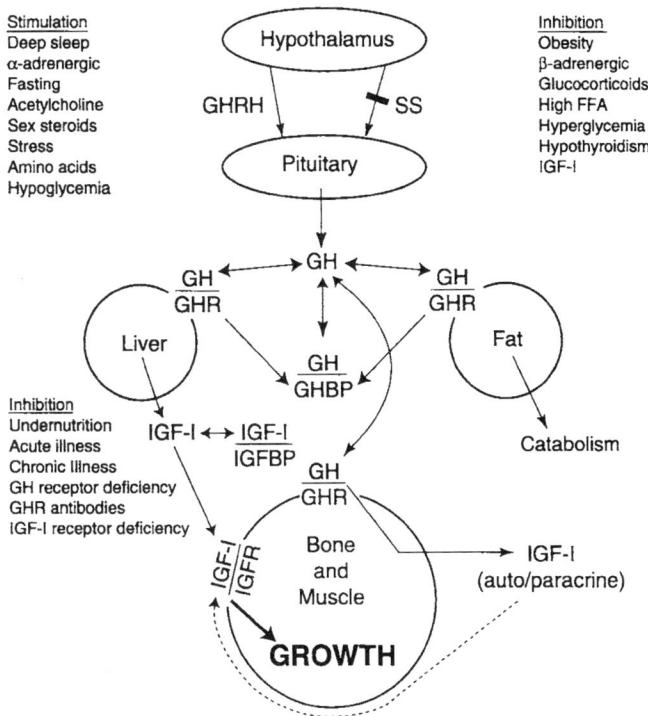

Fig. 1. Simplified diagram of the GH-IGF-I axis involving hypophysiotropic hormones controlling pituitary GH release, circulating GH binding protein and its GH receptor source, IGF-I and its largely GH-dependent binding proteins, and cellular responsiveness to GH and IGF-I interacting with their specific receptors. Reprinted from *Trends Endocrinol Metab*, vol 5, Rosenbloom AL, Guevara-Aguirre J, Rosenfeld RG, Pollock BH. Growth in growth hormone insensitivity, pp 296–303, 1994, with kind permission from Elsevier Science Ltd, The Boulevard, Langford Lane, Kidlington OX5 1GB, UK.

related to increased concentrations of IGF binding proteins (IGFBP) with normal or elevated GH and usually normal total IGF-I levels *(5)*. Malnutrition and other catabolic states that have been associated with GHI may be teleologically similar to the nonthyroidal illness (sick euthyroid) syndrome *(6)*.

THE GH-IGF-I AXIS

GH synthesis and secretion by the anterior pituitary somatotrophs is under the control of stimulatory GH releasing hormone (GHRH) and inhibitory somatostatin (SST) from the hypothalamus (Fig. 1). The stimulation and suppression of GHRH and SST result from a variety of neurologic, metabolic, and hormonal influences. Of particular importance to discussions of GHI is the feedback stimulation of SST by IGF-I, with resultant inhibition of GH release *(1,7)*.

GH bound to the soluble GH binding protein (GHBP) in the circulation is in equilibrium with approximately equal amounts of free GH. Because the binding sites for the radioimmunoassay of GH are not affected by the GHBP, both bound and unbound GH are measured *(8)*. GHBP is the proteolytic cleavage product of the full-length membrane bound receptor molecule in humans *(9)*. This characteristic permits the assay of circulating GHBP as a measure of cellular bound GHR, which usually correlates with GHR function *(2,10)*.

The GH molecule binds to a molecule of cell surface GHR at a unique binding site, which then dimerizes with another GHR molecule at a second binding site in the extracellular domain, so that a single GH molecule is enveloped by two GHR molecules *(11)*. The intact receptor lacks tyrosine kinase activity, but is closely associated with JAK2, a member of the Janus kinase family. JAK2 is activated by binding of GH with the GHR dimer, which results in self phosphorylation of the JAK2 and a cascade of phosphorylation of cellular proteins. Included in this cascade are signal transducers and activators of transcription (STATs), which couple ligand binding to the activation of gene expression, and mitogen activated protein kinases (MAPK). Other effector proteins have also been examined in various systems. This is a mechanism typical of the growth hormone/prolactin/cytokine receptor family that includes receptors for erythropoietin, interleukins, and other growth factors *(8)*

The effect of GH on growth is indirect, via stimulation of IGF-I production, primarily in the liver *(12)*. Hepatic IGF-I circulates almost exclusively bound to IGFBPs, less than 1% being unbound. The IGFBPs are a family of six structurally related proteins with a high affinity for binding IGF. At least four other related proteins with lower affinity for IGF peptides have been identified and are referred to as IGFBP-related proteins *(13)*. IGFBP-3 is the most abundant IGFBP, binding 75–90% of circulating IGF-I in a large (150–200 kDa) complex which consists of IGFBP-3, an acid labile subunit (ALS), and the IGF molecule. Both ALS and IGFBP-3 are produced in the liver as a direct effect of GH. The remainder of bound IGF is in a 50-kD complex largely with IGFBP-1 and IGFBP-2. IGFBP-1 production is highly variable, with the highest concentrations in the fasting, hypoinsulinemic state. The circulating concentration of IGFBP-2 is less fluctuant and is partly under the control of IGF-I; levels are increased in GHR deficient states, but increase further with IGF-I therapy of such patients *(7,14)*.

The IGFBPs modulate IGF action by controlling storage and release of IGF-I in the circulation, by influencing the binding of IGF-I to its receptor, by facilitating storage of IGFs in extracellular matrices, and by independent actions. IGFBPs 1, 2, 4, and 6 inhibit IGF action by preventing binding of IGF-I with its specific receptor. The binding of IGFBP-3 to cell surfaces is thought to decrease its affinity for IGF-I, effectively delivering the IGF-I to the type 1 IGF receptor. IGFBP-5 potentiates the effects of IGF-I in a variety of cells; its binding to extracellular matrix proteins allows fixation of IGFs and enhances IGF binding to hydroxyapatite. IGFs stored in such a manner in soft tissue may enhance wound healing. IGF independent mechanisms for IGFBP-1 and IGFBP-3 proliferative effects have been demonstrated in vitro and nuclear localization of IGFBP-3 has been reported. Cell surface association and phosphorylation of IGFBP determine the influence of IGFBPs. Specific protease activity, particularly affecting IGFBP-3, is also important in the modulation of IGF action in target tissues. IGFBP-3 specific proteolytic activity may alter the affinity of the binding protein for IGF-I, resulting in release of free IGF-I for binding to the IGF-I receptor *(7,12)*.

Autocrine and paracrine production of IGF-I occurs in tissues other than the liver. In growing bone, GH stimulates differentiation of pre-chondrocytes into chondrocytes able to secrete IGF-I, stimulating clonal expansion and maturation of the chondrocytes, with growth. It is estimated that approximately 20% of GH stimulated growth results from this autocrine-paracrine IGF-I mechanism *(15)*.

DISCOVERY OF LARON SYNDROME AND PRE-MOLECULAR STUDY

Following the initial report *(16)* of three Yemenite Jewish siblings, "with hypoglycemia and other clinical and laboratory signs of growth hormone deficiency, but with abnormally high concentrations of immunoreactive serum growth hormone," 22 patients were reported from Israel, all Oriental Jews, with an apparent autosomal recessive mode of transmission in consanguineous families *(17)*. These reports preceded the recognition of the critical role of cell surface receptors in hormone action and it was postulated that the defect was in the GH molecule that these patients produced. This impression was substantiated by the observation of free-fatty acid mobilization, nitrogen retention, and growth in patients being administered exogenous GH *(16,17)*. These effects may have been due to other pituitary hormones in the crude extracts administered or to nutritional changes in the investigative setting.

In the first patient reported outside of Israel, in 1968, there was no response to exogenous GH, leading to the hypothesis that the defect was in the GH receptor *(18)*. This hypothesis was substantiated by the failure to demonstrate sulfation factor activation (subsequently identified as IGF-I) with exogenous GH administration, reported in 1969 *(19)* and reports in 1973 and 1976 that the patients' GH was normal on fractionation, normal in its binding to antibodies, and normal in its binding to hepatic cell membranes from normal individuals *(20–23)*. In vitro demonstration of cellular unresponsiveness to GH was demonstrated by the failure of erythroid progenitor cells from the peripheral blood of two patients to respond to exogenous GH *(24)*. The failure of radioiodine labelled GH to bind to liver cell microsomes obtained from biopsy of two patients with Laron syndrome confirmed that the defect was in the GHR *(25)*.

Just before the report that human circulating GHBP was the extracellular domain of the cell surface GHR (9), two reports appeared indicating that GHBP was absent from serum of patients with Laron syndrome *(26,27)*.

THE MOLECULAR BASIS OF GHI

The GHR Gene

The GHR gene is on the proximal short arm of chromosome 5, spanning 86 kilobase pairs. The 5' untranslated region (UTR) is followed by 9 coding exons. Exon 2 encodes the last 11 base pairs of the 5'-UTR sequence, an 18 amino acid signal sequence, and the initial 5 amino acids of the extracellular hormone binding domain. Exons 3–7 encode the extracellular hormone binding domain, except for the terminal 3 amino acids of his domain, which are encoded by exon 8. Exon 8 further encodes the 24 amino acid hydrophobic transmembrane domain and the initial 4 amino acids of the intracellular domain. Exons 9 and 10 encode the large intracellular domain. Exon 10 also encodes the 2 kb 3'-UTR *(10)*.

GHR Gene Mutations

The initial report of the characterization of the GHR gene described non-contiguous deletion of exons 3, 5, and 6 in two Israeli patients with Laron syndrome *(28)*. The deletion of exon 3 has subsequently been shown to be an alternatively spliced polymorphism, rather than a functional component of the defect *(29)*. Only four Israeli patients have been described as homozygous for this mutation and a fifth was heterozygous (with, apparently, a different mutation of the other allele), among over 30 Oriental Jewish patients in Israel, indicating heterogeneity for the genetic defect in the GHR within an ethnically homogeneous population *(30)*. No other exon deletions have been described in patients with GHI, but 38 additional defects of the GHR gene have been described in association with GHI, including 8 nonsense mutations, 14 missense mutations, 5 frame shift mutations, 10 splice mutations, and a unique intronic mutation resulting in insertion of a pseudo-exon *(10,31)*. The functional insignificance of exon 3 is emphasized by the fact that no mutations affecting this exon have been associated with GHI. Neither have functional mutations been described in exon 2. A number of other mutations have been described which are either polymorphisms or have not occurred in the homozygous or compound heterozygous state *(30)*.

Only 3 of the homozygous or compound heterozygous defects that have been described thus far do not result in the expected absent or extremely low levels of GHBP. The D152H missense mutation occurs at the GHR dimerization site, with normal production and GH binding of the extracellular domain, but failure to dimerize at the cell surface. Thus, despite failure of GHR function, circulating concentrations of GHBP are normal. High concentrations of GHBP in serum occur with the splice mutations that are close to (G223G) or within (R274T) the transmembrane domain. These defects interfere with the normal splicing of exon 8, which encodes the transmembrane domain; the mature GHR transcript is translated into a truncated protein that retains GH binding activity but cannot be anchored to the cell surface *(30)*.

Several heterozygous mutations of the GHR have been proposed as causative of moderate growth failure with absence of other clinical characteristics of GHI *(32–35)*, but the heterozygous effects of only two cytoplasmic domain defects have been supported by biochemical findings and in vitro experimentation. A Caucasian mother and daughter and Japanese siblings and their mother with moderate short stature were heterozygous for an intronic splice mutation preceding exon 9 and a point mutation of the donor splice site in intron 9 of the GHR gene, respectively, resulting in an extensively attenuated, virtually absent intracellular domain *(36,37)*. Individuals with these heterozygous defects produce both normal and abnormal GHR protein, giving three possible types of GHR dimerization: a fully functional unit formed from two normal GHR molecules, a heterodimer of unknown functional capacity comprised of a mutant and normal molecule, or a nonfunctional homodimer formed by two mutant GHR molecules lacking a cytoplasmic domain. The normal function of some of these dimers was demonstrated in the affected Japanese mother and her two children by a substantial increase in the subnormal IGF-I levels following 3 d of GH injection *(37)*.

When these heterozygote GHR mutants were transfected into permanent cell lines, they demonstrated increased affinity for GH compared to the wild-type full-length GHR and markedly increased the production of GHBP. A dominant negative effect occurred when the mutant was co-transfected with full-length GHR, the result of overexpression of the mutant GHR and inhibition of GH-induced tyrosine phosphorylation and transcription activation *(36,38)*. Naturally occurring truncated isoforms have also shown this dominant negative effect in vitro *(39–41)*.

There is no convincing clinical or experimental evidence for any mutation involving the extracellular or transmembrane domains of the GHR having a deleterious effect in the heterozygous state, either as an isolated occurrence, or in the carrier relatives of individuals with GHI *(7,32,33,42–44)*.

In the largest cohort of GHI due to GHRD, that from Ecuador comprising 71 patients, all but one subject have the E180 splice mutation, which is shared with at least one Israeli patient of Moroccan heritage (45). Only four of the other reported defects are not family- or ethnicity-specific. The R43X mutation, two other nonsense mutations (C38X, R217X), and the intron 4 splice mutation have been described in disparate populations, on different genetic backgrounds, indicating that these are mutational hotspots *(30)*.

A novel intronic point mutation was recently described in a highly consanguineous family with two pairs of affected cousins with GHBP-positive GHI. This mutation resulted in a 108 bp insertion of a pseudoexon between exons 6 and 7, predicting an in-frame, 36 residue amino acid sequence. This is a region critically involved in receptor dimerization *(31)*.

Mutation of the GHR has been identified in fewer than half of the patients with GHRD outside of Ecuador; thus, it is likely that the list of mutations will continue to grow and provide further insight into the function of the GHR.

GH-GHR Signal Transduction Abnormality

The full clinical picture of Laron syndrome, with elevated circulating concentrations of GH, was seen in Arab siblings with apparently normal binding of GH to the GHR, inferred from normal serum concentrations of GHBP and IGFBP-3 *(46)*. A failure of GH-GHR signal transduction was also been proposed to explain short stature in four GHBP positive children from two unrelated Pakistani families *(47)*. The Pakistani patients differed from the Arab children in having low serum concentrations of IGFBP-3. In one family, there were severe and typical phenotypic features of GH deficiency, and the defect was thought to be close to the GHR, preventing activation of both the STAT and MAPK pathways demonstrated in cultured fibroblasts. In the other family, there was a less marked phenotype and a defect in activation of MAPK, but not the STAT pathway in cultured fibroblasts from the patients *(48)*.

EPIDEMIOLOGY

Geographic and Ethnic Distribution

Ethnic origin is known for over 90% of the ~260 reported cases of GHRD; it is likely that an equal number are not reported *(30)*. Nearly 50% are Oriental Jews as described in the original reports *(15,16)*, or known descendants of Iberian Jews who converted to Catholicism during the Spanish Inquisition. The latter comprise the largest ($n = 71$) and only genetically homogenous patient group. The finding of a Jewish patient of Moroccan origin with the same mutation as the Ecuadorian patients supports the hypothesis that this mutation was brought to the New World by Spanish conversos (new Christians) fleeing the Inquisition *(45)*. Thus far, there is no explanation for the middle eastern predominance of this condition, although the high frequency of consanguinity in Arab and traditional Jewish populations is certainly a factor. Nearly 90% of patients are either Oriental Jews, Arabs, or other middle easterners, from elsewhere in the Mediterranean area, or from the Indian subcontinent. Many of those from other parts of the world may have middle eastern Semitic origins. The small numbers of non-Semitic, non-Mediterranean, non-Indian patients include a genetic isolate of Anglo-Saxons from a Bahamian island, five Africans, five Japanese, two siblings from Cambodia, a Vietnamese, and several from northern Europe *(10)*.

Morbidity and Mortality

The only available report of the effect of GHRD on mortality comes from the Ecuadorian population *(49)*. Because families in the relatively small area from which the Ecuadorian patients originate had intensive experience with this condition, lay diagnosis was considered reliable. Of 79 affected individuals for whom information could be obtained, 15 (19%) died under 7 yr of age, as opposed to 21 out of 216 of their unaffected siblings (9.7%, $p < 0.05$). The kinds of illnesses resulting in death, such as pneumonia, diarrhea, and meningitis, were no different for affected than for unaffected siblings.

The complete lifespan included in the Ecuadorian cohort provided an opportunity to look at adult mortality risk factors. This is of interest because GHD in adults is associated with premature atherosclerosis and increased cardiovascular mortality, with GH replacement therapy improving the risk factors of hyperlipidemia and obesity *(50)*. Twenty-three adults with GHD had elevated cholesterol levels, normal HDL-cholesterol (HDL-C) levels, elevated LDL-cholesterol (HDL-C) levels, and normal triglycerides compared to relatives and non-related community controls. It was postulated that the effect of IGF-I deficiency due to GHRD was to decrease hepatic clearance of LDL-C, since the triglyceride and HDL-C levels were unaffected. This effect was independent of obesity or IGFBP-1 levels, which were used as a surrogate for insulinemia *(50)*. The key pathogenic factor was thought to be the absence of GH induction of LDL receptors in the liver *(51)*.

Of 8 Ecuadorian patients over 50 yr of age followed for greater than 7 yr, 2 died of heart disease, an uncommon problem in the Andean setting *(48)*. This might suggest comparable increased cardiovascular risk to that seen with GHD in adults.

CLINICAL FINDINGS (TABLE 2)

Growth

Many, if not most, patients with GHI due to GHRD have normal intrauterine growth *(1)*. Children with GH gene deletion also have normal intrauterine growth despite total absence of endogenous GH *(4)*. Nonetheless, IGF-I is required for normal intrauterine growth as demonstrated by patients with intrauterine growth retardation with a proven IGF-I gene defect *(2)* or IGF receptor mutation *(3)*. Thus, this intrauterine IGF-I synthesis does not appear to be GH dependent.

Standard deviation score (SDS) for length declines rapidly after birth (Fig. 2) indicating the GH dependency of extra-uterine growth. Growth velocity with severe GHD or GHI is approximately half normal (Fig. 3). Occasional periods of normal growth velocity may be related to improved nutrition.

Despite normal sexual maturation, the pubertal growth spurt is minimal or absent, as documented in the most extensive available data, from Israel and Ecuador *(1,53)*. The adolescent growth spurt is GH dependent, reflected in significantly elevated circulating levels of GH and IGF-I compared to preadolescence and adulthood *(54)*. Among 24 Israeli patients followed from infancy to adulthood, persistent growth beyond the normal time of adolescence was seen only in boys. In the Ecuadorian population, girls also showed this phenomenon (Fig. 3). Adult stature in GHRD varies from –12 to –5.3 SDS in Ecuadorian patients and –9 to –3.8 SDS in others in the literature, using the US standards *(1)*. This is a height range of 95–124 cm for women and 106–141 cm for men

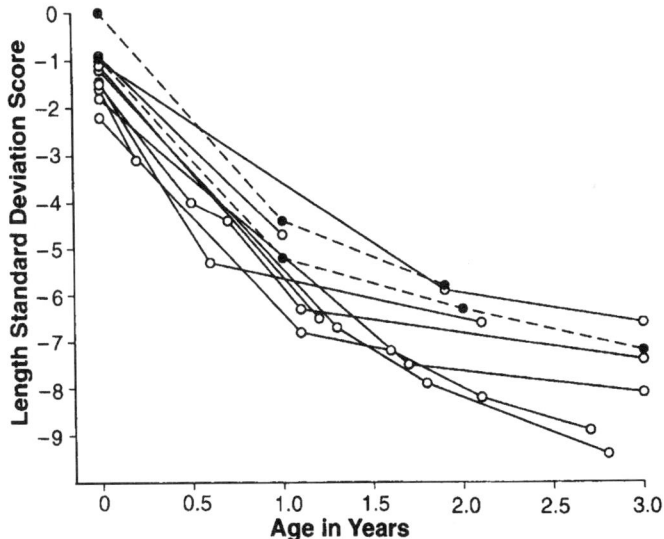

Fig. 2. Length standard deviation scores of nine girls from Ecuador (open circles, solid lines) and two brothers from southern Russia (solid circles, dashed lines) with known birth lengths, followed over the first 2–3 yr of life. Reprinted from *Trends Endocrinol Metab*, vol 5, Rosenbloom AL, Guevara-Aguirre J, Rosenfeld RG, Pollock BH. Growth in growth hormone insensitivity, pp 296–303, 1994, with kind permission from Elsevier Science Ltd, The Boulevard, Langford Lane, Kidlington OX5 1GB, UK.

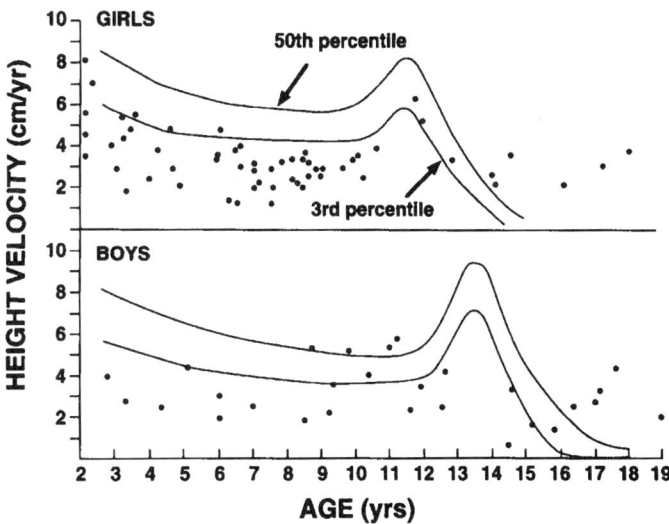

Fig. 3. Growth velocities of 30 Ecuadorian patients (10 males) with GH receptor deficiency; repeated measures were at least 6 mo apart. Third and 50th percentiles are from: Tanner JM, Davies PSW: Clinical longitudinal standards for height and height velocity for North American children. J Pediatr 1985;107:317–328. Reprinted from *Trends Endocrinol Metab*, vol 5, Rosenbloom AL, Guevara-Aguirre J, Rosenfeld RG, Pollock BH. Growth in growth hormone insensitivity, pp 296–303, 1994, with kind permission from Elsevier Science Ltd, The Boulevard, Langford Lane, Kidlington OX5 1GB, UK.

Table 2
Clinical Features of Severe IGF-I Deficiency
Resulting from GH Deficiency or GH Receptor Deficiency

Growth
- Birth weight - normal; birth length - usually normal
- Growth failure, from birth, with velocity 1/2 normal
- Height deviation correlates with (low) serum levels of IGF-I, -II and IGFBP-3
- Delayed bone age, but advanced for height age
- Small hands or feet

Craniofacial Characteristics
- Sparse hair before age 7; frontotemporal hairline recession all ages
- Prominent forehead
- Head size more normal than stature with impression of large head
- "Setting sun sign" (sclera visible above iris at rest) 25% < 10 yr of age
- Hypoplastic nasal bridge, shallow orbits
- Decreased vertical dimension of face
- Blue scleras
- Prolonged retention of primary dentition with decay; normal permanent teeth, may be crowded; absent 3rd molars
- Sculpted chin
- Unilateral ptosis, facial asymmetry (15%)

Musculoskeletal/Body Composition
- Hypomuscularity with delay in walking
- Avascular necrosis of femoral head (25%)
- High pitched voices in all children, most adults
- Thin, prematurely aged skin
- Limited elbow extensibility after 5 years of age
- Children underweight to normal for height, most adults overweight for height; markedly decreased ratio of lean mass to fat mass, compared to normal, at all ages
- Osteopenia indicated by DEXA

Metabolic
- Hypoglycemia (fasting)
- Increased cholesterol and LDL-C
- Decreased sweating

Sexual Development
- Small penis in childhood; normal growth with adolescence
- Delayed puberty
- Normal reproduction

in the Ecuadorian population. This wide variation in the effect of GHRD on stature was not only seen within the population but also within affected families, and this intrafamilial variability has also been described with severe GHD due to GH gene deletion *(4)*.

Some patients with GHRD may have an appetite problem in addition to their IGF-I deficiency. Crosnier et al. *(55)* studied a child aged 3 1/2 yr with GHRD who had severe anorexia. With his usual intake of approx 500 kcal/d, he grew at a rate of 2 cm/yr. With moderate hyperalimentation to approx 1300 kcal/d, growth rate increased to 9 cm/yr without significant change in plasma IGF-I level. The hyperalimentation period was associated with an increase in the IGFBP-3 bands on Western ligand blots, from total absence in the anorexic period to levels comparable to those seen in GHD. The catch-up growth noted could not be explained by hyperinsulinism, which has provided the explanation for accelerated or normal growth in children with GHD and obesity following removal of a craniopharyngioma. There was no appreciable increase in circulating basal or stimulated insulin during the hyperalimentation. In this patient, there was speculation that a nutrition dependent autocrine/paracrine increase in IGF-I concentration at the cartilage growth plate might have occurred independent of the GHR. Not considered at the time was the possibility that IGFBP-3 itself might have growth promoting effects. The importance of adequate nutrition for catch-up growth was emphasized by this study, reinforcing the notion that normal periods of growth in patients with GHRD without IGF-I replacement therapy, as noted in Figure 3, might be explained by periods of improved nutrition alone.

Craniofacial Characteristics

Affected children are recognized by knowledgeable family members at birth because of craniofacial characteristics of frontal prominence, depressed nasal bridge, and sparse hair, as well as small hands or feet, and hypoplastic fingernails (Fig. 4). Decreased vertical dimension of the face is demonstrable by computer analysis of the relationships between facial landmarks and is present in all patients when compared with their relatives (Fig. 5) including those with normal appearing facies (Fig. 6) *(56)*. Blue scleras, the result of decreased thickness of the scleral connective tissue, permitting visualization of the underlying choroid, were originally described in the Ecuadorian population, and subsequently recognized in other populations with GHRD, as well as in GHD *(57,58)*. Unilateral ptosis and facial asymmetry may reflect positional deformity due to decreased muscular activity *in utero*, although mothers do not recognize decreased fetal movement in pregnancies with affected infants *(59)*.

Musculoskeletal and Body Composition

Hypomuscularity is apparent in radiographs of affected infants, and is thought to be responsible for delayed walking despite normal intelligence and timing of speech onset *(59)*. Radiographs of the children also suggest osteopenia; dual photon absorptiometry and dual energy x-ray absorptiometry in children and adults confirm this. A study of dynamic bone histomorphometry in adults with GHRD demonstrated normal bone volume and formation rate, with reduction in trabecular connectivity. This study suggested that some of densitometry findings were artifactual, based on small bone size *(60)*.

Limited elbow extensibility seen in most patients over 5 yr of age in the Ecuadorian population is an acquired characteristic, absent in younger children and increasing in severity with age *(57,59)*. This feature is not peculiar to the Ecuadorian population or to IGF-I deficiency due to GHRD, recently confirmed by a Brazilian patient with GHRD with limited elbow extension *(61)* and observing this finding in all but the youngest patient in a family with eight individuals affected by multiple pituitary deficiencies *(58)*. The cause of this elbow contracture is unknown.

Although children appear overweight, they are actually underweight to normal weight for height, while most adults, especially females, are overweight with markedly decreased lean to fat ratios *(59)*.

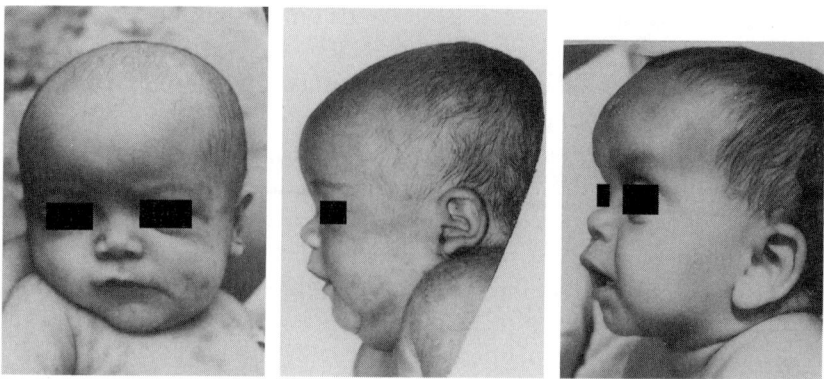

Fig. 4. Front and profile views of 4-mo-old girl, homozygous for the E180 splice mutation of the GHR, demonstrating paucity of hair, prominent forehead, hypoplastic nasal bridge, shallow orbits, and reduced vertical dimension of the face, and profile view of a three-year-old patient from the initial report of Laron syndrome *(6)*, demonstrating persistence of these features, and striking similarity with different genetic mutations. Reprinted from *Trends Endocrinol Metab*, vol 9, Rosenbloom, AL, Guevara-Aguirre J. Lessons from the genetics of Laron syndrome, pp 276–283, 1998, with kind permission from Elsevier Science Ltd, The Boulevard, Langford Lane, Kidlington OX5 1GB, UK.

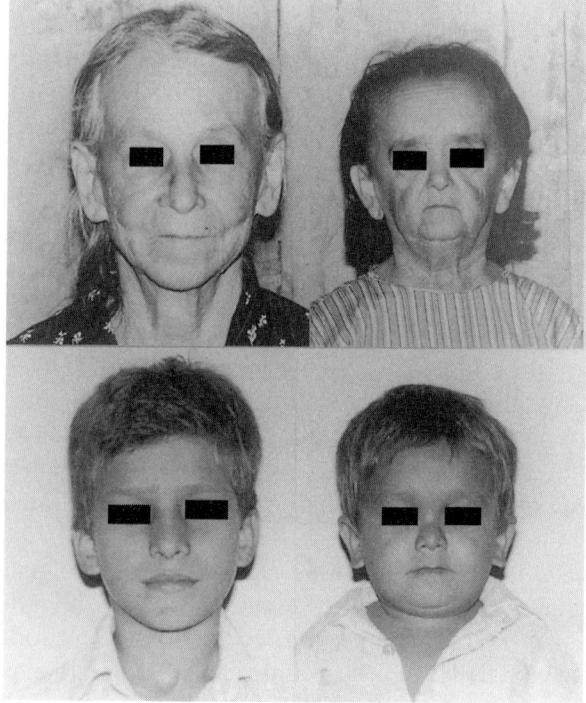

Fig. 5. Comparisons of facial appearance between 52-yr-old patient (right upper panel) and her 76-yr-old mother (left upper panel) and 9-yr-old patient (right lower panel) and his 11-yr-old unaffected brother (left lower panel). Photos were taken at exactly the same distances. Note strong familial similarity but marked difference in facial dimensions. Reproduced from *(59)* with permission from Karger AG, Basel, Switzerland.

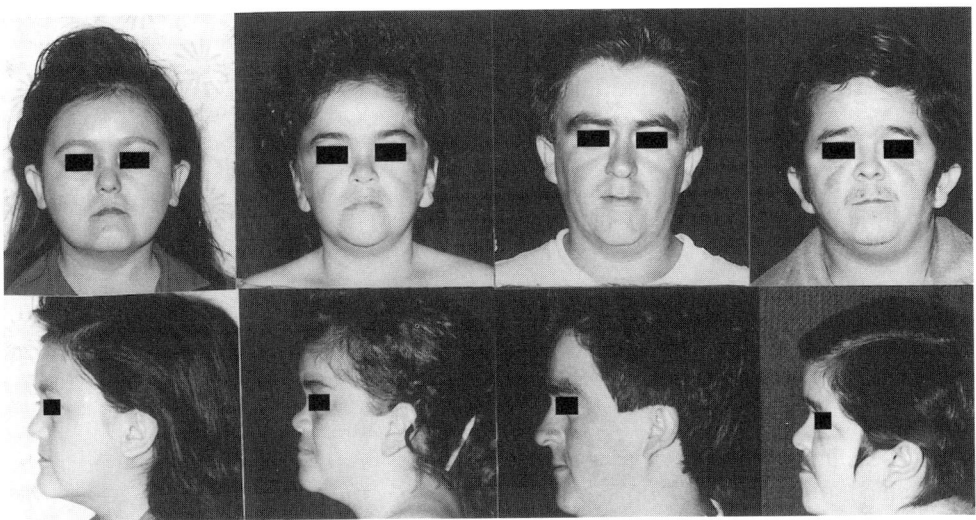

Fig. 6. Two women and two men from Ecuador with growth hormone receptor deficiency resulting from the E180 splice mutation of the GH receptor, demonstrating variation in craniofacial effects. From left to right, a 17-yr-old woman with height standard deviation score (SDS) –7.8, two years after menarche and a year after she stopped growing, a 19-yr-old woman 4 yr postmenarcheal with height SDS –6.5 (tallest female in the cohort), a 21-yr-old man with height SDS –7.6, and a 28-yr-old man with height SDS –9.2. Reprinted from Hormone and Metabolic Research, Volume 31. Rosenbloom AL. IGF-I deficiency due to GH receptor deficiency. Pages 161–171. Copyright 1999, with permission from Georg Thieme Verlag Stuttgart-New York.

Reproduction

Severe GHD is associated with small penis size with normal penile growth at adolescence or with testosterone treatment in childhood. This is also true of GHRD. Although puberty may be delayed 3–7 yr in some 50% of individuals, there is normal adult sexual function with documented reproduction by males and females *(49)*. Females require C-section delivery.

Intellectual and Social Development

Intellectual impairment was originally considered a feature of the Laron syndrome *(62)*. Among 18 affected children and adolescents administered the Wechsler Intelligence Scale for Children, only 3 had IQs within the average range *(90–110)*; of the remaining 15 subjects, 3 were in the low average range *(80–89)*, 3 in the borderline range *(70–79)* and 9 in the intellectually disabled range (<70). These studies were done without family controls, so that the possibility of other factors related to consanguinity that might affect intellectual development could not be addressed. In a followup study 25 years later, the investigators re-examined 8 of the original 18 patients and 4 new patients with GHRD, excluding 5 patients with mental disabilities who were in the original study *(63)*. This group had mean verbal and performance IQs of 86 and 92 on the Wechsler scale without evidence of visual motor integration difficulties noted in the earlier group, but a suggestion of deficient short term memory and attention. The investigators hypothesized that early and prolonged IGF deficiency might impair normal development of the central nervous system, or that hypoglycemia common in younger patients may have had a deleterious effect.

The recent description of intellectual impairment with severe IGF-I deficiency due to partial deletion of the IGF-I gene added concern about potential effects of severe IGF-I deficiency *in utero* (2). Nonetheless, patients with GH gene deletion and severe IGF-I deficiency have not been intellectually impaired (4), nor have those with severe IGF-I deficiency due to molecular defects in the GHRH-R (64). Sporadic anecdotal reports of patients with GHRD suggested a normal range of intelligence. The collective data from the European IGF-I treatment study group, which includes a wider range of clinical abnormality than either the Ecuadorian or Israeli population, notes a mental retardation rate of 13.5% among 82 patients, but formal testing was not carried out (65). Here again, the high rate of consanguinity was proposed as a possible explanation; hypoglycemia could not be correlated with these findings.

In the Ecuadorian population, exceptional school performance was reported among 51 affected individuals of school age or older who had attended school, with 44 typically in the top 3 places in their classes and most thought to be as bright or brighter than the smartest of their unaffected siblings (66).

The first controlled documentation of intellectual function in a population with GHRD was in the Ecuadorian patients, a study of school age individuals compared to their close relatives and to community controls. No significant differences in intellectual ability could be detected among these groups, using non-verbal tests with minimal cultural limitations. It was hypothesized that the exceptional school performance in this population might have been related to the lack of social opportunities due to extreme short stature, resulting in greater devotion to studies and superior achievement in school for IQ level (67).

The clinical findings of intellectual impairment with IGF-I gene deletion (2) and intellectual normality with GHRD is consistent with gene disruption studies in mice. The IGF-I deleted mouse is neurologically impaired, while the GHRD mouse is behaviorally normal (68,69). Thus, GHD dependent IGF-I production is not necessary for normal brain development and function.

BIOCHEMICAL FEATURES

Growth Hormone

Affected children have random GH levels that are greater than 10 ng/ml and may be as high as 200 ng/mL, with enhanced responsiveness to stimulation and paradoxical elevations following oral and intravenous glucose, as is seen in acromegaly (7,48). The GH levels show normal diurnal fluctuation. Twenty-four-h profiles demonstrate marked GH variability among adult patients with suppression by exogenous recombinant human IGF-I (14). Thus, the normal sensitivity of the GH secretion is preserved, despite lifelong elevated GH levels and lack of feedback suppression from IGF-I.

Postpubertal patients may have normal or elevated basal levels of GH but invariably demonstrate hyper-responsiveness to stimulation, which is all the more impressive considering their obesity, which suppresses GH responses in normal individuals. In the Ecuadorian population, mean basal GH level in adults was significantly lower than that in children (11 ± 11 ng/mL vs 32 ± 22 ng/mL, $p < 0.0001$). This is thought to be related to the greater, though still markedly abnormal, IGF-I levels in the adults, resulting in some feedback inhibition of GH secretion (7,49).

Growth Hormone Binding Protein

Absence of GHBP in the circulation was initially considered a requirement for the diagnosis of GHRD, along with the clinical phenotype, very low concentrations of IGF-I and IGFBP-3, and elevated (in children) or normal to elevated (in adults) GH levels. Chromatographic analysis for serum GHBP, however, showed measurable though reduced levels in a number of patients. The ligand mediated immunofunction assay (LIFA) used to measure GHBP serum levels since 1990, uses an anti-GH monoclonal antibody to measure the amount of GH bound to GHBP. As a largely functional assay, this should not detect structurally abnormal though expressed GHBP *(7)*.

As noted above, certain genetic defects in the GHR, those affecting dimerization or anchoring of the GHBP to the cell membrane and dominant negative mutations of the cytoplasmic domain, can result in normal or elevated GHBP levels. In the Ecuadorian population, despite in vitro evidence for failure of production of normally spliced receptor, 4 children and 4 adults out of 49 patients had serum GHBP levels higher than 40% of the sex specific lower limit for controls and 1 adult male had a level in the lower portion of the normal adult male range. The presence or amount of GHBP measured did not relate to stature *(59)*. There were no age-dependent changes, indicating that the difference in IGF values between children and adults was not related to the GHBP levels and the GHBP levels did not correlate with stature or with serum IGF-I levels. Although finding extremely low or undetectable levels of GHBP serves as an important diagnostic feature, it is not a *sine qua non* for the diagnosis of GHRD.

Insulin-Like Growth Factors

The lowest serum levels of IGF-I are seen in severe congenital defects in GH synthesis (GH gene deletion, GHRH-R deficiency), with deletion of the IGF-I gene, and with GHRD. IGF-II is not as severely suppressed, its reduction likely related to diminution of GHBP-3 rather than to decreased synthesis. In chronic disease states associated with acquired GHI, IGF-I levels are more likely to be reduced than are concentrations of IGF-II and IGFBP-3 *(7)*.

Among 50 Ecuadorian patients homozygous for the E180 splice-site mutation, IGF-I levels were significantly greater in adults 16–67 yr of age ($n = 31$, 25 ± 19 µg/L) than in the 19 subjects under 16 y of age (3 ± 2 µg/L, $p < 0.0001$), although still markedly below the normal range of 96–270 µg/L. The children's levels were too low to correlate with stature, but in the adults IGF-I levels correlated inversely with statural SDS with a coefficient of 0.64 ($p < 0.001$). IGF-II levels in adults were also significantly greater than in children (151 ± 75 µg/L vs 70 ± 42 µg/L, normal 388 to 792 µg/L, $p < 0.0001$). The correlation between serum IGF-I and IGF-II levels was highly significant, $r = 0.53$, $p < 0.001$. With no indication of age difference in GHBP levels, the increased levels of IGF-I and -II with adulthood suggest effects on synthesis of these growth factors which are not mediated through the GHR and are presumably under the influence of sex steroids. This hypothesis was challenged by findings in patients with GHRH resistance due to mutation of the GHRH receptor. Sexually mature individuals with severe short stature from GH deficiency resulting from GHRH receptor mutation and affected children have comparably very low IGF-I (and IGFBP-3) serum concentrations *(64)*. The correlation of IGF-I levels with stature in adults with GHRD indicates that, despite the markedly low levels, the influence of IGF-I on stature remains important in these subjects.

IGF Binding Proteins

In IGF deficiency states that are the result of GHD or GHRD, IGFBP-3 is reduced, and in children and adults with GHRD this reduction correlates with statural impairment (1). In renal disease, elevated IGFBP-3, as well as IGFBP-1 and IGFBP-2, are thought to impair the delivery of normal levels of IGF-I (5).

Short term and extended treatment of GHI with IGF-I has failed to result in increases in IGFBP-3 (14,70–74), whereas treatment of GHD with recombinant human GH restores levels to normal. This indicates that IGFBP-3 production is under the direct influence of GH.

IGFBP-I is elevated in GHD and GHRD; in GHRD it is the most abundant IGFBP and is strongly inversely related to insulinemia. IGFBP-2 is present at a mean 300% of control concentrations in children with GHRD and 175% of control in affected adults, a significant difference. The IGFBP-3 levels in adults with GHRD are significantly greater than those in affected children (75).

DIAGNOSTIC ISSUES IN GH RESISTANCE

GHI/GHRD is readily diagnosed in its typical and complete form because of: severe growth failure; the somatic phenotype of severe GHD; elevated serum GH levels; and marked reduction in IGF-I, IGF-II, and IGFBP-3 concentrations, with increased concentrations of IGFBP-1 and IGFBP-2. Most such individuals will also have absent to very low concentrations of GHBP, although the less common GHBP positive forms make absence of GHBP an important but not essential criterion. As noted in Table 1, some of the biochemical features of GHRD may be shared by conditions associated with acquired GH insensitivity, such as malnutrition and liver disease. In a large multinational study designed to identify patients for replacement therapy with recombinant human IGF-I (rhIGF-I), a scoring system was developed which assigned one point for each of the following:

- Height > 3 SD below mean height for age
- Basal GH > 2.5 µg/L
- Basal IGF-I <50 µg/L
- Basal IGFBP-3 < –2 SD
- IGF-I rise with GH (0.05 mg/kg/d × 4 d) < 15 µg/L
- IGFBP-3 rise with GH stimulation < 0.4 mg/L
- GH binding < 10% (based on binding of ^{125}I-hGH)

A score of 5 out of the possible 7 was considered diagnostic for GHR deficiency. This standard resulted in identification of 82 patients from 22 countries who reflect a wide variability for each criterion. Particularly noteworthy was that height SDS range was up to –2.2 (76). These criteria recognize the age and sex (after age 7 yr) variation of IGFBP 3 by using a standard of < –2 SD but, oddly, designate a fixed standard for IGF-I which is within the range of normal for children under age 7 (Table 3).

As noted above, the presence of a homozygous mutation or a compound heterozygous mutation affecting the GHR usually provides definitive diagnosis. Thirty-one of the 82 patients reported by Woods et al. (65) had a genetic study of the GHR, of whom 27 had abnormalities affecting both alleles of the GHR gene, in association with clinically and biochemically unequivocal GHRD. Identification of heterozygous mutations, however,

Table 3
Reference Values (ng/mL) for IGF-I
and IGFBP-3 According to Age and Sex (After Age 7 yr-F/M)[a]

Age (yr)	Mean IGF-I	−2 SD IGF-I	Mean IGFBP-3	−2 SD IGFBP-3
0	27	5	1874	1040
1	35	8	2058	1107
2	56	20	2153	1248
3	59	20	2203	1180
4	69	25	2321	1578
5	97	37	2628	1789
6	119	45	2862	1862
7	172/170	44/54	3913/3329	2190/1699
8	236/170	50/52	3840/3478	2497/2371
9	227/192	44/64	3413/3604	575/2265
10	270/131	94/37	3982/3244	2371/3244
11	308/137	93/30	4540/3396	2494/2041
12	387/219	126/63	4413/3666	2074/2167
13	459/329	216/83	4134/4334	2260/2616
14	481/519	271/183	4246/4354	2592/1946
15	473/518	254/335	4332/4028	2710/1495
16	431/519	192/401	4570/4842	3225/3435
17	412/372	253/210	4001/4152	2183/2065
18	408/499	223/206	4078/4810	1846/3235
19	335/397	182/168	4218/4752	2049/2495
20	255/434	86/267	4398/4554	2446/3214

[a] Adapted from the Meet-the-Professor session handouts for The Endocrine Society 81st Annual Meeting, June 12–15 1999. Clinical Utility of IGF and IGFBP Measurements by Ron G. Rosenfeld, MD.

is not necessarily helpful because, as noted earlier, polymorphisms have been described that appear to have no phenotypic consequences.

Partial GH Resistance

It is reasonable to consider that, as with GH deficiency, GH resistance might be expected to occur in an incomplete form, as is also seen with insulin resistance, androgen insensitivity, and thyroid hormone resistance. Affected children might have growth failure with normal or slightly increased GH secretion, low normal or slightly decreased GHBP levels, decreased IGF-I concentrations, but not as severely reduced as in complete GHD or GHRD, and they might respond to supraphysiologic doses of GH. It might also be expected, given the need for dimerization of the GHR for signal transduction, that certain mutations could have a dominant negative effect in the heterozygous state. As noted above, two such defects have been described. GHBP concentrations are low in children with idiopathic short stature (ISS, i.e., short children without a recognizable syndrome or GHD). Using a ligand mediated immunofunction assay Goddard et al. *(35)* studied a large number of short children with known causes of growth failure such as GHD and Turner syndrome, or ISS, and compared their GHBP concentrations in serum to those of normal controls. Ninety percent of the children with ISS had GHBP concentrations below the control mean and nearly 20% had concentrations that were two standard deviations or more below the normal mean for age and sex. To explore the possibility that these low GHBP concentrations might indicate partial GHI, molecular genetic analysis was done in 14 children with ISS who had low GHBP concentrations and normal GH secretion. Five GH receptor mutations were detected in four children. In one patient, there was compound heterozygosity involving mutations in exons 4 and 6. The other 3 patients were heterozygous for mutations in the GHR with no defects in the other allele. The method used could have missed additional mutations and there might also be involvement of the regulatory domains of the GHR. None of these patients had the clinical phenotype of GHD. Three of the four patients were treated with GH and had modest improvement in growth velocity in the first year. This modest response could be due to GH resistance or simply to the fact that they were not IGF-I deficient.

Whether the distribution of GHBP concentrations in ISS indicates that partial GHI is an important cause of short stature remains to be demonstrated. The 14 subjects studied by Goddard et al. *(35)* were selected from the large US National Cooperative Growth Study database. Thus, if other heterozygous mutations of the GHR besides those described as having a dominant negative effect ultimately prove to be one cause of partial GHI, this would explain only a very small proportion of ISS.

TREATMENT

Soon after the cloning of the human IGF-I cDNA, human IGF-I was synthesized by recombinant DNA techniques (rhIGF-I) and physiologic studies undertaken with intravenously administered rhIGF-I *(77)*. Subcutaneous preparations of rhIGF-I became available in 1990.

Short Term Effects of IGF-I Treatment in GHRD

INTRAVENOUS (IV) ADMINISTRATION

The hypoglycemic effect of an iv bolus of IGF-I (75 µg/kg) following an overnight fast was demonstrated in 9 patients with GHRD aged 11–33 yr. The hypoglycemia was symptomatic and associated with a fall in plasma insulin level with recovery only after food was taken at 2 h post-injection. Marked increase in serum GH concentration in the seven older individuals reflected the overriding effect of hypoglycemia stimulation, despite the expected SS response to the increased levels of free IGF-I *(78)*. Suppression of TSH levels provided indirect evidence of SS stimulation *(79)*. The elimination time for iv injected IGF-I was found to be markedly reduced in 3 children and 7 adults with GHRD compared to 3 healthy children and 3 healthy adults, presumably due to the absence of IGFBP-3 in the patients *(80)*. IGF-I given iv to a 9-yr-old child for 11 d demonstrated substantial anabolic effects, including decreased serum urea nitrogen, increased urinary calcium excretion, and decreased urinary phosphate and sodium excretion. As previously noted with iv IGF-I in normals, IGF-II levels were suppressed and asymptomatic hypoglycemia noted *(81)*.

SUBCUTANEOUS (SC) ADMINISTRATION

There was no significant hypoglycemia with IGF-I in a dose of 120–150 µg/kg/d sc for 7 d, followed by breakfast. Plasma GH was markedly reduced, and type 3 procollagen (a growth marker) increased *(82)*. Hypoglycemia did not occur with IGF-I sc at a dose of 40 µg/kg every 12 h over 7 d in 6 Ecuadorian adults with GHRD, although insulin levels were suppressed. There was a two-fold increase in urinary calcium excretion without a change in serum calcium levels. Mean integrated 24 h GH levels were suppressed, as were the number of peaks, the area under the curve, and clonidine stimulated GH release. The mean peak serum IGF-I levels were 253 ± 11 ng/mL reached between 2–6 h after injection and mean trough levels were 137 ± 8 ng/mL before the next injection, values not significantly different from those of normal control Ecuadorian adults. As previously noted, IGF-II levels decreased and correlated inversely with IGF-I levels, indicating that IGF-I was displacing IGF-II from available IGFBPs. There were no significant changes in the half-life or metabolic clearance of IGF-I between d 1 and 7, although the distribution volume did increase over this time. Although IGFBP-3 levels did not increase, elevated baseline IGFBP-2 levels (153% of control) increased 45% ($p < 0.01$) *(14)*.

The short-term studies demonstrated that there was an insignificant risk of hypoglycemia in the fed state with sc administration of IGF-I, despite low levels of IGFBP-3. There remained, however, concern whether the low IGFBP-3 levels would result in more rapid clearance of IGF-I *(80)*, with blunting of the therapeutic effect. Four children and 4 adults with GHRD treated for 7 d with a single daily subcutaneous injection of IGF-I in a dose of 120–150 µg/d experienced a significant *decrease* in serum IGFBP-3 levels measured by specific RIA (83). As noted above, Vaccarello et al. *(14)* did not find a significant change in IGFBP-3 levels following 7 d of twice daily sc injection of doses of IGF-I sufficient to raise serum levels to normal in adults with GHRD. Further studies found that the two forms of IGFBP-3 associated with IGF and ALS, which are able to form the ternary 150-kDa complex were abnormally distributed in these GHRD patients. This distribution was unchanged by IGF-I treatment that, in addition to not increasing the IGFBP-3, did not increase ALS levels *(70)*. Although it was hoped that chronic treatment would result in stimulation of ALS and IGFBP-3, this did not seem likely in view of the experience with GH treatment of GHD. In this situation, where serum IGFBP-3 levels are also reduced, exogenous GH rapidly increases IGFBP-3 levels *(84)*.

Long-Term Treatment with IGF-I in GHI

In addition to concerns regarding the failure of short-term therapy to increase IGFBP-3 levels, there was concern whether catch-up growth in children with GHI due to GHRD or to GH antibodies would be as substantial as occurs with GH replacement therapy in patients with GHD in the absence of a direct effect of GH on bone *(15)*. Growth acceleration comparable to that seen with GH treatment of GHD was reported in 5 children aged 3.3–14.5 yr with GHRD treated for 3–10 mo with single daily doses of 150 µg/kg. Baseline growth velocities of 2.8–5.8 cm/yr increased by approx 1.5–4 fold to 8.8–13.6 cm/yr, with the youngest patients responding most impressively. A reduction of subcutaneous fat, measured by skin-fold thickness, was noted in the four patients who were considered obese. In contrast to the single daily dosage of 150 µg/kg administered by Laron et al. *(85)*, Walker et al. *(86)* gave 120 µg/kg twice daily to a 9.7-yr-old child with GHRD with a change in growth velocity from 6.5 to 11.4 cm/yr over a 9 mo period. Although mean pre-treatment IGF-I levels of 9 ± 2 µg/L increased to 347 ± 26 µg/L after 2 h, serum concentrations of IGF-II were unchanged, contrasting with earlier short term studies. Serum and urinary urea nitrogen decreased while creatinine clearance, urine volume, and urinary calcium increased. There were no abnormalities in glucose metabolism.

The first report of treatment for longer than 10 mo was in two children with GHRD with pre-treatment growth velocities (GV) of 4.3 and 3.8 cm/yr at 8.4 and 6.8-yr of age, respectively. They had suppression of greatly elevated serum GH levels and increase in procollagen I levels shortly after starting treatment; 6 mo GV increased to 7.8 and 8.4 cm/yr, without side effects. In the second 6 mo of treatment GV decreased to 6.6 and 6.3 cm/yr and in the subsequent 5 mo growth rate returned to pre-treatment values. Improvement in bone density was documented by dual photon absorptiometry. These patients were treated with a dose of 40 µg/kg sc twice daily and the waning of their growth response after a year indicated that this dosage was not adequate for sustained effect (87).

Since 1995, data have become available on 70 patients with GHI treated with subcutaneous injections of IGF-I for 12 mo or longer. Seven of these patients were resistant to GH because of GH inhibiting antibodies developing after treatment with GH injections for GHD due to GH gene deletion. The rest of the patients had abnormalities in GH receptor function, including Pakistani and Arab patients thought to have post-receptor defects (46–48). The largest group of patients was recruited for the international multicenter study which included 33 patients from 12 countries, 3.7–23 yr-of-age, 2 with GH gene deletion and the rest with GHRD. 1-yr growth data were reported for 26 of these patients and 2-yr data for 18. The 7 patients not reported include 2 who stopped treatment before 12 mo because of insufficient growth response and 5 because of adverse events. 3 did not continue for a full 24 mo because of poor compliance, headache, and weight gain. In the entire group treated for 1-yr, average height SDS gain was 0.7; for the subgroup treated for more than 12 mo, first-year average gain was 0.8 SDS and over 2 yr, 1.2 SDS. Serum IGF-II levels decreased and IGFBP-3 concentrations remained constant during this long term therapy (74). The most recent report of the European study provided data on 17 patients treated for 48 mo or more. The overall increase in height SDS was 1.67 ± 1.16 (from -6.52 ± 1.34 to -4.85 ± 1.81) with an increase in BMI-SDS from 0.59 ± 1.82 to 1.83 ± 1.50. Interestingly, gain in BMI correlated with improvement in SDS for height in this group. The gain in BMI was postulated to be the result of insulin like effects during the peak times following IGF-I injection; fat cells lack IGF-I receptors, but high doses of IGF-I can have an insulin like effect by binding to the insulin receptor (88). The adverse events noted were headache, hypoglycemia, papilledema (1 instance), Bell's palsy (1 instance), lipohypertrophy, and tonsillectomy/adenoidectomy (3 instances).

The first IGF-I treatment report from the large Ecuadorian cohort was of growth and body composition changes in two adolescent patients treated with a combination of IGF-I (120 µg/kg bid) and LRH analog to forestall puberty. A girl age 18 and boy age 17.5 yr, with bone ages of 13.5 and 13 yr experienced an approximate tripling of growth velocity, increased bone mineral density, and maturation of facial features on IGF-I for one year. There was initial loss of fine straight hair followed by recovery of denser and curly hair with filling of the fronto-temporal baldness, the appearance of axillary sweating, loss of deciduous teeth, and appearance of permanent dentition. The boy had coarsening of his facial features (Fig. 7). Submaxillary gland enlargement was also noticed in one patient and fading of premature facial wrinkles, commonly associated with GHD, noted in the other patient. Serum IGF-I levels were seen to increase into the normal range during the first 2–8 h following IGF-I injection (89). Studies were done at doses of 40, 80, and 120 µg/kg with pharmacokinetic profiles suggesting a plateau effect between 80 and 120 µg/kg per dose. It was considered that the carrying capacity of the IGFBPs was saturated at this level (71). As previously noted, mean serum IGF-II levels decreased

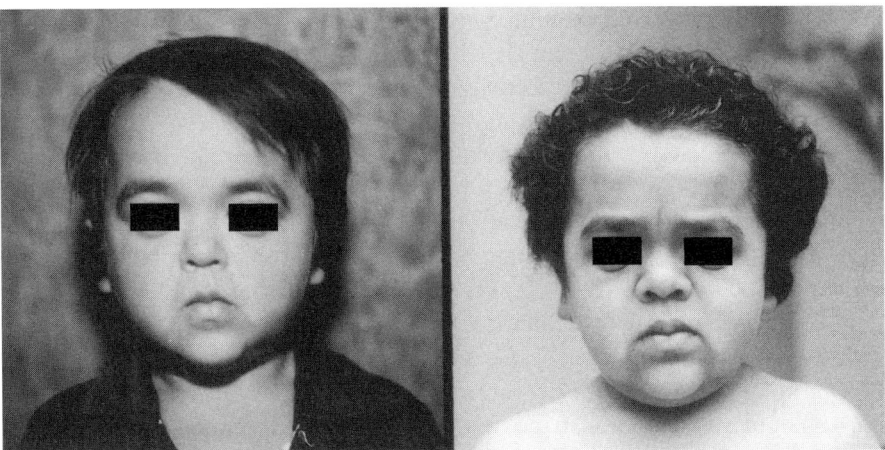

Fig. 7. Face and hair changes in 17.7-yr-old patient (bone age 13-yr) with GHRD during 6 mo treatment with IGF-I, 120 µg/kg bid and depot GnRH agonist begun at age 16.5-yr. Reproduced from Rosenbloom AL. IGF-I treatment of growth hormone insensitivity. In: Rosenfeld RG, Roberts CT (eds.) The IGF System: Molecular Biology, Physiology, and Clinical Applications. Copyright 1999, with permission from Humana Press, Totowa, NJ; pp. 739–769.

concurrently with the increase in IGF-I and serum IGFBP-3 levels did not respond to prolonged IGF-I treatment. There was no apparent change in the half-life of IGF-I during the treatment period, indicating no alteration of IGF-I pharmacokinetics induced by prolonged treatment *(71)*.

Tachycardia was noted in these adolescent patients and further studied in 16 prepubertal Ecuadorian patients during induction of treatment at progressive dosages of 40, 80, and 120 µg/kg bid. Both repeated palpation of the radial artery and continuous portable Holter monitoring were used. There was a direct dose related increase to approx 25% of baseline rate at the highest dosage. This was unrelated to glucose or electrolyte changes which were not significant *(90)*.

Seventeen prepubertal Ecuadorian patients were entered into a randomized double blind, placebo controlled trial of IGF-I at 120 µg/kg sc bid for 6 mo, following which all subjects received IGF-I. Such a study was considered necessary because of the observation of spontaneous periods of normal growth in these youngsters, the suggestion that nutritional changes that might accompany intervention would be an independent variable, and the need to control for side effects, particularly hypoglycemia, which occur in the untreated state. The 9 placebo-treated patients had a modest but not significant increase in height velocity from 2.8 ± 0.3 to 4.4 ± 0.7 cm/yr, entirely attributable to 3 individuals with 6-mo velocities of 6.6–8 cm/yr. Although this response was thought to be the result of improved nutritional status, there was no accompanying increase in IGFBP-3 as noted with nutrition-induced catch up growth by Crosnier et al. *(55)* in their GHRD patient with anorexia. For those receiving IGF-I, the height velocity increased from 2.9 ± 0.6 to 8.8 ± 0.6 cm/yr and all 16 patients had accelerated velocities during the second 6 mo period when all were receiving IGF-I. No changes or differences in IGFBP-3 were noted. There was no difference in the rate of hypoglycemia events, nausea or vomiting, headaches, or pain at the injection site between the placebo and IGF-I treated groups. One patient had asymptomatic papilledema developing one month after beginning IGF-I therapy that spontaneously resolved over several weeks without interrupting treatment. Six of the seven IGF-I treated patients experienced hair loss (72).

Two-yr treatment results in the Ecuadorian group have been reported, with comparison of the 120 mg/kg bid dosage to 80 mg/kg bid and also comparison of growth responses to those of GH treated GHD in the same population. There were no baseline differences between the low and high-dose groups for growth velocity, bone age, SDS for height, or mean % body weight for height (MBWH). No significant differences in GV or changes in height SDS, height age, or bone age between the 2 dosage groups were seen and a group of 6 subjects receiving the higher dose followed for a third year continued to maintain second year growth velocities. Improvement in mean height SDS over the 2-yr period was 1.5 for the higher dose and 1.3 for the lower dose, compared to 1.2 in the international study; in both the international and Ecuadorian cohorts, two-thirds of the 2-yr height SDS gain was in the first year. The annual changes in height age in both the first and the second year of treatment of the Ecuadorian children correlated with IGF-I trough levels which tended to be in the low normal range despite a failure of serum IGFBP-3 levels to increase (Fig. 8). The comparable growth responses to the two dosage levels and the similar IGF-I trough levels were thought to confirm the plateau effect at or below 80 µg/kg body weight twice daily (73).

Comparison of the growth responses of the 22 IGF-I treated GHRD patients to those of 11 GH treated GHD subjects in the same setting demonstrated GV increments in those with GHRD to be 63% of those achieved with GH treatment of GHD in the first year and less than 50% in the second and third years of IGF-I treatment. The GHRD group, however, did not differ from those with GHD in the change in bone age or in the ratio of height age to bone age changes over the 2-yr period. There was a greater change in % MBWH in the GHRD group treated with IGF-I, which, as noted by Ranke et al. (88), might reflect the insulin like action of the levels of IGF-I, contrasting with the lipolytic effect of GH replacement therapy. The difference in growth response between IGF-I treated GHRD and GH treated GHD was consistent with the hypothesis that 20% or more of GH influenced growth is due to the direct effects of GH on bone (15). Nonetheless, the comparable ratios of height age change to bone age change suggested similar long term effects for replacement therapy in these two conditions (73).

The Israeli report of 3 yr treatment of 9 patients, including the 3 with a presumed postreceptor defect, is the only one in which patients were given IGF-I as a single daily dosage (150–200 µg/kg). While the European and Ecuadorian study groups noted mean height SDS improvement of 0.7–1.0 over 1 yr and 1.2–1.5 over 2 yr, the Israeli patients had an improvement of only 0.4 over 1 yr and for the 6 with 2 yr data, 0.2 over 1 yr and 0.4 over 2 yr (91). The kinetic studies that originally formed the rationale for twice daily administration are supported by these observations. Of the 5 patients completing 3 yr of IGF-I treatment in the Israeli report, 3 were growing at slower rates than before treatment while the other 2 remained at comparable velocities to the second year of treatment. The subgroup with normal IGFBP-3 levels is particularly interesting, because the growth responses do not differ from those of the rest of the group, suggesting that the IGFBP-3 deficiency is not the explanation for the relatively deficient growth response to replacement therapy with IGF-I when compared to GH treatment of GHD (46). 2 prepubertal girls and 2 adult women with GHRD in Israel developed clinical features of hyperandrogenism and elevated androgen levels during treatment with IGF-I (92).

Five children with GHRD and 3 with growth attenuating antibodies to GH have been treated for 4 yr by Backeljauw and colleagues (93). The 2 yr data are comparable to data

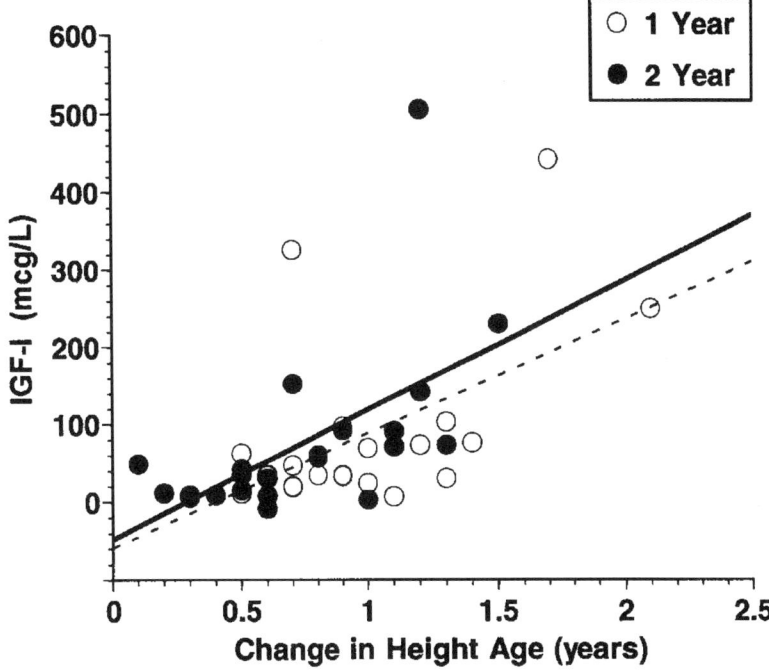

Fig. 8. Correlation of annual changes in height age and differences between baseline and trough levels of serum IGF-I with rhIGF-I treatment in 22 children with GHRD. The dashed line represents the one-year correlation ($r = 0.54$, $p = 0.009$) and the solid line represents the two-year correlation ($r = 0.58$, $p = 0.005$). Reproduced from *(73)* with permission from The Endocrine Society, Bethesda, MD.

in the European and Ecuadorian populations, with an improvement in height SDS over the 2 yr period of 1.1. Bone age was noted to advance consistent with chronologic age. There was rapid growth of the spleen and kidney, as determined by ultrasound during the first year with a slowing of spleen growth but a continued rapid kidney growth during the second year. In a preliminary report, the third year and fourth year results of treatment in this group were reported; a further decrease in height velocity to a mean 5.1 cm/yr occurred during the third year, but the fourth year mean height velocity was 5.7 cm/yr. Kidney growth continued in 5 of the 8 patients who had renal length for height at or above the 95th percentile. There were no functional or structural abnormalities of the kidneys, however *(94)*. In 5 of these patients, craniofacial growth has been monitored with the suggestion of mandibular overgrowth, most noticeable in the last 2 yr of treatment *(95)*.

A Vietnamese girl treated by Walker et al. *(96)* with IGF-I and LHRH analog had modest improvement of growth over the first 3 yr of treatment, a height SDS increase of 1.2 with dramatic slowing of growth response thereafter. As with the patient in Fig. 7, facial coarsening was noted.

CONCLUSION

If the tissue dose of IGF-I in patients with GHI treated with IGF-I is supraphysiologic, as indicated by increases in body fat and acromegaloid facial changes, why then do we not see sustained growth acceleration as in GH treated GHD? The administration of IGF-I with recombinant IGFBP-3 would be an important clinical study to determine how much of this deficit is due to IGFBP 3 deficiency. The dual effector hypothesis remains the best explanation for inadequate growth response *(15)*. With diminished ability to stimulate prechondrocyte differentiation and local IGF-I production, children with GHI can expect only partial recovery of normal growth with IGF-I replacement. The comparable ratios of change in height age to change in bone age over 2 yr of treatment in GHI children treated with IGF-I and GHD children treated with GH, however, suggest that the absence of a direct GH effect in GHI may have a temporal, rather than absolute effect on long-term response to treatment *(73)*. Thus, IGF-I replacement therapy of GI may need to continue longer than GH treatment of GHD to achieve normal height. This goal will likely require suppressing adolescence in most children with GHI, using GnRH analogs *(89)*.

In addition to statural attainment, goals of replacement therapy with IGF-I in GHI include improvement in body composition, normalization of facial appearance, and possible reduction of risk factors for childhood and adult mortality. All studies that have monitored body composition have verified lean mass increases, including increased bone density. Normalization of craniofacial features has also been apparent *(97)*. Voice change has not been remarked on, but can be expected. It is likely that maintenance of body composition changes will require continued treatment in adulthood.

The reduction of risk factors for the higher mortality in infancy and childhood with GHRD is to be expected with IGF-I therapy, but the reason for this increased risk is unknown. Leukocytes share in the general up regulation of IGF-I receptors in GHRD, and appear to function normally in this condition *(98)*. In a study of one affected infant (who died at 7 mo with bronchitis) and 5 adults with GHRD from Ecuador, Diamond et al. *(99)* demonstrated a variety of immune disturbances in the infant and 3 of the adults. The pathologic significance of these findings remains uncertain *(100)*.

The ability to resolve the many remaining questions about treatment to attain normal stature and body composition in GHI is thwarted by the decision of the few manufacturers to no longer synthesize IGF-I. This decision was based on the inability to identify a substantial market to justify the costs of manufacture and regulatory clearance.

REFERENCES

1. Rosenbloom AL, Guevara-Aguirre J, Rosenfeld RG, Pollock BH. Growth in growth hormone insensitivity. Trends Endocrinol Metab 1994;5:296–303.
2. Woods KA, Camacho-Hübner C, Savage MO, Clark AJL. Intrauterine growth retardation and postnatal growth failure associated with deletion of the insulin-like growth factor I gene. N Engl J Med 1996;335:1363–1367.
3. Abizzajab MJ, Goddard A, Grigorescu F, Lautier C, Smith RJ, Chernausek SD. Human IGF-I receptor mutations associated with intrauterine and post-natal growth retardation. Proc Endocr Soc 82nd Ann. Mtg 2000 abstract #1947, p. 470.
4. Rivarola MA, Phillips JA III, Migeon CJ, Heinrich JJ, Hjelle BJ. Phenotypic heterogeneity in familial isolated growth hormone deficiency type I-A. J Clin Endocrinol Metab 1984;59:34–40.
5. Powell DR. Effects of renal failure on the growth hormone-insulin-like growth factor axis. J Pediatr 1997;131:S13–516
6. De Groot LJ. Dangerous dogmas in medicine: the nonthyroid illness syndrome. J Clin Endocrinol Metab 1999;84:151–164.
7. Rosenfeld RG, Rosenbloom AL, Guevara-Aguirre J. Growth hormone (GH) insensitivity due to primary GH receptor deficiency. Endocr Rev 1994;15:369–390.
8. Postel-Vinay M-C, Kelly PA. Growth hormone receptor signalling. Bailliere's Clin Endocrinol Metab 1996;10:323–326.
9. Leung DW, Spencer SA, Cachianes G. Growth hormone receptor and serum binding protein: purification, cloning and expression. Nature 1987;330:537–543.

10. Rosenbloom AL. Physiology and disorders of the growth hormone receptor (GHR) and GH-GHR signal transduction. Endocrine 2000;12(2):107–119.
11. de Vos AM, Ultsch M, Kossiakoff AA. Human growth hormone and extracellular domain of its receptor: crystal structure of the complex. Science 1992;255:306–312.
12. Rajaram S, Baylink DJ, Mohan S. Insulin-like growth factor-binding proteins in serum and other biological fluids: regulation and functions. Endocr Rev 1997;18:801–831.
13. Baxter RG, Binoux MA, Clemmons DR, et al. Recommendations for nomenclature of the insulin-like growth factor binding proteins superfamily. J Clin Endocrinol Metab 1998;83:3213.
14. Vaccarello MA, Diamond FB Jr, Guevara-Aguirre J, et al. Hormonal and metabolic effects and pharmacokinetics of recombinant human insulin-like growth factor-I in growth hormone receptor deficiency/Laron syndrome. J Clin Endocrinol Metab 1993;77:273–280.
15. Daughaday WH, Rotwein P. Insulin-like growth factors I and II: peptide, messenger ribonucleic acid and gene structures, serum and tissue concentrations. Endocr Rev 1989;10:68–91.
16. Laron Z, Pertzelan A, Mannheimer S. Genetic pituitary dwarfism with high serum concentration of growth hormone–a new inborn error of metabolism? Isr J Med Sci 1966;2:152–155.
17. Laron Z, Pertzelan A, Karp M. Pituitary dwarfism with high serum levels of growth hormone. Isr J Med Sci 1968;4:83–94.
18. Merimee TJ, Hall J, Rabinovitz D, McKusick VA, Rimoin DL. An unusual variety of endocrine dwarfism: Subresponsiveness to growth hormone in a sexually mature dwarf. Lancet 1998;2:191–193.
19. Daughaday WH, Laron Z, Pertzelan A, Heins JN. Defective sulfation factor generation: a possible etiological link in dwarfism. Trans Assoc Am Physicians 1969;82:129–138.
20. Bala RM, Beck JC. Fractionation studies on plasma of normals and patients with Laron dwarfism and hypopituitary gigantism. Can J Physiol Pharmacol 1973;91:845–852.
21. Eshet R, Laron Z, Brown M, Arnon R. Immunoreactive properties of the plasma hGH from patients with the syndrome of familial dwarfism and high plasma IR-hGH. J Clin Endocrinol Metab 1973;37:819–821.
22. Tsushima T, Shiu. RPC, Kelly PA, Friesen HG. Radioreceptor assay for human growth hormone and lactogens: structure-function studies and clinical applications. In: Raiti S (ed) Advances in Human Growth Hormone Research. USPHS, Bethesda, MD. USPHS-DHEW Publication 74–612,1973, pp. 372–387.
23. Jacobs LS, Sneid DS, Garland JT, Laron Z, Daughaday WH. Receptor-active growth hormone in Laron dwarfism. J Clin Endocrinol Metab 1976;42:403–406.
24. Golde DW, Bersch N, Kaplan SA, Rimoin DL, Li CH. Peripheral unresponsiveness to human growth hormone in Laron dwarfism. N Engl J Med 1980;303:1156–1159.
25. Eshet R, Laron Z, Pertzelan A, Arnon R, Dintzman M. Defect of human growth hormone receptors in the liver of two patients with Laron-type dwarfism. Isr J Med Sci 1984;20:8–11.
26. Daughaday WH, Trivedi B. Absence of serum growth hormone binding protein in patients with growth hormone receptor deficiency (Laron dwarfism). Proc Natl Acad Sci USA 1987;84:4636–4640.
27. Baumann G, Shaw MA, Winter RJ. Absence of plasma growth hormone-binding protein in Laron-type dwarfism. J Clin Endocrinol Metab 1987;65:814–816.
28. Godowski PJ, Leung DW, Meacham LR, et al. Characterization of the human growth hormone receptor gene and demonstration of a partial gene deletion in two patients with Laron-type dwarfism. Proc Natl Acad Sci USA 1989;86:8083–8087.
29. Pantel J, Machinis K, Sobrier ML, Duquesnoy P, Goossens M, Amselem S. Species-specific alternative splice mimicry at the growth hormone receptor locus revealed by the lineage of retroelements during primate evolution. A novel mechanism accounting for protein diversity between and within species. J Biol Chem 2000;275:18,664–18,669.
30. Rosenbloom AL, Guevara-Aguirre J. Lessons from the genetics of Laron syndrome. Trends Endocrinol Metab 1998;9:276–283.
31. Metherell LA, Munroe PB, Bjarnson R, et al. Proc Endocr Soc 82nd Ann Mtg 2000 absract #1994, p. 482.
32. Attie KM, Carlsson LMS, Rundle AC, Sherman BM. Evidence for partial growth hormone insensitivity among patients with idiopathic short stature. J Pediatr 1995;127:244–250.
33. Sanchez JE, Perera E, Baumbach L, Cleveland WW. Growth hormone receptor mutations in children with idiopathic short stature. J Clin Endocrinol Metab 1998;83:4079–4083.
34. Kou K, Lajara R, Rotwein P. Amino acid substitutions in the intracellular part of the growth hormone receptor in a patient with the Laron syndrome. J Clin Endocrinol Metab 1993;76:54–59.

35. Goddard AD, Covello R, Luoh S-M, et al. Mutations of the growth hormone receptor in children with idiopathic short stature. N Eng J Med 1995;333:1093–1098.
36. Ayling RM, Ross R, Towner P, et al. A dominant-negative mutation of the growth hormone receptor causes familial short stature. Nature Genet 1997;16:13–14.
37. Iida K, Takahashi Y, Kaji H, et al. Growth hormone (GH) insensitivity syndrome with high serum GH binding protein levels caused by a heterozygous splice site mutation of the GH receptor gene producing a lack of intracellular domain. J Clin Endocrinol Metab 1998;83:531–537.
38. Iida K, Takahashi Y, Kaji H, et al. Functional characterization of truncated growth hormone (GH) receptor (1–277) causing partial GH insensitivity syndrome with high GH-binding protein. J Clin Endocrinol Metab 1999;84:1011–1016.
39. Dastot F, Sobrier ML, Duquesnoy P, Duriez B, Goosens M, Amselem S. Alternative spliced forms in the cytoplasmic domain of the human growth hormone (GH) receptor regulate its ability to generate a soluble GH binding protein. Proc Natl Acad Sci USA 1996;93:10,723–10,728.
40. Ross RJM, Esposito N, Shen XY, et al. A short isoform of the human growth hormone receptor functions as a dominant negative inhibitor of the full-length receptor and generates large amounts of binding protein. Mol Endocrinol 1997;11:265–273.
41. Amit T, Bergman T, Dastot F, Youdim MBH, Amselem S, Hochberg Z. A membrane-fixed, truncated isoform of the human growth hormone receptor. J Clin Endocrinol Metab 1997;82:3813–3817.
42. Iida K, Takahashi Y, Kaji H, et al. The C422F mutation of the growth hormone receptor gene is not responsible for short stature. J Clin Endocrinol Metab 1999;84:4214–4219.
43. Chujo S, Kaji H, Takahashi Y, Okimura Y, Abe H, Chihara K. No correlation of growth hormone receptor gene mutation P561T with body height. Eur J Endocrinol 1996;134:560–562.
44. Rosenbloom AL, Guevara-Aguirre J, Berg MA, Francke U. Stature in Ecuadorians heterozygous for the growth hormone receptor (GHR) gene E180 splice mutation does not differ from that of homozygous normal relatives. J Clin Endocrinol Metab 1998;83:2373–2375.
45. Berg MA, Peoples R., Perez-Jurado L, et al. Receptor mutations and haplotypes in growth hormone receptor deficiency: a global survey and identification of the Ecuadorian E180 splice mutation in an oriental Jewish patient. Acta Paediatr 1994;399(Suppl):112–114.
46. Laron Z, Klinger B, Eshet R, Kaneti H, Karasik A, Silbergeld A. Laron syndrome due to a post-receptor defect: response to IGF-I treatment. Isr J Med Sci 1993;29:757–763.
47. Freeth JS, Ayling RM, Whatmore AJ, et al. Human skin fibroblasts as a model of growth hormone (GH) action in GH receptor-positive Laron's syndrome. Endocrinology 1997;138:55–61.
48. Freeth JS, Silva CM, Whatmore AJ, Clayton PE. Activation of the signal transducers and activators of transcription signaling pathway by growth hormone (GH) in skin fibroblasts from normal and GH binding protein-positive Laron syndrome children. Endocrinology 1998;139:20–28.
49. Rosenbloom AL, Francke U, Rosenfeld RG, Guevara-Aguirre J. Growth hormone receptor deficiency in Ecuador. J Clin Endocrinol Metab 1999;84:4436–4443.
50. Jorgensen JO, Müller J, Moller J, Wolthers T, Vahl N, Juul A, Skakkebaek NE, Christiansen JS. Adult growth hormone deficiency. Horm Res 1994;42:235–241.
51. Rosenbloom AL, Martinez V, Kranzler J, Bachrach LK, Rosenfeld RG, Guevara-Aguirre J. Natural history of growth hormone receptor deficiency. Acta Paediatr Suppl 1999;428:153–156.
52. Rudling M, Norstedt G, Olivecrona H, Reihnér E, Gustafsson J-A, Angelin B. Importance of growth hormone for the induction of hepatic low density lipoprotein receptors. Proc Natl Acad Sci 1992;89:6983–6987.
53. Laron Z, Lilos P, Klinger B. Growth curves for Laron syndrome. Arch Dis Child 1993;68:768–770.
54. Rose SR, Municchi G, Barnes KM, et al. Spontaneous growth hormone secretion increases during puberty in normal girls and boys. J Clin Endocrinol Metab 1991;73:428–435.
55. Crosnier H, Gourmelen M, Prévot C, Rappaport R. Effects of nutrient intake on growth, insulin-like growth factors, and their binding proteins in a Laron-type dwarf. J Clin Endocrinol Metab 1993;76:248–250.
56. Schaefer GB, Rosenbloom AL, Guevara-Aguirre J, et al. Facial morphometry of Ecuadorian patients with growth hormone receptor deficiency/Laron syndrome. J Med Genet 1994;31:635–639.
57. Rosenbloom AL, Guevara-Aguirre J, Rosenfeld RG, Fielder PJ. The little women of Loja. Growth hormone receptor-deficiency in an inbred population of southern Ecuador. N Engl J Med 1990; 323:1367–1374.
58. Rosenbloom AL, Selman-Almonte A, Brown MR, Fisher DA, Baumbach L, Parks JS. Clinical and biochemical phenotype of familial anterior hypopituitarism from mutation of PROP-1 gene. J Clin Endocrinol Metab 1999;84:50–57.

59. Rosenbloom AL, Guevara-Aguirre J, Fielder PJ, et al. Growth hormone receptor deficiency/Laron syndrome in Ecuador: Clinical and biochemical characteristics. Pediatr Adolesc Endocrinol 1993;24:34–52.
60. Bachrach LB, Marcus R, Ott SM, et al. Bone mineral, histomorphometry, and body composition in adults with growth hormone receptor deficiency. J Bone Mineral Res 1998;3:415–421.
61. Bandeira F, Camargo K, Caldas G, Rosenbloom AL, Stabler B, Underwood LE. Primary growth hormone insensitivity: case report. Arq Bras Endocrinol Metab 1997;41:198–200.
62. Frankel JJ, Laron Z. Psychological aspects of pituitary insufficiency in children and adolescents with special reference to growth hormone. Isr J Med Sci 1968;4:953–961.
63. Galatzer A, Aran O, Nagelberg N, Rubitzek J, Laron Z Cognitive and psychosocial functioning of young adults with Laron syndrome. Pediatr Adolesc Endocrinol 1993;24:53–60.
64. Maheshwari HG, Silverman BI, Dupuis J, Baumann G. phenotype and genetic analysis of a syndrome caused by an inactivating mutation in the growth hormone-releasing hormone receptor: dwarfism of Sindh. J Clin Endocrinol Metab 1998;83:4065–4074.
65. Woods KA, Dastot F, Preece MA, et al. Extensive personal experience. Phenotype: genotype relationships in growth hormone insensitivity syndrome. J Clin Endocrinol Metab 1997;82,3529–3535.
66. Guevara-Aguirre J, Rosenbloom AL. Psychosocial adaptation of Ecuadorian patients with growth hormone receptor deficiency/Laron syndrome. Pediatr Adolesc Endocrinol 1993;24:61–64.
67. Kranzler JH, Rosenbloom AL, Martinez V, Guevara-Aguirre J. Normal intelligence with severe IGF-I deficiency due to growth hormone receptor deficiency: a controlled study in genetically homogeneous population. J Clin Endocrinol Metab 1998;83:1953–1958.
68. Zhou Y, Xu BC, Maheshwari HG, et al. A mammalian model for the Laron syndrome produced by targeted disruption of the mouse growth hormone receptor/binding protein gene (the Laron mouse). Proc Natl Acad Sci USA 1997;94:13,215–13,220.
69. Beck KD, Powell-Braxton L, Widmer H-R, Valverde J, and Hofti, F. IGF-I gene disruption results in reduced brain size, CNS hypomyelination, and loss of hippocampal granule and striatal parvalbumin-containing neurons. Neuron 1995;14:717–730.
70. Gargosky SE, Wilson KF, Fielder PJ, et al. The composition and distribution of insulin-like growth factors (IGFs) and IGF-binding proteins (IGFBPs) in the serum of growth hormone receptor-deficient patients: effects of IGF-I therapy on IGFBP-3. J Clin Endocrinol Metab 1993;77:1683–1689.
71. Wilson KF, Fielder PJ, Guevara-Aguirre J, et al. Long-term effects of insulin-like growth factor (IGF)-I treatment on serum IGFs and IGF binding proteins in adolescent patients with growth hormone receptor deficiency. Clin Endocrinol 1995;42,399–407.
72. Guevara-Aguirre J, Vasconez O, et al. A randomized, double blind, placebo controlled trial on safety and efficacy of recombinant human insulin-like growth factor-I in children with growth hormone receptor deficiency. J Clin Endocrinol Metab 1995;80:1393–1398.
73. Guevara-Aguirre J, Rosenbloom AL, Vasconez O, Martinez V, Gargosky SE, Rosenfeld RG. Two year treatment of growth hormone receptor deficiency (GHRD) with recombinant insulin-like growth factor-I in 22 children: Comparison of two dosage levels and to GH treated GH deficiency. J Clin Endocrinol Metab 1997;82:629–633.
74. Ranke MB, Savage MO, Chatelain PG, et al. Insulin-like growth factor I improves height in growth hormone insensitivity: two years' results. Horm Res 1995;44:253–264.
75. Rosenbloom AL, Guevara-Aguirre J, Fielder PJ, Gargosky S, Cohen P, Rosenfeld RG. Insulin-like growth factor binding proteins-2 and -3 in Ecuadorian patients with growth hormone receptor deficiency and their parents. Pediatr Adolesc Endocrinol 1993;24:185–191.
76. Woods KA, Savage MO. The Laron syndrome: typical and atypical forms. Bailliere's Clin Endocrinol Metab 1996;10:371–387.
77. Rosenbloom AL. IGF-I treatment of growth hormone insensitivity. In: Rosenfeld RG, Roberts CT, eds. The IGF System: Molecular Biology, Physiology, and Clinical Applications. Totowa NJ; Humana Press, 1999, pp. 739–769.
78. Laron Z, Erster B, Klinger B, Anin S. Effect of acute administration of insulin-like growth factor I in patients with Laron-type dwarfism. Lancet 1988;2:1170–1172.
79. Laron Z, Klinger B, Silbergeld A, Lewin R, Erster B, Gil-Ad I. Intravenous administration of recombinant IGF-I lowers serum GHRH and TSH. Acta Endocrinologica 1990;123:378–382.

80. Klinger B, Garty M, Laron Z. Elimination characteristics of intravenously administered rIGF-I in Laron-type dwarfs. Dev Pharmacol Ther 1990;15:196–199.
81. Walker JL, Ginalska-Malinowska M, Romer TE, Pucilowska JB, Underwood LE. Effects of the infusion of insulin-like growth factor I in a child with growth hormone insensitivity syndrome (Laron syndrome). N Engl J Med 1991;324:1483–1488.
82. Laron Z, Klinger B, Jensen LT, Erster B. Biochemical and hormonal changes induced by one week of administration of rIGF-I to patients with Laron type dwarfism. Clin Endocrinol 1991;35:145–160.
83. Laron Z, Klinger B, Blum WF, Silbergeld A, Ranke MB. IGF binding protein 3 in patients with Laron type dwarfism: effect of exogenous rIGF-I. Clin Endocrinol 1992;36:301–304.
84. Lee PDK, Durham SK, Martinez V, Vasconez O, Powell DR, Guevara-Aguirre J. Kinetics of insulin-like growth factor (IGF) and IGF-binding protein responses to a single dose of growth hormone. J Clin Endocrinol Metab 1997;82:2266–2274.
85. Laron Z, Anin S, Klipper-Aurbach Y, Klinger B. Effects of insulin-like growth factor on linear growth, head circumference, and body fat in patients with Laron-type dwarfism. Lancet 1992;339:1258–1261.
86. Walker JL, Van Wyk JJ, Underwood LE. Stimulation of statural growth by recombinant insulin-like growth factor I in a child with growth hormone insensitivity syndrome (Laron type). J. Pediatr 1992;121:641–646.
87. Heinrichs C, Vis HL, Bergmann P, Wilton P, Bourguignon JP. Effects of 17 months treatment using recombinant insulin-like growth factor-I in two children with growth hormone insensitivity (Laron) syndrome. Clin Endocrinol 1993;38:647–651.
88. Ranke MB, Savage MO, Chatelain PG, Preece MA, Rosenfeld RG, Wilton P. Long- term treatment of growth hormone insensitivity syndrome with IGF-I. Results of the European Multicentre Study. The Working Group on Growth Hormone Insensitivity Syndromes. Horm Res 1999;51:128–134.
89. Martinez V, Vasconez O, Martinez A, et al. Body changes in adolescent patients with growth hormone receptor deficiency receiving recombinant human insulin-like growth factor I and luteinizing hormone-releasing hormone analog: preliminary results. Acta Paediatr 1994;399(Suppl):133–136.
90. Vasconez O, Martinez V, Martinez AL, et al. Heart rate increase in patients with growth hormone receptor deficiency treated with insulin-like growth factor I. Acta Paediatr 1994;399(Suppl):137–139.
91. Klinger B, Laron Z. Three year IGF-I treatment of children with Laron syndrome. J Ped Endocrinol Metab 1995;8:149–158.
92. Klinger B, Anin S, Sibergeld A, Eshet R, Laron Z. Development of hyperandrogenism during treatment with insulin-like growth factor-I (IGF-I) in female patients with Laron syndrome. Clin. Endocrinol. 1998;48:81–87.
93. Backeljauw PF, Underwood LE, The GHIS Collaborative Group. Prolonged treatment with recombinant insulin-like growth factor-I in children with growth hormone insensitivity syndrome–a clinical research center study. J Clin Endocrinol Metab 1996;81:3312–3317.
94. Backeljauw PF, Kissoondial A, Underwood LE, Simmons KE. Effects of 4 years treatment with recombinant human insulin-like growth factor-I (rh IGF-I) on craniofacial growth in children with growth hormone insensitivity syndrome (GHIS). Horm Res 1997;48(Suppl 2):40(Abstract 243).
95. Backeljauw PF, Underwood LE. The GHIS collaborative group. Prolonged treatment with recombinant insulin-like growth factor-I (rh IGF-I) in children with growth hormone insensitivity syndrome (GHIS): 4 year update. Horm Res 1997;48(Suppl 2):15(Abstract 58).
96. Walker JL, Crock PA, Behncken SN, et al. A novel mutation affecting the interdomain link region of the growth hormone receptor in a Vietnamese girl, and response to long-term treatment with recombinant human insulin-like growth factor-I and luteinizing hormone-releasing hormone analog. J Clin Endocrinol Metab 1998;83:2554–2561.
97. Leonard J, Samuels M, Cotterill AM, Savage MO. Effects of recombinant insulin-like growth factor I on craniofacial morphology in growth hormone insensitivity. Acta Paediatr 1994;399(Suppl):140–141.
98. Bjerknes R, Vesterhus P, Aarskog D. Increased neutrophil insulin-like growth factor-I (IGF-I) receptor expression and IGF-I-induced functional capacity in patients with untreated Laron syndrome. Eur J Endocrinol 1997;136:92–95.

99. Diamond F, Martinez V, Guevara-Aguirre J, et al. Immune function in patients with gorwth hormone receptor deficiency (GHRD). Proc Endocrinol Soc 78th Ann Mtg, 1996, vol 1, p. 276.
100. Le Roith D, Blakesley VA. The yin and the yang of the IGF system: immunological manifestations of GH resistance. Eur J Endocrinol 1997;136:33–34.

3
Growth Hormone Treatment of Children with Idiopathic Short Stature or Growth Hormone Sufficient Growth Failure

Jean-Claude Desmangles, MD, John Buchlis, MD, and Margaret H. MacGillivray, MD

Contents

> Introduction
> Definition of ISS
> Height Outcomes of ISS Patients After GH Therapy
> Ethical Considerations
> Psychosocial Considerations
> Adverse Effects
> Growth Regulatory Genes: Their Influence on Childhood Growth
> Conclusion
> References

INTRODUCTION

The efficacy of growth hormone (GH) treatment in children with idiopathic growth failure has been the subject of controversy because of ethical concerns *(1,2)*, financial considerations *(3)* and variable adult height outcomes *(4,5)*. Much of the disagreement about the benefits of GH treatment relates to the heterogeneity of the study populations receiving therapy. Ideally, the efficacy of GH therapy should be based on the height outcomes of homogeneous populations of pathologically short children rather than the adult heights of children with variable shortness of differing etiologies. Published studies have sometimes combined children who had constitutional delay of growth and adolescence with subjects who had either severe genetic short stature or significant growth failure growth failure based on abnormal heights and growth rates for chronological age. These short children have been classified by various terminologies: Normal Variant Short Stature (NVSS), Idiopathic Short Stature (ISS), Constitutional Delay of Growth and Puberty (CGDP), GH neurosecretory dysfunction, idiopathic growth fail-

From: *Contemporary Endocrinology: Pediatric Endocrinology: A Practical Clinical Guide*
Edited by: S. Radovick and M. H. MacGillivray © Humana Press Inc., Totowa, NJ

ure, and non-GH deficient short stature. Without treatment, the height outcomes in most studies have failed to reach mid-parental target height. In contrast, GH therapy has resulted in mixed height outcomes; some patients reached or exceeded genetic target height whereas others did not. Given the high cost and potential risk of adverse events, some authors have criticized the use of GH in healthy very short children without a documented endocrine disorder *(1)*. Some of this disagreement may be resolved as we improve our ability to identify mutations in various growth regulating genes such as *SHOX, GHRH, Ghrelin, GHRP, Pit-1, Prop-1, GH* and their receptors.

Linear growth is a complex process influenced by many genetic and environmental factors *in utero* and during childhood. A normal pattern of growth is sound evidence of good health during childhood or adolescence. Innocent causes of short stature include genetic short stature and constitutional delay of growth and adolescence; occasionally these entities occur together. When abnormal growth is present, the evaluation must include a complete history, individualized hormone and biochemical tests as well as genetic analyses when necessary. Treatment decisions depend on identifying the etiology of the child's growth problem. At present, access to molecular testing is limited; hence the clinician often has to use clinical judgment when an etiology is not identified. The differential diagnoses of growth disorders include intrauterine growth disturbances (IUGR or small for gestational age [SGA]), malnutrition, chronic disease, endocrine dysfunction, skeletal dysplasias, emotional deprivation and genetic syndromes. In the absence of a specific etiology, the child is classified as having ISS or idiopathic growth failure. The following are the main clinical criteria: abnormally slow growth velocity for chronologic age and/or height more than 2–2.5 standard deviations (SD) from the mean for chronological age. Suboptimal growth during puberty (< 6 cm/yr) is another clue to a growth abnormality.

This chapter will review the current opinions and options regarding the etiology, evaluation, diagnosis, prognosis and treatment of idiopathic short stature.

DEFINITION OF ISS

Despite the availability of established standards for normal height, weight, and growth velocity, there is considerable diversity of opinion regarding the definition of 'abnormal" growth in children. Some investigators have used heights that are less than the 5th or the 3rd percentile to select short children for therapeutic intervention trials. Others have required a more rigid cut-off, i.e., height that is more than 2.5 SD below the mean for age. Another entry criterion is slow growth velocity that is less than the 25th percentile for age. Pathologically short children may grow at either a normal or subnormal velocity for age. Opinions differ on the management of the former group of short subjects who are sometimes classified "normal short."

In some GH treatment studies, children with ISS were required to have heights less than the 3rd percentile, peak GH response after pituitary provocative testing of >10 ng/mL, absence of dysmorphic features, concomitant disease or low birth weight *(5–7)*, and abnormal growth velocity for age as well as delayed bone age. Our current diagnostic tests for GH deficiency are pharmacologic not physiologic: they will identify severely GH deficient children if a cut off of 5 ng/mL is used. However, they do not detect suboptimal spontaneous GH secretion, bioactive GH, or GH insensitivity due to mild GH receptor dysfunction. Other indicators of inadequate GH secretion such as IGF-1 and

IGFBP-3 are frequently uninformative. Consequently, we are left with uncertainty about the true cause of the growth disorder in most pathologically short children who have normal GH stimulation tests and IGF 1 levels. The heterogeneity of this population has been a major reason for the current debate as to whether GH treatment is or is not beneficial based on height outcomes *(8)*.

One approach to reducing the heterogeneity has involved subdividing the ISS children according to genetic background. Those with familial short stature (FSS) include short children growing according to their genetic potential and those with non-familial short stature (NFSS) include children growing below their genetic potential. This approach does not take into account the possible genetic transmission of a growth regulatory gene mutation within families with familial short stature. More recently other experts *(9)* have recommended the following definition of idiopathic short stature: "ISS is a heterogeneous state that encompasses individuals of short stature, including those with FSS, for which there is no currently recognized cause." This definition is likely to persist until we improve our ability to identify specific mutations within the family of growth regulating genes.

HEIGHT OUTCOMES OF ISS PATIENTS AFTER GH THERAPY

Following the approval of recombinant GH in 1985, many studies have examined the growth responses of short GH sufficient children treated with GH. Growth velocity and height improved in the short term but height outcomes were mixed with little or no long term gains. None of the early studies were randomized or placebo controlled, and outcomes were judged on the basis of whether the participants reached predicted height or genetic target height. Given the heterogeneous nature of this population, the ambiguous outcomes are not surprising. It was also apparent that it was not possible to predict accurately which patient would respond well to GH.

GH treatment did not improve adult height over predicted height in a number of published studies *(7,10,11)*. However, when adult heights *(12,13)* after GH treatment were compared to the final heights of untreated historical controls, the GH treated patients had heights very close to genetic target height and significantly better than the untreated group (Table 1).

The height outcomes of untreated patients varies among the studies; some investigators have reported that final height was lower than both predicted adult height and target height *(12–15)*, while others have reported final adult heights equal to predicted adult heights *(16)*. The clinical significance of these results is uncertain, given the heterogeneity of the populations studied and the relatively small number of patients (Table 2).

The largest analysis of GH treated ISS children was the KABI International Growth Study (KIGS) which divided its population (36.9% of the total population) into those with familial short stature (FSS) versus those with non-familial short stature (NFSS). Analysis of these two groups revealed that GH-treated patients with FSS reached both their mid-parental height and target height while patients with NFSS did not. Nevertheless, the NFSS group had adults heights which exceeded those of the FSS group. One randomized trial studying GH therapy in ISS females near final adult height showed that the GH treated girls reached a significantly higher final height than the control group *(17)*. It is clear from these studies that GH therapy seems to improve height outcome in some children, but not in all. In 1987, the NIH started a randomized placebo controlled

Table 1
Height Outcomes of Treated Patients

Author (ref)	GH dose U/lg/wk	N sex	Baseline age (yr)	Baseline Ht SDS	Predicted HT SDS (PH)	Final Ht SDS (FH)	Target Ht SDS (TH)	Comments
Bierich (10)	0.5	15 M + F	12.7	−3.2	−1.6	−1.6	−0.7	FH = PH; FH < TH
Zadik (15)	0.75	11 M	12.8	−3.3	−1.8	−1.5	−2.1	FH = PH; FH > TH
Guyda (4)	0.75	60 M	12.0	−2.9	−2.1	−1.7	−0.6	FH > PH; FH < TH for both sexes
		39 F	11.0					
Wit (12)	0.5–1.0	7 M	11.2	−3.5	−2.7	−2.6	−1.1	FH = PH; FH < TH
Hintz (20)	1.0	48 M	10.4	−2.7	−2.6	−1.5	−0.9	FH > PH; FH < TH
		21 F						
Buchlis (5)	1.0	30 M	12.4	−2.9	−1.7	−1.5	−1.2	FH = PH; FH = TH
		6F	9.7	−2.7	−2.0	−1.3	−0.9	FH > PH; FH = TH
Lopez–Seguerro (47)	0.5–0.7	35 M	11.1	−2.78	−2.09	−1.31	−1.6	FH > PH; FH > TH
Loche (7)	G₁: 0.5	G₁: 4 M–3 F	10.5	−2.5		−1.6		FH = PH; FH = TH for both sexes
	G₂: 1.0	G₂: 6 M–2 F	11.8	−2.4		−1.4		
Mc Caughey (48)	30 /m²	7 F	8.07	−2.52	−1.73	−1.14	−1.47	FH > PH; FH > TH

FH = final height; PH = predicted height; TH = genetic target height or mid-parental height

Table 2
Height Outcomes of Untreated Patients

Author (ref)	N sex	Baseline age (y)	Baseline Ht SDS	Predicted Ht SDS (PH)	Final Ht SDS (FH)	Target Ht SDS (TH)	Comments
Ranke (41)	20 M	11	−2.1	−0.8	−1.1	−0.6	FH + PH; FH < TH for both sexes
	5 F	8.4	−2.7	−2.5	−2.4	−0.9	
Blethen (42)	27 M	12.8	−1.9	−1.7	−1.7		FH = PH
Crowne (43,44)	43 M	14	−3.4	−1.3	−1.6	−0.6	FH + PH; FH < TH for both sexes
	15 F	14.2	−3.4	−1.3	−1.5	−0.6	
Bramswig (45)	37 M	14.8	−2.2	−0.2	−0.7	−0.4	FH < PH; FH = TH
	32 F	12.9	−2.1	−0.8		−0.6	FH = PH; FH = TH
LaFranchi (46)	29 M		−2.0	−0.9	−1.2	−0.2	FH = PH; FH < TH for both sexes
	13 F		−2.0	−1.4	−1.3	−0.4	
Albanese (14)	78 M	14.3	−2.7	−1.4	−2.0	−0.5	FH < PH; FH < TH for both sexes
	14 F	13	−3.2	−1.7	−2.3	−0.8	
Zadik (15)	17 M	12.5	−3.1	+1.8	−2.7	−1.9	FH < PH; FH < TH
Wit (12)	16 M –11 F	10.5	−3.0		−2.4	−1.0	FH < PH
Sperlich (16)	49 M	13.3	−2.3	−1.0	−1.0	−0.3	FH = PH; FH < TH
Buchlis (5)	41 M	12.7	−2.9	−1.7	−1.9	−0.9	FH = PH; FH < TH for both sexes
	17 F	12.2	−3.0	−2.5	−2.5	−1.1	

FH = final height; PH = predicted height; TH = genetic target height or mid-parental height study of GH treatment in healthy, short, GH sufficient children. They observed that the height outcomes of those given GH therapy were significantly greater than those given placebo. This is the best evidence to date of a beneficial effect of GH therapy in healthy, pathologically short, GH-sufficient children. The efficacy of GH treatment in this population was probably underestimated because many of the participants were in puberty at entry into the study.

Another new approach to the treatment of ISS involves the combined use of GH and a gonadotropin releasing hormone (GnRH) analog in pubertal short children. In a non-randomized, concurrent, non-placebo-controlled study, the adult heights (18) were markedly improved by the combination of GnRH analog and GH treatment. The rational of combined treatment is based on using GH treatment to prevent the growth decelerating effects of the analog (19) and using the analog to prevent the pubertal progression of bone maturation. This therapy appears to be more effective if it is started when bone age is young.

ETHICAL CONSIDERATIONS

There is general agreement that children with normal variants of short stature do not need GH treatment. However, opinions differ about the use of GH in healthy, pathologically short children with normal GH provocative tests. Decisions about the use of GH in this population cannot be based exclusively on serum GH concentrations, but must include clinical, auxological, biochemical, and psychological considerations. Because of our limited ability to evaluate each of the growth regulating genes and because we lack a gold standard for diagnosing GH deficiency, we must be careful to distinguish between short normal children and those with pathologic growth of unknown etiology. Most authors have combined these two groups in their discussion about the ethical issues of GH therapy. Lantos and colleagues (2) have suggested that short stature is not a disease, and therefore it is unethical to use GH since we are exposing these subjects to the potential risks of GH administration. Others have advocated a more flexible approach based on the severity of the growth disorder as well as auxological and psychological variables (1). Would the ethical arguments be altered if GH treatment restored normal adult height in these children without compromising their general health? Recent data from controlled studies show that adult heights were improved by GH treatment of ISS with most subjects achieving stature in the lower part of the normal height range (5,7,10,11,20–22).

PSYCHOSOCIAL CONSIDERATIONS

While some studies have shown that patients with severe short stature are psychologically disadvantaged because of frequent teasing, academic under-achievement, and behavioral problems such as anxiety, somatic complaints, impulsivity, and distractibility (23), other studies have shown that a great majority of short children adopt satisfactory coping strategies. Recent evidence suggests that the psychosocial adaptations of short children are comparable to controls in the general population regardless of whether or not they were referred for medical evaluation (24,25). In the Wessex Growth Study, short children below the 3rd percentile did not differ from classmates on measures of self-esteem, self-concept, or teacher's report of behavioral problems (26). However, these short children were more dissatisfied with their height than the control group. A similar school based study reported no adverse effects of short stature on popularity or friendships, but student peers viewed them as looking younger. Among 522 children and adolescents, ages 4–18, referred to a pediatric endocrinology clinic, more than half reported being teased weekly *(27)* and being treated younger than their chronological age (juvenilization). Nevertheless, the overall psychological adaptations of these short children were generally comparable to community norms *(27,28)*. Moreover, GH treatment of ISS patients did not appear to have any long term beneficial effect on either psychological adjustment or quality of life during young adulthood *(26,29)*. The potential exists for a negative psychological effect of GH treatment if expected height is not achieved. Although psychosocial morbidity is not generally associated with short stature, the results of behavioral studies should not be applied to children or parents who believe that pathologic short stature interferes with lifestyle and psychological well-being. Ideally, these children would benefit from psychological support with or without GH therapy. If GH treatment is used, families should be informed that treatment may or may not accelerate linear growth and that adult heights are likely to be normal but below average.

An experienced psychologist is an important member of the health care team; they can reassure parents that most healthy short children do as well psychologically and academically as individuals of average height and can advise if psychological support services are needed regardless of the medical decision.

At present, opinions differ about the use of psychological assessments in the decision making process pertaining to therapy for ISS. Should psychological maladjustment be a prerequisite for medical treatment of pathological short stature, or should the decision to use GH be based mainly on the severity of the growth disturbance and clinical criteria? For example, healthy adolescent boys with exaggerated gynecomastia are not required to be psychologically compromised in order to undergo corrective surgery. Therefore, we recommend that auxological considerations be the primary basis for therapeutic intervention. We also emphasize that concomitant psychological support be provided.

ADVERSE EFFECTS

Careful monitoring of any child receiving GH therapy is mandatory, especially when administered in non-GHD patient. Adverse effects associated with GH treatment have been relatively uncommon. From the safety data obtained from two large post marketing databases (NCGS and KIGS), it appears that GH therapy is remarkably safe. Indeed, the KIGS database *(30)* reported that the most common side effect from GH in 3499 children with ISS was headache (0.71%). Other rare adverse events included convulsions (0.34%), arthralgias (0.22%), edema (0.02%), Osgood-Schlater disease (0.02%), slipped capital femoral epiphysis (0.05%), and scoliosis (0.05%). No malignancies or any metabolic side effects of clinical significance were reported *(31)*. Nevertheless, long term safety monitoring is strongly recommended.

GROWTH REGULATORY GENES: THEIR INFLUENCE ON CHILDHOOD GROWTH

At present, the diagnostic approach to growth disorders of childhood has focused mainly on measuring the serum GH responses to pharmacologic stimulation of the pituitary gland (insulin-induced hypoglycemia, L-Arginine, L-Dopa, Clonidine and the like) and quantitation of serum concentrations of IGF-1 and IGFBP-3. Short girls usually have their karyotypes analyzed for the possibility of an X chromosome abnormality. The presence of disproportionate short stature requires a skeletal survey to check for one of the chondrodystrophies. When growth failure is associated with dysmorphic features, genetic syndromes must be considered (Down Syndrome, Prader-Willi Syndrome, and the like). Prenatal growth disturbances which result in IUGR or SGA may cause persistent growth failure throughout childhood and adolescence. Psychosocial stress, malnutrition, or chronic diseases may also impact on childhood growth. In addition, oral glucocorticoids are known to cause deceleration or even growth arrest when used as anti-inflammatory or immunosuppressive medications. To a less extent this holds true for inhaled glucocorticoids in many children. Major gains have been made in visualizing the hypothalamus, stalk and pituitary gland using magnetic resonance imaging (MRI). This study is an essential part of evaluation of the growth evaluation even in the absence of neurologic symptoms. In the absence of any detectable abnormality in the diagnostic assessment, a pathologically short child is considered to have idiopathic growth failure or idiopathic short stature (ISS).

Currently, increasing attention is being given to the contribution of important genes that influence childhood growth. As time goes by, access to genetic analyses of these genes will be facilitated when commercial laboratories offer molecular diagnoses. The following are members of an expanding family of growth regulatory genes:

- The growth hormone releasing hormone (GHRH) and the GHRH receptor genes are critical stimulators of GH production by the somatotrophs of the anterior pituitary *(32)*. Mutations of the GHRH receptor (GHRH-R) gene causes GH deficiency and dwarfism *(33)*. Children with this disorder fail to increase serum GH concentrations after administration of recombinant GHRH. GH therapy is highly efficacious.
- Growth Hormone Releasing peptides (GHRP) are small synthetic molecules which act through an orphan G-protein coupled receptor, GHRP-R to stimulate GH release from the pituitary *(34)*. The GHRPs and their receptors are also referred to as GH secretagogs (GHS) and GHS-R respectively. The GHRP-R was cloned in 1996 *(35)*. In 1999, the natural GHRP was identified and given the name Ghrelin *(36)*. GHS-Rs are located on pituitary somatotrophs and on neuropeptide (NPY) in the hypothalamus. Ghrelin is mainly generated by the stomach and secreted into the circulation. This peptide increases feeding and weight gain in addition to stimulation of GH release from the anterior pituitary cell. It is hypothesized that Ghrelin has a positive effect on energy balance and thereby facilitates the anabolic actions of GH *(34)*. The clinical significance of GHS and GHS-R is being evaluated.
- Prop-1 and Pit-1 genes are essential for the differentiation of precursor cells into somatotrophs. The Prop-1 gene is said to be the prophet of the Pit-1 gene because it plays a critical role in Pit-1 gene differentiation. A mutation of Prop-1 causes gonadotropin, GH, TSH, and prolactin deficiencies, whereas a mutation of the Pit-1 gene is associated with intact gonadotropin production but failure of the somatotroph, thyrotroph, and lactotroph lineage. The pituitary gland is enlarged in children with the Prop-1 gene mutation whereas it is small in those with a Pit-1 gene mutation. GH treatment and thyroid hormone replacement are needed for normal growth in these children. Testosterone treatment of males with a Prop-1 mutation may be needed during infancy if micropenis is present, and during adolescence for induction of pubertal development.
- GH gene mutations may be inherited as homozygous autosomal recessive mutations, which lead to absence of GH production during fetal life (Type 1A IGHD). Affected

infants are short at birth and experience severe hypoglycemia. GH therapy is transiently beneficial, but treatment fails after the affected child develops antibodies to exogenous GH. Consanguinity is likely in the parents
- GH gene mutations are not found in children with Type 1B IGHD, which is also inherited as an autosomal recessive condition. GH deficiency rather than total absence is characteristic of this defect and response to GH treatment is good.
- Type 2 IGHD is caused by autosomal dominant disorder in families with an affected parent and an affected sib. In one family, a missense mutation in the GH gene resulted in a bioinactive GH product which failed to activate the GH receptor and also inhibited the action of exogenous GH by a dominant negative effect *(37)*.
- Type 3 IGHD is an X-linked disorder associated with immunoglobulin deficiencies.
- GH-R gene mutations may result in complete or partial GH insensitivity. Patients with complete GH insensitivity have homozygous mutations of the GH-R gene leading to the absence of the extracellular domain of GH-R and very low or absent Growth Hormone Binding Protein (*[38]*; (*see* Chapter 2). Partial GH insensitivity is associated with variable levels of GHBP and is the result of a heterozygous mutation of the GH-R gene which interferes with GH signal transduction.
- IGF-1 gene deletion was documented in an infant with IUGR and post natal growth failure *(39,40)*. In addition, a partial deletion *(40)* was reported in a boy with severe growth retardation, undetectable serum IGF-1 level, elevated GH concentration, and insulin resistance. GH treatment was not effective, even though the GH receptor was normal, because the IGF-1 gene was mutated. However, recombinant IGF-1 treatment improved linear growth, reduced GH levels, and improved insulin sensitivity.
- SHOX gene (Short Stature HOmeoboX-containing gene) is located in the pseudo-autosomal region of the short arms of the X and Y chromosomes *(39)*. Loss of one active gene or a mutation leads to haploinsufficiency and short stature. The short stature of Turner syndrome is explained by the loss of SHOX gene combined with aneuploidy. Tall stature in girls with Turner syndrome is associated with 46, X i (Xp). Increased height in Klinefelter's syndrome (47 XXY) results from the presence of 3 active SHOX genes. A deficiency of one SHOX gene causes Leri-Weill dyschondrosteosis syndrome (mesomelic dysplasia, short forelegs, and Madelung deformity of the forearms). The latter has been termed the dinner fork deformity because the dorsal dislocation of the ulna and triangulation of the radial epiphysis. Loss of both SHOX genes is responsible for Langer syndrome (homozygous Leri-Weill dyschondrosteosis syndrome), associated with extraordinarily mesomelic dwarfism, rudimentary fibula, and micrognathia. A SHOX mutation accounts for a minority of patients with ISS.

CONCLUSION

GH therapy in patients with ISS results in mixed outcomes because of the heterogeneity of the study populations. When molecular diagnostic tests become more available, it is likely that the ISS population will be subdivided into homogenous groups and fewer short children will be diagnosed with idiopathic short stature. It is also likely that we will be able to distinguish GH responsive from GH unresponsive forms of short stature. Eventually, newer therapeutic agents will become available such as the *SHOX* gene product. In the meantime, we recommend that the guidelines outlined in this chapter be used to distinguish healthy children with innocent short stature from equally healthy, pathologically short children with poorly understood disorders of growth. Therapeutic intervention in the latter group must continue to be based on sound auxological and clinical criteria, and is likely to remain a subject of ongoing debate.

REFERENCES

1. Underwood LE, Rieser PA. Is it ethical to treat healthy short children with growth hormone? Acta Paediatr Scand 1989;362(Suppl):18–23.
2. Lantos J, Siegler M, Cutler L. Ethical issues in growth hormone therapy. JAMA 1989;261(7): 1020–1024.
3. Finklestein BS, Silvers JB, Marrero U, Neuhauser D, Cuttler L. Insurance coverage, physician recomendations and access to emerging treatments. JAMA 1998;279(9):663–668.
4. Guyda HJ. Four Decades of growth hormone therapy: what have we achieved? J Clin Endocrinol Metab 1999;84(12):4307–4316.
5. Buchlis JG, Irizarry L, Crotzer BC, Shine BJ, Allen L, MacGillivray MH. Comparison of Final Heights of growth hormone-treated vs Untreated Children with Idiopathic Growth Failure. J Clin Endocrinol Metab 1998;83(4):1075–1079.
6. Genentech Collaborative Study Group. Idiopathic Short Stature 2. J Pediatr 1989;115:713–719.
7. Loche S, Cambiaso P, Setzu S, et al. Final height after growth hormone therapy in non-deficient children with short stature. J Pediatr 1994;125(2):196–200.
8. Ranke MB. Toward a consensus on the definition of short stature. Horm Res 1996;45(Suppl 2): 64–66.
9. Kelnar CJH, Albertsson-Wikland K, Hintz RL, Ranke MB, Rosenfeld RG. Should we treat children with idiopathic short stature? Horm Res 1999;52:155–157.
10. Bierich JR, Nolte K, Drew K, Brugman G. Constitutional delay of growth and adolescence. Result of a short term treatment with growth hormone. Acta Endocrinol (Copenh) 1992;127:392–396.
11. Zadik Z, Mira U, Landau H. Final height after growth hormone therapy for peripubertal boys with a subnormal integrated concentration of growth hormone. Horm Res 1992;37(4–5):104–105.
12. Wit JM, Kamp GA, Rikken B, et al. Spontaneous growth and response to growth hormone in children with growth hormone deficiency or idiopathic short stature (review). Pediatr Res 1996;39(2):295–302.
13. Wit JM, Boersma B, de Muink, et al. Long term results of growth therapy in children with short stature, subnormal growth rate and normal growth hormone response to secretagogues. Dutch growth hormone working group. Clin Endocrinol 1995;42(4):365–372.
14. Albanese A, Standhope R. Does constitutional delayed puberty cause segmented disproportion and short stature. Eur J Pediatr 1993;152:293–296.
15. Zadik Z, Chalew S, Lhlekrhzk A. Effect of long term growth hormone therapy on bone age and pubertal maturationin boys with and without classic growth hormone deficiency. J Pediatr 1994;125(2):189–195.
16. Sperlich M, Butenandt O, Schwarz HP, Butenandt O. Final height and predicted height in boys with untreated constitutional growth delay. Eur J Pediatr 1995;154(8):627–632.
17. Rekers-Momberg LT, Wit JM, Massa GG, et al. Spontaneous growth in idiopathic short stature. European Study Group. Arch Dis Child 1996;75(3):175–180.
18. Tanaka T, Horikawa R, Mari S, et al. Increased pubertal height in non-GHD short children treated with combined GH and GnRH analogs. Abstract presented at the 6th joint meeting of the LWPES, and ESPE, Montreal, Canada July 6–10, 2001.
19. Kaplowitz PB. If gonadotropin-releasing hormone plus growth hormone (GH) really improves growth outcomes in short non-GH-deficient children, then what? (Editorial). J Clin Endocrinol Metab 2001;86(7):2695–2698.
20. Hintz RL, Attie KM, Baptista J, Roche A. Effect of growth hormone treatment on adult height of children with idiopathic short stature. N Engl J Med 1999;340(7):502–507.
21. Leshek EW, Rose SR, Yanovski JA, et al. Effect of growth hormone treatment on the final height of children with non-growth hormone-deficient short stature: a randomized, double-blind, placebo-controlled trial. abstract presented at the 6th joint Meeting of the LWPES and ESPE, Montreal Canada, July 6–10, 2001.
22. Guyda HJ. Growth Hormone treatment of Non-Growth hormone deficient Children with Short Stature. Clin Pediatr Endocrinol 1996;5(Suppl 7):11–18.
23. Stabler B, Clopper RR, Stoppani C, Compton PG, Underwood LE. Academic achievement and psychological adjustment in short children. The National Cooperative Growth Study. J Dev Behav Pediatr 1994;15(1):1–6.
24. Sandberg DE. Should short children who are not deficient in growth hormone deficient be treated? West J Med 2000;172:186–189.

25. Zimet GD, Cutler M, Litvene M, Dahms W, Owns R, Cuttler L. Psychosocial Adjustment of Children Evaluated for short stature: a preliminary report. J Dev Behav Pediatr 1995;16(4):264–270.
26. Downie B, Mulligan J, McCaughey ES, Stratford RJ, Betts PR, Voss LD. Psychological response to growth hormone treatment in short normal children. Arch Dis Child 1996;75(32):35.
27. Sandberg DE, Michael P. Psychosocial stresses related to short stature: does their presence imply psychiatric dysfunction? In: Drotar D, ed. Assessing pediatric health-related quality of life and functionnal status: implication for research, practice and policy. Lawrence Erlbaum, New Jersey 1998, pp. 287–312.
28. Sandberg DE, Brook AE, Campos SP. short stature: A psychosocial burden requiring growth hormone therapy? Pediatr 1994;94(6):832–840.
29. Rekers-Mombarg, Busschbach JJ, Dicke J, Wit JM. Quality of life of young adults with idiopathic short stature: effect of growth hormone treatment. Dutch Growth Hormone Working Group. Acta Paediatrica 1998;87(8):865–870.
30. Wilton P. Adverse events during GH treatment: 10 years' experience in KIGS, a pharmaco-epidemiological survey. Growth hormone therapy in KIGS- 10 years' experience. Johann Ambrosius Barth Verlag, 1999:349–364.
31. Saenger P, Attie KM, DiMartino-Nardi J, Frahm L, Frane JW. Metabolic consequences of 5 year growth hormone (GH) therapy in children treated with GH for idiopathic short stature. J Clin Endocrinol Metab 1998;83(9):115–120.
32. Giustina A, Veldhuis JD. Pathophysiology of the Neuroregulation of growth Hormone Secretion in Experimental Animals and the Human. Endocrine Rev 1998;19(6):717–797.
33. Salvatori R, Hayashida CY, Aguiar-Oliveira MH, et al. Familial dwarfism due to a novel mutation of the growth hormone-releasing hormone receptor gene. J Clin Endocrinol Metab 1999;84(3):917–923.
34. Bowers CY. Growth hormone releasing peptides (GHRP). Cellular and molecular life sciences. 1998;54(12):1316–1329.
35. Howard AD, Feighner SD, Cully DF, et al. A Receptor in pituitary and hypothalamus that functions in growth hormone release. Science 1996;273:974–977.
36. Takaya K, Ariyasu H, Kanamoto N, et al. Ghrelin strongly stimulates growth hormone (GH) release in humans. J Clin Endocrinol Metab 2000;85:4908–4911.
37. Takahashi Y, Hidesuke K, Okimura Y, Goji K, Abe H, Chihara K. Brief report:Short stature caused by a mutant growth hormone 29. N Engl J Med 1996;334(7):432–436.
38. Carlsson LM, Attie K, Compton PG, Vitangcol RV, Merimee TJ. Reduced concentration of growth hormone binding protein in children with idiopathic short stature J Clin Endocrinol Metab 1994;78:1325–1330.
39. Woods KA, Camacho-Hubner C, Savage MO, Clark AJL. Brief report: intrautrine growth retardation and post-natal growth failure asssociated with deletion of the insulin-like growth factor 1 gene. N Engl J Med 1996;335(18):1363–1367.
40. Camacho-Hubner C, Woods KA, Miraki-Moud F, et al. Effects of recombinant human insulin-like growth factor (IGF-1) therapy on the growth hormone-IGF system of a patient with partial IGF-1 deletion. J Clin Endocrinol Metab 1999;84(5):1611–1616.
41. Ranke MB, Aronson AS. Adult height in children with constitutional short stature. Acta Paediatr Scand 1989;362:27–31.
42. Blethen SL, Gaines S, Weldon V. Comparison of predicted and adult heights in short boys: effect of androgen therapy. Pediatr Res 1984;467–469.
43. Crowne ED, Shalet SM, Wallace WHB, Eminson DM, Price DA. Final height in boys with untreated constitutional delay of growth and puberty. Arch Dis Child 1990;65:1109–1112.
44. Crowne ED, Shalet SM, Wallace WHB, Eminson DM, Price DA. Final height in girls with untreated constitutional delay of growth and puberty. Eur J Pediatr 1990;150:708–712.
45. Bramswing JH, Frasse M, Holthoff ML, Von Lengerke HJ, Petrykowski W, Schellong G. Adult height in boys and girls with untreated short stature and constitutional delay of growth and puberty: accuracy of five different methods of height prediction. J Pediatr 1990;117:886–891.
46. LaFranchi S, Hanna C, Mandel S. Constitutional delay of growth: expected vs final adult height. Pediatr 1991;87:82–86.
47. Lopez-Siguerro JP, Garcia-Garcia E, Carralero I, Martinez-Aedo MJ. Adult height in children with idiopathic short stature treated with growth hormone 9. J Pediatr Endocrinol Metab 2000;13(9):1595–1602.
48. McCaughey ES, Mulligan J, Voss LD, Betts PR. Randomised trial of growth hormone in short normal girls. Lancet 1998;351:940.

4
Growth Hormone Treatment of Children Following Intrauterine Growth Failure

Steven D. Chernausek, MD

CONTENTS

INTRODUCTION
MECHANISM OF IUGR
CLINICAL PRESENTATION
DIAGNOSITIC EVALUATION
GROWTH HORMONE THERPAY
FUTURE DIRECTIONS
REFERENCES

INTRODUCTION

Intrauterine growth retardation (IUGR) is a pathologic condition where fetal growth is restrained by either extrinsic (maternal) factors or a disorder intrinsic to the fetus itself. Each year, nearly fourteen million infants are born with IUGR worldwide *(1)*; rates are especially high in developing countries because of poor nutrition and limited prenatal care. This is a significant problem because of the morbidity that accompanies IUGR. Complications in the immediate post-partum period include hypoglycemia, necrotizing enterocolitis, and persistence of the fetal circulation, to name a few *(2)*. Moreover, the first year survival rate is substantially reduced in infants who have had IUGR *(3)*.

There are long-term sequelae of IUGR as well. Affected patients may have poor school performance and attenuated intellectual development *(4)*. There is evidence that intrauterine nutrient deprivation leads to obesity, insulin resistance, and hyperlipidemia later in life, an effect thought to be due to *in utero* "programming" of metabolic status *(5)*. Postnatal growth is also affected adversely. Somewhere between 10–40% of children who are born following IUGR remain growth-retarded in childhood *(6,7)*. Many never reach normal adult size. The effect of IUGR on subsequent growth and its amelioration by growth hormone (GH) is the focus of this chapter.

The percentage of patients said to have had IUGR depends on the definition applied, but generally is ca. 3% in the United States and 10% in developing countries. It is important to consider definitions used to define IUGR as they have some bearing on interpretation of published reports. Intrauterine growth retardation (or intrauterine

From: *Contemporary Endocrinology: Pediatric Endocrinology: A Practical Clinical Guide*
Edited by: S. Radovick and M. H. MacGillivray © Humana Press Inc., Totowa, NJ

growth restriction) is a failure to grow at a normal rate in the *in utero* environment. Sequential measurements of fetal size *in utero* are usually not available, and therefore IUGR is infrequently documented with precision. Additionally, the phase of pregnancy during which the growth aberration occurred is rarely defined. The more commonly used definition is small-for-gestational-age (SGA), which is simply a statistical definition for low birth weight at the calculated gestational age. Typical lines of demarcation are –2 SDs or the 3rd percentile. Though patients who fall below this are assumed to have had a period of IUGR, in some cases they simply represent the end of the normal spectrum of birth size. Similarly, patients may have had IUGR, especially in the last trimester, but have a birth weight that surpasses the minimal standards. These patients may have other features of IUGR such as decreased subcutaneous tissue, hypoglycemia, etc.

After birth, most patients increase their growth velocity significantly and eventually catch up *(6,7)*. However, it should be noted that there is a relationship between birth weight and size that is maintained for several years of childhood, with patients being born especially small remaining short on the average *(8)*. The etiologies of IUGR are as varied as those for short stature as adults and are summarized in Table 1.

MECHANISMS OF IUGR

A deficiency of insulin secretion (such as occurs in pancreatic agenesis) or action (e.g., insulin receptor deficiency/leprauchanism) in humans severely impairs fetal growth and though specific, is a rare cause of IUGR *(9)*. More common fetal insults that produce IUGR are hypoxia, which occurs in placental insufficiency, high altitude living, maternal hypertension, etc and nutrient deprivation. Restriction of oxygen or nutrient results in adaptive responses on the part of the fetus, which tend to preserve organ differentiation and maturation at the expense of physical growth and energy stores (fat and glycogen). It is clear that the insulin-like growth factor (IGF) axis is intimately involved in these adaptive responses. Because this chapter deals predominantly with practical aspects of diagnosis and treatment of short stature in patients born SGA, detailed review of the components of the IGF system and their roles in control of fetal growth is beyond its scope (for reviews, *see* works by Rosenfeld *[10]* and Efstratiadis *[11]*). However, it is worthwhile to consider the in vivo experiments using mouse mutant models that have defined major hormonal influences on prenatal and postnatal growth (Table 2). The physiology is summarized as follows: IGF-1 and IGF-2 are the major hormonal regulators of fetal growth and can compensate, at least partially, for deficiency of each other. The growth-promoting effects of the IGFs are principally mediated by the type I or IGF-1 receptor, a homolog of the insulin receptor. The IGF-2 "receptor," in contrast, serves a clearance mechanism of tissue IGF-2 and thereby modulates tissue IGF-2 abundance. During fetal life, the IGF system operates largely independently of GH, which has little influence on body size before birth in humans and before 2 wk in rodents. Thereafter, the influence of IGF-2 declines and IGF-1, under the control of GH, becomes the dominant growth regulator of postnatal life.

Though much of our insight into mechanisms comes from studies of rodents, many of the experimental findings have been confirmed in man. Humans with GH insensitivity due to receptor deficiency are near normal size at birth, indicating a modest role for GH in prenatal growth *(12)*. In contrast, children with genetic lesions in the IGF-1 gene *(13)* and IGF-1 receptor gene *(14)* show severe intrauterine growth retardation and subse-

Table 1
Causes of Fetal Growth Retardation

Locus	Classification/cause	Example
Maternal	Low oxygen/nutrients	Severe maternal undernutrition, multiple gestation, cigarette smoking, high altitude living
	Infection	CMV, Toxoplasmosis, AIDS
	Toxin	Alcohol
Placental	Vascular anomalies	Velamentous cord insertion, placental hemangioma
	Placental deficiency	Sub-optimal implantation site, placental undergrowth, infarction
Fetal	Defects in insulin secretion or action	Leprechaunism, pancreatic agenesis
	Chromosome aneuploidy	Turner S, Trisomy 13, Trisomy 18
	Genetic syndromes	Bloom, Dubowitz, Fanconi, Seckel, Russel-Silver Syndromes

Table 2
Effects of Deletion of Murine Genes on Growth

Deleted gene(s)	Prenatal growth (% Normal BW)	Postnatal growth	Comments	Ref.
IGF-1	60	Retarded		(52,53)
IGF-2	60	Normal		(54)
IGF-1 & IGF-2	30	NA	Neonatal Death	(55)
IGF-1 R	45	NA	Neonatal Death	(52)
IGF-2/Man-6-P R	140	NA	Neonatal Death, anomalies	(56,57)
Insulin R	90	NA	Develop Diabetes	(58)
IRS-1	60–80	Normal		(59,60)
GH R	100	Retarded		(61)

IGF-1 = Insulin-like growth factor-1, IGF-2 R/ Man-6-P R is IGF-2/manose-6 phosphate receptor. Data are compiled from several sources.

quent postnatal growth deficiency, just as predicted from murine deletion mutants. Such data, when considered in the context of the reports describing positive correlation between cord blood IGF-1 concentration and birth size *(15–17)*, illustrate the pivotal role of the IGF axis in controlling prenatal and postnatal growth.

Though changes in the IGF axis appear to mediate the alterations in growth, primary disturbances of GH/IGF are unlikely to be the root cause for most cases of IUGR with poor postnatal growth. Certainly classical GH deficiency is uncommon as an explanation for poor growth following IUGR. Why then would one expect that GH treatment would be beneficial in patients with short stature associated with IUGR? The most straightforward answer is that GH administered at pharmacological dosages stimulates the system sufficiently to overcome whatever cellular condition has not allowed the expected "catch-up growth" that would restore age-appropriate size. Studies reported by Lupu, et al. *(18)* detail the extent to which the GH-IGF axis influences growth in the rodent. In mature animals, approximately 70% of body size is due to the actions of IGF, of which about half relate to GH-mediated changes in IGF concentration while the remainder reflects IGF direct effects (i.e., not related to GH stimulation of IGF production). GH appears to have direct effects, independent of IGFs, on body size. When these elements are accounted, only about 17% of body size in the adult mouse relates to factors other than GH or IGF. This means that diseases or conditions that alter growth significantly likely will impact the GH-IGF system at some point, either limiting the production of the IGFs, reducing the abundance or function of the IGF receptor, or perturbing specific steps along the intracellular signal transduction pathway.

CLINICAL PRESENTATION

Patients generally present to the endocrinologist in one of two ways. The first is immediately following birth, when categorized as small for gestational age. The questions that arise at this time relate to potential causes of intrauterine growth retardation and whether patient will have normal growth thereafter. The extent of the evaluation will depend on the severity of growth retardation, whether the patient is experiencing other medical problems or has dysmorphic features, and whether the cause is evident.

A more common presentation is that of the short child between ages 3 and 8. The child was born with a low birth weight and was expected to "catch up". However, catch up never occurred and he has had the same relative degree of short stature for many years. That is, when plotted on the growth chart, his trajectory seems to parallel the norm, just 3–5 SDS below average. The child has otherwise been healthy and his parents are concerned that the short stature will become increasingly problematic as the patient ages, and wonder whether anything can be done to improve his stature. It is not always evident that the persistent small size is related to a growth disorder that began prior to birth. Only by reviewing the birth weight and history of pregnancy and delivery does this information come to light.

DIAGNOSTIC EVALUATION

The causes of growth failure are many, as are the tests that can be applied to such patients. One should consider the likely possibilities and apply the diagnostic tests that are reasonably expected to be helpful. There are important reasons for establishing a diagnosis. However, it should be emphasized that in many cases it is impossible to ascertain the precise of cause of the prenatal growth failure. Since this chapter deals primarily with the use of GH in augmenting growth in such children, the diagnostic discussion is directed towards determining whether GH therapy is warranted. The diagnostic approach is framed under several relevant questions.

1. *Does the patient have a disorder that limits both pre- and postnatal growth?* Certain common endocrine disorders such as hypothyroidism and GH deficiency only affect postnatal growth substantially even when the condition is congenital. Thus, these are simply eliminated as diagnostic possibilities when prenatal growth restriction is evident. The same applies for common, acquired causes of growth failure such as celiac disease,

Table 3
Useful Tests for IUGR-Associated Short Stature

General	Specialized
Complete Blood Count	Karyotype (Turner Syndrome)
Erythrocyte Sedimentation Rate	Cytogenetic Studies to assess chromosome stability
BUN/Creatinine	(Bloom Syndrome, Fanconi Syndrome)
Serum Electrolytes	
IGF-1/IGFBP-3	
T4, TSH	
Radiological Skeletal Survey	

and the like. Patients who are born SGA frequently show catch-up growth during the first year and do not require further evaluation. Patients being evaluated for IUGR who are still in the first few months of life should simply be tracked in terms of growth if they have no dysmorphic features, malformations, or suspicious symptoms. It is clear that most patients destined to catch up will demonstrate increased growth velocity and during the first 6 mo of life and have caught up by the end of the first year *(6,19,20)*. Patients who have shown no evidence for improved growth following birth need further evaluation.

2. *Is the cause of IUGR obvious?* Careful history and physical exam can be very helpful in explaining the intrauterine growth retardation. Maternal hypertension, poor weight gain during pregnancy all suggest a maternal factor. Dysmorphic features in the baby imply a syndrome associated with IUGR may be present. Diagnostic tests that may be particularly helpful for evaluating patients with IUGR are listed in Table 3. A karyotype is particularly important for females since Turner syndrome may show mild prenatal growth restriction. Patients with dysmorphic features should have karyotyping as well, or be considered for other specialized genetic tests and further evaluation by a geneticist/dysmorphologist. It is particularly important to recognize Bloom syndrome, a recessive disorder associated with severe IUGR and poor postnatal growth. These patients have increased chromosomal breakage and usually develop malignancies later in childhood. For these reasons, GH therapy would seem contraindicated. The diagnosis of Bloom syndrome is often suspected with routine chromosome studies in which there is increased chromosome breakage and formation of triradial chromosomes. Confirmation requires specialized chromosomal studies which examine rates of sister chromatid exchange. Assessment of renal function is required because mild forms of renal dysplasia can produce IUGR and moderate postnatal growth failure that is otherwise not evident. These patients may manifest oligohydramnios as a clue to the diagnosis.

3. *Why has the patient not shown catch-up growth?* If more were known of the mechanisms involved in catch-up growth, it would be easier to explain why, in some cases, it does not occur. In some situations, the fetal growth retardation may have been so severe and the cellular mass at birth is so low that overall somatic size is ultimately restricted. Even with normalization of nutritional and hormonal factors, simply restoring normal growth (body size doubling at normal intervals) still leaves a person small relative to the peers. In other cases, patients do not reach normal size following birth because of persistence of a defect in growth regulation or cellular growth and replication. From a practical point of view, it is important to consider that catch-up growth may be impaired in patients whose nutritional status is compromised. A careful dietary history and review by a nutritionist can be helpful, and is especially indicated in a patient with low weight for height.

There is also evidence that GH secretion is reduced and limiting catch-up growth in some patients. Though absence of GH clearly cannot explain intrauterine growth retardation, studies by Boguszewski et a.l *(21)* and de Waal et al. *(22)* have suggested that there is an increased incidence of low GH secretion in patients with short stature following IUGR. The data imply that reduced pituitary GH secretion contributes to the relatively poor postnatal growth in some cases. However, the ability of indices of GH secretion to predict response to GH therapy for this group of patients is not clear. Earlier reports suggested low overnight GH concentrations or low IGF-1 concentrations were associated with an improved response *(23,24)*, whereas later reports examining greater numbers found no predictive value in these measures *(25–27)*. However, such studies frequently differ in the patient selection (e.g., severity of IUGR and short stature), the dosing of GH, and the tests of GH release. Studies that examine larger numbers of patients only slightly SGA, likely include a significant proportion that do not necessarily have disorders of prenatal growth and/or have differing etiologies from those patients who are –4 to –5 SD below average for birth size. In addition, large doses of GH administered could obscure underlying differences in sensitivity to GH. Thus, the heterogeneous nature of this patient population continues to confound efforts to grasp all the variables of their growth and GH response. It is not surprising then that efforts to model predictors of response to GH treatment are least successful for the group with IUGR-associated short stature *(28)*.

Most patients do not meet biochemical criteria for classic GH deficiency or other known endocrine disorders, and thus the most likely explanation for their poor postnatal growth is the persistence of a problem intrinsic to the fetus. There may be a specific genetic defect that continues to limit growth or the early growth restriction has, in some way, reprogrammed the growth regulating system so that the child remains small. Indeed, most animal models of prenatal growth restriction do not show postnatal catch-up growth following birth.

GROWTH HORMONE THERAPY

Effects on Somatic Growth

The earliest reports of GH administration to patients with IUGR-associated short stature indicated that short-term linear growth was stimulated by GH *(29–31)*. However, enthusiasm was diminished by the suggestion that the growth stimulation was not sustained *(32)*, and that undesirable bone age advancement was negating the effect *(33)*. Such data implied that patients were unlikely to have meaningful benefit from long-term GH therapy in terms of final height. However, the doses employed were modest by today's standards, being similar to those given to patients with GH deficiency at the time. Data from the last decade shows clearly that exogenous GH stimulates growth in children with IUGR-associated short stature and that such growth can be sustained for several years (Fig 1.). Table 4 displays results from several large, intermediate-term studies indicating that 4–6 yr of therapy increases height by 2–2.5 SDS, depending on the dose employed. Though there are no randomized, controlled studies that define the effect on final height, it is likely that GH treatment leads to gains in adult height, given what we know about final height in untreated patients and the effects of GH therapy in other non-GH deficient conditions such as Turner syndrome *(34)* and idiopathic short stature *(35)*. In one of the few studies to report final height, Coutant et al. *(36)*, (Table 4) showed only

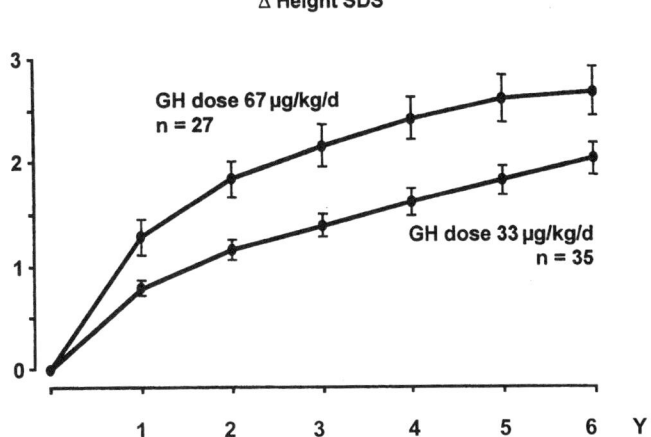

Fig. 1. Height SD score in patients with IUGR-associated short stature randomized to receive GH daily at two distinct doses. Patients were approx 5 yr of age on average at the start of treatment. Note the clear dose response relationship most apparent in the first years of treatment. Reproduced with permission from ref. (37).

very modest effect on final height, but the GH dose was low and the patients began treatment at age 10 yr on average. Thus, it appears that doses need to be higher than those used for treatment of GH deficiency and that treatment needs to be started during early childhood, perhaps in the 3–8 yr age range, to achieve satisfactory results.

Though the growth promoting effect of GH on such patients is clear, many questions remain in terms of patient selection criteria, dosage and dosing schedules, and monitoring for side effects. As previously noted, there are data suggesting that patients have an increased frequency of GH deficiency, measured by overnight sampling (21,22). Furthermore, as a group, they have lower than average IGF-1 concentrations. (22). Thus, even though GH stimulation testing does not appear to predict response to GH therapy (26), it is possible that individualization of dosing based on endogenous GH secretion may be helpful; this remains to be proven.

Continuous versus intermittent schedules have also been evaluated (37). Short-term treatment makes some sense since the underlying growth rate of patients may be near normal. In theory, therapy that could boost a patient to a higher percentile growth channel might be all that is needed for long-term benefit. Data thus far supports this concept, but suggests that the effect is not complete. Figure 2 shows results from a study that compared a short high dose period of treatment with a more moderate sustained therapy. The high-dose group lost some ground in the years following GH withdrawal, such that after 5 yr heights were equivalent. Data such as these has led some to propose intermittent dosing schedules for treatment.

An important issue facing the treating physician is the possibility of adverse effects. Even though used for over three decades in large numbers of children, GH rarely causes any serious morbidity (38). However, use in IUGR-associated short stature presents new issues. First, the dose of GH used in several studies is higher than that used for most patients in the past. Clearly, GH is being used as a pharmacological agent to stimulate seemingly reluctant biologic pathways involved in somatic growth. Hence, the side-effect profile of GH may be altered with the increased dose. Second, this patient popu-

Table 4
Summary of Selected Trials of GH Given Continuously for at Least 4 Years to Patients with IUGR-Associated Short Stature

Study format	N	Treatment duration (Yr)	GH dote (mg/kg/wk) (approx)	SDS start	SDS end	Comments	Ref.
Clinical Trial	58	4	0.30	−3.6	−1.6	No difference in response based on GH stimulation test result.	26
Composite of Clinical Trial	35	6	0.23	−3.4	−1.4		37
Clinical Trial	27	6	0.46	−4.0	−1.3		27
	41	5	0.23	−3.0	−0.8		
	38	5	0.46	−3.1	−0.5		
Clinical Trial	70	4.6 ± 2.5	0.14	−2.9	−2.0	Subjects followed until final height. Untreated "controls" had normal GH stimulation test; Treated patients had GH peak < 10 ng/mL.	
	40	0	NA	−2.8	−2.2	Control Group	36
Registry analysis (NCGS)	270	4	0.29	−3.6	−1.8	Uncontrolled Survey with 46 patients in 4th year.	62

Dosage of GH is approximate because in some cases doses were given on basis of body surface area or described in international units rather than mass. Conversion employed was 1 mg = 3 IU.

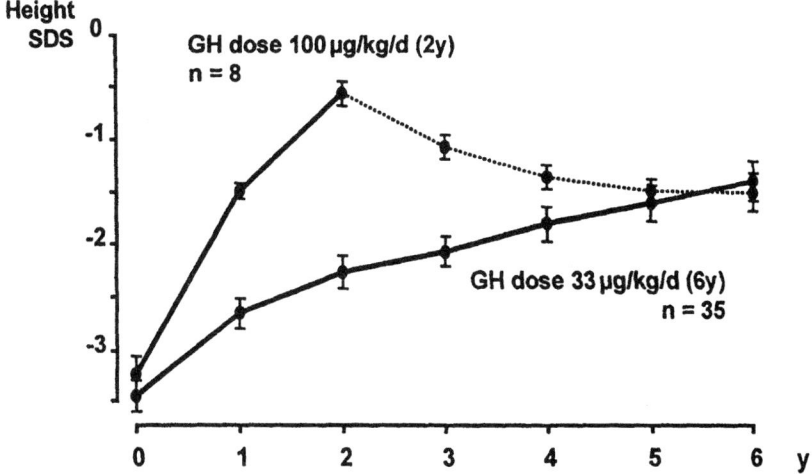

Fig. 2. Height SD score in patients treated with a 2 year course of high dose (100 μg/kg) daily GH and followed for 4 additional years untreated (dotted line). They are compared to patients treated with a lower dose of GH continuously for 6 yr. Note that patients on high dose grew very well during GH therapy but that height SD score was not maintained when GH supplementation was withdrawn. Reproduced with permission from ref. *(37)*.

lation may have unique susceptibilities to certain pharmacological properties of GH. The issue of insulin resistance is most pertinent. Epidemiological and experimental data indicate that humans born small for gestational age have an increased incidence of obesity and type II diabetes as adults, with the implication that the period of fetal undernutrition results in a resetting of intrinsic insulin sensitivity *(39)*. Patients with IUGR already show evidence of decreased insulin sensitivity as children *(40)*. Could GH, which diminishes insulin sensitivity, add to the risk of developing obesity, hyperlipidemia, and insulin resistance (syndrome X) later in life? Though data from patients treated thus far show only modest effects on basal insulin levels *(41)* and no clinically significant impact on glucose or lipid metabolism *(42)*, the observation period may not be long enough, and the numbers of patients treated with the highest doses still too few to detect significant long-term sequelae.

Additional important theoretical or potential complications of pharmacological GH therapy include orthopedic problems, such as carpel tunnel syndrome in adults, and scoliosis and slipped capital femoral epiphysis in children, and the possible promotion of malignancy risk *(43,44)*. The latter has been difficult to define. Analysis of risk of GH treatment in patients who developed GH deficiency as a consequence of tumor treatment do not indicate much of a role for GH in the development of relapse *(45,46)*. However, large epidemiological studies find that risks for prostate cancer *(47)* and breast cancer *(48)* are increased for people with serum IGF-I concentrations in the upper normal ranges. The studies do not prove cause and effect, but tumor cells in culture frequently express IGF-1 receptors and replicate in response to IGF-1 *(49)*. This raises the question as to whether the high IGF-1 levels that generally accompany high dose GH therapy might have adverse consequences over the long term.

Therapeutic Considerations

Growth Hormone has only recently been approved by the US Food and Drug Administration for treatment of non-GH deficient short stature in children born SGA. Experience with treatment of this patient group is therefore limited. However, based on the data described above, administration of GH to significantly short patients with IUGR-associated short stature should be considered in certain clinical situations. The author's approach to such patients is outlined, representing one way of dealing with the complex and controversial issues that surround the topic.

CRITERIA FOR GH THERAPY

Treatment should presently be limited to those patients in whom short stature is at least moderately severe (probably –2.5 SDs or less) and where there is little expectation of meaningful catch-up growth over the next several years. If significant catch-up is going to occur, it is usually evident during the first year of life. Since patterns can be variable, however, careful measures over at least 6 mo (preferably 12) should be performed to assess underlying growth velocity. Patients that present after age 2 with persistent short stature typically have a growth rate in the low normal range and are unlikely to show substantial improvement in height SDS over the next several years. Assessing final height prognosis with a bone age measure is not helpful because the patients are generally quite young and may have a pathological condition, both of which render the prediction inaccurate. Since younger patients appear to respond better, treatment can be initiated once it is clear that the current growth velocity will be insufficient to normalize height. Patients in mid-childhood would likely benefit as well, but those well into puberty may not be helped unless they have concomitant GH deficiency.

Measures of GH secretion, though frequently performed, do not appear to predict growth response and may only be helpful in dealing with reimbursement issues. I presently measure IGF-1 and IGFBP-3 and perform standard GH stimulation testing if these parameters are subnormal. If the IGFs and measures of GH release are all low, this suggests that a lack of GH is limiting the patients current skeletal growth and the need for supplementation seems clear. Baseline IGF-I also may be useful to help interpret serum concentrations during therapy. However, since many with apparently normal GH secretion respond to therapy, the testing does not necessarily alter the intention to treat.

GH DOSING AND MONITORING

Though relatively high doses may be ultimately required for the best growth response (the FDA approved dose is 0.48 mg/kg/wk, 0.07 mg/kg/d), beginning therapy at a dose around 0.04–0.05 mg/kg/d (a common dose for GH deficiency) offers certain advantages. Since the response of patients is highly variable, acceptable improvement may be observed on such a regimen. After 6–12 mo of therapy the dose may be increased if the growth rate is insufficient to produce catch-up and the medication is being tolerated without safety concern. Alternatively, one could begin therapy at the relatively higher dose in order to achieve more rapid growth initially, keeping the absolute dose constant and allowing the patient to "grow into" a more modest weight-based dose once a satisfactory height percentile is reached. Each approach has its advantages and more experience in needed with various treatment regimens.

Patients should have re-evaluation at a minimum of six-mo intervals with careful history and physical examination, seeking signs and symptoms of scoliosis, other orthopedic abnormalities, pseudotumor cerebri and assessment of growth response to therapy. Periodic measurement of glucose tolerance and/or insulin sensitivity seems wise, and monitoring of circulating IGF-1 have been recommended as an additional safety parameter *(50)*. Yet there are few data that define the extent of the risk and clearly specify in what ways the physician should deal with abnormalities. A simple measure of glucose insulin pairs in the fasting and fed (post CHO challenge) performed shortly after initiating GH therapy and periodically thereafter would easily identify those who develop diabetes or severe insulin resistance. The testing could be repeated every few years or when there are substantial increments in GH dose. This represents a conservative approach and the yield is likely to be quite low in the youngest patients at the start of therapy. However, the changes that might be observed after therapy of longer duration into the pubertal years are more difficult to predict.

Periodic assessment of circulating IGF-1 during GH therapy has been recommended for patients receiving GH. It is perhaps most valuable in for determining dose replacement of GH for adults with GH deficiency *(44)*, but has been advocated as a safety measure for other conditions where GH is used *(50)*. The notion is that doses of GH the produce supranormal levels of IGF-1 may be hazardous to the patient, perhaps increasing the risk of future malignancy or portending other GH-related side effects. The theory is reasonable, but its value is unproven and for individual patients with IUGR-associated short stature is particularly problematic since it is possible that a degree of IGF-1 resistance plays a role in growth limitation in certain patients. In that circumstance, raising IGF-1 concentrations above normal may be desirable. Furthermore the ranges of IGF-1 are very wide, suggesting varied sensitivity of individuals to IGF or that circulating IGF-1 is a poor reflection of signal strength at the cellular level. Clearly much more work needs to be done to define how measures of GH secretion and action can be used in the selection of therapeutic regimens for patients.

FUTURE DIRECTIONS

There is little doubt that GH will be used more frequently to ameliorate short stature that follows IUGR. Future studies need to clarify the issues discussed above, defining for physicians how the drug can be used with the greatest safety and efficacy. Whether all patients should receive the same, relatively high dose, or whether dosing can be tailored using markers of GH action that reflect individual sensitivity should be explored. The effects that GH therapy might have on the propensity to develop insulin resistance needs to be examined and assessed over time in larger numbers of patients. Though there is a presumption that GH may aggravate the problem, the opposite might be observed since IGF treatment improves insulin sensitivity in a rat model of "syndrome X" produced by fetal caloric restriction *(51)*.

The response of individuals is highly variable and must relate to the variety of conditions that initiated the growth problem and the different mechanisms involved in restraining subsequent growth. Improved methods to establish molecular-genetic diagnoses in IUGR patients are expected to ultimately be helpful in selecting the patients who will benefit from therapy and defining individuals at risk for specific sequelae. Though patients with specific genetic syndromes have rarely been evaluated in detail, there is really no reason to believe that for some the responses to GH would not equal that of non-syndromic patients. The ability to assess the growth regulatory components of specific patients on a molecular-genetic and functional basis to explain and categorize the growth anomalies, and to use the information to design and optimize therapy should enhance pediatrician of the future's ability to care for children born SGA.

REFERENCES

1. de Onis M, Blossner M, Villar J. Levels and patterns of intrauterine growth retardation in developing countries. Eur J Clin Nutr 1998;52(Suppl 1):S5–15.
2. Kliegman RM, Das UG. Intrauterine growth retardation. In: Fanaroff AA, Martin RJ, eds. Neonatal-Perinatal Medicine: Diseases of the Fetus and Infant. 7th ed. St. Louis, MO. Mosby, Inc., 2002, pp. 228–262.
3. McIntire DD, Bloom SL, Casey BM, Leveno KJ. Birth weight in relation to morbidity and mortality among newborn infants. N Engl J Med 1999;340(16):1234–1238.
4. Bos AF, Einspieler C, Prechtl HF. Intrauterine growth retardation, general movements, and neurodevelopmental outcome: a review. Dev Med Child Neurol 2001;43(1):61–68.
5. Godfrey KM, Barker DJ. Fetal nutrition and adult disease. Am J Clin Nutr 2000;71(Suppl 5): 1344S–1352S.
6. Albertsson-Wikland K, Karlberg J. Natural growth in children born small for gestational age with and without catch-up growth. Acta Paediatr 1994;399(Suppl):64–70; discussion 71.
7. Fitzhardinge PM, Steven EM. The small for date infant I. Later growth patterns. Pediatrics 1972;49:671–681.
8. Binkin NJ, Yip R, Fleshood L, Trowbridge FL. Birth weight and childhood growth. Pediatrics 1988;82(6):828–834.
9. Fowden AL. Insulin deficiency: effects on fetal growth and development. J Paediatr Child Health 1993;29(1):6–11.
10. Rosenfeld RG, Roberts CT. The IGF System: molecular biology, physiology, and clinical applications. Humana Press, Totowa, NJ: 1999.
11. Efstratiadis A. Genetics of mouse growth. Int J Dev Biol 1998;42(7):955–976.
12. Rosenfeld RG, Rosenbloom AL, Guevara-Aguirre J. Growth hormone (GH) insensitivity due to primary GH receptor deficiency. Endocr Rev 1994;15:369–390.
13. Woods KA, Camacho-Hubner C, Savage MO, Clark AJL. Intrauterine growth retardation and postnatal growth failure associated with deletion of the insulin-like growth factor I gene. N Engl J Med 1996;335:1363–1367.
14. Abbuzzahab MJ, Goddard AD, Grigorescu F, Lautier C, Smith RJ, Chernausek SD. Human IGF-1 receptor mutations associated with intrauterine and post-natal growth retardation. Program and Abstracts of the 82nd Annual Meeting of The Endocrine Society 2000:Abstract 1947.
15. Reece EA, Wiznitzer A, Le E, Homko CJ, Behrman H, Spencer EM. The relation between human fetal growth and fetal blood levels of insulin-like growth factors I and II, their binding proteins, and receptors. Obstet Gynecol 1994;84:88–95.
16. Fant M, Salafia C, Baxter RC, et al. Circulating levels of IGFs and IGF binding proteins in human cord serum: relationships to intrauterine growth. Regul Pept 1993;48:29–39.
17. Lassarre C, Hardouin S, Daffos F, Forestier F, Frankenne F, Binoux M. Serum insulin-like growth factors and insulin-like growth factor binding proteins in the human fetus: relationships with growth in normal subjects and in subjects with intrauterine growth retardation. Pediatr Res 1991;29:219–225.
18. Lupu F, Terwilliger JD, Lee K, Segre GV, Efstratiadis A. Roles of growth hormone and insulin-like growth factor 1 in mouse postnatal growth. Dev Biol 2001;229(1):141–162.
19. Hokken-Koelega ACS, De Ridder MAJ, Lemmen RJ, De Muinck Keizer-Schrama SMPF, Drop SLS. Children born small for gestational age: Do they catch up? Pediatr Res 1995;387:267–271.
20. Fitzhardinge PM, Inwood S. Long-term growth in small-for-date children. Acta Paed Scand 1989;349:27–33.
21. Boguszewski M, Rosberg S, Albertsson-Wikland K. Spontaneous 24 hour growth hormone profiles in prepubertal small for gestational age children. J Clin Endocrinol Metab 1995;80:2599–2606.
22. de Waal WJ, Hokken-Koelega AC, Stijnen T, de Muinck Keizer-Schrama SM, Drop SL. Endogenous and stimulated GH secretion, urinary GH excretion, and plasma IGF-I and IGF-II levels in prepubertal children with short stature after intrauterine growth retardation. The Dutch Working Group on Growth Hormone. Clin Endocrinol (Oxf) 1994;41(5):621–630.

23. Frank GR, Cheung PT, Horn JA, Alfaro MP, Smith EP, Chernausek SD. Predicting the response to growth hormone in patients with intrauterine growth retardation. Clin Endocrinol 1996;44:679–685.
24. Hindmarsh PC, Smith PJ, Pringle PJ, Brook CGD. The relationship between the response to growth hormone therapy and pre-treatment growth hormon secretory status. Clin Endocrinol 1988;28:559–563.
25. Boguszewski M, Albertsson-Wikland K, Aronsson S, Gustafsson J, Hagenas L, Westgren U, et al. Growth hormone treatment of short children born small-for-gestational- age: the Nordic Multicentre Trial. Acta Paediatr 1998;87(3):257–63.
26. Azcona C, Albanese A, Bareille P, Stanhope R. Growth hormone treatment in growth hormone-sufficient and -insufficient children with intrauterine growth retardation/Russell-Silver syndrome. Horm Res 1998;50(1):22–27.
27. Sas T, de Waal W, Mulder P, et al. Growth hormone treatment in children with short stature born small for gestational age: 5-year results of a randomized, double-blind, dose- response trial. J Clin Endocrinol Metab 1999;84(9):3064–3070.
28. Ranke MB, Guilbaud O, Lindberg A, Cole T. Prediction of the growth response in children with various growth disorders treated with growth hormone: analyses of data from the Kabi Pharmacia international growth study. Acta Paediatr 1993;391(Suppl):82–88.
29. Grunt JA, Enriquez AR, Daughaday WH. Acute and long term responses to hGH in children with idiopathic small-for-dates dwarfism. J Clin Endocrinol Metab 1972;35:157–168.
30. Foley TP Jr, Thompson RG, Shaw M, Baghdassariam A, Nissley SP, Blizzard RM. Growth responses to human growth hormone in patients with intrauterine growth retardation. J Pediatr 1974;84:635–641.
31. Lanes R, Plotnick LP, Lee PA. Sustained effect of human growth hormone therapy on children with intrauterine growth retardation. Pediatrics 1976;63:731–735.
32. Tanner JM, Lejarraga H, Cameron N. The natural history of the Silver-Russell syndrome: a longitudinal study of thirty-nine cases. Pediatr Res 1975;9(8):611–623.
33. Stanhope R, Preece MA, Hamill G. Does growth hormone treatment improve final height attainment in children with short stature and intrauterine growth retardation? Arch Dis Child 1991;66:1180–1183.
34. Rosenfeld RG, Attie KM, Frane J, et al. Growth hormone therapy of Turner syndrome: beneficial effect on adult height. J Pediatr 1998;132:319–324.
35. Hintz RL, Attie KM, Baptista J, Roche A. Effect of growth hormone treatment on adult height of children with idiopathic short stature. Genentech Collaborative Group. N Engl J Med 1999;340(7):502–507.
36. Coutant R, Carel JC, Letrait M, et al. Short stature associated with intrauterine growth retardation: final height of untreated and growth hormone-treated children. J Clin Endocrinol Metab 1998;83(4):1070–1074.
37. de Zegher F, Albertsson-Wikland K, Wollmann HA, et al. Growth hormone treatment of short children born small for gestational age: growth responses with continuous and discontinuous regimens over 6 years. J Clin Endocrinol Metab 2000;85(8):2816–2821.
38. Maneatis T, Baptista J, Connelly K, Blethen S. Growth hormone safety update from the National Cooperative Growth Study. J Pediatr Endocrinol Metab 2000; 2(Suppl 13):1035–1044.
39. Barker DJ. The fetal origins of type 2 diabetes mellitus. Ann Intern Med 1999;130(4 Pt 1):322–324.
40. Hofman PL, Cutfield WS, Robinson EM, et al. Insulin resistance in short children with intrauterine growth retardation. J Clin Endocrinol Metab 1997;82(2):402–406.
41. Sas T, Mulder P, Aanstoot HJ, et al. Carbohydrate metabolism during long-term growth hormone treatment in children with short stature born small for gestational age. Clin Endocrinol (Oxf) 2001;54(2):243–251.
42. Sas T, Mulder P, Hokken-Koelega A. Body composition, blood pressure, and lipid metabolism before and during long-term growth hormone (GH) treatment in children with short stature born small for gestational age either with or without GH deficiency. J Clin Endocrinol Metab 2000;85(10):3786–3792.
43. Consensus guidelines for the diagnosis and treatment of growth hormone (GH) deficiency in childhood and adolescence: summary statement of the GH Research Society. GH Research Society. J Clin Endocrinol Metab 2000;85(11):3990–3993.
44. Anonymous. Consensus guidelines for the diagnosis and treatment of adults with growth hormone deficiency: summary statement of the Growth Hormone Research Society Workshop on Adult Growth Hormone Deficiency. J Clin Endocrinol Metab 1998;83(2):379–381.
45. Shalet SM, Brennan BM, Reddingius RE. Growth hormone therapy and malignancy. Horm Res 1997;48(Suppl 4):29–32.

46. Swerdlow AJ, Reddingius RE, Higgins CD, et al. Growth hormone treatment of children with brain tumors and risk of tumor recurrence. J Clin Endocrinol Metab 2000;85(12):4444–4449.
47. Chan JM, Stampfer MJ, Giovannucci E, et al. Plasma insulin-like growth factor-I and prostate cancer risk: a prospective study. Science 1998;279(5350):563–566.
48. Hankinson SE, Willett WC, Colditz GA, et al. Circulating concentrations of insulin-like growth factor-I and risk of breast cancer. Lancet 1998;351(9113):1393–1396.
49. Khandwala HM, McCutcheon IE, Flyvbjerg A, Friend KE. The effects of insulin-like growth factors on tumorigenesis and neoplastic growth. Endocr Rev 2000;21(3):215–244.
50. Wetterau L, Cohen P. Role of insulin-like growth factor monitoring in optimizing growth hormone therapy. J Pediatr Endocrinol Metab 2000;13(Suppl 6):1371–1376.
51. Vickers MH, Ikenasio BA, Breier BH. IGF-I treatment reduces hyperphagia, obesity, and hypertension in metabolic disorders induced by fetal programming. Endocrinology 2001;142(9):3964–3973.
52. Liu J-P, Baker J, Perkins AS, Robertson EJ, Efstratiadis A. Mice carrying null mutations of the genes encoding insulin-like growth factor I (Igf-1) and the type 1 IGF receptor (Igf1r). Cell 1993;75:59–72.
53. Powell-Braxton L, Hollingshead P, Warburton C, et al. IGF-I is required for normal embryonic growth in mice. Genes Dev 1993;7:2609–2617.
54. DeChiara TM, Efstratiadis A, Robertson EJ. A growth-deficiency phenotype in heterozygous mice carrying an insulin-like growth factor II gene disrupted by targeting. Nature 1990;345:78–80.
55. Baker J, Liu J-P, Robertson EJ, Efstratiadis A. Role of insulin-like growth factors in embryonic and postnatal growth. Cell 1993;75:73–82.
56. Wang Z-Q, Fung MR, Barlow DP, Wagner EF. Regulation of embryonic growth and lysosomal targeting by the imprinted *IGF2/Mpr* gene. Nature 1994;372:464–467.
57. Lau MMH, Stewart CEH, Liu Z, Bhatt H, Rotwein P, Stewart CL. Loss of the imprinted IGF2/cation-independent mannose 6-phosphate receptor results in fetal overgrowth and perinatal lethality. Genes Dev 1994;8:2953–2963.
58. Accili D, Drago J, Lee EJ, et al. Early neonatal death in mice homozygous for a null allele of the insulin receptor gene. Nat Genet 1997;12:106–109.
59. Araki E, Lipes MA, Patti ME, et al. Alternative pathway of insulin signalling in mice with targeted disuption of the IRS-1 gene. Nature 1994;372:186–190.
60. Tamemoto H, Kadowaki T, Tobe K, et al. Insulin resistance and growth retardation in mice lacking insulin receptor substrate-1 [see comments]. Nature 1994;372(6502):182–186.
61. Zhou Y, Xu BC, Maheshwari HG, et al. A mammalian model for Laron syndrome produced by targeted disruption of the mouse growth hormone receptor/binding protein gene (the Laron mouse). Proc Natl Acad Sci USA 1997;94(24):13,215–13,220.
62. Chernausek SD, Breen TJ, Frank GR. Linear growth in response to growth hormone in children with short stature associated with intrauterine growth retardation: the National Cooperative Growth Study experience. J Pediatr 1996;128:S22–27.

5 Growth Suppression by Glucocorticoids

Mechanisms, Clinical Significance, and Treatment Options

David B. Allen, MD

Contents

INTRODUCTION
MECHANISMS OF GROWTH SUPPRESSION BY GLUCOCORTICOIDS
EFFECTS OF INHALED CORTICOSTEROIDS ON GROWTH
TREATMENT OPTIONS FOR GROWTH FAILURE
    IN GC-TREATED CHILDREN
SUMMARY
REFERENCES

INTRODUCTION

Long-term treatment with glucocorticoids (GC) frequently results in growth failure in children. While most disorders requiring such treatment (e.g., organ transplantation, inflammatory bowel disease, rheumatoid diseases, severe asthma) are relatively rare, the expanding use of inhaled GC preparations for treatment of mild-to-moderate asthma has greatly increased the numbers of children chronically exposed to exogenous GC. This chapter reviews the mechanisms of GC effects on growth, current information about effects of inhaled corticosteroids (ICS) on growth of children with asthma, and preliminary investigations into reversal of GC-induced growth failure with human growth hormone (GH) therapy.

MECHANISMS OF GROWTH SUPPRESSION BY GLUCOCORTICOIDS

The pathogenesis of growth suppression by GC involves several steps in the cascade of events leading to linear growth. (Fig. 1; *1*) During childhood, the primary known mediator of epiphyseal growth and maturation is GH. Pulsatile, primarily nocturnal release of pituitary GH occurs under the influence of interwoven hypothalamic stimulation (via growth-hormone-releasing hormone, GHRH) and inhibition (via somatosatin,

From: *Contemporary Endocrinology: Pediatric Endocrinology: A Practical Clinical Guide*
Edited by: S. Radovick and M. H. MacGillivray © Humana Press Inc., Totowa, NJ

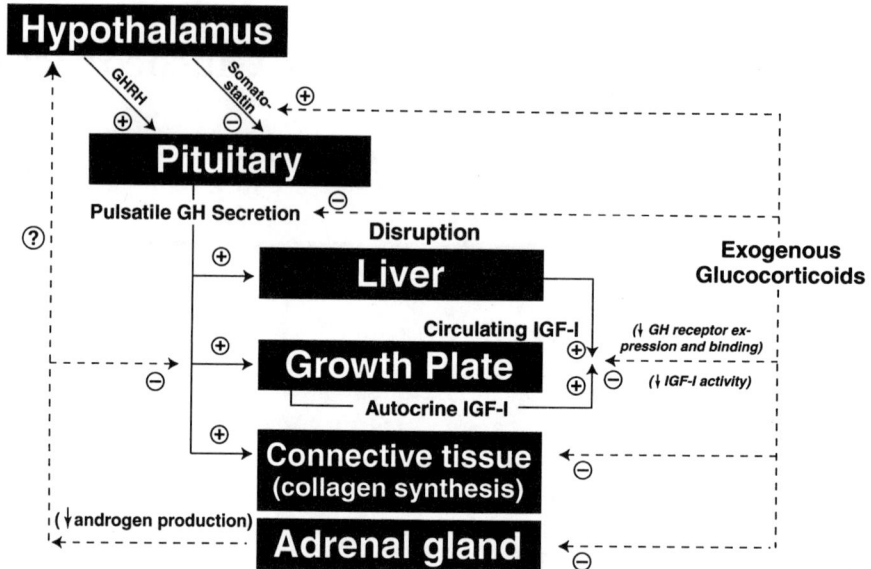

Fig. 1. Mechanisms of linear growth inhibition by glucocorticoids (derived from both in vivo and in vitro studies). Reproduced with permission from *(1)* The Endocrine Society.

SRIF). In late childhood and adolescence, GH secretion is augmented by sex steroids produced by the adrenal glands and gonads. Growth-promoting effects of GH in epiphyseal cartilage are mediated both directly and indirectly through insulin-like-growth-factor 1(IGF-1). Linear growth also requires synthesis of new type 1 collagen.

Glucocorticoids have dichotomous action at the level of the pituitary and hypothalamus. Cortisol facilitates pituitary GH synthesis by altering the affinity and density of pituitary GHRH receptors and interacting with a GC-responsive element on the GH gene *(2)*. Thus, a minimum level of cortisol is essential for normal GH manufacture. On the other hand, GC administration *inhibits* GH release through enhancement of hypothalamic SRIF release *(3)*, possibly due to enhanced beta-adrenergic responsiveness of hypothalamic SRIF neurons *(4)*.

In children with renal transplants, a reverse relationship between daily dose of GC and peak amplitude or mean levels of GH was noted, whereas the GH pulse frequency was not changed. In the clinical setting, this attenuation of GH secretion associated with exposure to exogenous GC can be both rapid and profound *(5)*. In spite of these observations, spontaneous and stimulated GH levels are not invariably low in GC-treated subjects; results vary according to the dose and timing of GC administration and the methodology of GH testing

Glucocorticoids reduce GH receptor expression and uncouple the receptors from their signal transduction mechanisms *(6)*. Hepatic GH receptor binding and plasma levels of GH binding protein (GHBP, derived from the GH receptor) are markedly reduced in dose-dependent fashion by GC treatment, an effect accompanied by growth failure in treated animals *(6)*. Significant reductions in circulating GHBP levels have been reported in GC-treated children compared with age-matched controls *(7)*. While not yet proven, it is likely that these effects on GH receptor synthesis and expression occur in non-liver tissues such as chondrocytes or muscle.

Circulating IGF-1 levels can be decreased, normal, or increased in GC-treated patients. Both IGF-1 mRNA content in liver and other tissues and a GH-induced rise in serum IGF-1 is inhibited by dexamethasone (DEX) *(8)*. IGF-1 *activity* falls precipitously within hours of oral GC administration due to IGF-1 "inhibitors" in serum fractions of molecular weight 12,000–32,000 *(9)* that clearly differ from IGF-binding proteins. In renal allograft and post-liver transplant patients, elevated levels of IGF binding protein-3 (IGFBP-3) are accompanied by normal IGF-1 levels, suggesting reduced bioavailability of IGF-1 *(10,11)*.

Multiple additional effects of GC contribute to the profound impairment in linear growth associated with supraphysiologic GC therapy. Glucocorticoids inhibit chondrocyte mitosis and collagen synthesis within growth plates. Addition of GH to DEX-treated chondrocyte cultures restores proliferation rates to normal *(12)*, suggesting that GH and/or IGF-1 could partially overcome the growth suppressive effects of GC *(13)*. GC interfere directly with post-translational modifications of the precursor procollagen chains and increase collagen degradation. In children with inflammatory bowel disease, type I procollagen levels decrease during administration of GC *(14)*. Glucocorticoids also interfere with nitrogen and mineral retention required for the growth process. Under the influence of GC excess, energy derived from protein catabolism is increased and the contribution from lipid oxidation is decreased. Glucocorticoids inhibit bone formation directly through inhibition of osteoblast function, and indirectly, by decreasing sex steroid secretion (in older children and adolescents). They also decrease intestinal calcium absorption (partially reversible with vitamin D therapy), increase urinary calcium excretion, and promote bone resorption due to secondary hyperparathyroidism. Osteopenia is particularly prominent in trabecular bone, such as the vertebrae. Skeletal maturation is delayed by long-term GC therapy, and impaired mineralization can cause delay in bone age maturation in excess of delay of height age advancement *(15)*.

Dose, type of GC preparation, and timing of GC exposure each influence the degree of growth suppression observed. Large amounts of exogenous GC are not required for this adverse effect; relatively modest doses of prednisone (3–5mg/m^2/d) or hydrocortisone (12–15mg/m^2/d) can impair growth, particularly in prepubertal children. Alternate day GC therapy reduces, but does not eliminate, the chances for growth failure *(16,17)*. Children exposed to GC excess just prior to puberty may be particularly susceptible to growth suppression; childhood growth velocity and endogenous GH secretion is often transiently reduced during this period. Suppression of adrenal sex steroid secretion (adrenarche) by exogenous GC at this time may also contribute to slowed growth (Fig. 1).

Effects of GC treatment on final height are difficult to evaluate owing to the inability to distinguish between medication effects from the natural history of the underlying disease. In one study of children with nephrotic syndrome, high-dose GC therapy for >18 mo led to significant loss in height percentiles *(18)*, whereas alternate-day or intermittent GC therapy was not associated with diminished final height *(19)*. Nevertheless, as shown by a recent meta-analysis, chronic treatment with prednisone is highly correlated with a statistically significant reduction in height achieved *(20)*.

EFFECTS OF INHALED CORTICOSTEROIDS ON GROWTH

Inhaled corticosteroid (ICS) administration now represents the most common mode of exposure of children to therapeutic GC. Although physical properties shared by ICS (e.g., rapid inactivation of absorbed drug) increase the ratio of topical anti-inflammatory to systemic activity, questions remain about the systemic effects of ICS. In children, the major controversy regarding ICS use in children is the issue of growth impairment.

Adverse effects from ICS should be anticipated if daily systemic exposure exceeds normal endogenous cortisol production or if the pattern of drug bioavailability significantly disrupts normal diurnal hormonal rhythms. Systemic GC effect reflects not only the amount of ICS absorbed into circulation through airway and intestinal routes, but also the drug's binding affinity and plasma half-life, the volume of distribution, the potency and half-lives of its metabolites, the patient's sensitivity to and metabolism of the medication, and newly described factors such as the duration of GC contact with the cell or the rate of rise in steroid concentration. Consequently, individual risk for adverse effects from ICS varies widely.

Systemic bioavailability of ICS results from a combination of oral (swallowed fraction) and lung components. ICS are absorbed unaltered into the circulation from the pulmonary vasculature, and the amount reaching that site is influenced by delivery vehicle (e.g., deposition of dry powder generally exceeds pressurized metered-dose inhalation) and technique. The bioavailability of swallowed drug varies significantly; beclomethasone dipropionate (BDP), (FLU), and triamcinolone acetonide (TA) 20–22%, BUD 10–15% *(21)* and fluticasone propionate (FP) 1% *(22)*. These differences in inactivation of swallowed drug (which exerts little or no therapeutic effect) appear to be critical in determining a drug's therapeutic effect vs systemic effect profile. Plasma half-lives of most ICS are brief (e.g.,1.5–2 h) primarily owing to extensive first pass hepatic metabolism. Intrapulmonary metabolism of ICS is also variable; BDP differs from other ICS because it is metabolized to potent active metabolites in the lung, which prolong the half-life of "BDP-effect" (~15 h) and account for most of the systemic GC effect of inhaled BDP *(23)*.

Properties which make ICS extremely potent might increase risk for adverse effects as well. Two such factors are relative binding affinity for the glucocorticoid receptor compared with DEX (e.g., 8:1 for racemic BUD and 20:1 for FP) and increased fat solubility (i.e., lipophilicity) The ranked order of lipophilicity among currently used ICS is FP > BDP > BUD > TA > FLU, with FP being 3-fold and 300-fold more lipophilic than BDP and BUD, respectively *(24)*. Receptor pharmacokinetics and lipophilicity roughly predict differences in clinical drug potency: e.g., when compared µg to µg, FP is approximately 2–3 times as potent as BDP. However, precise comparisons of different ICS are confounded by complexities of determining the *clinical therapeutic* equivalence of each compound and its delivery system. For instance, BUD delivered by metered-dose inhaler approximates BDP in potency, while delivery of BUD by dry powder inhaler may compare µg-for-µg in GC effect with FP, presumably due to greater lung deposition of the drug *(25)*.

Do ICS impair growth? A critical analysis of this question is complicated by two central factors: first, children with chronic asthma frequently exhibit growth retardation, primarily in proportion to severity of pulmonary disease *(26)*. Second, substantial differences exist between specific ICS, and results obtained by studying one should not be extrapolated to another. Until recently, most studies of growth in asthmatic children treated with ICS have suffered from flaws in study design. These include lack of evaluation of pubertal status, inappropriate stratification of pubertal status by age alone, lack of an adequate untreated control group, lack of baseline growth rate data, and baseline differences in age and height between treatment groups. However, during the past several years, prospective and, in some cases, well-controlled studies have overcome these confounding factors.

During the last 10 yr, 4 consecutive studies have demonstrated annual growth reductions of ~1.5 cm/yr in pre-pubertal children treated with 400 µg/d of BDP compared with children treated with theophylline *(27)*, placebo *(28,29)*, or salmeterol *(29,30)*. Thus, it has been clearly shown that conventional dose treatment with inhaled BDP, administered without interruption, is *capable* of suppressing linear growth. On the other hand, asthma exacerbations are increased and quality of life measures are decreased in the absence of ICS therapy *(29)*.

The question arises whether this effect on growth is peculiar to BDP or consistently observed with other ICS preparations. ICS which have greater first-pass inactivation by the liver (e.g., BUD and FP) would theoretically be expected to have reduced effect on the growth axis for a given degree of airway anti-inflammatory effect. One noncontrolled observational study of children treated with BUD for 3–6 yr (mean daily dosage decreased from 710 to 430 µg over the course of the study) showed no significant changes in growth velocity *(31)*. A controlled study of asthmatic adolescents showed that BUD treatment was not associated with a significant effect on growth velocity compared to placebo. Males treated with either BUD or placebo showed similar slowing of growth rates, indicating a likely confounding effect of delayed puberty *(32)*. With regard to FP, a recent double-blind, randomized, parallel-group study of prepubertal children showed no significant difference in one-year mean height increase (6.15 cm in the placebo group, 5.94 cm in the FP 50 µg bid group, and 5.73 cm in the FP 100 µg bid group). Thus, at clinically equivalent dosages, any potential growth effect of FP appeared to be ~25% that associated with BDP *(33)*. Available information regarding effects of ICS on growth derives from studies using low-to-medium doses of ICS. With the exception of anecdotal reports, there is a lack of information regarding the effect of high dose ICS for treatment of severe asthma, on growth rates and final stature.

Other factors, including age and growth pattern of the child, underlying disease severity, and timing of drug administration affect risk of growth suppression by ICS. Susceptibility to growth suppression by a variety of influences appears increased during the 2–3 yr prior to puberty, when growth rates are low and the resiliency of the growth hormone axis is transiently, physiologically low. Most studies of growth effects of ICS have focused on children of this age, so that results cannot confidently be extrapolated to infants or adolescents. Contributions of asthma disease itself can be over- and underestimated. Since children with mild-moderate persistent asthma recruited into recent prospective trials have normal mean heights and skeletal ages for chronological age, it appears that at least moderate-to-severe asthma is required to significantly slow the tempo of childhood growth *(34)*. Finally, selectively eliminating nighttime administration of ICS might also avoid GC-mediated blunting of nocturnal pituitary GH secretion and/or ACTH-induced adrenal androgen production *(35)*. Preliminary studies of treatment of infants and toddlers with BDP 200 µg daily via a metered dose inhaler (MDI) and spacer plus mask (Aerochamber, *36*), or nebulized BUD (1–4 mg/d, *37*) reported no reduction in mean linear growth rates. However, a recent controlled study of children with ages 6 mo to 8 yr treated with BUD inhalation suspension (0.5 mg once or twice daily) revealed a small, statistically significant decrease in growth velocity *(38)*. Potential benefit of early intervention with ICS is supported by one long-term study that showed improvement in lung function was significantly greater in children who started BUD treatment within 2 yr of diagnosis of asthma compared with those who started later *(39)*.

Traditionally, the *clinical relevance* of growth suppression by ICS has been judged more on ultimate effect on final height than short-term reductions in growth rate *(40)*. In two recent retrospective studies, final adult height was not significantly reduced in young adults treated with ICS during (actual mean numeric differences were 1.22 cm *(40)* and 1.4 cm *(41)*, p = NS for both). It could not be determined whether a small difference in *adult height minus target height* (statistically significant in one study) in ICS-treated patients was due to ICS treatment or differences in asthma. A meta-analysis of 21 studies indicated that growth impairment was linked to oral corticosteroid treatment whereas inhaled BDP treatment was associated with reaching normal height *(20)*.

How can recent prospective studies showing growth suppression by inhaled BDP be reconciled with retrospective studies showing minimal or no effect on growth rate or height? One likely explanation stresses the differences between therapeutic efforts to achieve *disease control* vs *symptom control (42)*. Outside clinical trials, most patients reduce drug exposure by titrating medication to control symptoms alone *(43)*. It remains unknown whether long-term administration of ICS at doses sufficient to maintain control of inflammation could affect an asthmatic child's final height. In addition, long-term final height data should be extrapolated with caution to today's children, who are now receiving ICS treatment earlier in life for milder asthma for longer duration and with greater consistency than in the past *(43)*.

Studies cited above suggest the following conclusions regarding the significance and clinical relevance of ICS effects on childhood growth: 1) persistent asthma requires anti-inflammatory treatment, and ICS are the most effective available therapy; 2) detectable slowing of one-year growth in pre-pubertal children can occur with continuous, twice-daily treatment with BDP (400 μg/d); 3) effects of ICS on growth beyond one year of treatment or through adolescence remain unknown; 4) effects of ICS treatment during childhood on adult height appear minimal; 5) in contrast, oral corticosteroid treatment is associated with reduced adult stature; 6) use of ICS with more efficient first-pass hepatic inactivation of swallowed drug reduces risk of growth suppression; 7) risk for growth suppression can be increased when ICS therapy is combined with intranasal or dermal steroid therapy; and 8) titration to the lowest effective dose will minimize an already low risk of growth suppression by ICS.

TREATMENT OPTIONS FOR GROWTH FAILURE IN GC-TREATED CHILDREN

Recognition of GC-induced suppression of GH secretion combined with an unlimited supply of synthetic human GH has renewed interest in the potential reversal of GC-induced growth failure by GH therapy. In 1952, Selye demonstrated in rats that addition of crude bovine GH reversed growth inhibition caused by GC treatment. With increasing doses of GC, larger amounts of GH extract were required to sustain growth *(44)*. More recent animal studies have substantiated a dose-dependent compensation of growth depressing effects of methylprednisolone by GH *(45)*. IGF-1 is also able to partially counterbalance GC-mediated growth retardation *(46)*. Experimental evidence gleaned from rat models of uremia indicate that, while GH receptor expression and

GHBP levels may be reduced under these conditions, GH can still stimulate linear growth and anabolism *(45)*. Further, restoration of normal growth plate architecture *(45)* and increased vertebral and femoral bone mass *(47)* have been reported in GC-treated rats receiving GH. In piglets, DEX-related reductions in plasma osteocalcin, urinary N-telopeptide, and whole body and femoral mineral density could be prevented by concomitant treatment with GH *(48)*.

In slow-growing children with rheumatic diseases, asthma, and inflammatory bowel disease, GH therapy has been investigated to a limited degree. Early treatment efforts using relatively low-dose, thrice weekly, pituitary-derived GH revealed either insignificant growth velocity increments or acceleration in growth rate coincident with fluctuations in disease activity and GC dosage *(49,50)*. Subsequently, preliminary investigations of daily, conventional dose (0.3 mg/kg/wk) recombinant human GH therapy, in which GC dosages remained relatively constant, showed a return to normal growth rates in treated children over a 12–24 mo period. Markers of collagen synthesis were also increased by GH treatment *(51)*. As expected, persistence of disease activity and higher GC dosage (e.g., prednisone dose >0.35 mg/kg/d) *(52)* interfere with GH-responsiveness.

Recent analysis of larger numbers of GC-dependent children ($n = 83$) followed over a 12-mo period reveal a mean response to GH therapy (mean dose = 0.3 mg/kg/wk) of doubling of baseline growth rate (e.g., 3.0 ± 1.2 cm/yr to 6.3 ± 2.6 cm/yr) (Fig. 2, *53*) Responsiveness to GH was negatively correlated with the dose of GC. In a recent study of 14 severely growth-impaired children with rheumatoid arthritis (mean height SDS = –4.0, GH administered at a dose of 0.5 mg/kg/wk resulted in an increase in mean growth velocity from 1.9–4.5 cm/yr. Awareness of the fact that, *without intervention*, height SDS and predicted final adult height *continue to decline* with time in many GC-treated children, is important to an appropriate interpretation of results. While difficult to prove, *preservation of height SDS* most likely represents a beneficial therapeutic outcome. Long-term GH-responsiveness and effects of GH therapy on final height in these children remain unknown.

Several studies have reported a salutary effect of GH therapy (0.05 mg/kg/d administered daily) on the growth of children following renal transplantation, most of whom are treated with relatively low doses of GC (5–10 mg/d or 0.1–0.2 mg/kg/d of prednisone) and have stable allograft function *(54,55)*. Growth rates of prepubertal posttransplant children have generally increased two-to-three fold during the first 1–2 yr of GH therapy, decline subsequently but remain above baseline growth velocity *(56)*. Gains in height standard deviation (SD) scores approximate 1 SD following 2–4 yr of therapy, and approximately one-half of the children achieve "normal" heights (i.e., within 2 SD of the mean, *57*). Bone maturation tends to parallel chronological age *(58)*. IGF-1 levels are not particularly low in children with renal allografts; however, increases in IGF-1 levels which exceed changes in IGF-BP3 levels suggest greater bioavailability of IGF-1 during GH treatment *(59)*. Growth stimulation in pubertal children with renal allografts, while less consistent than that observed in younger patients, is still significant *(60)*.

In addition to restoring linear growth, GH therapy may counter some of the catabolic effects of GC. Studies using isotope tracer infusions have shown that the increased proteolysis and leucine oxidation caused by prednisone could be abolished by treatment with high doses of human GH *(61)*. Subsequent observations suggest that GH, directly or through IGF-1, counteracts GC-induced protein catabolism through independent stimulation of protein synthesis without altering protein breakdown *(62)*. Alternatively,

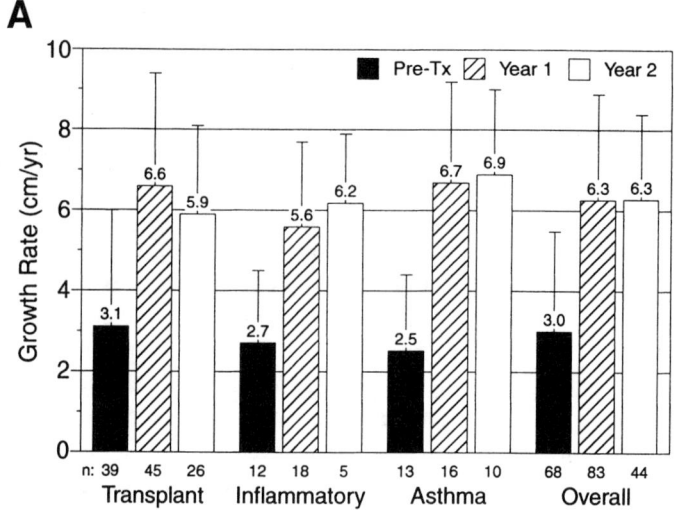
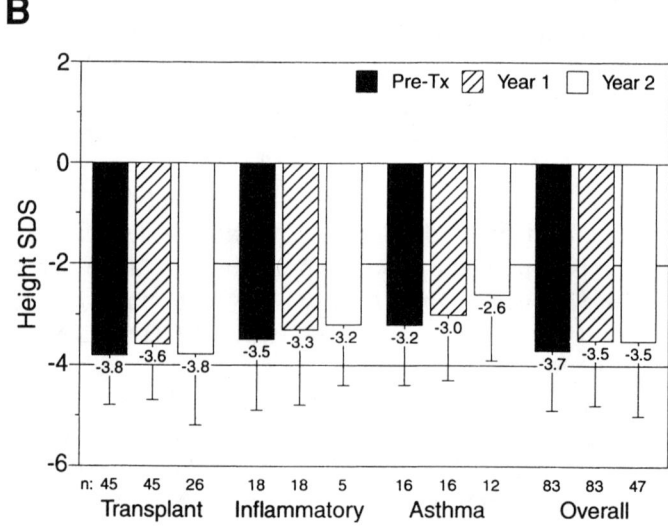

Fig. 2. A. Effect of GH and GC therapy on growth rate (mean ± SD) after 1 and 2 yr of treatment. Results are grouped by the therapeutic indication for GC therapy. B. Effect of GH and GC therapy on height SD score (mean ± SD) after 1 and 2 yr of treatment. Results are grouped by the therapeutic indication for GC therapy. Reproduced with permission from *(1)* The Endocrine Society.

accompanying hyperinsulinemia might contribute substantially to the observed protein anabolic effect by decreasing proteolysis *(63)*. Interestingly, twice daily injections of recombinant IGF-1, which also abolish GC-induced increases in proteolysis and reduce leucine oxidation in prednisone-treated individuals, do not elevate plasma glucose concentrations and actually reduce circulating insulin levels *(64)*. GH may also counteract the anti-anabolic effects of GC on bone. In a group of adults receiving chronic GC treatment, in whom GHRH-stimulated GH levels were suppressed, levels of osteocalcin and carboxy-terminal propeptide of type I procollagen rose with short term GH therapy *(65)*. Detailed studies of the metabolic effects of GH administration in children receiving long-term GC therapy have not yet been done.

Potential adverse effects of combined GH/GC therapy in children with GC-dependent disorders include altered carbohydrate metabolism, stimulation of autoimmune disease activity, increased cancer risk, and, in transplant recipients, graft dysfunction or rejection. Elevated fasting and stimulated insulin levels have been observed in renal allograft patients receiving GH; however, these changes frequently predate institution of GH therapy, correlate with prednisone dosage, and are not affected by the addition of GH *(66)*. Among all GH-treated GC-dependent children, detectable elevations in blood glucose concentrations have been rare. GH-induced exacerbations of chronic disease activity also appear to be very unusual, but the number of patient-years available for study of this question remains small.

With regard to renal allograft function and survival, there are theoretical reasons for concern. GH, through the action of IGF-1, affects glomerular hemodynamics and increases GFR *(67)*. In partially nephrectomized rats, prolonged GH administration is associated with the development of glomerulosclerosis *(68)*. In addition, the immunostimulatory effects of GH might reduce the effect of immunosuppression *(69)*. Nevertheless, most investigators report no difference between GH-treated and control renal allograft patients with regard to changes in glomerular filtration rate (GFR), effective plasma flow, other measures of renal function, and rates of allograft rejection *(58,60,70)*. Although preliminary analysis of one randomized prospective study suggested that GH might slightly increase allograft rejection rates *(71)*, final analysis indicated that biopsy-proven acute rejection episodes were not significantly more frequent in the group receiving GH *(72)*. Long-term and careful follow-up of children with renal transplants receiving GH therapy is still needed to resolve this important issue.

SUMMARY

Glucocorticoids exert multiple growth suppressing effects, interfering with endocrine (e.g., endogenous GH secretion) and metabolic (e.g., bone formation, nitrogen retention, collagen formation) processes essential for normal growth. Relatively small oral doses of daily exogenous GC, alternate-day oral GC therapy, and even inhaled GC are capable of slowing growth in some children. Treatment of asthma with ICS represents, by far, the most common therapeutic use of GC today. While systemic effects of these preparations are greatly reduced compared with oral GC treatment, suppression of growth can still occur when higher doses of ICS are used. Reduction of ICS dose to the lowest effective dose, selection of ICS preparations with minimal bioavailability of swallowed drug, and monitoring of growth of ICS-treated children is recommended.

Growth-inhibiting and catabolic effects of GC can be variably counterbalanced by GH therapy. With regard to linear growth, GH-responsiveness depends on the GC dose and severity of underlying GC-dependent disease. Short-term risks of combined GH and GC therapy appear low; longer term risks (e.g., reduced allograft function and/or survival, increased underlying disease activity, oncologic risk) require further study. GH therapy in GC-dependent children remains experimental; children considered for such treatment should be enrolled in studies that facilitate careful monitoring and collective data analysis.

REFERENCES

1. Allen DB, Julius JR, Breen TJ, Attie KM. Treatment of glucocorticoid-induced growth suppression with growth hormone. J Clin Endocrinol Metab 1998;83:2824–2829.

2. Moore DD, Marks AR, Buckley DI, Kapler G, Payvar F, Goodman HM. The first intron of the human growth hormone gene contains a binding site for clucocorticoid receptor. Proc Natl Acad Sci USA 1985;82:699–702.
3. Wehrenberg WB, Janowski BA, Piering AW, Culler PF, Jones KL. Glucocorticoids: potent inhibitors and stimulators of growth hormone secretion. Endocrinology 1990;126:3200–3203.
4. Miell JP, Corder R, Pralong FP, Gallard RC. Effects of dexamethasone on GHRH, arginine, and dopaminergic stimulated GH secretion and total plasma IGF-I concentrations in normal male volunteers. J Clin Endocrinol Metab 1991;72:675–681.
5. Kaufmann S, Jones KL, Wehrenberg WB, Culler FL. Inhibition by prednisone of growth hormone (GH) response to GH-releasing hormone in normal men. J Clin Endocrinol Metab 1988;67:1258–1261.
6. Gabrielsson BG, Carmignac DF, Flavell DM, Robinson ICAF. Steroid regulation of growth hormone (GH) receptor and GH-binding protein messenger ribonucleic acids in the rat. Endocrinology 1995;136:209–217.
7. Tonshoff B, Mehls O. In: Tejani AH, Fine RN, editors. Pediatric Renal Transplantation. John Wiley & Sons, New York, NY: 1994, pp. 441–459.
8. Luo J, Reid R, Murphy L. Dexamethasone increases hepatic insulin-like growth factor binding protein-1 (IGFBP-1) mRNA and serum IGFBP-1 concentrations in the rat. Endocrinology 2000;125:165–171.
9. Unterman TG, Phillips LS. Glucocorticoid effects on somatomedins and somatomedin inhibitors. J Clin Endocrinol Metab 1985;61:618–626.
10. Hokken-Koelega ACS, Stijnen T, deMuinckKeizer-Schrama SMPF, Blum WF, Drop SLS. Levels of growth hormone, insulin-like growth factor I (IGF-I) and -II, IGF binding protein-1 and -3, and cortisol in prednisone-treated children with growth retardation after renal transplantation. J Clin Endocrinol Metab 1993;77:932–938.
11. Sarna S, Sipila I, Vihervuori E, Koistinen R, Holmberg C. Growth delay after liver transplantation in childhood: studies of underlying mechanisms. Pediatr Res 1995;38:366–372.
12. Jux C, Leiber K, Hugel U, et al. Dexamethasone impairs growth hormone (GH)-stimulated growth by suppression of local insulin-like growth factor (IGF)-I production and expression of GH- and IGF-I-receptor in cultured rat chondrocytes. Endocrinology 2000;139:3296–3305.
13. Robinson ICAF, Gabrielsson B, Klaus B, Mauras N, Holmberg C, Mehls O. Glucocorticoids and growth problems. Acta Paediatr 1995;411:81–86.
14. Hyams JS, Moore RE, Leichtner AM, Carey DE, Goldberg BD. Relationship of type I procollagen to corticosteroid therapy in children with inflammatory bowel disease. J Pediatr 1988;112:893–898.
15. Morris HG. Growth and skeletal maturation in asthmatic children: effect of corticosteroid treatment. Pediatr Res 1975;9:579–583.
16. Sadeghi-Nelad A, Semor B. Adrenal function, growth, and insulin in patients treated with corticoids on alternate days. Pediatrics 1969;43:277–283.
17. Reimer LG, Morris HG, Ellis EE. Growth of asthmatic children during treatment with alternate-day steroids. J Allergy Clin Immunol 1975;55:224–231.
18. Lam CN, Arneil GC. Long-term dwarfing effects of corticosteroid treatment for childhood nephrosis. Arch Dis Child 1968;43:589–594.
19. Foote KD, Brocklebank JT, Meadow SR. Height attainment in children with steroid responsive nephrotic syndrome. Lancet 1985;2:917–976.
20. Allen DB, Mullen M, Mullen B. A meta-analysis of the effects of oral and inhaled glucocorticoids on growth. J Allergy Clin Immunol 1994;93:967–976.
21. Ryrfeldt A, Edsbacker S, Pouwles R. Kinetics of epimeric glucocorticoid budesonide. Clin Pharmacol Therapeut 1984;35:525–530.
22. Harding SM. The human pharmacology of fluticasone propionate. Respir Med 1990;84(Suppl A):25–29.
23. Johansson SA, Andersson KE, Brattsand R. Topical and systemic glucocorticoid potencies of budesonide and beclomethasone dipropionate in man. Eur J Clin Pharmacol 1982;22:523.
24. Johnson M. Pharmacokinetics and pharmacodynamics of inhaled glucocorticoids. J Clin Allergy Immunol 1996;98:169–176.
25. Agertoft L, Pedersen S. A randomized, double-blind dose reduction study to compare the minimal effective dose of budesonide Turbuhaler and fluticasone propionate Diskhaler. J Allergy Clin Immunol 1997;99(6):773–780.

26. Ninan T, Russell G. Asthma, inhaled corticosteroid treatment, and growth. Arch Dis Child 1992;67:703–705.
27. Tinkelman DG, Reed CE, Nelson HS, Offord KP. Aerosol beclomethasone dipropionate compared with theophylline as primary treatment of chronic mild to moderately severe asthma in children. Pediatrics 1993;92:64–77.
28. Doull IJM, Freezer NJ, Holgate ST. Growth of prepubertal children with mild asthma treated with inhaled beclomethasone dipropionate. Am J Respir Crit Care Med 1995;151:1715–1719.
29. Simons FER. A comparison of beclomethasone, salmeterol, and placebo in children with asthma. N Engl J Med 1997;337:1659–1665.
30. Verberne AAPH, Frost C, DipStat MA, Roorda RJ, van der Laag H, Kerribijn KF. One year treatment with salmeterol compared to beclomethasone in children with asthma. Am J Resp Crit Care Med 1997;156:688–695.
31. Agertoft L, Pederson S. Effects of long-term treatment with an inhaled corticosteroid on growth and pulmonary function in asthmatic children. Respiratory Med 1994;88:373–381.
32. Merkus PJFM, VanEssenZandvliet EEM, Duiverman EJ, VanHouwelingen HC, Kerrebijn KF. Long term effect of inhaled corticosteroids on growth rate in adolescents with asthma. Pediatrics 1993;91:1121–1126.
33. Allen DB, Bronsky EA, LaForce CF, et al. Growth in asthmatic children treated with fluticasone propionate. J Pediatr 1998;132:472–477.
34. Martin AJ, Landau LI, Phelan PD. The effect on growth of childhood asthma. Acta Paediatr Scand 1981;70:683–688.
35. Allen DB. Systemic effects of intranasal steroids: an endocrinologist's perspective. J Clin Allergy Immunol 2000;106(Suppl 4):S179–S190.
36. Teper AM, Kofman CD, Maffey AF, Vidaurreta S, Bergadi I, Heinrich J. Effect of inhaled beclomethasone dipropionate on pulmonary function, bronchial reactivity and longitudinal growth in infants with bronchial asthma. Asthma 1995;95:13–13.
37. Reid A, Murphy C, Steen HJ, McGovern V, Shields MD. Linear growth of very young asthmatic children treated with high-dose nebulized budesonide. Acta Paediatr 1996;85:421–424.
38. Skoner DP, Szefler SJ, Welch M, Walton-Bowen K, Cruz-Rivera M, Smith JA. Longitudinal growth in infants and young children treated with budesonide inhalation suspension for persistent asthma. J Allergy Clin Immunol 2000;105:259–268.
39. Pedersen S, Warner JO, Price JF. Early use of inhaled steroids in children with asthma. Clin Exper Allergy 1997;27:995–1006.
40. Silverstein MD, Yunginger JW, Reed CE, et al. Attained adult height after childhood asthma: Effect of glucocorticoid therapy. J Allergy Clin Immunol 1997;99:466–474.
41. Van Bever HP, Desager KN, Lijssens N, Weyler JJ, Du Caju MVL. Does treatment of asthmatic children with inhaled corticosteroids affect their adult height? Pediatr Pulmonol 1999;27:369–375.
42. Lemanske RF, Allen DB. Choosing a long-term controller medication in childhood asthma: the proverbial two-edged sword. Am J Respir Crit Care Med 1997;156:685–687.
43. Milgrom H, Bender B, Ackerson L, Bowry P, Smith B, Rand C. Noncompliance and treatment failure in children with asthma. J Allergy Clin Immunol 1996;98:1051–1057.
44. Selye H. Prevention of cortisone overdosage effects with the somatotropic hormone (STH). Am J Physiol 1952;171:381–384.
45. Kovacs G, Fine RN, Worgall S. Growth hormone prevents steroid-induced growth depression in health and uremia. Kidney Int 1991;40:1032–1040.
46. Tomas FM, Knowles SE, Owens PC. Insulin like growth factor I (IGF-I) variants are anabolic in dexamethasone treated rats. Biochemistry 1992;282:91–97.
47. Ortoft G, Gronbaek H, Oxlund H. Growth hormone administration can improve growth in glucocorticoid- injected rats without affecting the lymphocytopenic effect of the glucocorticoid. J Bone Mineral Res 1999;14:710–721.
48. Ward WE, Atkinson SA. Growth hormone and insulin-like growth factor-I therapy promote protein deposition and growth in dexamethasone-treated piglets. J Pediatr Gastroenterol Nutr 1999;28:404–410.
49. Morris HG, Jorgensen JR, Elrick H, Goldsmith RE, Subryan VL. Metabolic effects of human growth hormone in corticosteroid-treated children. J Clin Invest 1968;47:436–451.
50. McCaffery TD, Nasr K, Lawrence AM, Kirsner JB. Effect of administered human growth hormone on growth retardation in inflammatory bowel disease. Dig Dis 1974;19:411–416.

51. Allen DB, Goldberg BD. Stimulation of collagen synthesis and linear growth by growth hormone in glucocorticoid-treated children. Pediatrics 1992;89:416–421.
52. Rivkees SA, Danon M, Herrin J. Prednisone dose limitation of growth hormone treatment of steroid-induced growth failure. J Pediatr 1994;125:322–325.
53. Allen DB, Julius JR, Breen TJ, Attie KM. Reversal of glucocorticoid-induced growth failure by human growth hormone. Pediatr Res 1996;39:84A.
54. VanDop C, Jabs KL, Donohoue PA, Bock GH, Fivush BA, Harmon WE. Accelerated growth rates in children treated with growth hormone after renal transplantation. J Pediatr 1992;120:244–250.
55. Maxwell H, Dalton RN, Nair DR, et al. Effects of recombinant human growth hormone on renal function in children with renal transplants. J Pediatr 1996;128:177–183.
56. Hokken-Koelega ACS, VanZaal MAE, deRidder MAJ, et al. Growth after renal transplantation in prepubertal children impact of various treatment modalities. Pediatr Res 1994;35:367–371.
57. Fine RN, Sullivan EK, Kuntze J, Blethen S, Kohaut E. The impact of recombinant human growth hormone treatment during chronic renal insufficiency on renal transplant recipients. J Pediatr 2000;136:376–382.
58. Tonshoff B, Haffner D, Mehls O. Efficacy and safety of growth hormone treatment in short children with renal allografts. Kidney Int 1993;44:199–207.
59. Mehls O, Tonshoff B, Kovacs G. Interaction between glucocorticoids and growth hormone. Acta Pediatr Suppl 1993;388:77–82.
60. Hokken-Koelega ACS, Stijnen T, deRidder MAJ, et al. Growth hormone treatment in growth-retarded adolescents after renal transplant. Lancet 1994;343:1313–1317.
61. Horber FF, Haymond MW. Human growth hormone prevents the protein catabolic side effects of prednisone in humans. J Clin Invest 1990;86:265–272.
62. Bennet WM, Haymond MW. Growth hormone and lean tissue catabolism during long-term glucocorticoid treatment. Clin Endocrinol 1992;36:161–164.
63. Fukagawa NK, Minaker KL, Rowe W. Insulin-mediated reduction of whole body protein breakdown dose-response effects on leucine metabolism in postabsorptive man. J Clin Invest 1985;76:2306–2311.
64. Mauras N, Beaufrere B. rhIGF-I enhances whole body protein anabolism and significantly diminishes the protein catabolic effects of prednisone in humans without a diabetogenic effect. J Clin Endocrinol Metab 1995;80:869–874.
65. Guistina A, Bussie AR, Jacobello C, Wehrenberg WB. Effects of recombinant human growth hormone (GH) on bone and intermediary metabolism in patients receiving chronic glucocorticoid treatment with suppressed endogenous GH response to GH-releasing hormone. J Clin Endocrinol Metab 1995;80:122–129.
66. VanDop C, Donohoue PW, Jabs KL, Bock GH, Fivush BA, Harmon WE. Glucose tolerance in children with renal allografts and effect of growth hormone treatment. J Pediatr 1991;118:708–714.
67. Hirschberg R, Kopple JD, Blantz RC, Tucker BJ. Effects of recombinant human insulin-like growth factor I on glomerular dynamics in the rat. J Clin Invest 1991;87:1200–1206.
68. Allen DB, El-Hayek R, Friedman AL. Effects of prolonged growth hormone administration on growth, renal function, and renal histology in 75% nephrectomized rats. Pediatr Res 1996;31:406–410.
69. Manredi R, Tumietto F, Azzaroli L. Growth hormone (GH) and the immune system impaired phagocytic function in children with idiopathic GH deficiency is corrected by treatment with biosynthetic GH. J Pediatr Endocrinol 1994;7:245–251.
70. Johansson G, Sietnieks A, Janssens F. Recombinant human growth hormone treatment in short children with chronic renal disease, before transplantation or with functioning renal transplants: an interim report on five European studies. Acta Paediatr Scand 1990;370(Suppl):36–42.
71. Broyer M, Guest G, Crosnier H, Berard E. Recombinant growth hormone in children after renal transplantation. Lancet 1994;343:539–540.
72. Guest G, Berard E, Crosnier H, Chevallier T, Rappaport R, Broyer M. Effects of growth hormone in short children after renal transplantation. Pediatr Nephrol 1998;12:437–446.

6 Growth Hormone Therapy in Prader-Willi Syndrome

Aaron L. Carrel, MD and David B. Allen, MD

CONTENTS

    INTRODUCTION
    LINEAR GROWTH IN PWS
    BODY COMPOSITION IN PWS
    EFFECTS OF GH TREATMENT ON LINEAR GROWTH
    EFFECTS OF GH ON BODY COMPOSITION
    EFFECTS OF GH ON MUSCLE STRENGTH AND AGILITY
    SAFETY OF GH TREATMENT IN PWS
    ACKNOWLEDGMENTS
    REFERENCES

INTRODUCTION

Prader-Willi syndrome (PWS), initially described in 1956, is now known to be caused by a deletion of the paternal allele in position 15q11–13 (~70% of patients) or a uniparental (maternal) disomy, affecting the same region or the whole of chromosome 15 *(1)*. Thus, PWS is a manifestation of genomic imprinting; the critical region of chromosome 15 is active only in the paternally inherited chromosome. Affected children are characterized by distinct facies, obesity, hypotonia, short stature, hypogonadism, and behavioral abnormalities *(2)*. With an incidence of 1 in every 12,000 births, PWS is the most common syndromal cause of marked obesity.

Many features of PWS suggest hypothalamic dysfunction, some with endocrine implications including: hyperphagia, sleep disorders, deficient growth hormone (GH) secretion, and hypogonadism *(3–5)*. This article reviews current knowledge regarding causes of and potential treatments for impaired growth and physical function observed in children with PWS.

From: *Contemporary Endocrinology: Pediatric Endocrinology: A Practical Clinical Guide*
Edited by: S. Radovick and M. H. MacGillivray © Humana Press Inc., Totowa, NJ

LINEAR GROWTH IN PWS

Growth of children with PWS is characterized by moderate intrauterine (average –1 standard deviation score [SDS]) and postnatal growth delay. Usually after age 2 or 3 yr, when caloric intake increases and obesity begins to develop, growth rates become normal. However, catch-up in length/height relationship is less common. The hands and feet of these children tend to be particularly small. Childhood growth rates are close to normal, but lack of normal pubertal growth often results in reduced adult stature (mean 146 cm for adult PWS female, 152 cm for adult PWS male). The slow growth and delayed skeletal maturation observed in some, but not all PWS children contrasts with healthy obese children, in whom growth acceleration and bone age advancement are commonly seen with overnutrition.

Growth impairment in PWS cannot be attributed to any known intrinsic bone or cartilage abnormality. Consequently, attention has focussed on possible defective hypothalamic regulation of the growth process. Growth hormone responses to insulin, arginine, clonidine, L-dopa, or GH releasing hormone (GHRH) are reported to be low-normal or blunted in PWS, as are sleep-induced GH secretion and 24-h integrated GH concentrations *(3,4)*. One study of 54 consecutive patients with PWS revealed GH levels <10 ng/mL following clonidine provocation in all patients (mean peak GH was 1.1 ng/mL) *(5)*.

Interpretation of these results is complicated by the fact that GH secretion is often suppressed in non-GHD obese individuals, and is partially returned toward normal by weight loss *(6,7)*. The reason for this effect of obesity on GH secretion remains unclear, although negative feedback by insulin-like growth factor 1 (IGF-1) levels sustained by a state of over-nutrition has been proposed *(8)*. Nevertheless, substantial evidence supports the existence of a true GH deficient state in PWS. Children with PWS display borderline normal or diminished growth rates, in contrast to normal or accelerated growth typically seen in healthy non-PWS obese children. Elevated levels of insulin, considered a possible cause of growth acceleration, are not comparable in PWS and 'healthy' obese children. Insulin levels are lower in children with PWS than healthy obese children and rise to levels of obese children, suggesting relatively heightened insulin sensitivity compatible with reduced GH secretion *(9)*. It is possible that over-nutrition and hyperinsulinemia in children with PWS ameliorates growth retardation and skeletal maturation delay normally associated with severe GH deficiency, as it does in some children following craniopharyngioma surgery.

Levels of IGF-1 are relatively low in PWS children (mean ~ –1.5 SDS) when compared to normal-weight age-matched children, but not as low as in those with severe GHD *(5)*. This moderation in IGF-1 reduction likely reflects responsiveness of IGF-1 levels to food intake as well as GH secretion *(10)*; thus, moderately reduced IGF-1 levels in obese PWS children suggest underlying GHD. That nutrition-stimulated IGF-1 production is sustaining near-normal growth in children with PWS is supported by the observation that strict caloric restriction curtails growth more severely in PWS patients than in obese children (M Ritzen, unpublished observation).

Finally, even children with PWS with normal weight/height ratios show low GH responses to provocation. While a normal weight/height does not indicate normal body composition in PWS (which could theoretically affect GH secretion), these important

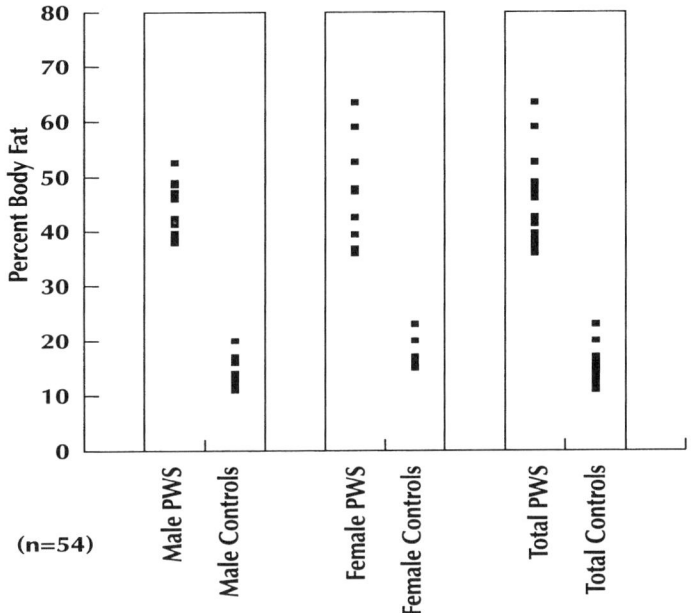

Fig. 1. Body composition in Prader-Willi Syndrome (PWS).

differences in body composition between PWS patients and individuals with "simple" obesity actually constitute the strongest indication of abnormal GH secretion in PWS.

BODY COMPOSITION IN PWS

Infants with PWS are hypotonic and often fail to thrive due to poor sucking and swallowing reflexes. Yet, body fat determined by skinfold measurements is elevated in underweight infants with PWS suggesting early alterations in body composition in the absence of obesity (11). Between the 2nd and 4th yr of life, progressive obesity usually commences primarily as a consequence of excessive caloric intake, but also due to decreased energy expenditure and reduced physical activity. The body composition of childhood PWS patients, illuminated by DXA scanning technology, is characterized by a marked reduction in lean body mass associated with increased fat mass (7,8) (Fig. 1), even in those subjects who appear less obese. Thus, while caloric restriction may minimize weight gain, the ratio between lean body mass and fat remains abnormal. Since resting energy expenditure (REE) is largely determined by the metabolic activity of lean body mass, REE is significantly reduced in individuals with PWS (~60% of predicted caloric utilization for non-PWS individuals with similar body surface area) (12). This extremely low "caloric tolerance" accounts for progressive weight gain in PWS children in whom caloric restriction has been successfully maintained.

The body composition of PWS resembles that of severely growth hormone deficient (GHD) individuals (i.e., reduced lean body mass and increased fat mass, bone mineral density, and energy expenditure) (12). This phenotype is clearly distinguishable from the parallel increase in lean body and fat mass observed in over-nourished obese but otherwise healthy individuals. The distinctive replacement of lean body mass by fat mass in PWS suggests that diminished GH secretion is secondary to hypothalamic dysfunction rather than obesity, and that abnormal body composition and reduced energy expenditure, linear growth, muscle strength, and pulmonary function might be improved in PWS by GH therapy *(11–14)*.

EFFECTS OF GH TREATMENT ON LINEAR GROWTH

Initial studies of the effect of GH treatment of children with PWS syndrome focussed on growth rate acceleration and improvement in stature as primary therapeutic goals. Early reports showing GH treatment increases growth rate in PWS children did not include control subjects and were relatively short term in duration *(13,14)*, and were viewed with skepticism *(15)*. Recent longer-term studies have provided additional evidence supporting a significant and sustained growth response to daily GH administration.

In a controlled study of 54 children with PWS, all of whom displayed subnormal peak GH levels in response to clonidine stimulation (peak GH level 2.0 ng/mL), mean first-year growth rates of GH-treated patients ($n = 35$; GH dose = 1mg/m^2/day, equivalent to 0.18–0.3 mg/kg/wk in the study group) were 10.1 ± 2.5 cm/yr (increase in mean growth velocity SDS from –1.1 to 4.6; $p < 0.001$), significantly greater than $5.0 + 1.8$ cm/yr observed in untreated control patients ($n = 19$). Mean bone age progressed 1.5 yr in the GH-treatment group compared with 1.4 yr in the non-GH-treatment group (p = NS) *(5)*. Over a 24 mo treatment interval, GH-treated subjects ($n = 35$) grew 17.9 ± 2.5 cm (10.1 ± 2.5 cm the first year and 6.8 ± 2.3 cm the second year, corresponding to a mean growth velocity SDS of 4.6 ± 2.9 and 2.2 ± 2.2, respectively ($p < 0.001$ for both years compared to pretreatment GV). Mean bone age progressed only 0.7 yr during the second year in the treatment group. Mean IGF-1 levels in GH-treated subjects were 522 ± 128 ng/mL at 1 year and 415 ± 153 ng/mL at 2 yr ($p < 0.0001$ for both compared to baseline values) *(16)*.

These observations have been confirmed in other studies. In 15 children with PWS, growth rate increased from –1.9 to +6.0 SDS during the first year of GH administration (0.1 IU/kg/d), compared to a decrease from –0.1 to –1.4 SDS in the control group ($n = 12$). For the treatment group, this corresponded to a mean growth rate of ~12 cm/yr, which exceeds that observed in most trials of treatment of children with isolated GHD *(17)*. Another (non-controlled) study of 23 PWS children treated with GH (24 U/m^2/wk) for a median of 3.5 yr showed an increase in mean height SDS of 1.8, and in children <6 yr, height predictions using the method of Bayley and Pinneau approached parental target height. Interestingly, hand length was also normalized by extended GH treatment in prepubertal PWS children *(18)*.

Our studies also adressed the issue of dose-responsiveness with respect to GH effect. We compared 0.3 mg/m^2/d, 1.0 mg/m^2/d, and 1.5 mg/m^2/d. GH-treatment with varied doses resulted in significantly different growth rates. Subjects treated with 0.3 mg/m^2/d grew an average 3.7 ± 1.9 cm/yr, while subjects treated with 1 mg/m^2/d grew 5.3 ± 2.8 cm/yr, and children treated with 1.5 mg/m^2/d grew 6.5 ± 3.1 cm/yr ($p < 0.05$ between each dose; Fig. 2). Mean bone age progressed 1.0 yr regardless of treatment group. Mean IGF-1 varied significantly between the low-dose and standard or high-dose groups, averaging 365 ± 111 ng/mL for the low dose, 567 ± 148 for standard dose, and 580 ± 190 for the high-dose group ($p < 0.05$).

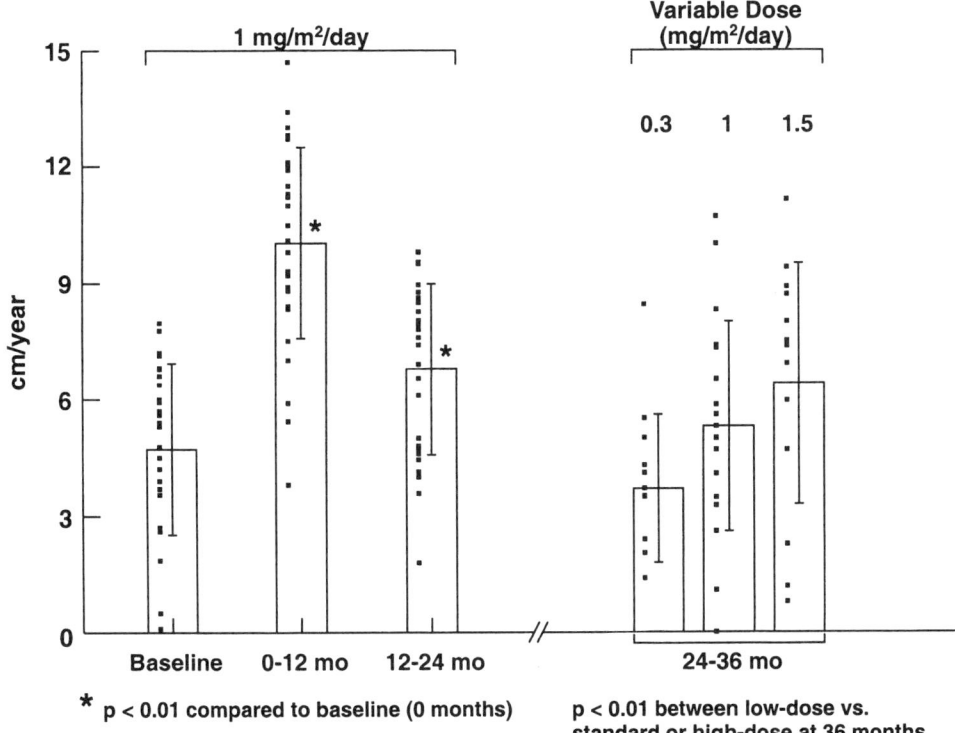

Fig. 2. GH Therapy in PWS: Growth Rate.

EFFECTS OF GH ON BODY COMPOSITION

Administration of exogenous GH to GHD children not only restores linear growth, but also promotes growth of lean body mass (muscle mass), decreases fat mass by increasing fat oxidation and total body energy expenditure, increases bone mineral density following an initial period of increased bone resorption, and improves cardiovascular risk factors *(19)*. Similarly, children with PWS respond to GH therapy with improvements in body composition. Previous uncontrolled short-term GH treatment trials in PWS reported improvements in body composition and muscle endurance and power *(11)*. Recent controlled studies of GH therapy in children with PWS confirm improvements in body composition following 6–12 mo of treatment. Our pretreatment body composition studies of children with PWS (utilizing DXA method) revealed markedly increased percent body fat ($45.2 \pm 8.3\%$ compared to non-PWS healthy children of the same age and sex [$16.7 \pm 3.5\%$]; $p < 0.0001$), even in children without obvious obesity (Fig. 1). Lean body mass was low (20.5 ± 6.1 kg, 50%) compared to normal mean lean body mass of ~80% in age-matched controls. During a period of 12 mo, mean percent body fat decreased by 8% overall ($46.3 + 5.8\%$ to $38.3 + 10.7\%$, $p < 0.01$) in GH-treated children, whereas no change was seen in the non-treated control PWS patients ($42.6 \pm 8.1\%$ to $45.8 \pm 8.8\%$; $p = $ NS). Lean body mass increased with GH treatment (to 25.6 ± 4.3 kg, $p < 0.01$) and remained unchanged in control subjects (21.7 ± 5.0 kg, $p = $ NS) *(5)*. Therapy for

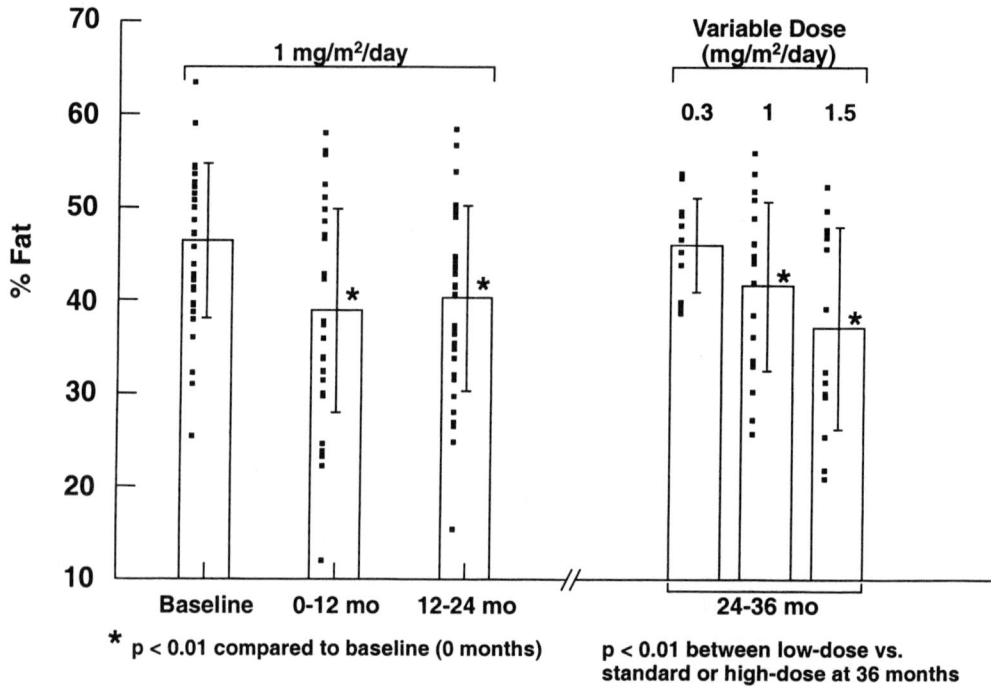

Fig. 3. GH Therapy in PWS: % Body Fat (DEXA).

24 mo of GH resulted in continued significant increases in lean body mass, with sustainment of the adipose loss during the initital 12 mo. Similar body composition changes have been reported in response to 12–24 mo of GH treatment by other investigators (17).

These remarkable changes in body composition attenuate but do not regress during more prolonged GH therapy. Recently reported data shows that, in contrast to marked reductions observed during the first 12 mo of GH treatment, percent body fat remains stable during months 12–24 of GH treatment ($40.3 \pm 10.0\%$, p = NS vs 12 mo measurement; $p < 0.001$ vs baseline); (Fig. 3). Importantly, lean body mass, which increased significantly after 12 mo of GH (25.2 ± 6.9 kg vs 22.9 ± 15.7 kg, $p < 0.01$), increased further during months 12–24. ($28.5 + 7.2$ kg at 24 mo, $0 < 0.01$ compared to 12 mo (Fig. 4). Our data regarding GH treatment, at different doses, resulted in significant differences with respect to body fat: 0.3 mg/m^2/d averaged $46 \pm 5.0\%$ body fat, while 1 mg/m^2/d averaged $41.0 \pm 9.0\%$, and 1.5 mg/m^2/d averaged 37.1 ± 10.9 % body fat ($p < 0.0001$; Fig. 4). In contrast, LBM remained unchanged in the low-dose group at 28.1 ± 8.2 kg, while increased LBM was observed in the 1 mg/m^2/d group (31.4 ± 7.8 kg), and 1.5 mg/m^2/d group (30.8 ± 7.1 kg) ($p = 0.06$; Fig. 4).

Given their reduced lean body mass, children with PWS would be expected to demonstrate markedly reduced REE (21). Prior to GH treatment, children with PWS showed reduced REE compared with predicted values for non-PWS children matched for surface area (22.4 ± 4.4 kcal/m^2/h vs 43.6 ± 3.2 kcal/m^2/h; $p < 0.0001$) (20). We predicted that REE would be increased by GH treatment. While only a trend toward increased REE was observed after 12 mo of GH therapy, changes in REE reached statistical significance after 24 mo compared with their own baseline measurements (16). While it is probable

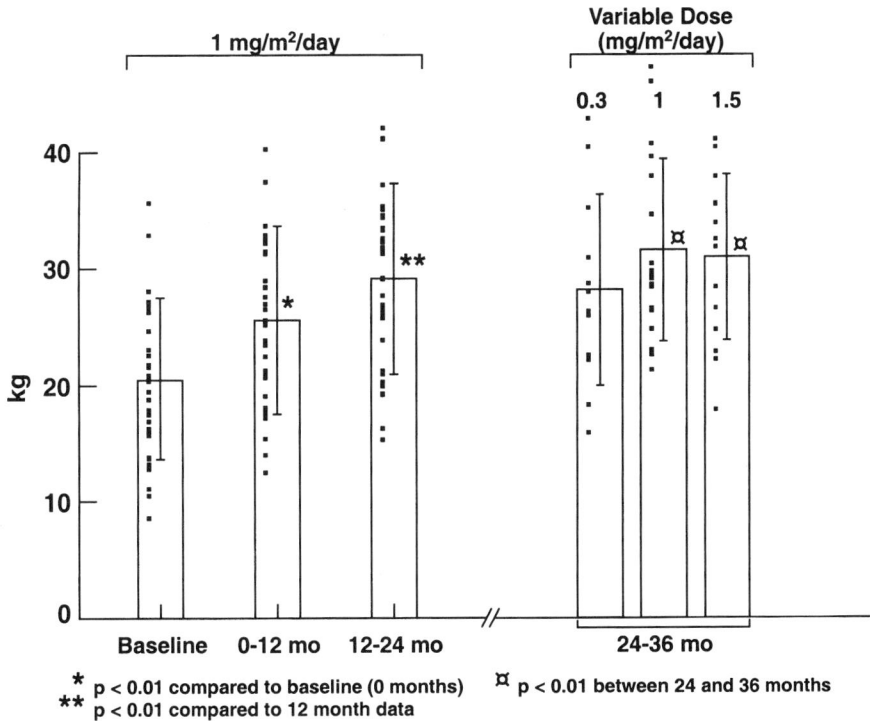

Fig. 4. GH Therapy in PWS: Lean Body Mass (DEXA). GH Therapy in PWS: Agility Run.

that GH effects on lean body mass accretion had positive effects on REE, it should also be noted that REE normally increases as children grow.

Deficiency of GH is associated with lipogenesis and fat storage predominating over the accretion of lean mass, even in the absence of overt obesity. Preference for fat utilization as an energy source is reflected in a reduction of respiratory quotient (RQ). The RQ normally ranges from 0.7 (strong predominance of fatty acid oxidation) to 1.0 (exclusive oxidation of carbohydrate) to <1.0 (indicating lipogenesis from carbohydrate). Two years of GH treatment in PWS children was associated with a decrease in RQ values ($0.81 + 0.07$ at baseline to $0.75 + 0.06$ at 24 mo, $p < 0.05$), indicating increased utilization of fat for energy. Thus, compared with non-GH-treated PWS controls, GH-treated PWS patients demonstrated a shift in energy derived from oxidation of fat, coinciding with reductions in fat mass shown by DXA scanning. Clinically, reduced body fat can be seen, consistent with an increase in fat utilization (Fig. 6).

Baseline total body BMD measurements were within the normal range (i.e., ± 2SD of normal reference data for childhood BMD provided by Lunar Inc, Madison, WI). In GH-treated PWS children, total body BMD increased from 0.89 ± 0.08 g/cm^2 at baseline to 0.92 ± 0.11 g/cm^2 at 12 months ($p < 0.001$) and 0.94 ± 0.11 g/cm^2 ($p < 0.001$) at 24 mo. Osteocalcin and procollagen levels continued to be significantly increased at 24 mo compared to baseline ($p < 0.01$), although lower than 12-mo levels. During months 24–36, no dosage effect was seen between various GH doses with respect to BMD accretion. BMD increased to 0.98 ± 0.09 g/cm^2 in the low- and standard-dose groups, and 0.97 ± 0.11 g/cm^2 in the high-dose group ($p = $ NS).

EFFECTS OF GH ON MUSCLE STRENGTH AND AGILITY

Substantial information is accumulating to support beneficial effects of 12–36 mo of GH therapy on improving body composition and linear growth in children with PWS. However, perhaps of greatest importance to patients and their families is the hope that GH therapy would improve the child's physical strength, activity, and developmental ability. Early reports included anecdotal reports of dramatic gains in physical activity abilities, and many parents of our subjects also claimed striking improvements in physical stamina, strength, and agility. Specifically, these included new gross motor skills (e.g., independently climbing up the school bus steps, carrying a gallon carton of milk at the grocery store, participating in a normal gym class without restrictions, being able to join a karate class).

The authors' research has included objective measures of changes in physical function during GH treatment, including a timed run, sit-ups, and weight lifting. Improvements in running speed, broad jump, sit-ups and arm curls after 12 mo of GH treatment compared to controls were documented *(5)*. Following 24 mo of GH treatment, improvements in broad jumping and sit-ups were maintained, while further improvement was found in running speed and arm curls (Table 1). Measurement of respiratory muscle forces was reliably obtained in a subset of subjects ($n = 20$). Increases in both respiratory muscle forces were seen after one year of therapy and maintained at 24 mo (Table 1)*(20)*. Further, no effect of dosage was noted between the various GH doses. Additionally, strength and agility data at 36 mo were not significantly different at any dose compared to 24 month data, although remained statistically improved from prior to GH therapy (Fig. 5).

In spite of these gains in physical function, PWS children still scored well below 2 SDS compared to non-PWS children for all parameters studied. While the lack of a blinded, placebo-controlled study design admittedly weakens the scientific validity of these findings, they do suggest that measured improvements in strength and agility were associated with "real-life" functional benefit to the children and their families.

SAFETY OF GH TREATMENT IN PWS

No significant adverse side effects have been observed by us or others during 12 *(17)* to 36 mo of GH treatment *(18)*. Specifically, our data indicate that, with regard to the predisposition of PWS children to developing scoliosis, mean change in spine curvature (12–13.8°) in GH-treated children was similar to that observed over 1 yr in the control group. Serum glucose and insulin levels obtained during an OGTT were slightly but nonsignificantly higher than baseline levels during GH treatment. Of aesthetic concern, the lower facial height became disproportionate with an SDS of 1.2 at 24 mo, supporting recent findings of accentuated growth of the high midface during GH therapy in PWS *(20)*. No abnormalities with respect to glucose homeostasis were determined.

Clearly the response of children with PWS to GH is greatest during the first 12 mo with regard to growth rate, decreases in body fat, increases in REE, improvements in physical function, and laboratory alterations in carbohydrate and lipid metabolism. Thus, the well-documented diminution in response to GH observed in virtually all growth studies during prolonged GH therapy appears to apply to other GH metabolic effects in children with PWS. On the other hand, study group regression toward baseline status did not occur during a second year of GH at a dose of $1 \text{ mg/m}^2/\text{d}$, while additional gains in BMD, fat utilization, and tests of muscle strength and agility were seen. In spite of these

Table 1
Strength and Agility Testing in PWS

	Treated Group n = 53			Non-treated Group n = 19	
	Baseline	12 mo	24 mo	Baseline	12 mo
Agility Run (s)	11.1 ± 6.1	9.4 ± 4.4[a,c]	8.9 ± 3.8[b]	10.3 ± 1.8	10.6 ± 0.4
Broad Jump (inch)	20.0 ± 11.1	24.4 ± 11.3[a,c]	26.3 ± 10.2[a]	17.5 ± 3.7	16.5 ± 3.3
Sit-ups (in 20 s)	9.1 ± 4.8	11.5 ± 4.7[a,c]	12.1 ± 4.8[a]	9.1 ± 3.4	9.3 ± 3.1
Weight Lifting (pounds x reps)	59 ± 28	73 ± 33[a,c]	95 ± 44	54 ± 25	64 ± 29
Inspiratory strength (cm/H_2O)	45.8 ± 23	55.7 ± 18.7[c]	60.1 ± 28.3	44.8 ± 13.2	40.4 ± 13.9
Expiratory strength (cm/H_2O)	54.6 ± 23.9	69.4 ± 24.8[c]	62 ± 26.4	58.8 ± 22.1	46 ± 13.3

[a] <0.01 compared to baseline.
[b] <0.01 compared to baseline and 12 mo.
[c] <0.01 compared to 12 mo control values.

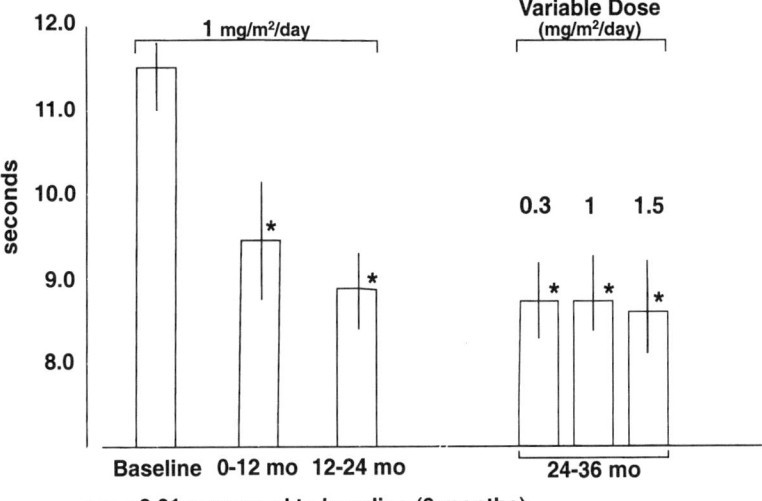

Fig. 5. GH Therapy in PWS: Agility Run.

encouraging results, current knowledge suggests that GH therapy is not capable of "normalizing" body composition in PWS. This could reflect the influence of other non-GH factors regulating body composition affected by the genetic mutation causing PWS and/or the relatively late institution of GH therapy following a critical period of abnormal adipose and muscle deposition in infancy. Future studies of earlier institution of GH therapy are needed to address these possibilities.

While these longer-term results of GH treatment in PWS children are encouraging, a cautious interpretation is still appropriate. Improvements in body composition and physical function, while marked during the first 12 mo of GH treatment, stagnated or slowed

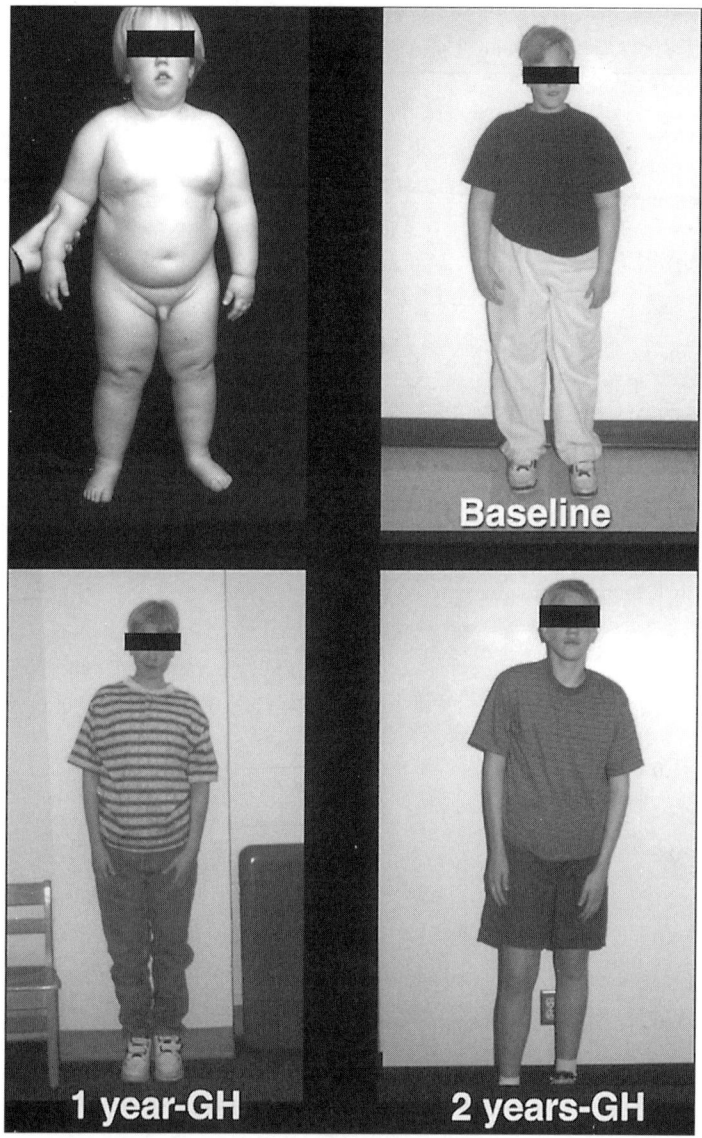

Fig. 6. The effect of two years of GH therapy in a child with Prader-Willi syndrome.

considerably during the second year. Preliminary data suggests that stabilization of fat mass and continued accretion of lean mass and bone mineral occur with three years of GH treatment when doses ≥ 1 mg/m^2/d are used. Still, body composition, while improved, remains significantly abnormal in PWS children following prolonged GH therapy. This observation, coupled with the fact that percent body fat in PWS children exceeds that observed in patients with severe GHD, makes it likely that factors other than deficiency of GH contribute to the accumulation of this extraordinary fat mass. Nevertheless, the work described above supports a possible extended and significant benefit of GH treatment in children with PWS, and provides impetus for further study of this question.

ACKNOWLEDGMENT

We wish to acknowledge the support of the children and their families for their enthusiastic participation in this study, and to the pediatric endocrine nurses and research associates who contributed to this study. This work is supported in part, by NIH Grant M01 RR03186-13S1, to Dr. Carrel, as well as funding from the Genentech Foundation for Growth and Development, and Eli Lilly.

REFERENCES

1. Carrel AL, Huber S, Voelkerding KV. Assessment of SNRPN expression as a molecular tool in the diagnosis of Prader-Willi syndrome. Mol Diagn 1999;4(1):5–10.
2. Prader A, Labhart A, Willi H. Ein syndrom von adipositas, kleinwuchs, kryptorchismus and oligophrenie. Schweiz Med Wochenschr 1956;86:1260–1261.
3. Angulo M, Castro-Magana M, Uy J. Pituitary evaluation and growth hormone treatment in Prader-Willi syndrome. J Pediatr Endocrinol 1991;167–173.
4. Costeff H, Holm VA, Ruvalcaba R, Shaver J. Growth Hormone Secretion in Prader-Willi Syndrome. Acta Paediatr Scand 1990;79:1059–1062.
5. Carrel AL, Myers SE, Whitman BY, Allen DB. Growth hormone improves body composition, fat utilization, physical strength and agility, and growth in Prader-Willi syndrome: A controlled study. J Pediatr 1999;134:215–221.
6. Williams T, Berelowitz M, Joffe SN, et al. Impaired growth hormone response to growth-hormone releasing factor in obesity. N Engl J Med 1984;311:1403–1407.
7. Dieguez C, Page MD, Scanlon MF. Growth hormone neuroregulation and its alterations in disease states. Clin Endocrin 1988;28:109–143.
8. Dieguez C, Casanueva FF. Influence of metabolic substrates and obesity on growth hormone secretion. Trends Endocrinol Metab 1995;6(2):55–59.
9. Ritzen EM, Bolme P, Hall K. Endocrine physiology and therapy in Prader-Willi syndrome. In: Cassidy SB, ed, Prader-Willi Syndrome and Other 15q Deletion Disorders. NATO ASI Series, vol. H61, 1992 Springer-Verlag, Berlin; 153–169.
10. Wabitsch M, Blum WF, Heinze E, et al. Insulin-like growth factors and their binding proteins before and after weight loss and their associations with hormonal and metabolic parameters in obese adolescent girls. Int J Obesity 1996;20:1073–1080.
11. Eilholzer U, Blum WF, Molinari L. Body fat determined by skinfold measurements is elevated despite underweight in infants with Prader-Labhart-Willi syndrome. J Pediatr 1999;134:222–225.
12. Carrel A:, Van Calcar S, Lattin L, Allen DB. Resting Energy Expenditure in children with Prader-Willi syndrome (abstract #P2-495). Proceedings from 1997 Meeting of the Endocrine Society, Minneapolis.
13. Angulo M, Castro-Magana M, Mazur B, Canas JA, Vitollo PM, Sarrantonio M. Growth hormone secretion and effects of growth hormone therapy on growth velocity and weight gain in children with Prader-Willi syndrome. J Pediatr Endocrinol Metab 1996;9:393–400.
14. Lee PDK, Wilson DM, Rountree L, Hintz RL, Rosenfeld RG. Linear growth response to exogenous growth hormone in Prader-Willi syndrome. Am J Med Genet 1987;28:865–867.
15. Connor EL, Rosenbloom A. Effects of growth hormone in Prader-Willi syndrome (editorial). Clin Pediatr 1993;32: 296–298.
16. Allen DB, Carrel AL, Myers S, Whitman B. Sustained benefit of 24 months of GH therapy on body composition, fat utilization, energy expenditure, bone mineral density, and physical strength and agility in children with Prader-Willi syndrome (oral presentation). Endocrine Society 81st meeting 1999, Abstract 035-1, p. 110.
17. Lindgren AC, Hagenas L, Muller J, et al. Growth hormone treatment of children with prader-Willi syndrome affects linear growth and body composition favourably. Acta Paediatr Scand 1998;87:28–31.
18. Eiholzer U. Long-term therapy with growth hormone in children with Prader-Willi syndrome normalizes height, weight and hand length, but not body composition and fat distribution. Horm Metab Res 1999;51;131.
19. Cuneo RC, Judd S, Wallace JD, et al. The Australian multicenter trial of growth hormone (GH) treatment in GH-deficient adults. J Clin Endocrinol Metab 1998;83:107–116.

20. Myers SE, Carrel AL, Whitman B, Allen DB. Sustained benefits after 2 years of growth hormone upon body composition, fat utilization, physical strength and agility, and growth in Prader-Willi syndrome. J Peadiatr 2000;137(1):42–50.
21. van Mil EA, Westerterp KR, Gerver WJ, Curfs LM, schrander-Stumpel CT, Kester AD. Energy expenditure at rest and sleep in children with Prader-Willi syndrome is explained by body composition. Am J Clin Nutr 2000;71:752–756.

7 Turner Syndrome

*Marsha L. Davenport, MD
and Ron G. Rosenfeld, MD*

CONTENTS

> INTRODUCTION
> PATHOGENESIS
> CLINICAL PRESENTATION
> DIAGNOSTIC GUIDELINES
> THERAPY
> REFERENCES

INTRODUCTION

Turner Syndrome (TS) is one of the most common human chromosome anomalies. It occurs in approximately 1:2000 female live births *(1)* regardless of ethnic background. Girls with TS have an abnormal or missing X chromosome that causes short stature and may cause lymphedema, cardiac abnormalities, gonadal dysgenesis, dysmorphic features and other problems *(2,3)*. Approximately 50–60% of girls with TS are reported to have a 45,X karyotype. These girls tend to have the severest phenotype and are frequently diagnosed as newborns *(4,5)*. Twenty to thirty percent ave structural abnormalities of the X chromosome such as rings, isochromosomes of the long arm, and partial deletions of the short arm. Thirty to forty percent have mosaic patterns (karyotypes having two or more distinct cell types) involving the X chromosome such as 45,X/46,XX, 45,X/46,X,i(X) and 45,X/46,XY. This is thought to result from chromosome loss after fertilization *(6)*.

PATHOGENESIS

Haploinsufficiency of X Chromosome Genes

The clinical features of TS appear to be primarily due to: 1) haploinsufficiency of X chromosome genes *(7)* 2) failure of chromosome pairing during germ cell development and 3) aneuploidy *(8)*. In normal females, either the maternal or paternal X chromosome is randomly inactivated in somatic cells during the late blastocyst stage and all descendants of that cell have the same inactive X. However, the X-inactivation process is not complete. Specific genes that have homologues on the Y-chromosome remain active on both X-chromosomes. Many of these "pseudoautosomal" genes, such as *SHOX* (Short Stature Homeobox-containing), are localized to the tip of the short arm of X. *SHOX* is expressed in the developing limbs (particularly at the elbow, knee, and wrist) and the first and second pharyngeal arches which form the maxillary shelves, mandible, auricular ossicles and the external auditory meatus *(9)*. Haploinsufficiency of *SHOX* expression in girls with TS results in short stature as well as developmental abnormalities of specific bones *(10,11)*.

It is likely, however, that haploinsufficiency of *SHOX* does not account for all phenotypic features of TS, and that haploinsufficiency of another pseudoautosomal gene causes maldevelopment of the lymphatics. Absence or hypoplasia of peripheral lymphatics causes generalized lymphedema, and a cystic hygroma may result from delayed connection of the lymphatic system to the jugular vein. It is estimated that >99% of 45,X conceptuses do not survive beyond 28 wk gestation *(12)* because severe lymphatic obstruction causes thoracic, pericardial and peritoneal effusions, and cardiac failure. A webbed neck, low upward sweeping hairline, and lowset prominent ears often result from a resolving cystic hygroma. Lymphedema and nail dysplasia may result from the more peripheral process *(12)*. Structural abnormalities of the heart and vascular system such as coarctation of the aorta and bicuspid aortic valve are much more common in girls with coexistent cystic hygroma or lymphedema, suggesting that dilated lymphatics encroaching on cardiac outflow or disordered intramyocardial lymphatic development may be responsible for their development.

The genes involved in other problems associated with TS such as nonverbal learning disability, metabolic disturbances, and autoimmune diseases have not been identified.

Abnormal Pairing During Meiosis

Gonadal dysgenesis occurs in the vast majority of individuals with TS and is caused by increased atresia of germ cells rather than a deficiency of germ cell formation. The rate of oocyte loss appears to correlate with the degree of pairing failure. Oocyte loss is rapid in X monosomy in which there is a generalized failure of normal meiotic pairing. Another factor contributing to gonadal dysgenesis is that both X chromosomes normally remain active in oocytes (in contrast to one normally being inactivated in somatic cells). Genes on both the short and long arms are important for maintenance of ovarian function, but their identities are unknown *(13)*.

Aneuploidy

Aneuploidy itself and chromosomal imbalance may disturb developmental fields, leading to global developmental defects. This may impair cell proliferation and cause growth retardation *(14)*.

Other Molecular Mechanisms

Other mechanisms that may be involved in the pathogenesis of TS include imprinting, abnormal X-inactivation, and X-linked recessive genes. Imprinting does not appear to play a significant role in gene expression on the X chromosome. For example, physical phenotype and response to GH do not differ in those with a paternal or maternal X *(15)*. Skuse and colleagues have suggested that an imprinted gene is involved in social cognition *(16)*, but these studies have not yet been confirmed *(17)*. Individuals with small ring X-chromosomes often have a severe phenotype that is not typical of TS and includes mental retardation *(18,19)*. In these cases, the loss of the *XIST* gene, which is involved in X-inactivation, may allow for normally inactivated genes to be expressed, thereby causing functional disomy. Finally, X-linked recessive disorders that are typically restricted to males may be seen in girls with TS.

CLINICAL PRESENTATION

Introduction

Clinical presentations vary widely and are responsible in part for the broad range of ages at which the diagnosis of TS is made *(3,20)*. For the majority of those diagnosed in prenatal life, the diagnosis is based upon an abnormal karyotype and/or ultrasound evidence of a cystic hygroma, hydrops fetalis, or cardiac defects. Since the ultrasound abnormalities are not specific for TS, the diagnosis should be confirmed by karyotype. Girls diagnosed during infancy almost invariably have lymphedema with or without a webbed neck and other dysmorphic features. In contrast, girls lacking these classic features are often not diagnosed until late childhood or adolescence when they are investigated for short stature and/or delayed puberty, or as adults when they develop premature ovarian failure *(21)*.

Lymphedema

Virtually all girls diagnosed during infancy have lymphedema secondary to maldevelopment of the lymphatic system. Lymphedema differs from that seen in congestive heart failure. It is most prominent over the metatarsals and metacarpals, with a crease across the wrist and ankle joints. Lymphedema usually improves over the first few months of life but may progress with puberty or hormonal therapy.

Dysmorphic Features

Most girls with TS have one or more dysmorphic features caused by lymphedema and/or skeletal abnormalities. However, the phenotype varies greatly and some girls with TS will have no apparent dysmorphic features. More than half of the girls have a high arched palate and/or retrognathia. Ears are often lowset and posteriorly-rotated with poor helix formation. The hairline tends to be low and upward sweeping, and in the minority, a webbed neck represents redundant skin that once stretched over a cystic hygroma. Ptosis, epicanthal folds, and downward slanting palpebral fissures are common eye findings. Some degree of nail dysplasia is found in three-quarters. Nails tend to be small, narrow, and inserted at an acute angle. Cubitus valgus and short 4th metacarpals are also common. About one-quarter of patients have pectus excavatum and a smaller number have inverted nipples *(3,21)*

Cardiovascular Abnormalities

Some individuals with TS are diagnosed in infancy secondary to cardiac lesions such as coarctation of the aorta or hypoplastic left heart. Aortic obstruction from a coarctation, usually periductal, may be minimal until the ductus arteriosus closes. Congestive heart failure can then develop rapidly. In older children, signs of coarctation generally consist of decreased pulse and blood pressure in the legs compared with the arms, and a systolic murmur heard well over the back.

Cardiac abnormalities in TS are most often left-sided. In one study of 244 individuals with TS, structural abnormalities were found in 40% *(22)*. A coarctation with or without a bicuspid valve was present in 14%, a bicuspid valve alone in 10%, aortic stenosis and/or regurgitation in 5%, and other structural defects such as hypoplastic left heart, ASD and VSD were present in 10%. In another study, partial anomalous pulmonary venous drainage was found in 2.9% of patients, giving it the highest relative risk compared to heart defects in the general population *(23)*. Aortic dissection is a rare but devastating complication of TS that usually occurs in adulthood. Although most cases have been associated with coarctation of the aorta, bicuspid aortic valve, hypertension and/or aortic root dilatation, 10% have had no known risk factors *(24–26)*.

Nonstructural abnormalities such as hypertension, conduction defects or mitral valve prolapse are also more common than in the general population, occurring in approximately 16% *(22)*. In a study of 62 patients with TS, age 5.4–22.4 yr, more than 30% were found to be mildly hypertensive, and over 50% had an abnormal diurnal blood pressure profile. Interestingly, the investigators were unable to correlate the presence of renal or cardiac abnormalities with hypertension, suggesting that other mechanisms are involved *(27)*.

Short Stature and Skeletal Abnormalities

Short stature is the single most common physical abnormality and affects virtually all individuals with TS. Untreated individuals achieve an average adult stature 20 cm shorter than that of their peers, resulting in a height about three standard deviations (SDs) below the mean *(28,29)*. This growth deficit is similar from country to country and the individual scatter around the mean height is not significantly different from that of the normal population *(30)*.

Growth failure is due to 1) mild to moderate growth retardation *in utero*; 2) slow growth during infancy; 3) delayed onset of the childhood component of growth; 4) slow growth during childhood; and 5) failure to experience a pubertal growth spurt *(31–33)*. Girls with TS average –0.5 to –1.2 SDs below the mean for birth weight. Although early cross-sectional studies suggested that growth velocity during the first few years of life is normal *(34)*, it is now clear that growth retardation during this period is relatively profound. In one study in which longitudinal measurements of height were obtained from full-term girls with Turner syndrome without other reasons for growth failure, mean height SDS fell from –0.5 at birth to –1.5 at age 1 yr and –1.8 at age 1.5 yr *(32)*. Using the infancy-childhood-puberty (ICP) model of growth, one can demonstrate that components of growth failure during this period include slow exponential growth during infancy as well as a significant delay in onset of the childhood component of growth *(31–33)*. Poor growth in the first year of life may be exacerbated in some by poor feeding and inadequate weight gain secondary to oral-motor dysfunction *(35)*. The height lost in the infancy and toddler years is not recovered. Growth during childhood is slow, there is no pubertal growth spurt, and growth is often prolonged into the early 20s.

Individuals with TS tend to appear stocky since they have a greater relative reduction in body height than in body width, and are often overweight. The increased relative width to height of the thorax accounts for a shieldlike chest and the illusion of widely spaced nipples. Hands and feet are also relatively large *(36)*. Developmental abnormalities of individual bones are responsible for many common findings such as short neck, cubitus valgus, genu valgum and short 4th metacarpals. The short neck is due in many cases to hypoplasia of one or more cervical vertebrae. Cubitus valgus occurs in almost 50% of patients and is caused by developmental abnormalities of the radial head. About 35–40% of patients has a short or borderline-short 4th metacarpal and many have abnormally acute angulation of their proximal row of carpals. A short 4th metacarpal causes a depression instead of a knuckle when the fist is clenched. Scoliosis develops in 12–20% of patients and although frequently idiopathic, may be associated with coalition of vertebrae or hemivertebrae *(3)*. Scoliosis often occurs in early childhood and may progress with growth spurts, including those induced with GH therapy *(37)*. Kyphosis also appears to be more prevalent (personal observation).

A delayed bone age is found in more than 85% of patients with TS but the degree of delay is not uniform amongst bones. The delay is greatest in the phalangeal bones, intermediate in the carpals and least in the metacarpals, radius and ulna *(38)*.

Osteoporosis and fractures are more frequent among women with TS *(39)*. Many girls have radiographic osteopenia and a coarse trabecular bone pattern even in the prepubertal years. Although interpretation of most studies of bone mineral density (BMD) in TS is difficult due to reporting of areal rather than volumetric BMD, some conclusions can be made. Prepubertal girls with TS have decreased levels of markers of bone formation, consistent with a low bone turnover state and decreased bone deposition. There is a deficit in radial BMD, a largely cortical site, during childhood. Osteopenia at predominantly trabecular sites develops during adolescence, progresses in adulthood, and is associated with increased bone turnover. The pathogenesis of the demineralization is unclear but is most likely an intrinsic bone defect that is exacerbated by suboptimal replacement of gonadal steroids *(40,41)*.

Orthodontic Problems

Individuals with TS have a posterior cranial base that is short and positioned at a shallow angle *(42)*. Because the mandible is pushed posteriorly and is relatively more hypoplastic than the rest of the face, retrognathia is common. There is an increased incidence of anterior open bite and lateral crossbite owing to a narrow maxillary arch *(43)*. The palate is high-arched with unusual palatal bulges on the medial aspect of the posterior alveolar ridges. Interestingly, girls with TS tend to have advanced dental age, rather than the delayed dental age expected for bone age-delayed individuals *(44)*. Tooth morphology is often abnormal and roots tend to be short, placing these girls at an increased risk for root resorption *(45)*.

Hearing Loss

Ear and hearing disorders are common problems among girls and women with Turner syndrome. The majority suffers from conductive hearing losses secondary to repeated attacks of otitis media during infancy and childhood. The high incidence of otitis media in this population (60–80%) *(46,47)* seems to result from a disturbed relationship between the middle ear and the Eustachian tube. A short, more horizontally-oriented Eustachian tube in TS girls results in poor drainage and ventilation of the middle ear space and may allow more nasopharyngeal microorganisms to reach the middle ear. Many girls require tympanostomy tube placement and a significant number develop complications such as mastoiditis and cholesteotoma. In a study in which 56 girls with TS between the ages of 4–15 yr were examined, 57% had eardrum pathology, such as effusion, myringosclerosis, atrophic scars, retraction pockets, and perforations. A conductive hearing loss (air-bone gap >10 dB HL) was found in 43%. In addition, a midfrequency sensorineural hearing loss

(SNHL) between 500–2000 Hz was present in 58% of the girls, 4 of whom required hearing aids *(47)*. This SNHL has been identified as early as age 5 and appears to be progressive *(48)*. By their mid-forties, more than 90% of women with TS have a hearing loss >20 dB, with greater than 25% requiring hearing aids. Audiometry has revealed high frequency (above that used for speech) SNHL in almost all individuals with TS studied (ages 6–38 yr), suggesting "premature aging" of the cochlea *(49)*.

Strabismus and Other Eye Problems

Strabismus is present in about one-third of the patients with TS, a frequency about 10 times greater than that in the general population, and usually develops between 6 mo and 7 yr *(50)*. Anterior chamber abnormalities have also been reported to be more common in girls with TS and may present as congenital glaucoma *(51)*. 10% of the patients are also red-green color blind, an X-linked recessive trait.

Renal Abnormalities

Renal malformations occur in approx 35–40% of individuals with TS *(52,53)*. Of those with malformations, about half have abnormalities of the collecting system and half have positional abnormalities, with the most common being horseshoe kidney. Interestingly, horseshoe kidney is more common in those with 45,X karyotypes, while collecting system malformations are more frequent in those with mosaic/structural X chromosome abnormalities *(52)*. Developmental abnormalities of the kidneys and collecting system predispose these individuals to urinary tract infections and hypertension *(53)*.

GI Disorders

Increased serum concentrations of liver enzymes are observed in as many as 31% of patients with TS, usually without clinical symptoms. An autoimmune pathogenesis may be operative in some cases, since many have elevated antinuclear and/or anti-smooth muscle antibodies. In others, mild hepatomegaly and increased echogenicity with fatty infiltration are associated with excess weight *(54)*. Fortunately, the hepatic disorder does not appear to progress. Celiac disease appears to be more prevalent in TS than in the general population and may be responsible for growth failure in some patients *(55)*. Gastric hemangiomas and telangiectasias are rare, but can produce massive gastrointestinal bleeding when present.

Keloids, Nevi, and Other Skin Problems

Patients with TS are at increased risk of hypertrophic scar or keloid formation. They also have an increased number of benign appearing melanocytic nevi that increase in size and number throughout childhood and particularly during adolescence *(56)*. Hemangiomas are more common than in the general population and may be related to lymphatic abnormalities. They usually enlarge during the first year of life, then undergo slow regression. Other common skin problems include atopic dermatitis, seborrheic dermatitis and keratosis pilaris.

Hypothyroidism and Other Autoimmune Disorders

Some autoimmune disorders are more prevalent in individuals with Turner Syndrome than in the general population. The most common of these is Hashimoto's thyroiditis, but girls with TS also appear to have a higher risk of celiac disease, inflammatory bowel disease (IBD) *(57)*, juvenile rheumatoid arthritis (JRA), and, perhaps, Type I diabetes mellitus *(39)*. In a study that evaluated 71 children with TS under 20-yr of age (mean age of 11.4 yr), 15.5% were hypothyroid, 17% were positive for thyroid peroxidase and/or thyroglobulin antibodies, and 33.8% had thyromegaly *(58)*. The frequency of thyroid abnormalities increased with age, with no abnormalities observed before 4-yr of age. Unlike previous reports, the risk of thyroid disease was not greater in those with structural rearrangements than those with a 45,X or mosaic karyotype. A survey of 15,000 JRA patients from pediatric rheumatology centers in the US, Europe and Canada revealed 18 girls with a diagnosis of TS. This represents a prevalence at least 6× greater than would be expected if the two conditions were only randomly associated. Patients had either polyarticular disease with early onset and progressive disabilities or oligoarticular arthritis with a benign course *(59)*.

Obesity, Lipids, and Glucose Homeostasis

Individuals with TS have a modestly decreased life span. In a study of the Danish TS population, approx 50% of all deaths were caused by cardiovascular disease, and these occurred 6–13 yr earlier than expected *(39)*. They were at increased risk for abnormalities constituting "the metabolic syndrome" including hypertension, dyslipidemia, Type 2 diabetes, obesity, hyperinsulinemia, and hyperuricemia *(39)*. For many of these short individuals, obesity becomes a major problem, especially during adolescence and adulthood. Body mass index (BMI) SDS begins to increase around age 9 yr *(60)* and may exacerbate a tendency towards Type 2 diabetes *(61)*. Even young TS patients with normal fasting plasma glucose and insulin levels have insulin responses during a hyperglycemic glucose-clamp that are nearly two fold greater than those of control subjects *(61)*. The increased insulin response appears to involve a defect in nonoxidative pathways of intracellular glucose metabolism. Adult women with TS have been demonstrated to have higher levels of apolipoprotein A-I and Lp(a), which are lowered with replacement of female sex hormones *(62)*.

Gonadal Failure

The majority of girls with TS have gonadal dysgenesis and pubertal delay. In those with gonadal dysfunction, follicle stimulating hormone (FSH) levels are increased during the first two years of life, decline gradually to reach low levels (often indistinguishable from those in normal girls) between 5–10 yr of age, and rise again to castrate levels around the usual age for puberty *(63,64)*. Measurement of FSH using an ultrasensitive assay is an inexpensive way to screen girls with short stature for gonadal failure and TS, especially for those who are younger than 5 yr or older than 10-yr of age. However, not all individuals with TS have gonadal dysgenesis and pubertal delay. In a recent Italian retrospective multicenter study of 522 patients older than 12 yr with TS, 32% of girls with cell lines containing more than one X and 14% of 45,X patients initiated puberty spontaneously *(65)*. Sixteen percent had spontaneous menarche that occurred at a mean age of 13.2 ± 1.5 yr and a similar bone age. Although some developed secondary amenorrhea, others had regular periods for many years. Unassisted pregnancy occurred in 3 patients (3.6%), of whom 2 had chromosomal abnormalities and malformations. Therefore, the diagnosis of TS should still be considered in girls with short stature, even if they are menstruating. In fact, TS should be considered in the differential diagnosis for women experiencing premature ovarian failure *(66)*.

When unassisted pregnancies occur, they are generally in patients with structural anomalies of the X chromosomes in which the Xq13–q26 region, containing the genes that are thought to control ovarian function, is spared; or in patients with a mosaic karyotype containing a 46,XX cell line, which preserves ovarian function. Of those who do achieve pregnancy, there is a high risk of spontaneous abortion (25–40%), chromosomal abnormalities in the offspring (20%), and perinatal death (7%) *(67)*.

Girls with karyotypes containing Y material, such as 45,X/46,XY, are at increased risk for developing gonadoblastomas. A gonadoblastoma is a gonadal tumor in which normal components of the ovary, such as oogonia, granulosa-Sertoli type cells, and Leydig-thecal type cells, are present in varying amounts within circumscribed nests. The latter may produce sex steroids, which may cause virilization or occasionally feminization, depending on the predominant sex steroid produced. Although the pure gonadoblastoma is not a malignant tumor, the germ cell component may invade the ovarian stroma, producing a potentially malignant germinoma. Occasionally a more malignant tumor, such as embryonal carcinoma or choriocarcinoma, may develop in a gonadoblastoma.

Using standard cytogenetic techniques, approx 5% of patients with TS have Y chromosomal materials, and of those, gonadoblastoma has been thought to develop in 15–25%. Recently, however, fluorescent *in situ* hybridization (FISH) studies using Y-specific DNA probes, have demonstrated that the percentage of girls with TS having Y chromosome material is probably higher. In a study of 114 females with TS who were examined for the presence of Y chromosome material by PCR, 14 patients (12.2%) had Y material *(68)*. Seven of the fourteen had Y material suggested by karyotype previously and had undergone ovariectomies, with 1 having a gonadoblastoma. Of the 7 patients with Y material diagnosed by PCR alone, 3 went on to have ovariectomies that did not reveal tumors, and the others (all more than 50-yr-old) had detailed ultrasonographies that did not suggest tumors *(68)*. Therefore, although the frequency of Y chromosome material detected by PCR is substantial, the occurrence of gonadoblastoma in this population seems to be low.

Learning Disabilities

Individuals with TS are at increased risk for specific neurocognitive deficits and problems in psychosocial functioning. These problems include deficits in visual-spatial/perceptual abilities, nonverbal memory function, motor function, executive function, attention, and social skills. These difficulties cut across all socioeconomic and ethnic boundaries *(17)*.

Although their distribution of IQs is relatively normal, lower full-scale IQs are more prevalent in this population due to lower scores on performance than verbal tasks. For example, results of Wechsler IQ tests in 226 women with TS revealed a 12-point discrepancy between mean verbal and performance IQs (101 vs 89). This verbal-performance IQ discrepancy, consistent with a non-verbal subtype of learning disability, has not been well correlated to age or karyotype *(69)*.

The neurocognitive deficits put them at a higher risk for educational problems. Rovet found that 48.2% of girls with TS vs only 20% of control subjects were recognized by their parents as having problems at school *(70)*. Mathematics is particularly problematic, and girls with TS score significantly lower than control subjects in overall arithmetic achievement. In Rovet's study, girls with TS obtained a mean global mathematics score

2.1 grades below their current placement level *(68)*. In a more recent study, a higher percentage of girls with TS made operation and alignment errors on a mathematics calculations test than did controls or another group with mathematic difficulties (fragile X syndrome) *(71)*. Although math is a consistent problem for girls with TS, hyperactivity, inattention, distractibility, and slowness may impair achievement in all educational disciplines. Many girls with TS repeat grades because of lagging cognitive and psychosocial skills.

Although individuals with TS do not appear to be at an overall higher risk for psychiatric problems, there is some evidence to suggest that obsessive-compulsive tendencies *(72)* and autism are more prevalent *(73)*.

Tumors and Miscellaneous

Besides gonadoblastoma, the risks for most cancers do not appear to be elevated in TS. Exceptions may include colon cancer *(39)* and neuroblastoma *(74)*.

DIAGNOSTIC GUIDELINES

A delay in diagnosis of TS is often the greatest obstacle to health care. In a recent study, the delay in diagnosis for those diagnosed in childhood or adolescence averaged more than 7 yr (based on the presence of dysmorphic features and/or growth failure). At the time of diagnosis, patients averaged 2.9 SD below the mean in height and had fallen below the 5th percentile for height an average of 5.3 yr earlier *(21)*.

In many girls with TS who have a delayed diagnosis, the TS phenotype is either absent or mild. This was the case when a systematic search for TS in 375 female children referred to a center with growth retardation (–2 SD) and/or decreased height velocity identified 18 cases of TS, an incidence of 4.8% *(75)*. To facilitate timely diagnoses, Savendahl and Davenport have suggested specific guidelines for screening girls for TS *(21)* (Table 1).

A karyotype should be performed in a reputable laboratory with a minimum of 25 cells in metaphase evaluated using giemsa trypsin (GTG-) banding. Any marker chromosomes should undergo further evaluation to determine whether or not Y material is present. Typically, laboratories perform the fluorescent *in situ* hybridization (FISH) technique using specific DNA probes to the Y chromosome *(76)*. Karyotypes that were performed more than 10 yr ago or had an inadequate number of cells examined should be repeated.

THERAPY

Introduction

The patient should be referred to a physician expert in the care of individuals with TS if at all possible. Primary care physicians and involved subspecialists should be aware of published consensus guidelines for their health supervision *(77,78)*.

Lymphedema

Lymphedema usually improves over the first few months of life. However, it may be severe or recur with puberty or hormone replacement therapy. Combined decongestive therapy (CDT) which uses manual lymphatic drainage, bandaging, exercises, skin care, and low stretch support garments is an effective and non-invasive treatment *(79,80)*.

Table 1
Guidelines: Screening Girls for Turner Syndrome[a]

Karyotype any girl with one or more of the following:[b]

Unexplained short stature (height <5th percentile)
- Webbed neck
- Peripheral lymphedema
- Coarctation of the aorta
- Delayed puberty

OR

Any girl with at least two or more of the following:
- Nail dysplasia
- High arched palate
- Short 4th metacarpal
- Strabismus

[a]Reproduced with permission, Savendahl L, Davenport ML. Delayed diagnoses of Turner's syndrome: proposed guidelines for change. J Pediatr 2000;137(4):458.

[b]Other suggestive features include a nonverbal learning disability, epicanthal folds, ptosis, cubitus valgus, multiple nevi, renal malformations, bicuspid aortic valve, recurrent otitis media and need for glasses.

Dysmorphic Features

Plastic surgery may be recommended for some individuals with severe webbed neck and/ or ear anomalies. With all surgeries, the risk of keloid formation must be considered *(81)*.

Cardiovascular Abnormalities

Although specific guidelines vary, there is no debate that the cardiovascular system should be monitored closely in individuals with TS. All patients should undergo a baseline cardiology evaluation at the time of diagnosis. This should include an imaging procedure, generally an echocardiogram. A cardiologist should direct the care of any patient in whom a cardiovascular malformation is detected. If appropriate, prophylactic antibiotics should be prescribed to prevent subacute bacterial endocarditis. Even in those with a normal baseline cardiovascular structure, a cardiology evaluation and imaging procedure should be repeated during adolescence and every 3–5 yr thereafter to rule out dilation of the aortic root, a process that can be advanced even in the absence of clinical findings. Patients should be counseled that aortic dissection presents with severe chest pain. A MRI is mandatory to rule out dissection, even if the chest pain was transient. Blood pressure should be closely monitored. Hypertension, whether idiopathic or associated with cardiac and/or renal disease, is common and may worsen with obesity and age. Any woman considering pregnancy should consult with a cardiologist and be monitored carefully throughout the pregnancy.

Short Stature and Skeletal Abnormalities

INTRODUCTION

Once the diagnosis of TS is made, growth should be assessed regularly using a TS-specific growth chart. Use of a TS-specific growth chart will facilitate detection of concurrent problems that affect growth, such as hypothyroidism, and aid in the evaluation of growth-promoting therapies. A growth chart for girls ages 2–18 is available based on growth data from 251 untreated European girls with TS *(82)*. These growth data are applicable to girls with TS from the US. Untreated patients are expected to follow a percentile on the TS curve throughout childhood and adolescence. As for the normal population, there is a strong genetic component to each individual's growth pattern. In fact, the height of any individual with TS is expected to be about 20 cm less than that of their midparental height (MPH).

The goals of hormonal therapies are to: 1) attain a normal height for age early in childhood; 2) progress through puberty at a normal age; 3) attain a normal adult height at a normal age; and 4) avoid the adverse effects of therapy *(83)*. The timing and administration of hormonal therapies for girls with TS are still evolving as experience is gained in their use. Growth hormone (GH) is the agent of choice. With the FDA approval of GH for use in TS in late 1996, the US joined other industrialized countries in recognizing GH therapy as the standard of care for girls with TS *(84)*. Clinical trials of GH have demonstrated that GH improves final height in girls with TS if administered appropriately *(2)*. When given in conjunction with GH therapy, anabolic steroids appear to have a beneficial effect *(85–87)*. However, anabolic steroids, including testosterone, oxandrolone, fluoxymesterone, and nandrolone, when used alone, increase short term height velocity but do not appear to improve final height.

Effects of GH on Linear Growth

Although most studies have not been randomized controlled trials, as a whole they demonstrate that GH increases growth velocity and improves final height of girls with TS. The magnitude of the benefit has varied tremendously depending upon study design *(85,86)*. However, it is now clear that with early diagnosis and initiation of treatment, a normal adult height is a reasonable goal for most girls with TS *(88)*. Factors now known to be important in determining the response include age at initiation of therapy, duration of therapy, GH dose, addition of anabolic steroids, and timing of estrogen replacement therapy. Most early studies reported height gains < 5 cm, but in these studies GH was started at a relatively late age and was given at low doses. In contrast, recent studies have documented height gains in the range of 5–16 cm *(88,89)*. In a multicenter, prospective, randomized trial in which patients began therapy at a mean age of 7–8 yr and received treatment for a mean of 6 yr, therapy with GH alone ($n = 17$) resulted in a height that was 8.4 ± 4.5 cm taller than the mean projected adult height at enrollment. Subjects receiving GH plus oxandrolone ($n = 43$) attained a mean height of 152.1 ± 5.9 cm, 10.3 ± 4.7 cm taller than their mean projected adult height *(88)*.

In the most encouraging study to date, GH therapy was initiated between the ages of 2–11 yr in Dutch girls with TS. After 7 yr, 85% had heights within the normal range. The mean height achieved in those who had completed therapy (either because adult height had been attained or they were satisfied with the height achieved) was dose-dependent. All girls received a GH dose of 4 IU/m^2/d (~ 0.045 mg/kg/d) in the first year. This dose was continued in group A, increased to 6 IU/m^2/d in the second year for groups B and C, and increased to 8 IU/m^2/d during the third year for group C. No estrogens were given to the girls in the first 4 yr of GH treatment. Thereafter, girls were given oral 17β-estradiol (5 μg/kg/d) for pubertal induction when they reached the age of 12 yr. The difference between predicted adult height before treatment and achieved height was 12.5 ± 2.1 cm, 14.5 ± 4.0 cm, and 16.0 ± 4.1 cm for groups A, B, and C, respectively *(89)*.

The patient's age at initiation of estrogen treatment is an important factor in determining growth response *(90)*. Chernausek et al. conducted a multicenter study in which 60 girls starting GH therapy were randomized to initiate estrogen therapy at either 12 or 15 yr of age. The patients were all less than 11 yr of age at entry (mean, 9.5 yr) and received 0.375 mg/kg/wk of GH for approx 6 yr. Patients in whom estrogen treatment was delayed until age 15 yr gained an average of 8.4 ± 4.3 cm over their projected height, whereas those starting estrogen at 12 yr gained only 5.1 ± 3.6 cm. Growth was stimulated for approx 2 yr after the initiation of estrogen, but then declined as bone age advanced.

Maximal height may not be attained if estrogen is initiated at a normal age. However, at least one study has demonstrated that treatment with relatively high doses of GH and low doses of estrogen can increase adult height significantly, even if GH is started at a relatively late age *(91)*. In a study of 19 girls <11 yr (mean age 13.6) with TS treated with 6 IU/m^2/d GH in combination with low dose estrogen (ethinyl estradiol 0.05 µg/kg/d, increased to 0.10 µg/kg/d after 2.25 yr), all girls exceeded their adult height prediction. The gain in height ranged from 1.6–12.3 cm and two-thirds gained more than 5 cm.

GH therapy should be optimized for each individual, given its high costs and potential risks. In one study, untreated patients with TS were treated initially with a GH dose of 0.23 mg/kg/wk that was doubled or tripled when growth velocity declined to less than twice that of its pretreatment level. The estimated final height benefit was 10.6 ± 3.8 cm compared to 5.2 ± 3.7 cm in a group who received a fixed dose of 0.3 mg/kg/wk. In the group receiving incremental increases in GH dose, 83% attained heights in the normal range *(92)*.

Ranke et al. have developed a mathematical model that can be used to predict the growth response to GH of patients with TS. In their model, GH dose is the most important predictor of height velocity in the first year of GH therapy. In yr 2–4 of therapy, height velocity during the previous year is the most important predictor. Additional predictors of height velocity in yr 1–4 of GH therapy include age (negative), weight SDS and additional treatment with oxandrolone *(93)*.

EFFECTS OF GH ON BODY PROPORTIONS

As expected, there are differences in the response of specific bones to GH treatment. On average, untreated girls with TS have relatively large trunks, hands, and feet, and broad shoulders and pelvis compared to height. GH treatment appears to exacerbate the disproportionate growth of feet and to modestly improve the disproportion between height and sitting height. There is no significant effect on relative width of the shoulders and pelvis *(94)*.

EFFECTS OF GH ON BONE MINERAL DENSITY

For girls with TS, GH therapy is likely to help maintain prepubertal bone mineral density (BMD) *(95)*. Preliminary BMD data on patients after long-term GH therapy show an absence of osteopenia *(40)*.

EFFECTS OF GH ON CRANIOFACIAL DEVELOPMENT

Thus far, GH therapy in girls with TS has not been demonstrated to have a significant effect on craniofacial growth *(41)*, with the possible exception of an increase in the length of the mandible *(96)*. However, in these relatively short term studies, the mean ages at initiation of GH therapy were 9 and 14 yr. The growth of the cranial base is largely complete by age 6, whereas the synchondrosis of the mandible does not close until late adolescence and can be reactivated in adulthood. The effect of early, prolonged and/or high-dose GH therapy is unknown.

EFFECTS OF GH ON PSYCHOSOCIAL FUNCTION

There is abundant anecdotal evidence that GH therapy improves psychosocial function, one of the principal goals of this therapy. Unfortunately, few studies have formally addressed this very important question, and controlled studies are unlikely in the future. However, there are some data confirming the observations of physicians, families and girls with TS that certain aspects of social interactions and behavior, but not cognition *(97)*, are improved with GH therapy. In a study of 38 girls with TS treated for 2 yr with GH, improvements were demonstrated in social and emotional functioning. The investigators reported that a quarter of the patients became more independent, happier and socially involved *(98)*. In a study in which girls with TS were evaluated after 3 yr of GH therapy, attention, social problems, and withdrawal were reported as improved *(99)*. In a Canadian study in which girls were randomized to either a GH or control group, analysis after 2 yr revealed that there was a correlation with higher growth rate and the girls' perceptions of themselves as more intelligent, more attractive, having more friends, greater popularity, and experiencing less teasing than the untreated group *(100)*. It is likely that earlier normalization of height will improve social functioning by allowing peers and adults to relate to the children in a more age-appropriate fashion. It also makes feminization at a normal time a viable option.

SAFETY OF GH THERAPY

Extensive postmarketing surveillance programs have documented that side effects of growth hormone therapy in children, including those with TS, are rare. However, families should be counseled to watch for the following potential complications and notify their physician immediately should symptoms occur:

1. Benign idiopathic intracranial hypertension (0.1–0.2%) is a potentially dangerous complication. GH should be discontinued for patients that complain of severe headache, visual changes, nausea and vomiting until papilledema has been excluded and/or has resolved.
2. Lymphedema may worsen or recur (0.4%).
3. Carpal tunnel syndrome has been reported in some children (<0.03%).
4. Slipped capital femoral epiphyses (SCFE) may present with limp, hip or knee pain (0.14%). Obesity, rapid growth and puberty are known risk factors.
5. Scoliosis may progress during periods of rapid growth, although GH does not increase the incidence of scoliosis.
6. An increase in the number, size, and degree of pigmentation of pigmented nevi may occur, but the risk of malignancy does not appear to be increased.
7. Insulin resistance increases, but there is generally no effect on glucose levels *(101,102)*. In girls with TS treated with GH for 7 yr, the prevalence of impaired glucose tolerance was low; all hemoglobin A1c levels were normal, and none of the girls developed diabetes mellitus. Insulin levels decreased to values close to or equal to pretreatment values after discontinuation of GH treatment *(103)*. In the National Cooperative Growth Study (NCGS) database, 21 children (0.1%) developed diabetes mellitus during GH treatment (2 with TS). Sixteen of the twenty-one had an identifiable factor other than GH that would be expected to increase their risk of diabetes substantially. These and other studies indicate that metabolic side effects of clinical significance are rare in girls with TS treated with GH.

8. Antibodies to GH may develop, but only two cases have been reported in which the antibodies made the GH ineffective. Recurrent or new tumors do not appear to be more frequent. In the NCGS, eight new cases of leukemia were diagnosed, five of whom had previous risk factors and none of whom had TS. By 1996, 200 patients with a previous history of leukemia and 1262 children with a history of previous brain tumors had been treated with GH and tumor recurrence rates were within the expected range.

SAFETY OF ANABOLIC STEROIDS

Side effects of anabolic steroids may include: 1) virilization with development of acne, deepening of the voice, and growth of facial hair; 2) transient elevation of liver function tests; 3) insulin resistance; and 4) premature skeletal maturation. Although mild virilization has occurred in girls treated with oxandrolone in a dose of 1.25 mg/kg/d *(104)*, treatment with lower doses (0.5– 0.75 mg/kg/d) appears to be safe.

GENERAL RECOMMENDATIONS FOR GROWTH-PROMOTING THERAPIES

GH should be offered as a therapy for all girls with TS who are predicted to have a subnormal height. The predicted response to GH should be carefully reviewed with patients and their families to help limit unrealistic expectations of future height. Routine evaluation of GH secretory status in girls with TS is not warranted, since GH secretion in this group is similar to that of the normal population and GH secretory responses do not correlate with responses to exogenous GH *(105)*. Because GH therapy for this population is a pharmacological one, it requires somewhat higher doses than those used for GH-deficient patients. Standard GH therapy in the US for TS is 0.375 mg/kg/wk divided into six or seven doses. Division of GH dosing into two shots per day does not appear to be advantageous over one shot per day *(91)*. GH is now available in depot form, but no testing has been performed in non-GH deficient populations, such as TS.

Although GH has been initiated at a mean age of 9–11 yr in most studies, it is becoming clear that girls who begin GH therapy at an earlier age and receive GH for a longer period of time will experience a greater increment in height *(89,106)*. Therefore, it is suggested that GH therapy be initiated once growth failure is documented. Normalization of height during childhood may improve psychosocial status and allow for more age-appropriate initiation of estrogen therapy.

Oxandrolone may be used as an adjunct to GH therapy. A dose of 0.5–0.75 mg/kg/d is recommended, since side effects are frequently demonstrated at higher doses. Many endocrinologists have chosen to initiate oxandrolone therapy around the age of 10–11 yr, the time at which these girls would normally be starting puberty and experiencing ovarian androgens.

Orthodontic Problems

Because many girls with TS have orthodontic problems, early evaluation by an orthodontist is suggested. The timing of any orthodontic treatment should take into consideration growth promoting therapies that may alter tooth and jaw alignment. In addition, because the dental roots are short, unnecessary tooth movement should be minimized to avoid root resorption and loss of teeth.

Hearing Loss

Ear and hearing function should be assessed as soon as the diagnosis of TS is made. Ideally, children with TS should have pneumatic otoscopy performed at every visit to the physician, and tympanometry should be performed if otoscopy is equivocal. Any child who has fluid in both middle ears for a period of 3 mo should undergo a complete hearing evaluation by a pediatric audiologist *(107)*. In general, tympanostomy tubes are recommended when bilateral conductive hearing deficiency of at least 20 dB HL is associated with bilateral effusions for a period of more than 3 mo. Chronic or recurrent middle ear disease should be managed aggressively to minimize the likelihood of middle ear damage and permanent hearing loss. In patients with TS, early tube placement may be justified since otitis media with effusion is less likely to resolve spontaneously than in the normal population. Because infection of the tonsils and adenoids may contribute to sinus and middle ear infections, tonsillectomy and/or adenoidectomy may be considered as additional therapeutic options for some patients. Patients should be warned to protect their hearing by avoiding exposure to loud noises unless appropriate ear protection is in use. In general, they should not be in environments in which they must shout to be heard.

Strabismus and Other Eye Problems

Children should be evaluated for strabismus at every clinic visit between the ages of 6 mo and 5 yr of age. Because early correction of visual alignment is critical for normal binocular vision to develop, any child with strabismus should be referred immediately to an ophthalmologist for further evaluation. In fact, it may be prudent for every child with TS to have an ophthalmology exam around 2 yr of age.

Renal Abnormalities

All patients with TS should be routinely screened by ultrasound for renal abnormalities. Both those with and without structural abnormalities seem to be at increased risk for chronic urinary tract infections.

GI Disorders

GI bleeding should be in the differential diagnosis of children with anemia. Celiac disease and IBD should be considered for those with unexplained weight loss.

Keloids and Other Skin Problems

Patients should be forewarned before having their ears pierced or undergoing surgical procedures that keloids may arise. The risk of keloid formation should certainly be discussed when cosmetic surgery is being considered. The patient, family and physician should examine nevi regularly to look for dysplastic features such as asymmetry, border irregularity, color variability, and diameter greater than 5 mm. Patients should also be advised to limit sun exposure.

Hypothyroidism and Other Autoimmune Disorders

Because autoimmune hypothyroidism may develop insidiously, thyroid function should be monitored yearly. For those growing poorer than expected, antibody studies for celiac disease should be considered.

Obesity, Lipids, and Glucose Homeostasis

Patients should be encouraged to maintain their weight within an appropriate range for height and receive early dietary counseling if necessary. Girls with risk factors for Type

2 diabetes mellitus should be screened with fasting blood glucoses or a modified, oral glucose tolerance test (OGTT).

Gonadal Failure

Ideally, the dosing and timing of estrogen replacement should mimic normal pubertal development *(108)*. Beginning estrogen replacement in early adolescence (10–12-yr of age) would allow puberty to begin and to progress at a normal age, and would also permit maximal bone accretion during adolescence. On the other hand, estrogen is also responsible for epiphyseal fusion, and premature use of estrogen replacement may lead to early termination of skeletal growth, thereby compromising adult height. Efforts to maximize growth prior to adolescence are, consequently, of great importance, since this would allow the patient both to attain a normal adult height and to progress through puberty at a relatively normal age. Ideally, GH and estrogen therapy should be customized for each patient to allow for both normal growth and puberty and to address the priorities of each child.

In general, estrogen replacement should not begin prior to 12-yr of age, nor be delayed beyond 15 years of age. Serum gonadotropin concentrations can be measured prior to onset of estrogen therapy, to document gonadal failure; sonographic evaluation may provide additional information about the status of the ovaries and uterus. Estrogen replacement should begin at a relatively low dose, typically one-sixth to one-fourth of the adult dose. Conjugated estrogens (Premarin) may be started at 0.3 mg/d, increasing to 0.625 mg/d after 6–12 mo. On this regimen, the majority of girls will be able to attain at least Tanner 3 breast development within 12 mo; and, if necessary, the estrogen dose can be increased to 1.25 mg/d. Alternative estrogen preparations include oral ethinyl estradiol (50–100 ng/kg/d), 17-beta-estradiol, or estrogen patches; the potential advantages of one preparation over another in TS have not been systematically evaluated. After 1–2 yr of unopposed estrogens, a progestin is added for 10–12 d each month to induce menses and diminish the risk of endometrial hyperplasia and/or carcinoma. One common regimen is to limit estrogen replacement to d 1–26 of each month, and give medroxyprogesterone acetate (Provera) 5–10 mg on d 17–26.

Long-term treatment with estrogen and progestin that is initiated during mid- to late adolescence and is continued throughout adulthood appears necessary for a normal peak bone mass to be achieved. Additional measures to prevent osteoporosis should be used, such as ensuring adequate calcium intake (>1000 mg of elemental calcium daily in the pre-teen years, and 1200–1500 mg daily after 11-yr of age), encouraging weight-bearing activities, and avoiding overtreatment with thyroid hormones *(40)*.

Because gonadoblastomas may occur as early as young childhood, prophylactic gonadectomies are recommended at the time of diagnosis for most girls with karyotypes containing Y chromosome material or marker chromosomes identified as Y material by FISH *(109)*. Recommendations for those found by PCR technique alone are less clear.

The reproductive options for women with TS continue to expand. For the rare woman who is fertile, prenatal amniocentesis is recommended because of the high rate of chromosomal abnormalities. Those who are sterile may choose to adopt children or undergo artificial fertilization. In a recent study, the clinical pregnancy rate achieved by embryo transfer in women with TS was similar to that of other oocyte recipients with primary ovarian failure; however, a greater percentage (40%) ended in miscarriage *(110)*. The greater miscarriage rate may be the result of uterine factors. Careful assessment before and during follow-up of pregnancy is important because of the increased risk of cardiovascular and other complications. Some physicians have recommended that only one embryo be transferred at a time to avoid the additional complications caused by twin pregnancy.

Learning Disabilities

Children with TS should undergo a baseline developmental evaluation at the time of initial diagnosis or at latest, during the preschool years. Academic tutoring, occupational therapy and training in problem solving strategies can help girls and women with TS cope with their visual-spatial and cognitive challenges. Individual psychotherapy may be required to address the social and emotional difficulties commonly experienced by individuals with TS *(111)*. Timely institution of estrogen therapy may be important since there is some evidence that some neurocognitive deficits such as memory, reaction time, and speeded motor function result from estrogen deficiency and are at least somewhat reversible with estrogen treatment *(17)*. Many patients and their families benefit tremendously from support group programs, such as those offered by the Turner Syndrome Society of the United States (TSSUS), which can be accessed at http://www.turner-syndrome.org.

REFERENCES

1. Nielsen J, Wohlert M. Chromosome abnormalities found among 34,910 newborn children: results from a 13-year incidence study in Arhus, Denmark. Hum Genet 1991;87:81–83.
2. Saenger P. Turner's Syndrome. N Engl J Med 1996;335(23):1749–1754.
3. Lippe BM. Turner Syndrome. In: Sperling MA, ed. Pediatric Endocrinology. W.B. Saunders Co., Philadelphia, PA 1996, pp. 387–421.
4. Hook EB, Warburton D. The distribution of chromosomal genotypes associated with Turner's syndrome: Livebirth prevalence rates and evidence for diminished fetal mortality and severity in genotypes associated with structural X abnormalities or mosaicism. Hum Genet 1983;64:24–27.
5. Neely EK, Rosenfeld RG. Phenotypic correlations of X-chromosome loss. In: Wachtel SS, ed. Molecular Genetics of Sex Determination. Academic Press, San Diego: 1994, pp. 311–339.
6. Leonova J, Hanson C. A study of 45,X/46,XX mosaicism in Turner syndrome females: a novel primer pair for the (CAG)n repeat within the androgen receptor gene. Hereditas 1999;131(2):87–92.
7. Zinn AR, Ross JL. Turner syndrome and haploinsufficiency. Curr Opin Genet Dev 1998;8(3):322–327.
8. Ogata T, Matsuo N. Turner syndrome and female sex chromosome aberrations: deduction of the principal factors involved in the development of clinical features. Hum Genet 1995;95(6):607–629.
9. Clement-Jones M, Schiller S, Rao E, et al. The short stature homeobox gene SHOX is involved in skeletal abnormalities in Turner syndrome. Hum Mol Genet 2000;9(5):695–702.
10. Blaschke RJ, Rappold GA. SHOX: Growth, Leri-Weill and Turner Syndromes. Trends Endocrinol Metab 2000;11(6):227–230.
11. Ellison JW, Wardak Z, Young MF, Gehron RP, Laig-Webster M, Chiong. PHOG, a candidate gene for involvement in the short stature of Turner syndrome. Hum Mol Genet 1997;6(8):1341–1347.
12. Kajii T, Ferrier A, Niikawa N, et al. Anatomic and chromosomal anomalies in 639 spontaneous abortuses. Hum Genet 1980;55:87–98.
13. Simpson JL, Rajkovic A. Ovarian differentiation and gonadal failure. Am J Med Genet 1999;89(4):186–200.
14. Haverkamp F, Wolfle J, Zerres K, et al. Growth retardation in Turner syndrome: aneuploidy, rather than specific gene loss, may explain growth failure. J Clin Endocrinol Metab 1999;84(12):4578–4582.
15. Tsezou A, Hadjiathanasiou C, Gourgiotis D, et al. Molecular genetics of Turner syndrome: correlation with clinical phenotype and response to growth hormone therapy. Clin Genet 1999;56(6):441–446.
16. Skuse DH, James RS, Bishop DV, et al. Evidence from Turner's syndrome of an imprinted X-linked locus affecting cognitive function. Nature 1997;387:705–708.

17. Ross J, Zinn A, McCauley E. Neurodevelopmental and psychosocial aspects of Turner syndrome. Ment Retard Dev Disabil Res Rev 2000;6(2):135–141.
18. Migeon BR, Luo S, Stasiowski BA, et al. Deficient transcription of XIST from tiny ring X chromosomes in females with severe phenotypes. Proc Natl Acad Sci U S A 1993;90:12,025–12,029.
19. Turner C, Dennis NR, Skuse DH, Jacobs PA. Seven ring (X) chromosomes lacking the XIST locus, six with an unexpectedly mild phenotype. Hum Genet 2000;106(1):93–100.
20. Massa GG, Vanderschueren Lodeweyckx M. Age and height at diagnosis in Turner syndrome: influence of parental height. Pediatrics 1991;88:1148–1152.
21. Savendahl L, Davenport ML. Delayed diagnoses of Turner's syndrome: proposed guidelines for change. J Pediatr 2000;137(4):455–459.
22. Sybert VP. Cardiovascular malformations and complications in Turner Syndrome. Pediatrics 1998;101(1):e11.
23. Mazzanti L, Cacciari E. Congenital heart disease in patients with Turner's syndrome. Italian Study Group for Turner Syndrome (ISGTS). J Pediatr 1998;133(5):688–692.
24. Bordeleau L, Cwinn A, Turek M, Barron-Klauninger K, Victor G. Aortic dissection and Turner's syndrome: case report and review of the literature. Journal of Emergency Medicine 1998;16(4):593–596.
25. Lin AE, Lippe B, Rosenfeld RG. Further delineation of aortic dilation, dissection, and rupture in patients with Turner Syndrome. Pediatrics 1998;102(1):e12.
26. Elsheikh M, Casadei B, Conway GS, Wass JA. Hypertension is a major risk factor for aortic root dilatation in women wtih Turner's syndrome. Clin Endocrinol (Oxf) 2001;54:69–73.
27. Nathwani NC, Unwin R, Brook CG, Hindmarsh PC. The influence of renal and cardiovascular abnormalities on blood pressure in Turner syndrome. Clin Endocrinol (Oxf) 2000;52(3):371–377.
28. Sybert VP. Adult height in Turner syndrome with and without androgen therapy. J Pediatr 1984;104:365–369.
29. Ranke MB, Pfluger H, Rosendahl W, et al. Turner syndrome: spontaneous growth in 150 cases and review of the literature. Eur J Pediatr 1983;141(2):81–88.
30. Rochiccioli P, David M, Malpuech G, et al. Study of final height in Turner's syndrome: ethnic and genetic influences. Acta Paediatrica 1994;83(3):305–308.
31. Even L, Cohen A, Marbach N, et al. Longitudinal analysis of growth over the first 3 years of life in Turner's syndrome. J Pediatr 2000;137(4):460–464.
32. Davenport ML, Punyasavatsut N, Gunther D, Savendahl L, Stewart PW. Turner syndrome: a pattern of early growth failure. Acta Paediatr Suppl 1999;88(433):118–121.
33. Karlberg J, Albertsson-Wikland K, Nilsson KO, Ritzen EM, Westphal O. Growth in infancy and childhood in girls with Turner's syndrome. Acta Paediatr Scand 1991;80(12):1158–1165.
34. Ranke MB, Stubbe P, Majewski F, Bierich JR. Spontaneous Growth in Turner's Syndrome. Acta Paediatr Scand Suppl 1988;343:22–30.
35. Mathisen B, Reilly S, Skuse D. Oral-motor dysfunction and feeding disorders of infants with Turner syndrome. Dev Med Child Neurol 1992;34(2):141–149.
36. Gravholt CH, Naeraa RW. Reference values for body proportions and body composition in adult women with Ullrich-Turner Syndrome. Am J Med Genet 1997;72:403–408.
37. Allen DB. Safety of human growth hormone therapy: current topics. J Pediatr 1996;128(5:Pt 2):Pt 2):S8–13.
38. Even L, Bronstein V, Hochberg Z. Bone maturation in girls with Turner's Syndrome. Eur J Endocrinol 1998;138:59–62.
39. Gravholt CH, Juul S, Naeraa RW, Hansen J. Morbidity in Turner syndrome. J Clin Epidemiol 1998;51(2):147–158.
40. Rubin K. Turner syndrome and osteoporosis: mechanisms and prognosis. Pediatrics 1998;102 2 Pt 3:481–485.
41. Hass AD, Simmons KE, Davenport ML, Proffit WR. The Effect of Growth Hormone on Craniofacial Growth and Dental Maturation in Turner Syndrome. Angle Orthod 2000;70(6):43–52.
42. Rongen-Westerlaken C, Van Den Born E, Prahl-Andersen B, et al. Shape of the craniofacial complex in children with Turner syndrome. J Biol Buccale 1992;20:185–190.
43. Laine T, Alvesalo L, Savolainen A, Lammi S. Occlusal morphology in 45,X females. J Craniofac Genet Dev Biol 1986;6(4):351–355.
44. Midtbo M, Halse A. Skeletal maturity, dental maturity, and eruption in young patients with Turner syndrome. Acta Odontol Scand 1992;50:303–312.

45. Townsend G, Jensen BL, Alvesalo L. Reduced tooth size in 45,X (Turner Syndrome) females. Am J PhysAnthrop 1984;65:367–371.
46. Sculerati N, Ledesma Medina J, Finegold DN, Stool SE. Otitis media and hearing loss in Turner syndrome. Arch Otolaryngol Head Neck Surg 1990;116:704–707.
47. Stenberg AE, Nylen O, Windh M, Hultcrantz M. Otological problems in children with Turner's syndrome. Hear Res 1998;124(1–2):85–90.
48. Roush J, Davenport ML, Carlson-Smith C. Early-onset sensorineural hearing loss in a child with Turner syndrome. J Am Acad Audiol 2000;11(8):446–453.
49. Gungor N, Boke B, Belgin E, Tuncbilek E. High frequency hearing loss in Ullrich-Turner syndrome. Eur J Pediatr 2000;159(10):740–744.
50. Chrousos GA, Ross JL, Chrousos GC, et al. Ocular findings in Turner Syndrome: A Prospective Study. Ophthalmology 1984;91:926–928.
51. Lloyd IC, Haigh PM, Clayton-Smith J, et al. Anterior segment dysgenesis in mosaic Turner syndrome. British Journal of Ophthalmology 1997;81(8):639–643.
52. Bilge I, Kayserili H, Emre S, et al. Frequency of renal malformations in Turner syndrome: analysis of 82 Turkish children. Pediatr Nephrol 2000;14(12):1111–1114.
53. Lippe B, Geffner ME, Dietrich RJ, Boechat MI, Kangarloo H. Renal malformations in patients with Turner syndrome: imaging in 141 patients. Pediatrics 1988;82:852–856.
54. Larizza D, Locatelli M, Vitali L, et al. Serum liver enzymes in Turner syndrome. Eur J Pediatr 2000;159(3):143–148.
55. Bonamico M, Bottaro G, Pasquino AM, et al. Celiac disease and Turner syndrome. J Pediatr Gastroenterol Nutr 1998;26(5):496–499.
56. Becker B, Jospe N, Goldsmith LA. Melanocytic nevi in Turner syndrome. Pediatr Dermatol 1994;11(2):120–124.
57. Hayward PA, Satsangi J, Jewell DP. Inflammatory bowel disease and the X chromosome.
58. Medeiros CC, Marini SH, Baptista MT, Guerra G Jr, Maciel-Guerra AT. Turner's syndrome and thyroid disease: a transverse study of pediatric patients in Brazil. J Pediatr Endocrinol Metab 2000;13(4):357–362.
59. Zulian F, Schumacher HR, Calore A, Goldsmith DP, Athreya BH. Juvenile arthritis in Turner's syndrome: a multicenter study. Clin Exp Rheumatol 1998;16(4):489–494.
60. Blackett PR, Rundle AC, Frane J, Blethen SL. Body mass index (BMI) in Turner Syndrome before and during growth hormone (GH) therapy. Int J Obes Relat Metab Disord 2000;24(2):232–235.
61. Caprio S, Boulware S, Diamond M, et al. Insulin resistance: an early metabolic defect of Turner's syndrome. J Clin Endocrinol Metab 1991;72:832–836.
62. Hojbjerg GC, Christian K, Weeke J, Sandahl CJ. Lp(a) and lipids in adult Turner's syndrome: impact of treatment with 17beta-estradiol and norethisterone. Atherosclerosis 2000;150(1):201–208.
63. Conte FA, Grumbach ME, Kaplan SL. A diphasic pattern of gonadotrophin secretion in patients with the syndrome of gonadal dysgenesis. J Clin Endocrinol Metab 1974;670–674.
64. Chrysis DC, Spiliotis BE, Stene M, Davenport ML. Ultrasensitive assay for gonadotropins: potential use in the dignosis of Turner syndrome. 80th Annual Meeting of the Endocrine Society 1998;169.
65. Pasquino AM, Passeri F, Pucarelli I, Segni M, Municchi G. Spontaneous pubertal development in Turner's syndrome. Italian Study Group for Turner's Syndrome. J Clin Endocrinol Metab 1997;82(6):1810–1813.
66. Crosignani PG, Rubin BL. Optimal use of infertility diagnostic tests and treatments. The ESHRE Capri Workshop Group. Hum Reprod 2000;15(3):723–732.
67. Tarani L, Lampariello S, Raguso G, et al. Pregnancy in patients with Turner's syndrome: six new cases and review of literature. Gynecological Endocrinology 1998;12(2):83–87.
68. Gravholt CH, Fedder J, Naeraa RW, Muller J. Occurrence of gonadoblastoma in females with Turner syndrome and Y chromosome material: a population study. J Clin Endocrinol Metab 2000;85(9): 3199–3202.
69. Rovet JF. The cognitive and neuropsychological characteristics of females with Turner Syndrome. In: Berch DB, Berger BG, editors. Sex Chromosome Abnormalities and Human Behavior. Boulder, CO: Western Press, 1990:38–77.
70. Rovet JF. The psychoeducational characteristics of children with Turner syndrome. J Learn Disabil 1993;26:333–341.
71. Mazzocco MM. A process approach to describing mathematics difficulties in girls with Turner syndrome. Pediatrics 1998;102(2 Pt 3):492–496.

72. El Abd S, Patton MA, Turk J, Hoey H, Howlin P. Social, communicational, and behavioral deficits associated with ring X turner syndrome. Am J Med Genet 1999;88(5):510–516.
73. Donnelly SL, Wolpert CM, Menold MM, et al. Female with autistic disorder and monosomy X (Turner syndrome): parent-of-origin effect of the X chromosome. Am J Med Genet 2000;96(3): 312–316.
74. Blatt J, Olshan AF, Lee PA, Ross JL. Neuroblastoma and related tumors in Turner's syndrome. J Pediatr 1997;131(5):666–670.
75. Gicquel C, Gaston V, Cabrol S, Le Bouc Y. Assessment of Turner's syndrome by molecular analysis of the X chromosome in growth-retarded girls. J Clin Endocrinol Metab 1998;83(5):1472–1476.
76. Abulhasan SJ, Tayel SM, al Awadi SA. Mosaic Turner syndrome: cytogenetics versus FISH. Ann Hum Genet 1999;63(Pt 3):199–206.
77. American Academy of Pediatrics. Health Supervision for Children With Turner Syndrome. Pediatrics 1995;96(6):1166–1173.
78. Rosenfeld RG, Tesch L, Rodreiguez-Rigau LJ, McCauley E, Albertsson-Wikland K, Asch R. Recommendations for Diagnosis, Treatment, and Management of Individuals with Turner Syndrome. The Endocrinologist 1994;4(5):351–358.
79. Lerner R. What's New in Lymphedema Therapy in America? Int J Angiol 1998;7(3):191–196.
80. The diagnosis and treatment of peripheral lymphedema. Consensus document of the International Society of Lymphology Executive Committee. Lymphology 1995;28(3):113–117.
81. Thomson SJ, Tanner NS, Mercer DM. Web neck deformity; anatomical considerations and options in surgical management. Br J Plast Surg 1990;43(1):94–100.
82. Lyon AJ, Preece MA, Grant DB. Growth curve for girls with Turner syndrome. Arch Dis Child 1985;60(10):932–935.
83. Saenger P. Growth-promoting strategies in Turner's syndrome. J Clin Endocrinol Metab 1999;84(12): 4345–4348.
84. Plotnick L, Attie KM, Blethen SL, Sy JP. Growth hormone treatment of girls with Turner syndrome: the National Cooperative Growth Study experience. Pediatrics 1998;102 2 Pt 3:479–481.
85. Carel JC, Mathivon L, Gendrel C, Chaussain JL. Growth hormone therapy for Turner syndrome: evidence for benefit. Horm Res 1997;48(Suppl 5):31–34.
86. Donaldson MD. Growth hormone therapy in Turner syndrome—current uncertainties and future strategies. Horm Res 1997;48(Suppl 5):35–44.
87. Haeusler G, Schmitt K, Blumel P, Plochl E, Waldhor T, Frisch H. Growth hormone in combination with anabolic steroids in patients with Turner syndrome: effect on bone maturation and final height. Acta Paediatr 1996;85(12):1408–1414.
88. Rosenfeld RG, Attie KM, Frane J, et al. Growth hormone therapy of Turner's syndrome: beneficial effect on adult height. J Pediatr 1998;132(2):319–324.
89. Sas TC, de Muinck K, Stijnen T, et al. Normalization of height in girls with Turner syndrome after long-term growth hormone treatment: results of a randomized dose-response trial. J Clin Endocrinol Metab 1999;84(12):4607–4612.
90. Chernausek SD, Attie KM, Cara JF, Rosenfeld RG, Frane J. Growth hormone therapy of Turner syndrome: the impact of age of estrogen replacement on final height. Genentech, Inc., Collaborative Study Group. J Clin Endocrinol Metab 2000;85(7):2439–2445.
91. Sas TC, de Muinck K, Stijnen T, et al. Final height in girls with Turner's syndrome treated with once or twice daily growth hormone injections. Dutch Advisory Group on Growth Hormone. Arch Dis Child 1999;80(1):36–41.
92. Carel JC, Mathivon L, Gendrel C, Ducret JP, Chaussain JL. Near normalization of final height with adapted doses of growth hormone in Turner's syndrome. J Clin Endocrinol Metab 1998;83(5): 1462–1466.
93. Ranke MB, Lindberg A, Chatelain P, et al. Predicting the response to recombinant human growth hormone in Turner syndrome: KIGS models. KIGS International Board. Kabi International Growth Study. Acta Paediatr Suppl 1999;88(433):122–125.
94. Sas TC, Gerver WJ, de Bruin R, et al. Body proportions during long-term growth hormone treatment in girls with Turner syndrome participating in a randomized dose-response trial. J Clin Endocrinol Metab 1999;84(12):4622–4628.
95. Sato N, Nimura A, Horikawa R, Katumata N, Tanae A, Tanaka T. Bone mineral density in Turner syndrome: relation to GH treatment and estrogen treatment. Endocr J 2000;47(Suppl):S115–S119.
96. Rongen-Westerlaken C, Van Den Born E, Prahl-Andersen B, et al. Effect of growth hormone treatment on craniofacial growth in Turner's syndrome. Acta Paediatr 1993;82(4):364–368.

97. Ross JL, Feuillan P, Kushner H, Roeltgen D, Cutler GB Jr. Absence of growth hormone effects on cognitive function in girls with Turner syndrome. J Clin Endocrinol Metab 1997;82(6):1814–1817.
98. Huisman J, Slijper FM, Sinnema G, et al. Psychosocial effects of two years of human growth hormone treatment in Turner syndrome. The Dutch Working Group: Psychologists and Growth Hormone. Horm Res 1993;39 Suppl 2:56–59.
99. Siegel PT, Clopper R, Stabler B. The psychological consequences of Turner syndrome and review of the National Cooperative Growth Study psychological substudy. Pediatrics 1998;102 2 Pt 3:488–491.
100. Rovet J, Holland J. Psychological aspects of the Canadian randomized controlled trial of human growth hormone and low-dose ethinyl oestradiol in children with Turner syndrome. The Canadian Growth Hormone Advisory Group. Horm Res 1993;39(Suppl 2):60–64.
101. Joss EE, Zurbrugg RP, Tonz O, Mullis PE. Effect of growth hormone and oxandrolone treatment on glucose metabolism in Turner syndrome. A longitudinal study. Horm Res 2000;53(1):1–8.
102. Saenger P. Metabolic Consequences of Growth Hormone Treatment in Paediatric Practice. Horm Res 2000;53(Suppl)S1:60–69.
103. Sas TC, Muinck Keizer-Schrama SM, Stijnen T, Aanstoot HJ, Drop SL. Carbohydrate metabolism during long-term growth hormone (GH) treatment and after discontinuation of GH treatment in girls with Turner syndrome participating in a randomized dose-response study. Dutch Advisory Group on Growth Hormone. J Clin Endocrinol Metab 2000;85(2):769–775.
104. Rosenfeld RG, Hintz RL, Johanson AJ, et al. Three-year results of a randomized prospective trial of methionyl human growth hormone and oxandrolone in Turner syndrome. J Pediatr 1988;113(2):393–400.
105. Cavallo L, Gurrado R. Endogenous growth hormone secretion does not correlate with growth in patients with Turner's syndrome. Italian Study Group for Turner Syndrome. J Pediatr Endocrinol Metab 1999;12(5 Suppl 2):623–627.
106. Saenger P. Growth-promoting strategies in Turner's syndrome. J Clin Endocrinol Metab 1999;84(12):4345–4348.
107. Stool SE, Berg AO, Berman S, et al. Quick Reference Guide for Clinicans, Managing Otitis Media with Effusion in Young Children, Quick Reference Guide for Clinicans. AHCPR Publication No 94-0623 1994.
108. Rosenfield RL, Perovic N, Devine N. Optimizing estrogen replacement in adolescents with Turner syndrome. Ann N Y Acad Sci 2000;900:213–214.
109. Damiani D, Guedes DR, Fellous M, et al. Ullrich-Turner syndrome: relevance of searching for Y chromosome fragments. J Pediatr Endocrinol Metab 1999;12(6):827–831.
110. Foudila T, Soderstrom-Anttila V, Hovatta O. Turner's syndrome and pregnancies after oocyte donation. Hum Reprod 1999;14(2):532–535.
111. Boman UW, Moller A, Albertsson-Wikland K. Psychological aspects of Turner syndrome. J Psychosom Obstet Gynaecol 1998;19(1):1–18.

8 Management of Adults with Childhood Growth Hormone Deficiency

David M. Cook, MD

CONTENTS

    INTRODUCTION
    WHICH PATIENTS REMAIN PERSISTENTLY GH DEFICIENT AFTER CHILDHOOD?
    WHY SHOULD WE REPLACE YOUNG ADULTS WITH GH?
    CONTRAINDICATIONS FOR CONTINUING GH THERAPY
    CLINICAL EXAMPLES OF YOUNG ADULTS REQUIRING GH THERAPY
    MONITORING THERAPY
    SUMMARY
    REFERENCES

INTRODUCTION

In August, 1996 the FDA approved growth hormone (GH) replacement therapy for growth hormone deficient adults in the US. This approval was based upon studies of growth hormone deficient adults treated with growth hormone in clinical trials in Europe *(1)*. Naturally, the Europeans familiar with these clinical trials and earlier approval developed experience with GH replacement therapy in adults sooner than American adult endocrinologists. Various learning curves had to be developed in the US before adult endocrinologists became comfortable with diagnosing, dosing, and monitoring these patients. Meanwhile, pediatric endocrinologists in the US, long familiar with GH replacement therapy for children, began to struggle with management of GH deficient children who received GH for growth reasons and had achieved their target growth and bone age development with GH therapy. Traditionally, these patients discontinued GH and were not further replaced. Because GH deficient adults were found to have increased mortality rates, fracture rates, and reduced quality of life, and that these parameters seemed to reverse with GH therapy *(2–6)*, questions began to surface concerning whether young adults who were GH deficient as children should be restarted. A number of questions were generated by these circumstances that will be addressed in this review.

From: *Contemporary Endocrinology: Pediatric Endocrinology: A Practical Clinical Guide*
Edited by: S. Radovick and M. H. MacGillivray © Humana Press Inc., Totowa, NJ

Table 1
Etiology of Adult GHD in 1034 Hypopituitary Adult Patients[a]

Cause	%
Pituitary tumor	53.9
Craniopharyngioma	12.3
Idiopathic	10.2
CNS tumor	4.4
Empty sella syndrome	3.1
Sheehan's Syndrome	3.1
Head trauma	2.4
Hypophysitis	1.6
Surgery other than for pituitary treatment	1.5
Granulomatous diseases	1.3
Irradiation other than for pituitary treatment	1.1
CNS malformation	1.0
Perinatal trauma or infection	0.5
Other	2.5

[a]Adapted with permission from ref. (7).

This review will also cover experience to date concerning the metabolic changes observed in previously treated GH-deficient children after they stop GH and how they respond to restarting therapy.

WHICH PATIENTS REMAIN PERSISTENTLY GH DEFICIENT AFTER CHILDHOOD?

The various causes of GH deficiency (GHD) in children differ dramatically from etiologies of GH deficiency in adults. Most adults, for example, have readily recognizable causes of pituitary insufficiency due to obvious insults such as a tumor of the pituitary, surgery to remove the tumor or irradiation as part of the therapy of that tumor. There are, of course, a variety of other causes, but they are less common Table 1 (7). In adults just the presence of the tumor may affect normal pituitary function. It is estimated that patients with pituitary tumors who have all other hormones of the anterior pituitary intact will still have 25–35% chance of being GH deficient (8). As increasing damage occurs to the pituitary from the tumor or therapy and other hormones are lost, there is an increased incidence of GH deficiency. If 3 or 4 anterior pituitary hormones are lost, there is 95–100% chance of GH deficiency. If we couple the diagnosis of GH deficiency in adults with a low serum IGF-1, and three or four anterior pituitary hormone deficiencies, the probability of proving GH deficiency improves to a virtual certainty. Hartman has suggested that if the IGF-1 serum concentration is less than 84 ng/mL with pituitary damage and 3–4 anterior pituitary hormones lost there is a 98% chance the patient is GH deficient (9).

Childhood causes of GH deficiency differ from adult etiologies. A majority of childhood etiologies are idiopathic and not associated with known injury to the anterior pituitary Table 2 (10). Many of the children with isolated GH deficiency of childhood, who do not have other anterior pituitary hormone deficiencies and have an idiopathic

Table 2
Etiology of Childhood GHD[a]

Idiopathic	1366	72.3 %
Organic	424	22.4 %
Infection	6	0.3 %
Craniopharyngioma	149	7.9 %
CNS Tumor	144	7.6 %
Trauma	34	1.8 %
Irradiation	73	3.8 %
CNS Defects	13	0.7 %
Histiocytosis	5	0.3 %
Septo optia dysplasia	100	5.3 %

[a]Adapted with permission from ref. *(10)*.

Table 3
Consequences of Stopping GH in Childhood GHD Patients

1) Weight gain
2) Body composition changes (more fat)
3) Decreased bone density
4) Decreased exercise performance
5) Decreased ability to concentrate or study

cause, do not remain persistently GH deficient *(11,12)*. For this reason laboratory testing of this latter group is suggested to reconfirm the diagnosis.

The laboratory documentation necessary to reconfirm GH deficiency after childhood depends first upon the physician's clinical suspicion that the young adult might be persistently deficient. Not only does the clinician have to be suspicious, he or she must suggest to the patient there is a need for continuous replacement therapy into adulthood. In the current medical climate, the patient or family may challenge the physician as to whether the child should be continued on GH therapy. Typical consequences of GH deficiency that occur after stopping GH therapy in the average 18 or 19-yr-old patient are listed in Table 3. The accumulation of weight, especially in the truncal area, and decreased exercise performance are the most commonly reported complaints. Occasionally the young adult will notice a decrease in the ability to concentrate or study. The major impetus to return to therapy will come from the patient. Unfortunately, the average child does not want to return to the daily routine of receiving GH injections. In the future, this pattern will certainly change as pediatricians begin to inform patients that GH may be lifelong therapy. More user-friendly forms of GH delivery such as depot preparations are now available, such as Nutropin Depot, a two-wk delivery preparation *(12a)*. New technology may also facilitate GH replacement therapy. This agent is not currently approved for adults, but clinical studies are underway to create an adult indication. It may be that young adults, in transition to adult therapy, may benefit from continuing a depot preparation until their requirements decrease or they are ready to accept a daily injection regimen again.

Once the patient agrees to resume therapy, the next step is to verify if the deficiency is persistent. For patients who are panhypopituitary from causes such as craniopharyngioma, the documentation necessary for insurance approval will usually only consist of a single IGF-1 subnormal serum concentration. For those with isolated idiopathic causes, the documentation must be more rigorous and include a low serum IGF-1 concentration coupled with one or two GH release stimulation tests to confirm the diagnosis. As in children, there is no foolproof magic stimulation test. Any of the standard tests are associated with responses that are 15–20% false negative in normal individuals *(13)*. This would include arginine, L-Dopa, insulin-induced hypoglycemia, or growth hormone releasing hormone (GHRH). Combining arginine with GHRH probably has fewer, if any, false negative results. However, it stimulates pituitary release of GH by inhibiting somatostatin with arginine and affects the pituitary directly with GHRH *(14)*. Data generated in studies of USA patients *(14a)* suggest a cut-off of 4.1 with arginine plus GHRH since GH stimulation test remains a controversial way to diagnose GHD. The standard 5 ng/mL is used in the USA for arginine plus GHRH testing and/or insulin-induced hypoglycemia. One theoretical problem associated with the combined arginine/GHRH test is the false negative rate observed in patients with neurosecretory deficiency of GH, which might be observed in patients who have received cranial irradiation for childhood leukemia. In the final analysis, laboratory diagnosis of GH deficiency in the adult or the child who has completed vertical growth is arbitrary, and stimulation testing is not foolproof. We have established criteria for GH deficiency as follows: 1) the patient should have a reasonable cause for the deficiency. The documentation during childhood with associated poor growth is sufficient to satisfy these criteria. 2) The second criteria is a low IGF-1 for age and sex, and 3) the third criteria is a poor response to a standard provocative stimulus. The only caveat for the latter criteria is to eliminate clonidine as a stimulation test, which is an adequate stimulus to GH release in children but not considered an adequate test in adults because of excessive false positives (suggesting GH deficiency when it doesn't exist) in normals *(18)*.

It is estimated that around 40% of patients with idiopathic GH deficiency in childhood will not be GH deficient as adults. This fact underscores the need for complete laboratory testing for this group of patients if they are to be considered for GH replacement therapy. The literature would suggest that approximately 35% of patients with isolated GHD would revert to normal upon retesting after they have stopped GH therapy *(19)*. For idiopathic deficiency associated with multiple hormones deficient the number drops to 11% and for X-ray induced cranial irradiation the rate drops to 3%. In craniopharyngioma the number of patients that have normal stimulation tests after GH therapy in childhood is close to zero. For this reason, many insurance companies will accept a low insulin-like growth factor (IGF-1) as adequate proof the patient is persistently GH deficient. Maghnie has looked at the predictive value of pituitary magnetic resonance imaging (MRI) findings with the thought that small pituitary volume might be more predictive of chronic GH deficient *(20)*. He separated patients into four groups. The first two groups consisted of one with small pituitary gland size and the second with normal size pituitary based upon MRI findings. The other two groups consisted of one with stalk agenesis and the last with craniopharyngioma. The pituitary size was not helpful for predicting persistent GH deficiency, and insulin or arginine testing results were quite variable. Combining arginine with insulin-induced hypoglycemia demonstrated almost complete responsiveness in the first two groups and no responsiveness in the latter two groups. The study underscored the difficulties in making the diagnosis of GHD in patients with isolated GH deficiency. In summary, more stringent testing of patients with idiopathic GHD of childhood onset is necessary. To this end, insulin-induced hypoglycemia or arginine plus GHRH is suggeted to provide convincing evidence of persistent GHD. Less stringent tests such as L-DOPA or arginine alone are not suggested since they are less stringent and release GH to a lower cut-off point than insulin or arginine plus GHRH *(14a)*.

WHY SHOULD WE REPLACE YOUNG ADULTS WITH GH?

The indications for return of GH therapy in children who have completed growth targets and are in transition to adulthood are the same for adults who have developed the deficiency later in life. GH deficiency in adults is associated with increased mortality, decreased quality of life and an increase in bone fracture rates. Other reasons include abnormal risk factors for accelerated atherogenesis, including increased cholesterol and decreased HDL cholesterol. Although these findings are compelling reasons to treat young adults who have completed vertical growth, the major impetus stems from the issues surrounding bone health. We now believe that the full bone maturation process continues to around age thirty. Stopping GH at age 17 or 18, could theoretically inhibit this process and leave these patients at risk for early age osteoporosis *(21,22)*. The evidence for this phenomena is indirect but convincing. Ter Maaten has looked at a group of 38 patients who were GH deficient as children and received subsequent GH therapy for a period of 3–5 yr *(23)*. This group showed marked improvement in leg muscle area, decreases in skin fold and intra-abdominal fat, and improvement in total bone mineral content. Kaufman has looked at the bone mineral content in GH-deficient males with isolated and multiple deficiencies *(24)*. In both groups bone density is decreased. Since mortality figures have to do with an older population and is only theoretically important when talking to an 18-yr-old young man or woman, it is really bone density and the risk for fracture that is the most important indication for continuing GH in the transitioning patient.

Various studies have reported decreased bone density in young adults who have been GH deficient as children. Not only are the bones decreased in density, they seem to be small bones with small bone volumes *(25)*. There is no current data to suggest that these bones are at risk for fracture, but the assumption seems valid. We do know that maximum development of bones continues until age 30. If the young adult stops GH at age 17 and GH is necessary for bone maturation and development, a strong case can be made for continuing GH not only until age thirty, but lifelong.

In adults, quality of life is dramatically improved with replacement of GH in GH-deficient adults *(26)*. In children, there does not seem to be this dramatic difference in quality of life change after replacing GH. The reasons for this are not clear. One suggested explanation is that adults remember their previous functioning level of energy they had before developing GH deficiency, and children do not. We do know that children who remain GH deficient after childhood may not achieve successful employment *(27)*.

In summary, quality of life issues do not emerge as an important reason to continue GH therapy after childhood. It must be kept in mind, however, just how important these quality of life questions can be when addressed not only to the patient but also to the spouse or parent. The individual patient may not recognize the subtle consequences of chronic GH deficiency as well as their mother, father, or cohabiting partner. It is only when the patient returns to GH therapy that they realize what was missing. Burman demonstrated this in a quality of life study in adults *(28)*. This author studied GH defi-

Table 4
Why Childhood Deficiency Young Adults
Do Not Return to Therapy

1) The patient does not want to return to "shots"
2) The patient "feels fine"
3) The patient was told he/she could discontinue after growth potential achieved
4) The patient lacks motivation
5) The patient is not currently insured
6) The patient is not going to any physician much less an endocrinologist

cient adults taking GH replacement therapy and questioning the spouse on what changes they noticed in the functioning level of the patient. The responses of the spouses were statistically significant compared to those from the individual patients. Whether this same situation exists for young adults is not clear. What does appear to be clear is that almost every reason that can exist is operative in keeping many young adults from returning to GH replacement. Some reasons are listed in Table 4. The most common reason appears to be that the young adult does not want to return to "shots". These young adults often fall into other categories of not returning. The second is that the pediatrician did not discuss the possibility of continuing therapy after growth potential has been reached. This is clearly not an indictment of the pediatric endocrinologist, but only a fact of historical note. This is a very new idea and there was no need to introduce this concept to children as early as 6 yr ago when GH was first approved for GH-deficient adults, and only in the last 10 yr has the syndrome of GH deficiency in GH deficient adults been recognized.

Another reason for not returning to GH therapy after childhood is the lapse of insurance coverage when the child leaves home. New insurance plans often have an exclusion of GH for adults, and patients may not realize that they signed up for a group plan with this exclusion. Lastly, there is the impression from clinicians, such as myself, that these patients lose energy and motivation after stopping GH and cannot coordinate whatever it takes to return to GH therapy.

CONTRAINDICATIONS FOR CONTINUING GH THERAPY

Before reinstating GH it is reasonable to consider the contraindications to GH that might exist or have developed since stopping GH therapy. The first and most important would be the development of a malignancy. This should be obvious by the history, but the clinician should be aware of this possibility. Some patients may have had a central nervous system tumor that was irradiated in childhood. This should be re-examined by an appropriate MRI image of the pituitary area. The tumor may have recurred, or more importantly, a new tumor may have developed because of irradiation to the area. Developing a second central nervous system tumor is a known risk to after cranial irradiation. Known pituitary tumors such as craniopharyngioma should be stable for a 6-mo period before initiating GH. For this reason, an MRI is suggested in the year preceding GH therapy if a tumor is causing GH deficiency. If the cause is idiopathic and the patient is proven in the laboratory to be GH deficient, we suggest an MRI if an anatomic cause has not been ruled out. The young patient may, for example, have had a lesser quality CT scan of their pituitary area. An MRI may reveal stalk agenesis not seen with a less sensitive

Table 5
Laboratory Data of a 19-yr-old GH Deficient Male Patient

Test	Normal	Patient
Luteinizing Hormone	0.2–9 mIu/mL	0.9
Testosterone	270–1070 ng/dL	25
IGF-1	182–780 ng/mL	42 ng/mL
TSH	0.23–4.0 mIu/mL	1.8
Free T4	0.7–1.8 ng/dL	1.5

technique. This finding may help to support the diagnosis and need for lifelong therapy. An anatomic abnormality of the pituitary, it will also boost insurance approval, and help endorse continued need for GH replacement therapy if an anatomic lesion is identified.

Diabetes mellitus is another contraindication to GH therapy, if the diabetes is associated with proliferative retinopathy. Types I and II diabetes are not contraindications. If the patient is diabetic and GH therapy has begun, the diabetic control will worsen before it becomes better because of the positive affect on body composition. The increase in body fat, especially visceral fat, is associated with insulin resistance in the untreated adult GH-deficient patient. Administration of GH will aggravate the insulin resistant state and aggravate glucose control. After a period of time, GH therapy will change body composition, improve insulin sensitivity, and return glucose control. This will usually translate to an increase in insulin requirements by about 20%, or double the oral hypoglycemic drug therapy required to control glucose. Individual patients will differ. However, the patient should be warned that diabetes control will get worse before it gets better.

Pregnancy is not a contraindication for GH therapy. The placenta will produce human somatomammotropin during the third trimester, and therefore, during the last three months GH is not necessary.

CLINICAL EXAMPLES OF YOUNG ADULTS REQUIRING GH THERAPY

The Young Adult who has Never Been Treated

A 19-yr-old man was referred to our clinic from a specialist in internal medicine. He is from the Gilbert Islands in the South Pacific. He was evaluated in Australia in 1990 and found to be GH deficient. He was not approved for GH therapy because he was not an Australian citizen. He was lost to follow up until American missionaries found a way to help a number of needy young people living in the Gilbert Islands. His growth history was one of lifelong slow growth and arrest of growth at age 17. He has never developed secondary sex characteristics. On physical exam he weighed 146 lbs, and his height was 59 in, span 61 in, and lower segment 31 in. He had gynecomastia with a diameter of 7 cm right and 8 cm left. His testes measure 8 mm by 6 mm right and left, and he had no body hair. He had mild scrotal wrinkling. He had very poor muscle development. Laboratory data is listed in Table 5. An insulin tolerance test is given in Table 6. He had virtually no GH reserve and limited adrenocorticotropin (ACTH) and Cortisol reserve. His serum IGF-1 was 38 ng/mL (normal 180–780). His bone density results are listed in Table 7. Of note, his body percentage of fat was 51.1%. This later figure was quite striking considering that his BMI was calculated to be 29.4. The MRI of his pituitary revealed partial septo-

Table 6
Insulin Tolerance Test in a 19-yr-old Young Man With GHD

Time (min)	Glucose (mg %)	Growth hormone (ng/mL)	ACTH pg/mL	Cortisol (µg %)
0	85	<0.1	15.0	10.0
+20	37	<0.1	13.0	7.0
+40	28	<0.1	20.0	9.0
+60	210	.20	112.0	14.0
+90	108	<0.1	15.0	16.0

Table 7
DEXA Bone Density and Body Fat Percentage of a 19-yr-old GHD Patient

Location	% Age and sex normals
Hip	58%
Spine	70%
Percent body fat	51.1 %

optic dysplasia. His previous CT taken in Australia in 1990 was normal. His bone age of his left hand was that of a 16-yr-old.

Because of the theoretical potential for some bone growth and development, our plan was to begin with growth hormone alone despite the androgen deficiency. We start such "transition age" patients on a dose of 800 µg/d and plan to advance the dose by 400 µg every 4–6 wk, until the IGF-1 is in the mid- to high normal range (180–780 ng/mL). After a year of GH therapy, we will add sex steroids. This case is representative of patients who may have never received GH and who may need larger doses than the average adult. He may have some potential for vertical growth and we do not want to jeopardize this potential by adding sex steroids too soon.

17-yr-old who Recently Stopped GH and Referred for Continuing Care by her Pediatrician

A 17-yr-old woman is sent to you by her pediatrician for continuing care of her growth hormone deficiency of childhood. The patient had been treated with growth hormone since age four. Since stopping growth hormone one year ago she has noticed a weight increase of 15 lbs, decrease in exercise capability, and has noticed an inability to walk up stairs as well as she had while on growth hormone. She has had one CAT scan at age four but no other imaging of her pituitary. She is on no other replacement. On physical exam, she weighed 122 lbs and her height was 64.5 in. Her IGF-1 was 34 ng/mL (nl 182–780 ng/mL). Her growth hormone was undetectable before and after growth hormone stimulation with arginine plus GHRH. Her bone density in her lumbar spine was 93% of age matched normals and 91% at her hip. Bone density should be reported as two scores or percent of normal for age and gender. Using t scores is not appropriate for young adults below age 25 since peak bone mass is still developing. Using t scores may overstimate bone deficiency. Despite looking fit, her body fat was 35.6%, unexpectedly high, especially considering that her BMI was calculated to be 20.3. Her MRI was repeated and found to be perfectly normal. She was begun on 800 µg/d and the plan is to titrate her dose until IGF-1 is in the mid- to high normal range for her age and sex. This case represents as example of marked fat deposition associated with growth hormone deficiency in a young adult. It underscores the body composition changes after stopping GH replacement therapy in young adults. Her history of muscle weakness is also consistent with GH deficiency. She should be encouraged to continue GH life long.

Twenty-yr-old Young Man with a Craniopharyngioma

A 20-yr-old man is sent to you by a neurosurgeon for evaluation of his endocrine status. He had normal growth and development but has recently been found to have a craniopharyngioma identified because of the development of visual field abnormalities. Because of the visual field abnormalities, he underwent pituitary surgery to remove the tumor. Subsequent to the surgery he was found to be growth hormone deficient. After a year of replacement therapy with testosterone, thyroid hormone, and cortisol, and stable MRI image of his pituitary tumor, he returns for followup care. On physical exam he weighed 327 lbs, and was 67 in tall. His IGF-1 concentration was undetectable and he had no GH response to arginine stimulation testing (all GH concentrations less than 0.1 ng/mL). His fasting insulin was 48 IU/mL and simultaneous glucose 115 mg%. Because we were concerned about his glucose status we proceeded with GH therapy cautiously. He was started on 0.3 mg sc daily. Immediately he began to have polyuria and polydipsia. This progressed to moderate ketoacidosis over a 1-wk period. Because of this rather dramatic and sudden appearance of type II diabetes he did not want to restart GH therapy for fear of going into ketoacidosis again. Very shortly thereafter he required oral hypoglycemic agents to control his blood sugar. This case represents the extreme of aggravation of diabetes after beginning GH therapy, or exposing latent diabetes after starting GH therapy. Physicians should be aware of this category of patient when beginning GH therapy or tell their diabetic patients their diabetic control will get worse before it gets better.

27-yr-old Woman who Received Cranial Irradiation for Childhood Leukemia

This young lady presented with leukemia at age six. She received cranial irradiation at that age. After a recurrence at age twelve, she underwent a second course of cranial irradiation. Her growth was not impaired but she did have gonadotropin deficiency develop at age 23, with cessation of her menses, low estradiol and low serum gonadotropins. She has been started on premarin 0.625mg and provera 2.5mg. Her IGF-1 concentration was 97mg/ml (nl 182–481 ng/mL), and she had no detectable GH in response to insulin-induced hypoglycemia. She was begun on 0.3 mg and her dose escalated to bring her IGF-1 into the mid- normal range (*see* Table 8). At a dose of 14 µg/kg/d (1.2 mg/d) she had muscle and joint pain and pedal edema which was uncomfortable. At a dose of 12 µg/kg/d (1.0 mg/d) she felt comfortable and has continued on that dose. This patient represents the typical course of patients in their late twenties who require doses somewhere in between patients in their late teens or early twenties. She also represents the typical patient whose dose is controlled more by symptom tolerance than an absolute IGF-1 concentration.

Table 8
Escalation of GH Dose in a 27-yr-old Woman
With Childhood Leukemia & CNS Irradiation

µg/kd/d	µg/d	182–481 IGF-1 ng/mL (nl/ng/mL)
none	none	97 ng/mL
4	300	132
8	700	204
14	1200	224
12	1000*	180

*Reduced because of muscle pain and edema

19-yr-old Woman with Autoimmune Hypophysitis

This 19-yr-old woman was referred for evaluation of persistent fatigue despite normalization of free T4 and TSH for primary hypothyroidism. Because of the known association of autoimmune thyroid disease and pituitary autoimmunity, an IGF-1 concentration was obtained which was low, i.e., 60 ng/mL (nl 182–780 ng/mL). She was proven to have GH deficiency on the basis of a poor response of GH to insulin induced hypoglycemia (peak GH 3.3 ng/mL with normal responses greater than 5 ng/mL). Her dose was titrated to a mid range IGF-1 concentration to a total dose of 2.4 mg/d, which she tolerated without side effects. This young lady represents dosing experience with patients in their late teen and early twenties. She has required and tolerated rather large doses of GH to normalize her IGF-1 concentration and to achieve sufficient bipolysis. She did not have side effects of GH therapy, and her maintenance dose was established by titrating to mid to high normal IGF-1 concentration.

MONITORING THERAPY

Successful monitoring of the patient receiving GH therapy requires an awareness of side effects, not only of GH excess, but also symptoms associated with starting GH and/or raising a dose. Patients can frequently have transient adverse symptoms (usually d 7–10) after starting or raising a dose. These consist of muscle or joint pain and disappear by d 14–16 after initiating or raising dose. If symptoms persist after this period of time, the dose is considered excessive and the dose should be reduced to the next lower tolerated dose. The symptoms of excess should be covered by a discussion with the patient prior to initiating therapy. These can consist of muscle or joint pain, headache, edema, or carpal tunnel syndrome. The latter is managed by a four-day holiday from drug therapy then resumption of the same dose.

The patient's weight should be followed and the patient cautioned that weight loss is not usually observed with GH therapy but body composition changes are. From a low technology (and low cost) standpoint, waist and hip circumference should be obtained at 6 mo intervals. Usually the waist circumference will change more quickly than the hips, or both may improve despite no significant change in weight. If insurance will allow, DEXA should be performed before GH therapy is begun. When ordering this

Table 9
GH Dose Requirements of a 19-yr-old Patient
With Autoimmune Hypophysitis

Date	µg/d	IGF-1 (nl 180–780 ng/mL)
8/97	800	60
10/97	1200	130
1/98	1600	204
3/98	2000	300
5/98	2400	480

procedure, the best parameters to follow are hip, spine, and body composition. The software for the latter determination is widely available and should be requested. Since bone density decreases after beginning GH therapy in the first 6 mo, returns to baseline at 12 mo, and increases from baseline at 18 mo, we suggest the second DEXA study be performed no sooner than 18 mo after beginning therapy, then yearly thereafter.

Serum IGF-1 concentrations should be followed at 4- to 6-wk intervals until the plateau or maintenance dose is reached, then every 6 mo. The serum IGF-1 is more of a safety guide than an absolute concentration that defines the target dose. The IGF-1 should be used primarily as a guide to over therapy. If the IGF-1 exceeds the normal range, the dose should be reduced. An IGF-1 in the mid normal range is the target, but it should be recognized that there is no magic level. In most adults, the maintenance dose is reached by pushing the dose to tolerance and the development of symptoms of excess, then backing off to a tolerable level. In following this format the serum IGF-1 concentration is seldom exceeded.

Lipid concentrations may be obtained yearly. However, if there are no lipid abnormalities at baseline, there is no need to repeat these since they will only improve and not deteriorate. Blood sugar should be obtained and followed at 6-mo intervals to make sure the patient does not develop hyperglycemia. The index of suspicion should be greatest in patients who were hyperglycemic if and when they were suffering from Cushing's Disease and later had successful pituitary surgery, or if they have a family history of type II diabetes, and are currently obese.

SUMMARY

The treatment of young adults who have been growth hormone deficient as children is an emerging clinical science. The first and foremost important rule is to confirm the patient is persistently deficient, especially in patients who carry the diagnosis of idiopathic GH deficiency. A number of issues surround therapy including dosing and monitoring. As time passes, there will be more young adult patients seeking therapy for a number of reasons. These include education of pediatricians, and adult endocrinologists who are familiar with the care of this group of patients and the patients themselves seeking a solution to their symptoms. For both patients and physicians, the process of getting patients back on therapy will be very satisfying because of the return of energy, physical performance and restoration of body composition.

REFERENCES

1. Attanasio AF, Lamberts, SWJ, Matranga AMC, et al. Adult growth hormone deficient patients demonstrate heterogenity between childhood onset and adult onset before and during human GH treatment. J Clin Endocrinol Metab 1997;82:82–88.
2. Rosen T, Bengtsson BA. Premature mortality due to cardiovascular disease in hypopituitarism. Lancet 1990;336:285–288.
3. Bates AS, Van't Hoff W, Jones PJ, et al. The effect of hypopituitarism on life expectancy. J Clin Endocrinol Metab 1996;81:1169–1172.
4. Rosen T, Wilhelmsen L, Landin-Wilhelmsen K, et al. Increased fracture frequency in adult patients with hypopituitarism and GH deficiency. Euro J Endocrinol 1997;137:240–245.
5. Bulow B, Hagmar L, Mikoczy Z, et al. Increased cerebrovascular mortality in patients with hypopituitarism. Clin Endocrinol 1997;46:75–81.
6. Wiren L, Bengtsson B, Johannsson G. Beneficial effects of long-term GH replacement therapy on quality of life in adults with GH deficiency. Clin Endocrinol 1998;48:613–620.
7. Adapted from Clin Endocrinol 1990;50:703–713.
8. Toogood AA, O'Neill P, Shalet S. The severity of growth hormone deficiency in adults with pituitary disease is related to the degree of hypopituitarism. Clin Endocrinol 1994;41:511–516.
9. Hartman ML, Crowe BJ, Biller BM, et al. Which patients do not require a GH stimulation test for the diagnosis of adult GH deficiency? J Clin Endocrinol Metab. 2002;87(2):477–485.
10. August GP, et al. J of Peds 1990;116:899.
11. DeBoer H, van der Veen EA. Why retest young adults with childhood-onset growth hormone deficiency. J Clin Endocrinol Metab 1997;82:2032–2036.
12. Nicolson A, Toogood A, Rahim A, et al. The prevalence of severe growth hormone deficiency in adults who received growth hormone replacement in childhood. Clin Endocrinol 1996;44:311–316.
12a. Cook DM, Bill BMK, Vance ML, et al. The pharmacokinetic and pharmacodynamic characteristics of a long-acting growth hormone (GH) preparation (nutropin depot) in GH-deficient adults. J Clin Endocrinol Metab. 2002;87(10):4508–4514.
13. Ghigo E, Bellone J, Aimaretti G, et al. Reliability of provocative tests to assess growth hormone secretory status. Study in 472 normally growing children. J Clin Endocrinol Metab 1996;81:3323–3327.
14. Aimaretti G, Corneli G, Razzore P, et al. Comparison between insulin-induced hypoglycemia and growth hormone (GH)-releasing hormone + arginine as provocative tests for the diagnosis of GH deficiency in adults. J Clin Endocrinol Metab 1998;83:1615–1618.
14a. Biller BM, Samuels MH, Zager A, et al. Sensitivity and specificty of six tests for the diagnosis of adult GH deficiency. J Clin Endocrinol Metab. 2002;87(5):2067–2079.
15. Growth Hormone Research Society. Consensus guidelines for the diagnosis and treatment of adults with growth hormone deficiency: summary statement of the Growth Hormone Research Society Workshop on adult growth hormone deficiency. J Clin Endocrinol Metab 1998;83:379–381.
16. Hoffman DM, O'Sullivan AJ, Baxter RC, et al. Diagnosis of growth hormone deficiency in adults. Lancet 1994;343:1064–1068.
17. Aimaretti G, Corneli G, Razzore P, et al. Comparison between insulin induced hypoglycemia and growth hormone (GH)-releasing hormone + arginine as provocative tests for the diagnosis of GH deficiency in adults. J Clin Endocrinol Metab 1998;83:1615–1618.
18. Rahim A, Toogood A, Shalet SM. The assessment of growth hormone in normal young adults using a vareity of provocative agents. Clin Endocrinol 1996;45:557–562.
19. Wacharasindhu S, Cotterill AM, Camacho-Hubner C, et al. Normal growth hormone secretion in growth hormone insufficient children retested after completion of linear growth. Clin Endocrinol 1996;45:553–556.
20. Maghnie M, Strigazzi C, Tinelli C, et al. Growth hormone (GH) deficiency (GHD) of childhood onset: Reassessment of GH status and evaluation of the predictive criteria for permanent GHD in young adults. J Clin Endocrinol Metab 1999;84:1324–1328.
21. Saggese G, Baroncelli G, Bertelloni S, et al. The effect of long-term growth hormone (GH) treatment on bone mineral density in children with GH deficiency. Role of GH in the attainment of peak bone mass. J Clin Endocrinol Metab 1996;81:3077–3083.
22. DeBoer H, Blok G, Van Lingen A, et al. Consequences of childhood-onset growth hormone deficiency for adult bone mass. J Bone Min Res 1994;9:1319–1322.
23. Ter Maaten J, DeBoer H, Kamp O, et al. Long-term effects of growth hormone (GH) replacement in men with childhood-onset GH deficiency. J Clin Endocrinol Metab 1999;84:2373–2380.

24. Kaufman JM, Taelman P, Vermeulen A, et al. Bone mineral status in growth hormone-deficient males with isolated and multiple pituitary deficiencies of childhood onset. J Clin Endocrinol Metab 1992;74:118–123.
25. Baroncelli G, Bertelloni S, Ceccarelli C, et al. Measurement of volumetric bone mineral density accurately determines degree of lumbar undermineralization in children with growth hormone deficiency. J Clin Endocrinol Metab 1998;83:3150–3154.
26. Wiren R, Wilhelmsen L, Wiklund I, et al. Decreased psychological well-being in adult patients with growth hormone deficiency. J Clin Endocrinol 1994;40:111–116.
27. Gartorio A, Molinari P, Grugni G, et al. The psychosocial outcome of adults with growth hormone deficiency. Acta Med Auxol 1986;18:123–128.
28. Burman P, Broman JE, Hetta J, et al. Quality of life in adults with growth hormone (GH) deficiency: response to treatment with recombinant human GH in a placebo-controlled 21-month trial. J Clin Endocrinol Metab 1995;80:3585–3590.

II HYPOTHALAMIC AND PITUITARY DISORDERS

9 Diabetes Insipidus

Frederick D. Grant, MD

CONTENTS

INTRODUCTION
NORMAL PHYSIOLOGY OF WATER BALANCE
CLINICAL PRESENTATION
CAUSES OF DIABETES INSIPIDUS
DIAGNOSIS
TREATMENT OF DIABETES INSIPIDUS
REFERENCES

INTRODUCTION

Diabetes insipidus (DI) is a syndrome of dysregulated free water balance resulting from vasopressin deficiency or insensitivity of the kidney to vasopressin action. In the absence of vasopressin-mediated urinary concentration, there is increased excretion (polyuria) of dilute (urine osmolality less than plasma osmolality) urine. The loss of free water leads to increased thirst and water intake (polydipsia). If the thirst is not quenched, the progressive free water deficit leads to a hyperosmolar state characterized by plasma hypernatremia. Diabetes insipidus may be characterized as central, when due to vasopressin deficiency, or nephrogenic, when the result of diminished renal responsiveness to the antidiuretic action of vasopressin. Central diabetes insipidus can be treated with vasopressin or vasopressin analogs such as desmopressin. Treatment of nephrogenic diabetes insipidus typically depends upon reversal of the underlying cause, but pharmacological treatment may be successful.

NORMAL PHYSIOLOGY OF WATER BALANCE

Vasopressin is the mammalian anti-diuretic hormone and regulator of free water balance and plasma osmolality. Vasopressin regulates plasma sodium concentration, but does not control total body sodium content, and thus has little effect on total body volume. Vasopressin is synthesized in neurons of the hypothalamus, then undergoes axonal transport through the pituitary stalk to the nerve endings that form the posterior pituitary gland. Regulated vasopressin secretion from the posterior pituitary occurs in response to physiological stimuli, such as hyperosmolality and volume depletion *(1)*. In the kidney, circulating vasopressin can bind to V2 vasopressin receptors located on the

From: *Contemporary Endocrinology: Pediatric Endocrinology: A Practical Clinical Guide*
Edited by: S. Radovick and M. H. MacGillivray © Humana Press Inc., Totowa, NJ

basolateral surface of epithelial cells in the distal tubule and collecting duct of the nephron. V2 receptor activation drives synthesis and translocation of aquaporin water channels to the luminal surface of the epithelial cells where these channels facilitate reabsorption of water *(2)*. This tubular reabsorption of water concentrates the urine and conserves total body water.

Plasma osmolality normally is regulated within a narrow range of approx 285–295 mosm/kg *(1)*. After water deprivation, increased plasma osmolality stimulates release of vasopressin from the posterior pituitary. Vasopressin-mediated urine concentration increases urine osmolality to greater than plasma osmolality, and with maximal urinary concentration, urinary osmolality can be as high as 1000 mosm/kg. If the action of vasopressin is not sufficient to maintain appropriate free water balance, a further increase in plasma osmoality stimulates thirst, which leads to intake of additional free water. With sufficient free water intake, plasma osmolality is maintained in the normal range *(4)*. However, if thirst is impaired or water is not available, continued dehydration results in the development of hyperosmolarity.

CLINICAL PRESENTATION

The clinical hallmarks of diabetes insipidus are polyuria of inappropriately dilute urine and hyperosmolarity. Polyuria can be defined as a urine output of greater than 2 L/m^2/d or approximately 40 mL/kg/d *(5)* and may be due to either a solute diuresis or water diuresis *(6)*. A solute diuresis can result from an excess excretion of either inorganic or organic solute. Filtration of exogenously administered sodium, such as after intravenous administration of large volumes of saline, will produce a solute diuresis as the excess sodium is excreted via the urine. Most diuretics produce a diuresis by increasing distal delivery of isotonic tubular filtrate to increase urine output. Excess delivery of other inorganic solutes, such as ammonia or bicarbonate also will induce a solute diuresis. Glucose will produce polyuria if plasma levels are sufficiently high (typically >180 mg/dL) so that the rate of glomerular filtration overwhelms the tubular reabsorption of glucose. Other organic solutes, such as mannitol, can be filtered, but do not undergo tubular reabsorption and will produce an osmotic diuresis *(6)*. Therefore, a solute diuresis will result in copious production of urine, but the presence of solute typically produces nondilute urine with urine osmolality greater than plasma osmolality.

A water diuresis is the production of large volume of dilute urine with osmolality less than plasma osmolality and typically less than 200 mosm/kg. A water diuresis can occur in response to a large water load such as the intentional intake of excess free water *(6)*. Primary polydipsia may be related to a pathophysiological disorder of thirst secondary to disruption of the thirst regulation in the hypothalamus (dipsogenic polydipsia) *(7)*. More typically, primary polydipsia is a volitional act with the volume of water drunk in excess of the needs of the body to maintain a normoosmolar state. Primary polydipsia may occur from habit or in response to social cues, but when severe is usually related to a psychiatric disturbance (psychogenic polydipisa). Patients with non-dipsogenic polydipsia do not have increased thirst, *per se*, but patients with psychogenic polydipsia have compulsive drinking that remits with resolution of psychiatric symptoms *(4)*. In contrast to primary polydipsia, patients with diabetes insipidus excrete dilute, hypoosmolar urine due to impaired urinary concentrating ability, and the resulting increased thirst and polydipsia is an appropriate physiological response to the loss of free water.

Hypernatremia is the most commonly measured manifestation of a hyperosmolar state. Sodium, with an equimolar amount of anions, accounts for most of the measurable and effective osmotic load of plasma. A free water deficit that results in a hyperosmolar state will produce hypernatremia, and therefore the plasma sodium level frequently serves as a clinical surrogate for osmolality. Hypernatremia can result from sodium excess or free water deficit (8). Most circumstances of excess sodium intake occur in situations where the individual has little control of intake. Examples of clinical situations with sodium excess include excess administration of hypertonic intravenous fluids, or excessive oral ingestion of hypertonic fluids such as seawater or hypertonic infant formula (9). Hypernatremia more commonly is the result of a free-water deficit. Water deprivation with persistent insensible losses leads to a free-water deficit that will cause a progressive increase in plasma osmolality. The normal response to hyperosmolality is increased secretion of vasopressin, which then acts on the kidney to concentrate the urine and facilitate free water conservation. After loss of both salt and water, impaired access to water or a relatively greater loss of water can lead to hypernatremia, even if total body sodium is also depleted. Thus, a diuresis can produce both hypernatremia and a decrease in blood volume. Diabetes insipidus is characterized by a defect in renal free water conservation. Patients with diabetes insipidus develop increased thirst and polydipsia to prevent development of hyperosmolality, but if free water intake is impaired, hyperosmolality and hypernatremia will develop.

Diabetes insipidus may occur acutely or may present as a more chronic condition. Non-traumatic central diabetes insipidus and most cases of nephrogenic diabetes insipidus present as chronic conditions. Hypothalamic or pituitary damage can lead to the acute onset of diabetes insipidus. The classic triphasic response has been described after injury to the pituitary or neurohypophysis (10). This is of particular note when managing the post-operative care of patients after surgery of the pituitary or hypothalamus. Within the first 12–48 h after acute trauma, vasopressin secretion may be severely impaired and result in diabetes insipidus. If the damage is severe enough to produce axonal degeneration in vasopressin secreting neurons, there will be unregulated secretion of vasopressin to the peripheral circulation. This can result in inappropriate anti-diuresis (SAIDH) and may lead to development of hyponatremia between 5–12 d after pituitary damage. If the trauma is so severe as to cause death of vasopressinergic neurons, then prolonged diabetes insipidus may ensue. Only some phases of this response may be clinically evident after acute damage to the pituitary or pituitary stalk, with no more than 10% of patients exhibiting all three phases (10).

The effect of diabetes insipidus on growth and development of children depends upon the age at which the disease becomes clinically apparent. With untreated diabetes insipidus, increased fluid intake will alter caloric intake. Children who drink water in preference to food or who have anorexia related to hypernatremia may show growth delay due to chronic derangement of water balance and caloric malnutrition (11). However, intake of large quantities of sweetened beverages in response to the increased thirst of diabetes insipidus can markedly increase caloric intake and lead to obesity. Nursing infants receive both caloric and free water intake from breast milk or formula. Chronic water deprivation in infants can lead to failure to thrive, irritability, constipation, and even fever (12). However, increased formula intake in response to increased thirst will provide calories in excess of needs and may result in the development of obesity in infants with diabetes insipidus (13).

Table 1
Causes of Central Diabetes Insipidus

Congenital
    Developmental Defects: septo-optic dysplasia, other mid-line defects
    Inherited Genetic Defects: Familial Diabetes Insipidus, Wolfram (DIDMOAD) syndrome

Pituitary Injury
    Head trauma
    Supra-sellar tumors: craniopharyngioma, germinoma
    Pituitary macroademona
    Surgery
    Vascular: cerebral aneurysm, intracranial hemorrhage, sickle cell disease

Infiltrative and Inflammatory Disorders
    Granulomatous Diseases: histiocytosis, sarcoidosis, Wegener's granulomatosis, syphillis
    Neoplasm: CNS lymphoma, leukemia, metastatic carcinoma (breast)
    Infections: bacterial meningitis, tubercular meningitis, viral encephalitis
    Autoimmune hypophysitis

CAUSES OF DIABETES INSIPIDUS

Diabetes insipidus results from an inadequate level of vasopressin or an impaired renal response to circulating vasopressin. Inadequate levels of vasopressin are nearly always associated with impaired pituitary secretion of vasopressin and can result from three main mechanisms: congenital deficiency of vasopressin, physical destruction of vasopressin secreting neurons, or the presence of an infiltrative or inflammatory process that inhibits vasopressin synthesis, transport, or secretion (Table 1).

Vasopressin deficiency may occur with a wide variety of congenital disorders, such as septo-optic dysplasia, that disrupt the normal development of the pituitary gland and other midline structures *(14)*. Diabetes insipidus is part of Wolfram's (DIDMOAD) Syndrome that is characterized by central Diabetes Insipidus, Diabetes Mellitus, Optic Atrophy, and sensorineural Deafness resulting from mutation of the *wolframin* gene *(15)*.

Familial diabetes insipidus is inherited as an autosomal dominant syndrome of vasopressin deficiency *(16)*. Infants are normal at birth, but between ages 2–10 yr they develop vasopressin deficiency and diabetes insipidus. The few reported autopsies in individuals with this disorder have suggested that there may be degeneration of vasopressin-secreting neurons *(17)*, but this has not been confirmed. Mutations have been identified at more than 30 sites within the vasopressin pre-prohormone *(18,19)*. All but two of these mutations are located in signal peptide or other regions of the vasopressin precursor. The mechanism by which this wide variety of mutations within the prohormone could cause vasopressin deficiency is not known. Vasopressin deficiency resulting from one identified point mutation within the vasopressin peptide sequence is inherited as an autosomal recessive disorder. This mutation produces leucine-vasopressin that has a limited ability to activate the vasopressin receptor in the kidney *(20)*.

Destruction of the pituitary gland, pituitary stalk, or hypothalamus can cause diabetes insipidus *(12,21–23)*. Head trauma can cause transection of the pituitary stalk to produce diabetes insipidus. However, the more common causes of pituitary destruction are tumors of the pituitary, hypothalamus, or surrounding structures. Suprasellar tumors such as craniopharyngioma and germinoma may present with diabetes insipidus. Surgical resection of pituitary or hypothalamic masses can cause temporary or permanent impairment of vasopressin secretion if there is damage to the pituitary gland or stalk. Radiation of the hypothalamus or pituitary can disrupt anterior pituitary function, but rarely has been reported to cause vasopressin deficiency.

A wide variety of infiltrative and infectious disorders have been associated with the development of central diabetes insipidus *(12,21–25)*. Infiltration of the pituitary stalk can disrupt transport of vasopressin to the posterior pituitary. Germinomas, sarcoidosis and histiocytosis X are the most commonly reported causes of diabetes insipidus due to disruption of the pituitary stalk. Acute bacterial meningitis and chronic meningeal processes such as tuberculosis and CNS lymphoma also can lead to central diabetes insipidus. "Idiopathic" central diabetes insipidus may represent a stalk lesion that is too small to visualize by magnetic resonance imaging (MRI). Although more common in adults, lymphocytic hypophysitis with involvement of the stalk of posterior pituitary has been reported in children *(26,27)*. One report has suggested a relationship between a prior viral infection and the onset of idiopathic diabetes insipidus *(23)*.

Diabetes insipidus occasionally may present during pregnancy, particularly in individuals with a pre-existing partial defect of vasopressin secretion. Circulating peptidases, synthesized in the placenta can participate in the degradation of vasopressin *(28)*. If the pituitary is unable to respond with an appropriate increase in vasopressin production and synthesis, the patient may develop diabetes insipidus. This syndrome should resolve after delivery, but occurrence of DI during pregnancy may indicate a need for further evaluation of water balance regulation and vasopressin action in the post-partum period *(29)*.

When the renal response to vasopressin is impaired, an individual develops nephrogenic diabetes insipidus. Inherited defects associated with nephrogenic diabetes insipidus have been identified in the V2 vasopressin receptor and in aquaporin 2, the water channel regulated by vasopressin *(30)*. Most mutations associated with abnormal V2 receptor function are inherited as X-linked recessive disorders and impair the receptor response to vasopressin *(31)* by decreasing vasopressin binding or downstream signaling *(32)*. Mutations of aquaporin 2 that are associated with nephrogenic diabetes insipidus are autosomal recessive. Most functional studies of these mutations have shown them to impair intracellular transport and subsequent vasopressin-mediated translocation of the aquaporin into the apical membrane of the renal tubular cell *(33,34)*. However, some of these mutations may impair the water channel function of the aquaporin *(35)* or prevent formation of aquaporin tetramers in the cell membrane *(36)*.

Acquired nephrogenic diabetes insipidus typically is not as severe as inherited forms and usually is related to underlying renal tubular or interstitial damage. Medullary or interstitial damage may affect water balance, not by inhibiting vasopressin action, but by disruption of the medullary gradient, which can prevent urinary concentration greater than plasma osmolality. Thus, interstitial disease can produce a relative vasopressin resistance *(37)*. A wide variety of agents and processes have been associated with development of nephrogenic diabetes insipidus (Table 2). The precise mechanism by which most of these agents inhibit vasopressin action and exert their effect is not known. Some drugs, such as demeclocycline, appear to impair post-receptor signaling of the V2 receptor. Nearly half of all cases of drug-induced nephrogenic diabetes insipidus are related to the long-term use of lithium salts *(38)*, which may inhibit post-receptor activation and

Table 2
Reported Causes of Nephrogenic Diabetes Insipidus

Congenital
- Inherited genetic disorders: mutations in V2 receptor or aquaporin 2
- Renal malformations: congenital hydronephrosis, polycystic kidney

Acquired Disorders
- Electrolyte Disorders: hypokalemia, hypercalcemia
- Renal Diseases: obstructive uropathy, chronic pyelonephritis, polycystic kidney disease
- Systemic Diseases: sickle cell disease, amyloidosis, multiple myeloma, sarcoidosis

Drugs
- Lithium salts
- Methoxyflurane
- Alcohol
- Demeclocycline and other tetracyclines
- Anti-infectious agents: foscarnet, amphotericin, methicillin, gentamicin
- Anti-neoplastic agents: cyclophosphamide, isophosphamide, vinblastine, platinum
- Other: phenytoin, acetohexamide, glyburide, tolazamide, colchicine, barbiturates

thereby decrease transcription of aquaporin mRNA, aquaporin synthesis, and translocation of aquaporin into the apical membrane of tubular cells. The reported prevalence of lithium-induced diabetes insipidus varies between 20–70% and may depend upon the dose and duration of therapy. The differentiation of acute and chronic lithium injury remains unclear. Short term exposure to lithium may impair urine concentrating ability in more than one-half of individuals. With discontinuation of lithium, renal function returns to normal. However, with prolonged exposure to lithium, irreversible changes occur with permanent renal tubule insensitivity to vasopressin and resulting impairment of urine concentration and free water preservation *(39)*.

DIAGNOSIS

The hallmarks of diabetes insipidus, polyuria, and hyperosmolality, can present with varying degrees of severity, and each can be caused by a wide variety of other conditions. Thus, the diagnosis of diabetes insipidus requires sufficient evaluation to characterize the polyuria and hyperosmolality and to rule out other conditions that could present with similar findings. It is important to confirm the diagnosis of diabetes insipidus before pursuing an extensive evaluation to determine the etiology or initiating therapy in an individual patient.

The diagnosis of diabetes insipidus depends upon confirmation of disrupted free water balance by characterizing polyuria and the potential hyperosmolar state. Other causes of polyuria, such as primary polydipsia or an osmotic diuresis must be ruled out by clinical evaluation and laboratory analysis. An osmotic diuresis can be identified by the presence of non-dilute urine. An individual with polydipsia and plasma sodium level that is low or low normal (and not near the upper range of normal) more likely has primary polydipsia and does not have diabetes insipidus. Conversely, in an individual with diabetes insipidus, polydipsia is driven by the free water deficit and resulting hyperosmolality, and it is unlikely that plasma sodium levels will be low.

The manner of diagnosing diabetes insipidus depends upon the presentation and clinical setting. A patient that slowly develops diabetes insipidus as an outpatient may be able to maintain sufficient oral intake of free water to maintain a normal plasma osmolality. This individual may present with complaints of excessive thirst and frequent urination. One clinical clue that these symptoms are not due to primary polydipsia may be bedwetting or frequent nocturia with high levels of urine output occurring during periods of decreased water intake. Patients with well-compensated DI are at risk for decompensation if they develop an acute medical illness or are otherwise limited in free water intake. In the same way, an individual developing acute DI after pituitary surgery or head trauma may not be able to respond to the need for increased free water intake and quickly will develop a hyperosmolar state.

The diagnosis of diabetes insipidus can be confirmed by observing the response to water deprivation (Table 3). The normal response to a free water deficit and mild increase in plasma osmolality is increased vasopressin secretion, which acts on the renal tubules to conserve free water and maintain plasma osmolality in the normal range. In an individual with diabetes insipidus, impaired free water conservation permits persistent excretion of an inappropriate volume of dilute urine. In the absence of increased water intake, this leads to a free water deficit and the development of hypernatremia.

The possibility of diabetes insipidus may be raised if a patient has a marked polyuria after head trauma or a surgical procedure in which the pituitary could be damaged. If access to *ad libitium* water intake is limited, excretion of inappropriately dilute urine (urine osmolality less than plasma osmolality) will lead to continued free water loss and development of hypernatremia. Careful assessment of documented fluid balance (I + O's) in the operating room and post-operative period and measurement of plasma and urine concentration will help in determining if persistent polyuria is driven by prior fluid overload or due to the development of diabetes insipidus. Development of hypernatremia with inappropriately dilute urine should be confirmed with laboratory measurement of plasma and urine osmolality. In the absence of hypernatremia, postoperative polyuria is more likely to represent a diuresis in response to intravenous fluid administered during or after surgery. Appropriate management of individuals with post-operative diuresis and possible diabetes insipidus should include serial measurement of plasma sodium and urine specific gravity every few hours until the diuresis resolves.

A clinical diagnosis of diabetes insipidus may be made in an individual with a likely cause for DI and acute development of dilute polyuria and hypernatremia. If this patient has hypernatremia in the presence of a dilute urine, then a formal water deprivation may not be required for the diagnosis of diabetes insipidus. In subjects with a clinical diagnosis of acute central diabetes insipidus, a therapeutic trial of desmopressin may be an appropriate diagnostic maneuver. However, pitfalls to this approach include the presence of a concurrent cause of polyuria and hypernatremia. For example, an osmotic diuresis following administration of mannitol during a neurosurgical procedure may produce polyuria and possibly mild hypernatremia if water access if impaired. Other medical problems may obscure the diagnosis of diabetes insipidus. For example, in patients with severe hypothalamic or pituitary destruction, centrally mediated cortisol or thyroid hormone deficiency may impair free water clearance *(10)*.

In individuals where the diagnosis of diabetes is not well documented, then a formal diagnostic test must be performed. One of the most common tests to confirm the diagnosis of diabetes insipidus is the water deprivation test *(5,12,24,40)*. As illustrated in

Table 3
Diagnostic Testing for Diabetes Insipidus (Summary)

I. Basal Testing:
    Diabetes Insipidus unlikely:
        serum osmolality <270 mosm/kg, urine osmolality >600 mosm/kg,
          or urine output <1 L/m^2
    Diabetes Insipidus likely:
        serum osmolality >300 (or serum sodium >150 meq/L)
          with urine osmolality <300 mosm/kg

II. Water Deprivation Study:
    A. Water Deprivation:
        1) Precede by overnight fast (if tolerated and if indicated by clinical circumstances)
        2) Continue complete water deprivation until:
            loss of >5% of basal body weight or
            plasma osmolality >300 mosm/kg or
            urine osmolality >600 mosm/kg
        3) Also discontinue if signs of hemodynamic compromise (blood pressure, heart rate)
    B. Vasopressin Administration:
        1) Parenteral administration of vasopressin analog
            Vasopressin (Pitressin) 1 U/m^2
            Desmopressin (DDAVP) 0.1 µg/kg (maximum 4 µg)
        2) Differential response to vasopressin
            Central Diabetes Insipidus:
                decrease in hourly urine output
                urine osmolality increases by 50%
            Nephrogenic Diabetes Insipidus:
                no decrease in urine output
                no increase in urine osmolality

III. Saline Infusion:
    1) Consider prior water load
    2) 3% saline at 0.1 mL/kg/h for up to 3 h or until plasma osmolality >300 mosm/kg
    3) Urine output decreases and urine osmolality increases when plasma osmolality
        reaches vasopressin secretory threshhold
    4) Analyze relationship between plasma osmolality, urine osmolality, and plasma/urine
        vasopressin levels using appropriate nomograms *(3,4,39,41)*

Table 3, the goal of the water deprivation test is to deprive the individual of sufficient free water so that vasopressin, if present, will be released and act on the kidney to promote urinary concentration. In the absence of vasopressin, free water deprivation will permit continued excretion of dilute urine, leading to a free water deficit and development of hyperosmolality. Subjects can be prepared for the formal water deprivation test, by an overnight fast. This decreases the osmotic load to the kidneys and begins the process of water deprivation. However, depending upon the clinical circumstances and age, some patients may require close observation during the entire period of deprivation. Up to 14 h of water deprivation may be required to complete an informative study in a patient with mild symptoms *(12)*.

Once the diagnosis of diabetes insipidus is confirmed, the response to administration of vasopressin (or a vasopressin analog such as desmopressin) demonstrates whether the

DI is due to vasopressin deficiency or an impaired renal response to vasopressin *(5,12,24,40)*. Patients with complete central diabetes insipidus typically have a greater than 50% increase in urinary osmolality. However, a urine osmolality greater than 600 mosm/kg is also an appropriate response and may be seen in cases of partial diabetes insipidus. Individuals with primary polydipsia should retain the ability to concentrate urine to greater than 600 mosm/kg even if little additional response is expected after desmopressin administration. In cases of nephrogenic diabetes insipidus, there will be less than 50% increase in urine osmolality. Urine osmolality will not increase greater than 400 mosm/kg and usually remains less than plasma osmolality *(24)*.

In some cases, the results of the formal water deprivation test may be inconclusive *(4,40)*. With a partial central deficiency of vasopressin, there may be some measurable response to water deprivation, but urinary concentration may not be normal. In cases of longstanding central DI, the response to exogenous vasopressin administration may be impaired due to washout of the renal medullary gradient. Patients without diabetes insipidus, including those with primary polydipsia, will maximally concentrate urine with adequate water deprivation and thus will not have a significant additional response to exogenous vasopressin. Therefore, endpoints need to be set for concluding a water deprivation study *(5,12,24,40)*. There are three: 1) persistent inappropriately low urinary osmolality despite a 3% loss of body weight, 2) hyperosmolarity and hypernatremia with an inappropriately low urinary osmolality, and 3) appropriate urinary concentration (>600 mosm/kg). Urine osmolality may appear to plateau at a submaximal concentration (<600 mosm/kg) without development of plasma hyperosmolarity. However, if the patient shows no signs of volume deficiency, then the water deprivation should be continued to determine if further concentration of urine to greater than 600 mosm/kg can be achieved. In some cases, it may be appropriate to use a therapeutic trial of desmopressin for a week. If the patient responds to therapy, this may confirm the diagnosis of central diabetes insipidus. If further testing is desired, the week of therapy should facilitate recovery of the concentrating gradient in the kidney, which may normalize the response to a test dose of desmopressin.

Other diagnostic tests may be needed to confirm the diagnosis of diabetes insipidus. Typically, urine or plasma vasopressin levels are not quickly available and usually are not required for the diagnosis of diabetes insipidus. However, in selected clinical circumstances, a vasopressin level may be helpful *(4,40,41)*. A plasma vasopressin level obtained after water deprivation will distinguish between central and nephrogenic diabetes insipidus *(41)* particularly is cases where there is only a partial defect in vasopressin secretion or action *(4,40)*. To be most informative, plasma vasopressin must be elevated as a function of plama osmolality *(40)*. Concurrent plasma osmolality and vasopressin levels obtained during a saline infusion also may help identify a partial defect in vasopressin secretion or may be useful when trying to study a patient that has a high likelihood of both central and nephrogenic diabetes insipidus. Vasopressin levels can be increased by hypotension, smoking, and nausea and these stimuli should be avoided during testing for diabetes insipidus *(23,40)*.

The saline infusion test *(4,23,42)* may be useful in patients in whom water deprivation can not be performed because of hemodynamic instability or in whom it would be difficult to obtain cooperation with water deprivation *(42)*. For example, infants can not tolerate an extended fast. A solution of 3% sodium chloride infused over 2–3 h at a dose of 0.1 mL/kg/h will provide a hyperosmolar stimulus to vasopressin secretion *(4,42)*.

When the threshold for vasopressin secretion is reached, urinary concentration will increase abruptly in response to increased vasopressin action on the kidney. Some authors suggest a water load (20 mL/kg of 5% dextrose intravenous over 2 h) prior to the saline infusion to ensure that vasopressin levels are suppressed at the beginning of the saline infusion test *(42)*. Comparison of plasma vasopressin levels with corresponding plasma osmolality can be used to determine if there is an appropriate relationship in the regulation of vasopressin secretion *(4,24,42)*. This test also is useful in identifying patients with normal vasopressin secretory ability, but an altered osmotic threshold for the release of vasopressin *(24)*.

Interpretation of the saline infusion test may be complicated by a number of issues. Vasopressin is highly labile and can degrade if the blood sample is not collected, processed, and stored correctly. Blood samples should be kept on ice, carefully processed immediately after the blood is obtained, and the plasma kept frozen until assayed *(43)*. Vasopressin levels rarely are assayed in hospital labs and require the sample to be sent to a reference laboratory, which may delay receipt of the results. Clinical laboratories do not always measure plasma osmolality with high precision and this may further complicate the interpretation of the saline infusion test *(4)*.

Once the diagnosis of diabetes insipidus is made, then efforts can be made to further identify the underlying cause if it is not clear from the clinical presentation. Patients with central diabetes insipidus should undergo imaging of the pituitary and hypothalamus. Unless a large intracranial mass is suspected, computed tomography (CT) scanning is of little use in determining the cause of diabetes insipidus. Magnetic resonance imaging (MRI) allows a more detailed study of the neurohypophysis, including the pituitary and the pituitary stalk *(44)*. Anterior pituitary microadenomas do not cause diabetes insipidus. The normal posterior pituitary typically has a characteristic bright spot on MRI and absence of this characteristic may suggest loss of vasopressin-secreting neurons or deficient vasopressin production. However, a bright spot may not be seen in up to one-fifth of normal individuals *(43)*.

Careful attention to the pituitary stalk may reveal a lesion disrupting vasopressin transport and secretion. Further evaluation of such a lesion will depend upon the clinical history of the patient. The previous diagnosis of a process, such as sarcoidosis, that can cause pituitary stalk infiltration may indicate that watchful observation while treating the underlying process is appropriate. Other tests may be needed to identify a systemic illness that may explain the infiltrative process. In rare circumstances, biopsy of the stalk lesion may be needed to rule out a diagnosis such as central nervous system lymphoma. However, this step should be undertaken with due consideration and guidance from experienced endocrinological and neurosurgical consultants, as the biopsy is likely to cause permanent damage to the pituitary stalk. If no lesion can be seen, then other causes, such as an inherited disorder or hypophysitis should be considered. If no cause for diabetes insipidus can be identified then the patient should be followed and re-assessed regularly. For example, germinomas may disrupt pituitary function and cause diabetes insipidus many years before they are apparent on MRI of the pituitary *(22,25)*. Follow-up should include periodic imaging for evidence of a growing mass and repeat assessment of anterior pituitary function as stalk lesions also may disrupt anterior pituitary function *(23,24)*.

Patients with nephrogenic diabetes insipidus should be evaluated to rule out an electrolyte disorder, such as hypercalcemia or hypokalemia that may contribute to renal insensitivity to vasopressin. Even in the absence mechanical urinary outlet obstruction, diagnostic imaging may reveal hydronephrosis as a result of the high flow of urine in the ureters. This seems to be more common in children and may represent functional urinary obstruction as result of the high urinary flow rate compared to the relative size of the urinary outflow system *(45)*. Treatment of the diabetes insipidus should help reverse the hydronephrosis.

With a family history of diabetes insipidus, genetic studies may be appropriate to confirm the cause of diabetes insipidus in an individual patient. Genetic studies also should be performed in an individual in whom there is no other apparent mechanism to cause diabetes insipidus. Identification of a genetic cause will eliminate the need for more invasive diagnostic evaluation and may be important if symptoms of diabetes insipidus appear in other family members.

TREATMENT OF DIABETES INSIPIDUS

Adequate free water intake is the first line of therapy for all cases of diabetes insipidus. Patients with an intact thirst mechanism will appropriately regulate plasma osmolality if allowed free access to water. If the patient is unable to drink by mouth, then intravenous administration of free water in the form of hypotonic fluids should be used to prevent development of a hyperosmolar state. If the patient has severe hypernatremia, intravenous administration of hypotonic fluid should be used to replenish the free water deficit.

Vasopressin and analogs such as desmopressin are the specific therapy for central diabetes insipidus *(46)* (Table 4). Because vasopressin must be administered parenterally and has a relatively short half-life, it is not an ideal drug for long-term treatment of diabetes insipidus. However, these same characteristics occasionally make it useful for short-term treatment of acute onset diabetes insipidus and for use in diagnostic testing. Other formulations of vasopressin were used in the past in an effort to overcome these two problems. An oil emulsion of vasopressin tannate (Pitressin Tannate) had a duration of action of up to 72 h. Although this allowed less frequent administration, the daily injections were painful and the bioavailability of vasopressin was variable. The unpredictable and prolonged duration of action also increased the risk of hyponatremia if combined with excessive fluid intake. This formulation is no longer marketed in the US. Lysine vasopressin had the advantage of being available for nasal administration, but still had a short half-life that required frequent dosing.

The synthetic vasopressin analog desmopressin (dDAVP) is now the standard therapy for central diabetes insipidus *(47,48)*. Desmopressin has two molecular alterations compared to native vasopressin: de-amidation of the amino terminal cysteine and replacement of arginine-8 with D-arginine. These two alterations result in a compound with a prolonged half-life of anti-diuretic activity and elimination of the pressor activity found in native vasopressin. Desmopressin can be administered parenterally, but also can be given by the nasal or oral route. Because of diminished delivery through the nasal or gastric mucosa and proteolysis by mucosal and gastric enzymes, these non-parenteral routes require higher doses of desmopressin than required with iv or sc administration (Table 4).

Table 4
Vasopressin Therapy for the Treatment of Central Diabetes Insipidus

Drug	Route	Concentration	Adult Dose	Onset	Duration
pitressin tannate in oil (Pitressin tannate[1])	IM	5 U/mL	2.5.–5 U qod		24–72 h
lysine vasopressin (Diapid[2])	nasal spray	50 U/mL	2 U	30 min	2–8 h
synthetic vasopressin (Pitressin)	SQ/IM	20 U/mL	2–10 U	minutes	2–8 h
desmopressin acetate (DDAVP) (Desmopressin)	IV/SQ	4 µg/mL	1–4 µg/d (divided doses)	minutes	6–12 h
	rhinal tube	100 µg/mL	5–40 µg/d	15–30 min	8–24 h
	nasal spray	100 µg/mL	10–40 µg/d (10 µg/spray)	15–30 min	8–24 h
	oral	100 µg/tab	100–800 µg/d (50–300 µg bid/tid)	1 h	8–12 h

[1]Production discontinued January, 1990
[2]Production discontinued June, 1999

Nasal administration can be accomplished using a rhinal tube or nasal spray. To use the rhinal tube, the patient draws the dose of desmopressin into the flexible plastic rhinal tube, places one end of the tube into the nose, and uses the mouth to blow through the tube to puff the medicine into the nose. Use of the rhinal tube requires that the patient have the dexterity and understanding to follow this technique, although parents can assist children with tube placement and providing the puff of air. Nasal administration of desmopressin can also be performed with a spray pump that administers a premeasured dose of 10 µg desmopressin per spray. However, utility of this form of nasal desmopressin can be limited in some situations. The fixed dose of the spray precludes small adjustments of dose and children may require doses smaller than 10 µg. Some authors suggest diluting rhinal tube desmopressin 1:10 in saline to facilitate administration of small doses by rhinal tube *(21)*. Nasal absorption of desmopressin can be affected by upper respiratory congestion.

Since 1995, an oral formulation of desmopressin has been marketed in the US. Because of ease of use, most patients initiating long-term desmopressin therapy opt for this form of administration. As most of an orally administered desmopressin dose is degraded before it can be absorbed, the oral dose is 10- to 20-fold greater than an equivalent nasal dose. Patients that previously have used the nasal formulation can be changed to the oral form of desmopressin. However, some individuals have become accustomed to rhinal tube administration and prefer to not change to the oral form of desmopressin. They report that they like the ability to make small adjustments in dose in response to changes in their daily routine and water intake. The duration of action of desmopressin has some variation among individuals and the appropriate dose and frequency must be determined for each individual patient. Although some patients may require only one dose per day, most find management of polyuria and polydipsia easier with twice daily nasal administration. Oral desmopressin usually requires administration two to three times a day. When initiating desmopressin therapy, it may be useful to start with one bedtime dose and then titrate the size and frequency of dosage based on the patient's response to therapy.

Administration of vasopressin or desmopressin requires careful attention to free water intake to prevent the development of hyponatremia. Oral intake of fluids may be driven by stimuli other than thirst, such as social cues and habitual drinking ingrained during a period of untreated diabetes insipidus. Providing a daily period of "break-through" with mild polyuria as the effect of the exogenous vasopressin decreases may be a convenient way to ensure that there is not excessive anti-diuresis with an accumulation of excess free water and progressive development of hyponatremia *(46)*.

In patients treated with diabetes insipidus, oral intake of fluids must be driven by and regulated by thirst. Management of diabetes insipidus in patients with an impaired thirst mechanism requires special attention to fluid balance. Daily measurement of intake and output as well as body weight may be needed to maintain fluid balance. Frequent monitoring of plasma sodium levels should be used to provide early identification of problems with water balance. However, management of diabetes insipidus in these individuals requires vigilance by both the patient and physician.

Peri-operative management of diabetes insipidus requires careful attention to fluid balance as assessed by intake and output, daily weight, and laboratory tests such as serum sodium and urine osmolality *(10,46)*. Careful measurement of urine volume and concentration may be facilitated by continuing the use of an indwelling urinary catheter for the

1–2 d after surgery. In patients with pre-existing diabetes insipidus, continuing desmopressin therapy will help maintenance of water balance. Care must be coordinated with other members of the healthcare team to ensure that fluid balance is carefully managed to prevent hyponatremia due to excess intravenous fluid administration.

Many approaches have been suggested for the management of acute post-operative diabetes insipidus. The first line of treatment remains adequate free water administration to prevent hyponatremia. Some clinicians prefer to use only fluids, while others initiate desmopressin therapy to help fluid balance and to improve patient comfort by decreasing thirst and decreasing the need to void. In this circumstance, parenteral administration of desmopressin is used because of the difficulty of nasal administration after trans-sphenoidal pituitary surgery. Parenterally administered desmopressin also has a shorter duration of action and decreases the chance of hyponatremia developing in response to excess fluid intake. Other clinicians use an intravenous infusion of vasopressin at a low dose (0.08–0.10 mU/kg) in the perioperative period or during other procedures, such as administration of chemotherapy, that have potential disruption of free water balance *(49)*.

Once a patient is taking oral fluids, fluid balance may be regulated by thirst. Depending upon the likely extent of pituitary and hypothalamic damage, the clinician must be sure that thirst is intact and that the patient is not responding to other cues, such as mouth dryness. Acute pituitary damage is likely to be accompanied by some or all of the classic triphasic response *(10)*. Patients are at risk for development of severe hyponatremia if desmopressin is continued into the period of SIADH or if a patient drinks to excess during therapy. Therefore, the decision as to whether to use desmopressin in the immediate post-operative period may depend upon the clinician's assessment as to the severity of polyuria, the likelihood that the patient will have permanent diabetes insipidus, the presence or absence of an intact thirst drive, other medical conditions that may be affected by hypernatremia (or hyponatremia), and patient comfort and convenience. Although symptoms may resolve, there should still be close monitoring of urine output volume, urinary osmolality (or specific gravity, which can be performed at the bedside), and plasma sodium levels to ensure that there is adequate, but not excessive, therapy. When patients are receiving intermittent desmopressin therapy, the onset of polyuria of dilute urine indicates the need for the next dose of desmopressin. Each subsequent dose of desmopressin should not be delayed until the patient again develops hypernatremia. However, patients should not be treated on an arbitrary fixed schedule, as the periodic breakthrough prevents the development of hyponatremia that may result with accumulation of excess free water *(46)*.

Infants are a special challenge in the management of DI as fluid intake is linked to caloric intake and usually is regulated by parents or other caregivers. Therefore, it is rarely appropriate to treat infants with vasopressin analogs. Satisfactory treatment requires that infants be given a combination of formula (or breast milk) and sufficient free water to maintain a normo-osmolar state. This can be accomplished by careful attention to intake and output and calculation of the volume of formula needed to meet the infant's caloric needs. If an infant is breastfeeding, it may be easier to have the mother use a breast pump so that the volume of milk can be measured accurately. Additional free water then is given to maintain water balance and normal plasma osmolality.

Other agents can have an anti-diuretic effect and could be used to treat diabetes insipidus. These include chlorpropamide, carbemazepine, and clofibrate. For example, chlorpropamide has been shown to be synergistic with vasopressin and has been proposed for use in the treatment of partial vasopressin deficiency. Chlorpropamide also has been reported to improve thirst sensation in patients with impaired thirst (50). Clofibrate (51) and carbamazepine (52) increase vasopressin release in patients with partial central diabetes insipidus. However, each of these agents has other metabolic actions and, with the availability of desmopressin, none is used for the routine treatment of central diabetes insipidus.

Treatment of nephrogenic diabetes insipidus frequently is an unsatisfying endeavor. Withdrawal of the precipitating drug may permit remission of the diabetes insipidus. However, this must be done in consultation with appropriate specialists that can help in management of the underlying disease and in identification of other agents that may be used without the development of diabetes insipidus. For example, use of other neuropsychiatric agents, such as valproic acid or carbamazepine, may permit a dose reduction or discontinuation of lithium. However, some clinical circumstances require continuation of the causative agent and subsequent management of the resulting diabetes insipidus.

Decreasing the solute load to the kidney, such as a low salt and low protein diet, will decrease the total urine volume and limit the degree of polyuria. Some patients with partial nephrogenic diabetes insipidus may respond to high doses of desmopressin (4). A variety of agents, including non-steroidal anti-inflammatory agents and diuretics, have been reported to improve the symptoms of diabetes insipidus. Indomethacin can decrease polyurina and polydipsia, while other agents such ibuprofen are much less effective (53). Diuretics, such as hydrochlorothiazide and amiloride (Midamor) probably ameliorate diabetes insipidus by producing a mild chronic volume depletion that leads to increased volume reabsorption in the proximal tubular of the kidney. With decreased distal delivery of filtrate, there is an overall decrease in urine volume. Combined therapy with hydrochlorothiazide and amiloride has been reported to be successful (54). Amiloride may decrease entry of lithium into tubular cells and thereby decrease the effect of lithium on vasopressin action, and sometimes amiloride therapy will provide complete resolution of lithium-induced nephrogenic diabetes insipidus (39). Amiloride may not be available in many community pharmacies, but should be available from a hospital pharmacy.

The use of diuretics for the treatment of nephrogenic diabetes insipidus is not risk-free. The persistent decrease in extracellular volume caused by diuretic therapy puts the patient at risk of hypovolemia and severe dehydration, particularly during an episode of febrile illness or water deprivation. Thiazide diuretics may cause hypokalemia, which can further impair renal responsiveness to vasopressin. Subjects with concurrent lithium-induced diabetes insipidus and hyperparathyroidism are particularly susceptible to water deprivation, as dehydration can precipitate hypercalcemia and the hypercalcemia can further exacerbate the diabetes insipidus. In patients treated with diuretics for lithium-induced diabetes insipidus, the resulting volume depletion and the effects on tubular function can decrease lithium clearance and may lead to increased plasma lithium levels.

Management of possible drug-induced nephrogenic diabetes insipidus should begin prior to the development of symptoms such as polyuria and polydipsia. When teenagers and young adults start lithium therapy, they should be informed of the possible development of diabetes insipidus and instructed to monitor urine volume. Progressive development of polyuria may be one indication to re-evaluate the need for chronic lithium therapy and consideration of substituting other therapies for lithium.

With attention to water balance and appropriate therapy, diabetes insipidus can be well controlled and have minimal impact on quality of life. Treatment of diabetes insipidus decreases sleep disruption and facilitates full participation in school and daily activities. Treatment of diabetes insipidus has been reported to improve school performance and behavior and allow normal growth *(6,11)*. With appropriate treatment, diabetes insipidus does not cause mental retardation *(55)*. Patients and families should understand that even short periods of non-compliance with therapy could lead to serious medical complications. However, intercurrent illness or stress can disrupt management of diabetes insipidus even in a well-controlled patient. Patients and caregivers should be instructed to closely follow water intake and urine output and to obtain daily weights during febrile or gastrointestinal illness. Evaluation of any change in mental status should include measurement of serum sodium to rule out hypernatremia due to exacerbation of the diabetes insipidus or hyponatremia secondary to water intoxication. If a patient or family is unable to communicate the history of diabetes insipidus, severe derangement in water balance could occur before the diagnosis of diabetes insipidus is recognized by emergency personnel or health providers unfamiliar with the patient. Thus, patients should be encouraged to wear a medical alert bracelet or other form of identification that provides a clear indication that they have diabetes insipidus.

REFERENCES

1. Vokes T, Robertson GL. Physiology of secretion of vasopressin. In: Czernichow P, Robinson AG, eds. Diabetes Insipidus in Man. Front Horm Res 1984;13:127–155.
2. Knepper MA, Verbalis JG, Nielsen S. Role of aquaporins in water balance disorders. Curr Opin Nephrol Hypertens 1997;6:367–371.
3. Schrier RW, Berl T, Anderson RJ. Osmotic and nonosmotic control of vasopressin release. Am J Physiol 1979;236:F321–F332.
4. Robertson GL. Differential diagnosis of polyuria. Ann Rev Med 1988;39:425–442.
5. Bayliss PH, Cheetham T. Diabetes insipidus. Arch Dis Child 1998;79:84–89.
6. Oster JR, Singer I, Thatte L, Grant-Taylor I, Diego JM. The polyuria of solute diuresis. Arch Intern Med 1997;157:721–729.
7. Hammond DN, Moll GW, Robertson GL, Chelmicka-Schorr E. Hypodipsic hypernatremia with normal osmoregulation of vasopressin. N Engl J Med 1986;315:433–436.
8. Adrogue HJ, Madias NE. Hypernatremia. N Engl J Med 2000;342:1493–1499.
9. Colle E, Ayoub E, Raile R. Hypertonic dehydration (hypernatremia): the role of feedings high in solutes. Pediatrics 1958;22:5–12.
10. Verbalis JG, Robinson AG, Moses AM. Postoperative and post-traumatic diabetes insipidus. in: Czernichow P, Robinson AG (eds). Diabetes insipidus in man. Front Horm Res 1984;13:247–265.
11. Kauli R, Galatzer A, Laron Z. Treatment of diabetes insipidus in children and adolescents. In: Czernichow P, Robinson AG, eds. Diabetes Insipidus in Man. Front Horm Res 1984;13:304–313.
12. Czernichow P. Pomerade R, Brauner R, Rappaport R. Neurogenic diabetes insipidus in children. In: Czernichow P, Robinson AG, eds. Diabetes Insipidus in Man. Front Horm Res 1984;13:190–209.
13. Brothers JA, Rogers DG. Morbid obesity in a young child. Clin Pediatric 2000;39:169–171.
14. Lees MM, Hodgkins P, Reardon W, et al. Frontonasal dysplasia with optic disc anomalies and other midline craniofacial defects: a report of six cases. Clin Dysmorphol 1998;7:157–162.
15. Strom TM, Hortnagel K, Hofman S, et al. Diabetes insipidus, diabetes mellitus, optic atrophy and deafness (DIDMOAD) caused by mutations in a novel gene (wolframin) coding for a predicted transmembrane protein. Hum Mol Genet 1998;7:2021–2028.
16. Pedersen EB, Lamm LU, Albertsen K, et al. Familial cranial diabetes insipidus: a report of five families. Genetic, Diagnostic and therapeutic aspects. Q J Med 1985;57:883–896.
17. Bergeron C, Kovacs K, Ezrin C, Mizzen C. Hereditary diabetes insipidus: an immunohistochemical study of the hypothalamus and pituitary gland. Acta Neuropathol 1991;81:345–348.

18. Rittig S, Robertson GL, Siggaard C, et al. Identification of 13 new mutations in the vasopressin-neurophysin II gene in 17 kindreds with familial autosomal dominant neurohypophyseal diabetes insipidus. Am J Hum Genet 1996;58:107–117.
19. Grant FD, Ahmadi A, Hosley CM, Majzoub JA. Two novel mutations of the vasopressin gene associated with familial diabetes insipidus and identification of an asymptomatic carrier infant. J Clin Endcrinol Metab 1998;83:3958–3964.
20. Willcutts MD, Felner E, White PC. Autosomal recessive familial neurohypophyseal diabetes insipidus with continued secretion of mutant weakly active vasopressin. Hum Mol Genet 1999;8:1303–1307.
21. Gregor NG, Kirkland RT, Clayton GW, Kirkland JL. Central diabetes insipidus: 22 years' experience. Am J Dis Child 1986;140:551–554.
22. Charmandari E, Brook CG. 20 years of experience in idiopathic central diabetes insipidus. Lancet 1999;353:2212–2213.
23. Maghnie M, Cosi G, Genovese E, et al. Central diabetes insipidus in children and young adults. N Engl J Med 2000;343:998–1007.
24. Moses AM. Clinical and laboratory observations in the adult with diabetes insipidus and related syndromes. In: Czernichow P, Robinson AG, eds. Diabetes Insipidus in Man. Front Horm Res 1984;13:156–175.
25. Mootha SL, Barkovich AJ, Grumbach MM, et al. Idiopathic hypothalamic diabetes insipidus, pituitary stalk thickening, and the occult intracranial germinoma in children and adolescents. J Clin Endocrinol Metab 1997;82:1362–1367.
26. Heinze HJ, Bercu BB. Acquired hypophysitis in adolescence. J Pediatr Endocrinol Metab. 1997;10:315–321.
27. Honegger J, Fahlbusch R, Bornemann A, et al. Lymphocytic and granulomatous hypophysitis: experience with nine cases. Neurosurgery 1997;40:713–723.
28. Durr JA, Hoggard JG, Hunt JM, Schrier RW. Diabetes insipidus in pregnancy associated with abnormally high circulating vasopressinase activity. N Engl J Med 1987;316:1070–1074.
29. Iwasaki Y, Oiso Y, Kondo K, et al. Aggravation of subclinical diabetes insipidus during pregnancy. N Engl J Med 1991; 324:522–526.
30. Fujiwara TM, Morgan K, Bichet D. Molecular biology of diabetes insipidus. Annu Rev Med 1995;46:331–343.
31. Schoneberg T, Schulz A, Biebermann H, et al. V2 vasopressin receptor dysfunction in nephrogenic diabetes insipidus caused by different molecular mechanisms. Hum Mutat 1998; 12:196–205.
32. Wildin RS, Cogdell DE, Valadez V. AVPR2 variants and V2 vasopressin receptor function in nephrogenic diabetes insipidus. Kidney Int 1998;54:1909–1922.
33. Kamsteeg EJ, Deen PM, van Os CH. Defective processing and trafficking of water channels in nephrogenic diabetes insipidus. Exp Nephrol 2000;8:326–331.
34. Tamarappoo BK, Yang B, Verkman AS. Misfolding of mutant aquaporin-2 water channels in nephrogenic diabetes insipidus. J Biol Chem 1999;274:34825–34831.
35. Goji K, Kuwahara M, Gu Y, Matsuo M, Marumo F, Sasaki S. Novel mutations in aquaporin-2 gene in female siblings with nephrogenic diabetes insipidus: evidence of disrupted water channel function. J Clin Endocrinol Metab 1998;83:3205–3209.
36. Kamsteeg EJ, Wormhoudt TA, Rijss JP, van Os CH, Deen PM. An impaired routing of wild-type aquaporin-2 after tetramerization with an aquaporin-2 mutant explains dominant nephrogenic diabetes insipidus. EMBO J 1999;18:2394–2400.
37. Leung AKC, Robson WLM, Halperin ML. Polyuria in childhood. Clin Pediatr (Phila) 1991;30: 634–640.
38. Bendz H, Aurel M. Drug-induced diabetes insipidus: Incidence, prevention and management. Drug Safety 1999;21:449–456.
39. Timmer RT, Sands JM. Lithium intoxication. J Am Soc Nephrol 1999;10:666–674.
40. Robertson GL. Diagnosis of diabetes insipidus. In: Czernichow P, Robinson AG, eds. Diabetes Insipidus in Man. Front Horm Res 1984;13:176–189.
41. Dunger DB, Seckl JR, Grant DB, Yeoman L, Lightman SL. A short water deprivation test incorporating urinary arginine estimstions in the investigation of posterior pituitary function in children. Acta Endocrinol (Copenh) 1988;117:13–18.
42. Mohn A, Acerini CL, Cheetham TD, Lightman SL, Dunger DB. Hypertonic saline test for the investigation of posterior pituitary function. Arch Dis Child 1998;79:431–434.

43. Kluge M, Riedl S, Erhart-Hofmann B, Hartmann J, Waldhauser F. Improved extraction procedure and RIA for determination of arginine8-vasopressin in plasma: role of premeasurement sample treatment and reference values in children. Clin Chem 1999;45:98–103.
44. Elster AD. Imaging of the sella: anatomy and pathology. Semin Ultrasound CT MR 1993; 14:182–194.
45. Uribarri J, Kaskas M. Hereditary nephrogenic diabetes insipidus and bilateral nonobstructive hydronephrosis. Nephron 1993;65:346–349.
46. Robinson AG, Verbalis JG. Treatment of central diabetes insipidus. In: Czernichow P, Robinson AG, eds. Diabetes Insipidus in Man. Front Horm Res 1984;13:292–303.
47. Cobb WE, Spare S, Reichlin S. Neurogenic diabetes insipidus: management with dDAVP (1-desamino-8-D arginine vasopressin). Ann Intern Med 1978;88:183–188.
48. Richardson DW, Robinson AG. Diagnosis and treatment, drugs five years later: Desmopressin. Ann Internal Med 1985;103:228–239.
49. Bryant WP, O'Marcaigh AS, Ledger GA, Zimmerman D. Aqueous vasopressin infusion during chemotherapy in patients with diabetes insipidus. Cancer 1994;74:2589–2592.
50. Bode HH, Harley BM, Crawford JD. Restoration of normal drinking behavior by chlorpropamide in patients with hypodipsia and diabetes insipidus. Am J Med 1971;51(3):304–313.
51. Moses AM, Howanitz J, Gemert M, Miller M. Clofibrate-induced anti-diuresis. J Clin Invest 1973;52:535–542.
52. Kimura T, Matsui K, Sato T, Yoshinoga K. Mechanisms of carbamazepine (Tegtretol)-induced antidiuresis: evidence for release of anti-diuretic hormone and impaired excretion of water load. J Clin Endocrinol Metab 1974;38:356–362.
53. Libber S, Harrison H, Spector D. Treatment of nephrogenic diabetes insipidus with prostaglandin synthesis inhibitors. J Pediatr 1986;108:305–311.
54. Kirchlechner V, Koller DY, Seidl R, Waldhauser F. Treatment of nephrogenic diabetes insipidus with hydrochlorothiazide and amiloride. Arch Dis Child 1999;80:548–552.
55. Hoekstra JA, van Lieburg AF, Monnens LA, Hulstijn-Dirkmat GM, Knoers VV. Cognitive and psychosocial functioning of patients with congenital nephrogenic diabetes insipidus. Am J Med Genet 1996;61:81–88.

10 Management of Endocrine Dysfunction Following Brain Tumor Treatment

Stuart Alan Weinzimer, MD
and Thomas Moshang Jr., MD

CONTENTS

INTRODUCTION
EFFECTS OF BRAIN TUMOR TREATMENT ON ENDOCRINE SYSTEMS
EVALUATION AND TREATMENT OF ENDOCRINE DISORDERS
CONCLUSION
REFERENCES

INTRODUCTION

Advances in modalities of treatment and improvements in long-term survival in children with brain tumors have resulted in a need to evaluate the late effects of cancer therapy on endocrine function in children. Long-term impairment of growth and sexual development are well-known complications of brain tumors and their treatments, although multiple endocrine systems may be altered following surgery, radiotherapy, and chemotherapy. In addition, co-morbidities of cancer therapy, such as nutritional deficiencies, psychosocial dysfunction, and the disease process itself, may amplify the deleterious effects of cancer treatment on the endocrine system. The aims of this review are to summarize the effects of brain tumors and their treatments on the endocrine system and to outline the management of endocrinopathies in survivors of childhood brain tumors.

EFFECTS OF BRAIN TUMOR TREATMENT ON ENDOCRINE SYSTEMS

Radiotherapy

Hypothalamic and pituitary hormone deficiencies are common after irradiation of the central nervous system (CNS), occurring usually at the level of the hypothalamus *(1,2)*. In children who receive radiation to the hypothalamus, the most common hormonal dysfunction is growth hormone deficiency (GHD), followed by hypogonadism *(3)*. The effects of irradiation on the hypothalamus and pituitary have been demonstrated to be dose-dependent. Above a dose of 18 Gy, the pubertal increase in spontaneous GH secretion is diminished, while above 24 Gy all spontaneous GH secretion is decreased. Above 27 Gy the GH response to provocative stimuli is blunted *(4)*. Production of adrenal hormones, thyroid hormones, and prolactin are not affected until cumulative radiation doses are above 30 Gy *(5)*.

The frequency of GH deficiency following cranial irradiation is dependent not only on cumulative dosage, but also on the fraction size, the age of the patient, and the interval between treatment and evaluation of GH production. A larger fraction size of radiation administered over a shorter time interval is more likely to cause GH deficiency than smaller fraction sizes administered over longer periods of time *(6)*. For example, Shalet demonstrated subnormal GH responses to provocative stimulation in 14 of 17 children treated with 25 Gy in 10 fractions over 2 wk, whereas only one of nine children treated with 24 Gy in 20 fractions over 4 wk failed GH testing *(7)*. Furthermore, in younger children, the same doses of radiation are more likely to cause GH deficiency *(8,9)*. The frequency of GH deficiency progressively increases as the time interval increases following irradiation. Duffner evaluated children with brain tumors treated with radiotherapy with serial provocative GH tests and demonstrated that within 3 mo of radiation, 28% failed provocative testing; at 6 mo, 82% failed, and at 1 yr, 88% failed *(10)*.

As mentioned earlier, GH deficiency is the most common endocrine dysfunction following radiotherapy, but in the doses commonly used to treat childhood brain tumors, multiple endocrinopathies of the hypothalamus and pituitary are typical. In a survey of 32 children and adults who received an average of 54 Gy radiation to the hypothalamus and pituitary as part of their brain tumor treatment, 28% had one hormone deficiency, 25% lacked two hormones, 25% lacked three hormones, and 12% lacked four hormones. Less than 10% of the subjects had all the hormone systems intact *(11)*. Gonadotropin deficiency is rarely seen following radiation doses less than 40 Gy, *(12,13)*, but increases progressively when doses in excess of 50 Gy are used, and may be present in 20–50% of patients over time *(14,15)*. The incidence of thyrotropin deficiency is uncommon (<10%) after radiation doses of less than 50 Gy *(16)*, but increases markedly at higher doses, approaching 65% in patients receiving a mean dose of 57 Gy *(14)*. Clinical adrenocorticotropin (ACTH) deficiency is uncommon in patients receiving less than 50 Gy to the hypothalamus and pituitary, but more subtle defects in the hypothalamic-pituitary-adrenal axis may be seen with doses over 35 Gy *(17)*. At doses greater than 50 Gy, ACTH deficiency has been reported in 18–35% of patients *(14,15)*.

In addition to the neuroendocrine effects of cranial irradiation on the hypothalamic-pituitary centers, radiotherapy also causes hormonal deficiency via direct cytotoxic effects on the endocrine glands. Irradiation to the head and neck for treatment of brain tumors produces permanent primary hypothyroidism in about 16–30% of patients receiving cranial or craniospinal irradiation *(14,18,19)*, or 60–80% of patients receiving direct neck irradiation *(20–22)*. The effect appears to be dose-related, with a threshold effect of approx 10 Gy *(23)* and clinically significant thyroid dysfunction at about 20 Gy *(12,24)*. The peak incidence of hypothyroidism following irradiation is about 2–4 yr, but thyroid dysfunction may develop after as many as 25 yr following radiotherapy *(25)*. Complicating risk factors for the development of hypothyroidism include younger patient age and the use of adjuvant chemotherapy *(16,26)*.

Although direct irradiation of the gonad is not a typical therapeutic modality of brain tumor treatment, a brief discussion on the cytotoxic effects of irradiation on the gonad follows. Direct gonadal irradiation typically results in permanent primary gonadal failure. In an ethically-questionable study on normal adult male incarcerated volunteers, spermatogonia were damaged at radiation doses as low as 200 cGy (27). Prepubertal gonads appear to be somewhat less radiosensitive; 11 of 31 boys and 16 of 16 girls who received gonadal radiation in prepubertal years demonstrated normal sexual development (28). However, even with doses less than 10 Gy, damage to testicular germ cells and ovarian follicular cells occurs (29,30).

While most of the endocrine dysfunction following cranial irradiation may be characterized as deficiency states, two forms of endocrine dysregulation manifest as excessive hormone production in children: precocious puberty and hyperprolactinemia. Precocious puberty may be seen as a complication of both low- and high-dose cranial irradiation (31–33), or as a manifestation of the brain tumor itself (34). Elevations in serum prolactin concentrations, due to the disruption of hypothalamic inhibitory centers, have been demonstrated in as many as 82% of males and 50% females after cranial radiotherapy with doses greater than 55 Gy (35).

Finally, radiotherapy may affect skeletal tissues directly and impair growth by a mechanism independent of hormonal dysfunction. Irradiation of the skeletal tissues causes arrest of chondrogenesis at the epiphyseal growth plate, impaired tubulation at the metaphysis, and faulty bone modeling at the diaphysis (36). Furthermore, radiation-induced damage of the blood vessels supplying the bones further impairs growth and active bone metabolism. Spinal irradiation, commonly employed in the treatment of some intracranial tumors to prevent metastasis, leads to loss of vertebral height, scoliosis, and muscle atrophy and produces disproportionate growth of the limbs relative to the trunk. Affected children develop increased upper to lower segment ratios and reduced sitting heights (37,38), particularly during puberty (39). The growth impairing effects of spinal irradiation are resistant to growth hormone therapy: growth hormone treatment failed to improve sitting height or promote catch-up growth in 19 children with growth hormone deficiency following craniospinal irradiation for brain tumors (18).

Chemotherapy

Chemotherapy also contributes to the poor growth and endocrine dysfunction seen in childhood survivors of brain tumors. Linear growth and skeletal maturation may arrest completely. The experience in treatment for childhood leukemia illustrates the effects of chemotherapy alone, without the confounding effects of intrinsic hypothalamic-pituitary disease. Poor growth and delayed skeletal maturation were seen in 30% of 21 children treated with intrathecal chemotherapy alone for leukemia (40). In children receiving both cranial irradiation and chemotherapy for leukemia, the greatest decline in growth velocity was seen during the first year of therapy, and catch-up growth and skeletal maturation did not occur until after the cessation of chemotherapy, independent of the radiation schedule (16,41). Furthermore, the severity of the growth impairment correlated with the intensity and duration of the chemotherapeutic regimen (42).

The deleterious effects of adjuvant chemotherapy on growth have been demonstrated in childhood brain tumor survivors as well. Children with medulloblastoma treated with chemotherapy in addition to craniospinal irradiation grew worse than similar patients treated with identical doses of radiation alone. The growth deceleration was noted in the

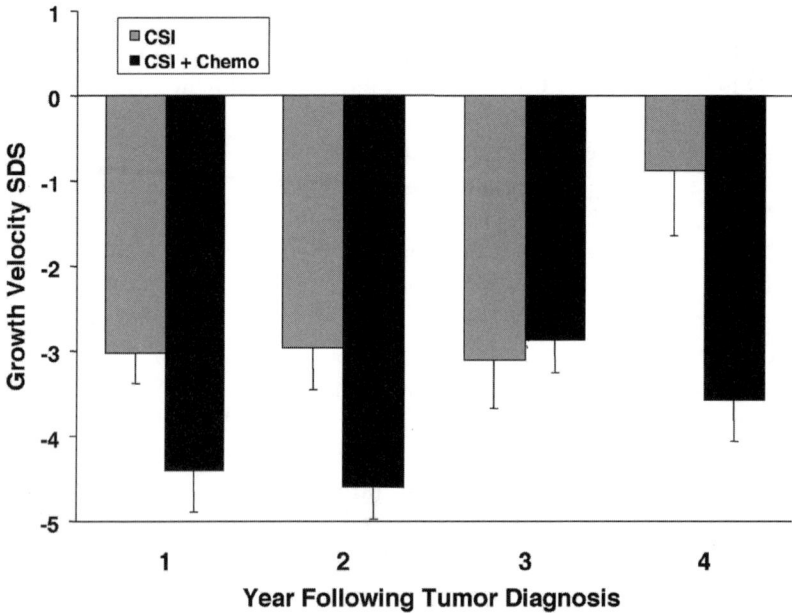

Fig. 1. A comparison of growth velocity, expressed as a standard deviation score (SDS) in children surviving medulloblastoma treated with craniospinal irradiation alone (CSI, gray bars) or combination craniospinal irradiation plus adjuvant chemotherapy (CSI + Chemo, black bars).

first year of treatment and persisted even after 4 yr *(43)* (Fig. 1). In a series of medulloblastoma survivors at the Children's Hospital of Philadelphia, the appearance of growth hormone deficiency after tumor treatment occurred earlier in patients who received both chemotherapy and radiation (3.5 yr) than in those who received radiation (5.1 yr). Furthermore, the spinal growth response to growth hormone treatment was attenuated in the children who received adjuvant chemotherapy *(44)*.

The growth failure seen during the acute phase of chemotherapy is related to the nausea, vomiting, malaise, cachexia and resultant poor nutrition. The mechanisms behind the prolonged deleterious effects of chemotherapy on growth are not well understood. Malnutrition states are associated with growth hormone resistance, wherein decreased circulating levels of insulin-like growth factors (IGF) and IGF binding proteins (IGFBP) prevail despite normal or even elevated pituitary production of growth hormone *(45)*. IGF and IGFBP deficiency have been demonstrated to precede growth hormone deficiency in children with medulloblastoma treated with craniospinal irradiation and chemotherapy *(46)*. Glucocorticoids and other chemotherapeutic agents have complex effects on the growth hormone-IGF-IGFBP axis, reducing growth hormone-stimulated IGF production and IGF responsiveness at the cartilage endplate *(47,48)*.

Chemotherapeutic agents, particularly aklylating agents, are well known to cause primary gonadal damage *(49–51)*. As with radiotherapy, prepubertal gonads appear to be somewhat more resistant to the damaging effects of chemotherapy than post-pubertal gonads, and ovaries may be somewhat more resistant than testes *(52)*.

Surgery

The nature and location of the brain tumor, as well as the need for direct surgical resection, greatly affects the risk of post-treatment endocrine dysfunction. Tumors of the hypothalamus, optic chiasm, or pituitary gland may cause pituitary damage directly by compression and invasion, and surgical resection may result in panhypopituitarism. In a series of 68 children with hypothalamic-chiasmatic glioma, surgical resection was associated with a twofold increase in growth hormone deficiency and five-fold increase in thyrotropin (TSH), ACTH, and vasopressin deficiency *(34)*. Transection of the infundibular stalk, even without complete pituitary resection, may result in permanent diabetes insipidus.

EVALUATION AND TREATMENT OF ENDOCRINE DISORDERS

It is critical that survivors of childhood brain tumors are monitored for the development of endocrine dysfunction. As mentioned previously, the effects of radiotherapy may not be evident initially; deficiencies may present years after initial treatment. The following discussion provides guidelines for the clinical and laboratory assessment of endocrine disorders and outlines basic treatment regimens. However, good clinical judgement is obviously paramount, and long-term monitoring must be individualized.

Growth Failure / Growth Hormone Deficiency

Children and adolescents should be monitored closely for growth deceleration, as growth failure is the most common endocrine complaint in this population *(53)*. Accurate determinations of standing height and weight should be made every 3–6 mo and plotted on standard growth charts for easy visual review. Ideally, sitting height and arm span measurements should be determined, and upper segment (sitting height) to lower segment (standing height minus sitting height) ratios should be calculated, since disproportionate growth frequently accompanies spinal irradiation *(54)*. Retardation of sitting height greater than standing height, decreasing upper segment to lower segment ratio, or decreasing standing height to arm span all suggest spinal height loss. This component of growth failure is resistant to growth hormone treatment, and families should be counseled that permanent loss of height is likely to occur. Interval growth velocity should also be calculated at each visit, as growth deceleration is frequently an earlier sign of growth hormone deficiency than short stature. It is important to consider the sexual development of the child when determining the adequacy of growth, as the contribution of pubertal levels of gonadal steroids may mask a true growth problem by maintaining a "normal" height or growth velocity. Comparison of actual growth velocity to standard growth velocity charts and attention to the timing and magnitude of the expected pubertal growth spurt are important factors in the clinical assessment of growth in adolescent brain tumor survivors.

Children who demonstrate a true growth deceleration, or in the case of pubertal children, who fail to mount a normal pubertal growth spurt in the presence of gonadal steroids, should be further evaluated for growth hormone deficiency. Initial screening studies should aim to exclude other medical causes of growth failure and include routine serum chemistry and hematologic profiles, erythrocyte sedimentation rate, thyroid function tests, and a hand and wrist radiograph for determination of skeletal age. Testosterone and ultrasensitive gonadotropin levels *(55)* should also be followed in boys and girls, respectively, of pubertal age or status. Assessment of growth hormone status should of course be considered in any child who has undergone cranial irradiation or who has had surgery directly to the hypothalamic-pituitary area.

The diagnosis of growth hormone deficiency is not straightforward; debate continues as to the most sensitive, specific, and reproducible test *(56)*. Reliance on purely anthropometric data ignores the multifactorial nature of growth failure in brain tumor survivors. Pituitary growth hormone secretion is pulsatile, rendering random serum growth hormone measurements useless for the evaluation of growth hormone deficiency. Repeated measurements of serum growth hormone levels over a 12 or 24-mo period increases the likelihood of "catching" peaks of growth hormone secretion but interpretation of these serial sampling tests is hampered by the absence of clear objective criteria for defining "normal" vs "growth hormone deficient" in terms of frequency and amplitude of peaks and pooled growth hormone concentrations.

Provocative testing with growth hormone secretagogues has been the traditional means of documenting growth hormone deficiency. The growth hormone secretagogues act to acutely stimulate pituitary growth hormone production, which can be assessed by serial serum measurements over a defined time period. Depending on the type of assay employed to measure serum growth hormone levels, a peak growth hormone response greater than 10 ng/mL is usually considered to be normal. Because many normally-growing children may fail to mount a normal response to one GH provocative test *(57)*, and repeated tests may yield divergent results in up to 25% of children *(58,59)*, a combination of two tests is usually suggested to reduce false failures. Growth hormone secretagogues include insulin, arginine, clonidine, L-Dopa, propranolol, glucagon, and growth hormone releasing hormone. These tests are technically difficult, require multiple blood sampling over longer periods of time, and in the case of the insulin test, may provoke dangerous side effects *(60)*. These tests are also "non-physiologic," in that children who have hypothalamic dysregulation due to cranial irradiation may mount a normal pituitary growth hormone response to these potent stimuli, but under normal basal conditions have subnormal spontaneous growth hormone secretion *(4)*.

In the last decade, measurement of the serum growth factors insulin-like growth factor-I (IGF-I) and IGF-binding protein-3 (IGFBP-3) has become standard in the evaluation of children with growth deceleration. Serum concentrations of IGF-I and IGFBP-3 exhibit little diurnal variation, accurately reflect spontaneous growth hormone secretion, and have been reported to be up to 95% sensitive and specific for diagnosing growth hormone deficiency in children *(61,62)*. However, serum IGF-I levels are often reduced in children with malnutrition and other catabolic diseases, and considerable overlap in IGF-I levels exists between short normal children and children with true growth hormone deficiency. Furthermore, we and others have demonstrated that IGF-I and IGFBP-3 concentrations may be less accurate in predicting growth hormone deficiency in children with brain tumors *(63)* and in children treated with cranial irradiation *(64,65)*. In our series of 72 children with brain tumors and growth hormone deficiency, normal IGF-I levels were found in 27% of patients and normal IGFBP-3 levels were found in 50% (Fig. 2). IGF-I and IGFBP-3 levels were particularly ineffective in predicting growth hormone deficiency in pubertal children and in children with hypothalamic-chiasmatic glioma, of which 33% had precocious puberty. Puberty, whether normal or precocious, may thus mask true growth hormone deficiency, because increased secretion of gonadal steroids improves growth velocity and increases serum concentrations of IGF-I and IGFBP-3 *(66–70)*.

Ultimately, the diagnosis of growth hormone deficiency is a clinical one, taking into account the location of the tumor, extent of pituitary resection or cranial irradiation, growth velocity of the patient, pubertal stage, bone age, IGF-I and IGFBP-3 levels, and response to one or more provocative stimuli. Brain tumor survivors should be monitored

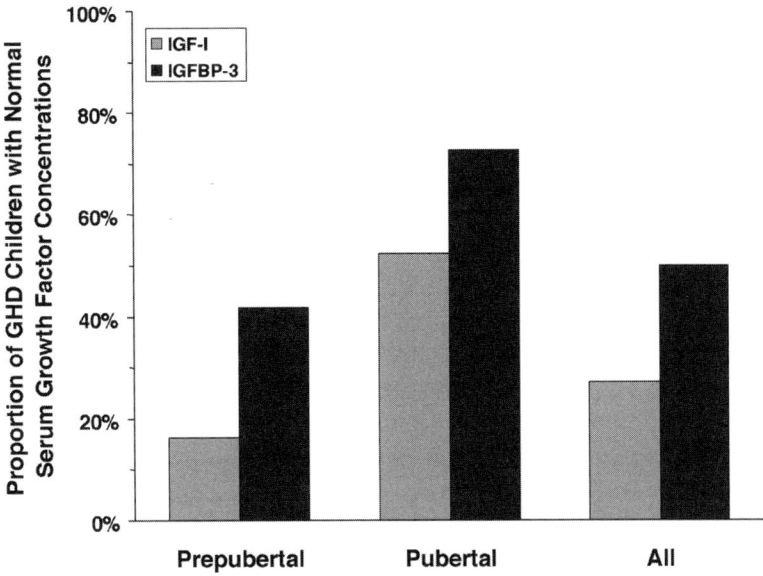

Fig. 2. Percentage of children with documented growth hormone deficiency (GHD) with normal serum conentrations of IGF-I (gray bars) and IGFBP-3 (black bars), in a series of 72 brain tumor survivors.

closely for deceleration in growth; accurate assessment of standing and sitting heights, upper and lower segment lengths, arm span, and weight should be determined every 3–6 mo, and height and weight measurements should be accurately plotted on standard growth curves. Pubertal stage should be recorded at each visit. Calculation of interval growth velocity should be determined at each visit, and plotted on standard growth velocity curves, particularly for adolescents, in whom a "normal" growth velocity may actually be blunted compared to typical velocities seen during the pubertal growth spurt. Children who demonstrate growth deceleration (or, for pubertal children, fail to demonstrate adequate growth acceleration) should have further evaluation, including routine blood chemistries and hematologic studies, thyroid function studies, and a radiograph of the hand and wrist for determination of the skeletal age. Provocative growth hormone testing should be considered if these preliminary studies do not identify another cause for poor growth. Furthermore, the clinician should continue to consider later-onset growth hormone deficiency in children who have received cranial irradiation, as the incidence of growth hormone deficiency progressively increases over time following irradiation *(10)*.

Once the diagnosis of growth hormone deficiency has been established, the initiation of replacement growth hormone therapy should proceed only after serial imaging studies, usually performed over 1–2 yr, demonstrate that there is no residual active tumor growth. Treatment is typically initiated at a dose of 0.3 mg/kg/wk, given as nightly subcutaneous injections. For families in whom adherence or needle phobia may be an issue, a depot form of growth hormone, given once or twice monthly, is a viable alternative to daily dosing *(71)*. Families should be counseled that although growth hormone therapy has been successful in improving growth in growth hormone deficient children following tumor treatment *(72,73)*, final height is still likely to fall short of midparental target height *(74)*. This is true especially for children who have received chemotherapy in addition to cranial irradiation *(43,44)* or who have received radiation to the spine, in whom direct skeletal injury is resistant to growth hormone therapy *(18)*.

A thorough discussion with the family of the risks and benefits of growth hormone therapy is critical before treatment is initiated. The potential mitogenic stimulation of tumor recurrence by growth hormone is a realistic concern. In single-institution studies *(75–77)* and in the two large international post-marketing surveillance databases (National Cooperative Growth Study and Kabi International Growth Study) *(78,79)*, however, the outcomes have been favorable. For craniopharyngioma, medulloblastoma, and hypothalamic glioma survivors, the three most common pediatric brain tumors, the incidence of tumor recurrence is no greater in children receiving growth hormone than in those who have not received growth hormone. Data is more limited on the less common tumors such as germinoma and ependymoma. Japanese investigators reported an increased risk of leukemia in children receiving growth hormone treatment *(80)*. However, a large international analysis demonstrated that the incidence of leukemia in children receiving growth hormone was no greater than the expected rate of leukemia in the population, when cases with known risk factors were excluded *(81)*. The most current data suggest that the increased frequency of leukemia in growth hormone treated patients is limited to those patients with known risk factors. It should be noted that children with prior tumors or radiation exposure do constitute a higher-risk group.

Ongoing surveillance of children receiving growth hormone for brain tumors necessarily requires serial brain imaging, typically at 6–12 mo intervals for the first several years. Quarterly clinical follow-up is recommended for assessment of growth, pubertal development, and for the development of such growth hormone-associated complications as scoliosis, slipped capital femoral epiphysis, and benign intracranial hypertension *(82)*.

There are currently no well-established criteria for titration of growth hormone dosage during therapy. Treatment is typically initiated with a standard dose based on weight, and doses are increased at subsequent visits for weight gain. Recently, investigators have promulgated the ideas of dose titration based on linear growth rate (the anthropometric argument) or by IGF-I level (the biochemical argument), although outcome data using these methods has yet to be collected and published. A recent study evaluated the use of higher doses of growth hormone, up to 0.7 mg/kg/wk, in pubertal subjects, to mimic the physiologic increase in growth hormone secretion during puberty, and demonstrated a modest increase in growth rate *(83)*.

Pubertal Disorders

As mentioned earlier, both delayed and precocious puberty may be seen in children treated with cranial irradiation for brain tumors. Accurate assessment of the pubertal stage should be made in all children at each visit to identify those with aberrant developmental patterns. Radiographs of the hand and wrist should be performed for the determination of the skeletal age in children with evidence either of sexual precocity (onset of breast budding in girls younger than 8-yr-old or testicular enlargement in boys younger than 9) or delay (lack of signs of puberty by age 13 in girls or 14 in boys).

Lack of pubertal development may be due to simple constitutional delay, a normal variant of growth frequently seen in children who have had a severe or chronic illness. These "late bloomers" will typically begin puberty when their bone age reaches 11–12.

No specific treatment is required other than reassurance, although treatment with short courses of gonadal steroids may accelerate pubertal development and ease the psychosocial adjustment of the adolescent.

True hypogonadism may be either primary (hypergonadotropic), due to radiation- or chemotherapy-induced gonadal failure, or secondary (hypogonadotropic), from surgical or radiation-induced injury to the hypothalamus or pituitary. The conditions are differentiated by the measurement of the gonadotropins lutenizing hormone (LH) and follicle stimulating hormone (FSH). Children with true hypogonadism should receive gonadal steroid replacement at an appropriate skeletal age. In children with co-existent hypogonadotropic hypogonadism and growth hormone deficiency, however, a later induction of puberty may provide a better final height outcome by delaying the closure of the epiphyseal plates.

Male hormone replacement is usually accomplished through monthly doses of intramuscular injections of testosterone enanthate or cypionate, starting at 50 mg and increasing gradually over 2–3 yr to 200 mg every 2–4 wk. Transdermal testosterone patches and gels have recently become available, and may produce more consistent serum levels of testosterone in the older adolescent on a stable replacement dose. Female hormone replacement is usually initiated with low doses of conjugated estrogens (Premarin, 0.3 mg) or ethinyl estradiol (20 µg) and increased over the next 1–2 yr, after which a progestin (medroxyprogesterone acetate, Provera) is added to the last 5 d of the cycle to induce bleeding. Once cycling has been induced, it is generally more convenient to use one of the estrogen-progestin combination oral contraceptive pills. Monitoring of gonadal steroid replacement is usually accomplished clinically, although mid-cycle or trough testosterone levels may provide useful information for dose titration in boys.

Precocious puberty in children with brain tumors is usually a complication of cranial irradiation and is typically more common in girls than boys *(33,84)*. However, precocious puberty due to tumor location may be seen in hypothalamic glioma and is a common presenting feature in boys with this tumor even before treatment *(34)* (Fig. 3). Sexual precocity further complicates the growth problems in children with brain tumor, by masking coexistent growth hormone deficiency and also by advancing skeletal maturation, reducing the time available for growth-promoting therapy. Treatment of sexual precocity with long-acting synthetic gonadotropin-releasing hormone (GnRH) agonists is effective in suppressing gonadal steroid production, and when initiated early, contributes to improvements in final height outcome *(85–87)*.

In children with precocious puberty, or in children with growth hormone deficiency in whom puberty will be delayed to maximize growth potential, treatment with GnRH agonists is usually initiated with depot leuprolide, 0.05 mg/kg given as a monthly intramuscular injection. Adequacy of suppression should be demonstrated by serial clinical assessment, bone age radiographs, and in boys, the documentation of prepubertal serum testosterone levels. In girls the LH level, as measured by a sensitive immunochemiluminometric assay *(55)*, should be suppressed to less than 0.3–0.5 mIU/mL *(88)*. If this test is not available, periodic documentation of a prepubertal LH response to GnRH during a standard GnRH provocative test may be indicated.

Hypothyroidism

Many of the symptoms and signs of hypothyroidism are non-specific and overlap with the side effects of cancer therapy, such as constipation, fatigue, increased sleep, and cold

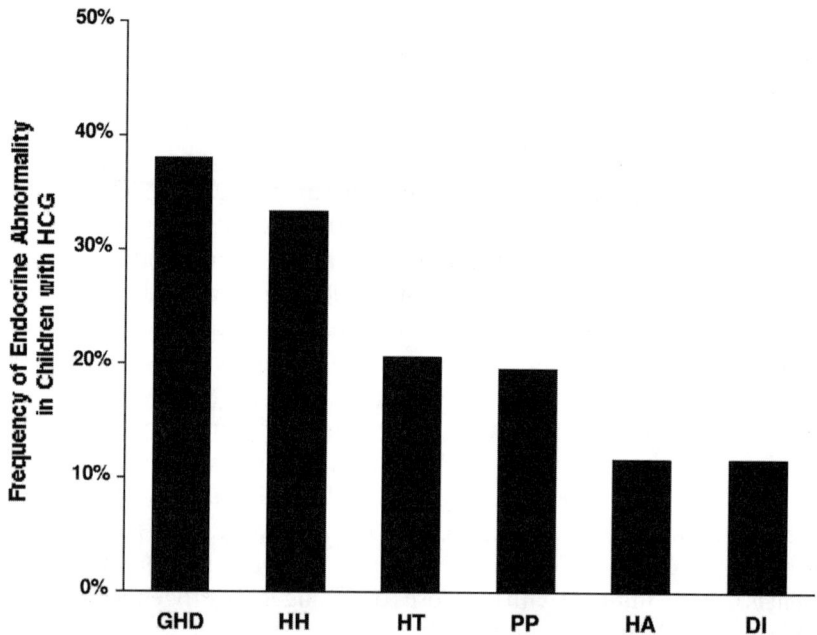

Fig. 3. Frequency of endocrine abnormalities occurring in children with hypothalamic-chiasmatic glioma (HCG). GHD, growth hormone deficiency; HH, hypogonadotropic hypogonadism; HT, hypothyroidism; PP, precocious puberty; HA, hypo-adrenalism; DI, diabetes insipidus.

intolerance. Frank myxedema is a late finding. Therefore, thyroid function should be monitored routinely. Primary hypothyroidism may occur following irradiation of the neck, and secondary hypothyroidism may be a complication of surgery or radiation to the pituitary. Children with a low T4 and elevated TSH obviously have primary hypothyroidism. However, in children who have received both cranial and neck irradiation and who are at risk for both primary and secondary hypothyroidism, the finding of a low or normal TSH does not preclude the existence of true hypothyroidism. In children who have received cranial irradiation or surgery, measurement of thyroid function should include not only T4 and TSH but also free T4 as well. Elevated TSH or depressed free T4 levels are indications for thyroid hormone supplementation. Central hypothyroidism may also be documented by a blunted or delayed response to TRH.

Treatment with levothyroxine is typically initiated at doses of 2–3 µg/kg/d, given as a daily dose. Repeat thyroid studies should be obtained 8–12 wk after the initiation of therapy or dose change, and in stable patients, once or twice yearly. Free and total T4 levels should be maintained in the upper half of the normal range. In children with primary hypothyroidism, maintenance of TSH levels in the lower half of the normal range is also sought.

Adrenal Insufficiency

Accurate assessment of adrenal function following brain tumor treatment is hampered by the diagnostic difficulty in evaluating the hypothalamic-pituitary-adrenal axis and the frequent use of high doses of glucocorticoids to reduce brain swelling in the immediate post-operative course, possibly inducing adrenal suppression in patients with normal adrenal function. Clinical symptoms of adrenal insufficiency (lethargy, nausea, vomiting, general malaise, and weight loss) may be attributed to surgery, chemotherapy, or cranial irradiation. However, adrenal insufficiency is a potentially life-threatening complication of cranial irradiation that should be investigated in all brain tumor survivors.

There is no clear consensus regarding the duration of adrenal suppression following high-dose glucocorticoid therapy and optimal protocol for weaning of hydrocortisone *(89)*. Maintenance hydrocortisone treatment, 10–15 mg/m^2 body surface area/d, should be initiated in all children treated with perioperative high-dose glucocorticoids. Once the high-potency glucocorticoids have been discontinued, the maintenance hydrocortisone may also be weaned slowly. Weaning is often accomplished with a gradual tapering of 10–20% of the total daily dose over 5–10 wk. During this time, families should be instructed to treat the appearance of symptoms of adrenal insufficiency or signs of intercurrent stress or illness with "stress" doses of hydrocortisone, 3–5 times the maintenance dose.

Once the child has been successfully weaned off hydrocortisone, adequacy of hypothalamic-pituitary-adrenal axis function may be tested. There are multiple tests of adrenal function, all with advantages and shortcomings *(90,91)*. Fasting 8 AM cortisol levels are generally neither sensitive nor specific for diagnosing adrenal insufficiency. Provocative testing, therefore, is indicated in most children. The "gold standard" test of adrenal function, the insulin tolerance test, may precipitate hypoglycemia or adrenal crisis and is generally avoided in this population. The metyrapone test is a very sensitive test of adrenal reserve during stress *(92)*, but is often limited in utility practically because of the tendency of children to vomit after receiving the dose. The standard 250 μg ACTH (Cortrosyn) stimulation test has been criticized as using an excessive "pharmacologic" dose of ACTH that fails to identify milder forms of adrenal insufficiency or adrenal insufficiency of recent onset. The low-dose (1 μg) ACTH stimulation test *(93,94)* may be more sensitive to the more subtle disturbances in the HPA axis, and is free of dangerous or unpleasant side-effects. The corticotropin releasing hormone (CRH) test has also demonstrated concordant results to insulin tolerance testing in 85% of patients tested for adrenal insufficiency *(95)*.

Patients who fail to demonstrate a cortisol response of at least 18 μg/dL on the low-dose ACTH test or CRH test should be initiated on maintenance hydrocortisone replacement and instructed for increasing the dose for periods of intercurrent illness or severe stress. The starting dose of maintenance hydrocortisone should approximate normal cortisol production rates in children, 6–8 mg/m^2/d *(96)*, although lower doses of hydrocortisone are frequently sufficient. Families should be instructed on techniques for parenteral injections of hydrocortisone for emergencies. Children should be monitored clinically for signs and symptoms of glucocorticoid excess as well as deficiency.

Disorders of Water Balance

Anti-diuretic hormone deficiency (diabetes insipidus) and excess (SIADH) are most frequently seen in the immediate post-operative period when the pituitary gland has been manipulated or resected. Diabetes insipidus unrelated to surgical trauma may also be a complication of the tumor itself. Symptoms of diabetes insipidus include excessive thirst and urination; the diagnosis is suggested by profuse dilute urine and elevated serum sodium levels. Formal water deprivation testing, in which a dehydrating stress is employed to stimulate the secretion of anti-diuretic hormone, is sometimes needed to confirm the diagnosis *(97)*. Normal individuals are typically able to prevent serum concentration to greater than 295 mOsm/L by concentrating the urine to greater than 800 mOsm/L *(98)*. Affected patients cannot adequately conserve water and concentrate the urine, and will thus continue to spill free water, reflected by an increase in the serum sodium and osmolarity. SIADH is characterized by oliguria, fluid overload, and hyponatremia. It is typically transient, occuring in the immediate post-operative period, in the setting of increased intracranial pressure or injury to the infundibular stalk. Treatment includes fluid restriction. Vigilant monitoring of fluid input and output and serum sodium is necessary, as the resolution of SIADH is often followed by the onset of diabetes insipidus.

Treatment of diabetes insipidus involves hormone replacement with long-acting synthetic forms of anti-diuretic hormone, DDAVP, either with an intranasal spray or an oral tablet. In patients with an intact thirst-sensing mechanism, the goal of treatment is to reduce urinary volume and frequency so that the child need not wake multiple times overnight to urinate or excuse him/herself from classes excessively. This is usually accomplished with once nightly or twice daily dosing of intranasal or oral DDAVP. Families are instructed to withhold subsequent dosing of DDAVP until the previous dose has worn off, readily noted by an increase in urination. Laboratory monitoring of the serum sodium and/or osmolarity is usually unnecessary. In infants, children with hypothalamic damage to the thirst center, or other brain injury resulting in the inability to communicate thirst, the management is more complex. Caregivers are typically asked to keep a log of fluid input and urinary output. Base water replacement is calculated, based on the child's age, body surface area, and clinical requirements, and supplemental water may is given for excessive urine output. Monitoring of the child's weight and serum sodium levels often aids in the clinical management.

An unusual but potentially dangerous water balance disorder in this population is cerebral salt-wasting. In this condition, brain natriuretic peptide is released inappropriately, resulting in excessive urinary losses of sodium and water, hyponatremia, and dehydration *(99,100)*. We have described coincident diabetes insipidus and cerebral salt-wasting in childhood survivors of brain tumors *(101)*. The danger of salt-wasting in children with diabetes insipidus is that the condition may not be recognized. Continued excessive urination may be interpreted as insufficient DDAVP replacement and repeated doses may be given inappropriately, worsening the hyponatremia and increasing the risk of hyponatremic seizures. A high index of suspicion must be maintained for salt-wasting, especially in the context of polyuria resistant to supplemental DDAVP administration. Urgent clinical and laboratory evaluation is indicated.

CONCLUSION

Children surviving brain tumor treatment are at a markedly increased risk of developing late endocrine complications. Regular evaluation is necessary to prevent hormonal disturbances that threaten the well being of these children. It is recommended that a child surviving brain tumor treatment be assessed soon after cancer therapy is completed (or earlier if clinical findings so dictate). The children should have regular interval (3–6 mo) visits, which include careful auxologic measurements as well as pubertal assessments. We routinely (yearly intervals) monitor bone age, IGF-I and IGFBP-3, free T4, TSH and morning cortisol concentrations. Clinical findings and symptoms dictate other tests, including gonadal steroids, or provocative tests, such as water deprivation, CRH, GnRH or growth hormone testing. Regular screening for hormonal disturbances and timely intervention has been successful in improving the general health and overall quality of life for this high-risk population.

REFERENCES

1. Ahmed SR, Shalet SM. Hypothalamic growth hormone releasing factor deficiency following cranial irradiation. Clin Endocrinol 1984;21;483–488.
2. Blacklay A, Grossman A, Ross RJM, et al. Cranial irradiation for cerebral and nasopharyngeal tumours in children: evidence for the production of a hypothalamic defect in growth hormone release. J Endocrinol 1986;108:25–29.
3. Rappaport R, Brauner R. Growth and endocrine disorders secondary to cranial irradiation. Pediatr Res 1989;25:561–567.
4. Shalet SM. Radiation and pituitary dysfunction. N Engl J Med 1993;328:131–133.
5. Sklar CA. Neuroendocrine complication of cancer therapy. In Schwartz CL, Constine LS, Hobbie WI, Ruccione KS, eds. Survivors of Childhood Cancer: Assessment and Management. Mosby, St. Louis, MO, 1994, pp. 97–110.
6. Withers HR. Biologic basis for altered fractionation schemes. Cancer 1985;55:2086–2091.
7. Shalet SM, Price DA, Beardwell CG, et al. Normal growth despite abnormalities in growth hormone secretion in children treated for acute leukemia. J Pediatr 1979;94:719–722.
8. Kirk JA, Stevens MM, Menser MA, et al. Growth failure and growth hormone deficiency after treatment for acute lymphoblastic leukemia. Lancet 1987;1:190–193.
9. Sklar CA. Growth and pubertal development in survivors of childhood cancer. Pediatrics 1991;18:53–60.
10. Duffner PK, Cohen ME, Vorhees ML, et al. Long-term effects of cranial irradiation on endocrine function in children with brain tumors, a prospective study. Cancer 1985;56:2189–2193.
11. Chapman RM. Effect of cytotoxic therapy on sexuality and gonadal function. Semin Oncol 1982;9:84–94.
12. Oberfield SE, Sklar C, Allen J, et al. Thyroid and gonadal function and growth of long-term survivors of medulloblastoma/PNET. In Green DM, D'Angio GJ (eds): Late Effects of Treatment for Childhood Cancer. New York, Wiley-Liss, 1992, p. 55.
13. Rappaport R, Brauner R, Czernichow P, et al. Effect of hypothalamic and pituitary irradiation on pubertal development in children with cranial tumors. J Clin Endocrinol Metab 1982;54:1164–1168.
14. Constine LS, Woolf PD, Cann D, et al. Hypothalamic-pituitary dysfunction after radiation for brain tumors. N Engl J Med 1993;328:87–94.
15. Lam KSL, Tse VKC, Wang C, et al. Effects of irradiation on hypothalamic-pituitary function: a 5 year longitudinal study in patients with nasopharyngeal carcinoma. Q J Med 1991;78:165–176.
16. Livesey EA, Brook CG. Thyroid dysfunction after radiotherapy and chemotherapy of brain tumours. Arch Dis Child 1987;64:593–595.
17. Oberfield SE, Nirenberg A, Allen JC, et al. Hypothalamic-pituitary-adrenal function following cranial irradiation. Horm Res 1997;47:9–16.
18. Clayton PE, Shalet SM, Price DA. Growth response to growth hormone therapy following craniospinal irradiation. Eur J Pediatr 1988;147:597–601.
19. Willi SM, Cooke K, Goldwein J, et al. Growth in children after bone marrow transplantation for advanced neuroblastoma compared with growth after transplantation for leukemia or aplastic anemia. J Pediatr 1992;120:726–732.
20. Fuks Z, Glatstein E, Marsa GW, et al. Long-term effects of external irradiation on the pituitary and thyroid glands. Cancer 1976;37:1151–1161.
21. Schimpff SC. Radiation-related thyroid dysfunction: implications for the treatment of Hodgkin's disease. Ann Intern Med 1980;92:91–98
22. Shalet SM, Rosenstock JD, Beardwell CG, et al. Thyroid dysfunction following external irradiation to the neck for Hodgkin's disease in childhood. Radiology 1977;28:511–515.
23. Kapalan MM, Garnick MB, Gelber R, et al. Risk factors for thyroid abnormalities after neck irradiation for childhood cancer. Am J Med 1983;74:272–280.

24. Devney RB, Sklar CA, Nesbit ME, et al. Serial thyroid function measurements in children with Hodgkin's disease. J Pediatr 1984;105:223–227.
25. Hancock SL, Cox RS, McDougall JR. Thyroid diseases after treatment of Hodgkin's disease. N Engl J Med 1991;325:599–605.
26. Oglivy-Stuart AL, Shalet SM, Gattamaneni HR. Thyroid function after treatment of brain tumors in children. J Pediatr 1991;119:733–737.
27. Rowley MJ, Leach DR, Warner GA, et al. Effect of graded doses of ionizing radiation on the human testis. Radiat Res 1974;59:665–678.
28. Sanders JE, Pritchard S, Mahoney P, et al. Growth and development following marrow transplantation for leukemia. Blood 1986;68:1129–1135.
29. Shalet SM, Beardwell CG, Jacobs HS, et al. Testicular function following irradiation of the human prepubertal testis. Clin Endocrinol 1978;9:483–490.
30. Stillman RJ, Schinfield JS, Schiff I, et al. Ovarian failure in long-term survivors of childhood malignancy. Am J Obstet Gynecol 1981;139:62–66.
31. Leiper AD, Stanhope R, Kitching P, Chessels JM. Precocious and premature puberty associated with treatment of acute leukemia. Arch Dis Chil 1987;62:1107–1112.
32. Sklar CA. Growth and pubertal development in survivors of childhood cancer. Pediatrics 1991;18:53–60.
33. Oglivy-Stuart AL, Clayton PE, Shalet SM. Cranial irradiation and early puberty. J Clin Endocrinol Metab 1994;78:1282–1286.
34. Collett-Solberg PF, Sernyak H, Satin-Smith M, et al. Endocrine outcome in long-term survivors of low-grade hypothalamic/chiasmatic glioma. Clin Endocrinol 1997;47:79–85.
35. Constine LS, Rubin P, Woolf PD, Daane K, Lush C. Hyperprolactinemia and hypothyroidism following cytotoxic therapy for central nervous system malignancies. J Clin Oncol 1987;5:1841–1851.
36. Goldwein JW. Effects of radiation therapy on skeletal growth in childhood. Clin Orthop 1991;262:101–107.
37. Oberfield SE, Allen JC, Pollack J, et al. Long-term endocrine sequelae after treatment of medulloblastoma: prospective study of growth and thyroid function. J Pediatr 1986;108:219–223.
38. Pasqualini T, Diez B, Domene H, et al. Long-term endocrine sequelae after surgery, radiotherapy, and chemotherapy in children with medulloblastoma. Cancer 1987;59:801–806.
39. Clayton PE, Shalet SM. The evolution of spine growth after irradiation. Clin Oncol 1991;3:220–222.
40. Hasle H, Helgestad J, Christensen JK, et al. Prolonged intrathecal chemotherapy replacing cranial irradiation in high-risk acute lymphatic leukemia: long-term follow-up with cerebral computed tomography scans and endocrinological studies. Eur J Pediatr 1995;154:24–29.
41. Tamminga RY, Zweens M, Kamps W, et al. Longitudinal study of bone age in acute lymphoblastic leukemia. Med Pediatr Oncol 1993;21:14–18.
42. Thun-Hohenstein L, Frisch H, Schuster E. Growth after radiotherapy and chemotherapy in children with leukemia or lymphoma. Horm Res 1992;37:91–95.
43. Olshan JS, Gubernick J, Packer RJ, et al. The effects of adjuvant chemotherapy on growth in children with medulloblastoma. Cancer 1992;70:2013–2017.
44. Moshang T, Grimberg A. The effects of irradiation and chemotherapy on growth. Endocrinol Metab Clin North Am 1996;25:731–741.
45. Counts DR, Gwirtsman H, Carlsson LMS, et al. The effects of anorexia nervosa and refeeding on growth-hormone binding protein, the insulin-like growth factors (IGFs) and the IGF-binding proteins. J Clin Endocrinol Metab 1992;75:762–767.
46. Nivot S, Benelli C, Clot JP, et al. Nonparallel changes of growth hormone (GH) and insulin-like growth factor-1, insulin-like growth factor binding protein-3, and growth hormone binding protein, after craniospinal irradiation and chemotherapy. J Clin Endocrinol Metab 1994;78:597–601.
47. Price DA, Morris MJ, Rowsell KV, et al. The effects of antileukaemic drugs on somatomedic production and cartilage responsiveness to somatomedin in vitro. Pediatr Res 1981;15:1553.
48. Baron J, Oerter Klein K, Colli MJ, et al. Catch-up growth after glucocorticoid excess: a mechanism intrinsic to the growth plate. Endocrinol 1994;135:1367–1371.
49. Chapman RM. Effect of cytotoxic therapy on sexuality and gonadal function. Semin Oncol 1982;9:84–94.
50. Jaffe N, Sullivan MP, Reid H, et al. Male reproductive function in long-term survivors of childhood cancer. Med Pediatr Oncol 1988;16:241–247.
51. Byrne J, Fears TR, Gail MH, et al. Early menopause in long term survivors of cancer during adolescence. Am J Obstet Gynecol 1992;166:788–793.

52. Siris ES, Leventhal BG, Vaitukaitis JL. Effects of childhood leukemia and chemotherapy on puberty and reproductive function in girls. N Engl J Med 1976;294:1143–1146.
53. Meacham LR, Ghim TT, Crocker IR, et al. Systematic approach for detection of endocrine disorders in children treated for brain tumors. Med Pediatr Oncol 1997;29:86–91.
54. Shalet SM, Gibson B, Swindell R, Pearson D. Effect of spinal irradiation on growth. Arch Dis Child 1987;62:461–464.
55. Neely EK, Hintz RL, Wilson DM, et al. Normal ranges for immunochemiluminometric gonadotropin assays. J Pediatr 1995;127:40–46.
56. Rosenfeld RG, Albertsson-Wikland K, Cassorla R, et al. Diagnostic controversy: the diagnosis of growth hormone deficiency revisited. J Clin Endocrinol Metab 1995; 80:1532–1540.
57. Marin G, Domene HM, Blackwell BJ. The effects of estrogen priming and puberty on the growth hormone response to standardized treadmill exercise and arginine-insulin in normal girls and boys. J Clin Endocrinol Metab 1994;79:537–541.
58. Tassori P, Cacciari E, Cau M, et al. Variability of growth hormone reponse to pharmacological and sleep tests performed twice in short children. J Clin Endocrinol Metab 1990;71:230–234.
59. Zadik Z, Chalew SA, Gilula Z, Kowarski AA. Reproducibility of growth hormone testing procedures: a comparison between 24-hour integrated concentration and pharmacological stimulation. J Clin Endocrinol Metab 1990;71:1127–1130.
60. Frasier D. A review of growth hormone stimulation tests in children. Pediatrics 1974;53:929–937.
61. Blum WF, Ranke MR, Kietzman K, Gauggel E, Zeisel HJ, Bierich JR. A specific radioimmunoassay for the growth hormone (GH)-dependent somatomedin-binding protein: its use for diagnosis of GH deficiency. J Clin Endocrinol Metab 1990;70:1292–1298.
62. Blum WF, Albertsson-Wikland K, Rosberg S, Ranke MB. Serum levels of insulin-like growth factor I (IGF-I) and IGF binding protein 3 reflect spontaneous growth hormone secretion. J Clin Endocrinol Metab 1990;76:1610–1616.
63. Weinzimer SA, Homan SA, Ferry RJ, Moshang T. Serum IGF-I and IGFBP-3 concentrations do not accurately predict growth hormone deficiency in children with brain tumors. Clin Endocrinol 1999;51:339–345.
64. Sklar C, Sarafoglou K, Whittam E. Efficacy of insulin-like growth factor binding protein-3 in predicting the growth hormone response to provocative testing in children treated with cranial irradiation. Acta Endocrinol 1993;129:511–515.
65. Tillmann V, Buckler JMH, Kibirige MS, et al. Biochemical tests in the diagnosis of childhood growth hormone deficiency. J Clin Endocrinol Metab 1997;82:531–535.
66. Rosenfield RL, Furlanetto R, Bock D. Relationship of somatomedin-C concentrations to pubertal changes. J Pediatr 1983;10:723–728.
67. Pescovity OH, Rosenfeld RG, Hintz RL, et al. Somatomedin-C in accelerated growth of children with precocious puberty. J Pediatr 1985;107:20–25.
68. Rosenfield RL, Furlanetto R. Physiologic testosterone or estradiol induction of puberty increases somatomedin-C. J Pediatr 1985;107:415–417.
69. Rosenfeld RG, Wilson DM, Lee PDK, Hintz RL. Insulin-like growth factors I and II in evaluation of growth retardation. J Pediatr 1986;109:428–433.
70. Juul A, Bang P, Hertel NT, et al. Serum insulin-like growth factor-I in 1030 healthy children, adolescents, and adults: relation to age, sex, stage of puberty, testicular size, and body mass index. J Clin Endocrinol Metab 1990;78:744–752.
71. Silverman B. Clinical trial results: sustained-release growth hormone given once or twice monthly in children with GH deficiency. National Cooperative Growth Study Thirteenth Annual Investigators Meeting, 1999, Charleston, SC.
72. Vassilopoulou-Sellin R, Klein MJ, Moore BD III, et al. Efficacy of growth hormone replacement therapy in children with organic growth hormone deficiency after cranial irradiation. Horm Res 1995;43:188–193.
73. Clayton PE, Shalet SM, Price DA. Response to growth hormone treatment in children with central nervous system malignancy. In: Ranke MB, Gunnarson R, eds. Progress in Growth Hormone Therapy - 5 Years of KIGS. J & J Verlag, Mannheim, 1994, pp. 173–189.
74. Oglivy-Stuart AL, Shalet S. Growth and puberty after growth hormone treatment after irradiation for brain tumours. Arch Dis Child 1995;73:141–146.
75. Moshang Jr T. Is brain tumor recurrence increased following growth hormone therapy? Trends Endocrinol Metab 1995;6:205–209.

76. Clayton PE, Shalet SM, Gattamaneni HR, Price DA. Does growth hormone cause relapse of brain tumors? Lancet 1987;1:711–713.
77. Oglivy-Stuart AL, Ryder WDJ, Gattamaneni HR, Clayton PE, Shalet SM. Growth hormone and tumour recurrence. BMJ 1992;304:1601–1605.
78. Moshang Jr T, Chen Rundle A, Graves DA, Nickas J, Johanson A, Meadows A. Brain tumor recurrence in children treated with growth hormone: The National Cooperative Growth Study experience. J Pediatr 1996;128(Supp):S4–S7.
79. Wilton P. Adverse events during growth hormone treatment: 5 years experience in the Kabi International Growth Study. In: Ranke MB, Gunnarsson R, eds. Progress in Growth Hormone Therapy: 5 Years of KIGS. J & J Verlag, Mannheim, 1994, pp. 291–307.
80. Watanabe S, Tsunematsu Y, Fumimoto J, et al. Leukemia in patients treated with growth hormone. Lancet 1988;1:1159–1160.
81. Fradkin JE, Mills JL, Schonberger LB, et al. Risk of leukemia after treatment with pituitary growth hormone. JAMA 1993;270:2829–2832.
82. Maneatis T, Baptista J, Connelly K, Blethen S. Growth hormone safety update from the National Cooperative Growth Study. J Pediatr Endocrinol Metab 2000;13:1035–1044.
83. Mauras N, Attie KM, Reiter EO, Saenger P, Baptista J. High dose recombinant human growth hormone (GH) treatment of GH-deficient patients in puberty increases near-final height: a randomized, multicenter trial. J Clin Endocrinol Metab 2000;85:3653–3660.
84. Oberfield SE, Soranno D, Niremberg A, et al. Age at onset of puberty following high dose central nervous system radiation therapy. Arch Pediatr Adolesc Med 1996;150:589–592.
85. Paul D, Conte FA, Grumbach MM, Kaplan SL. Long term effect of gonadotropin-releasing hormone agonist therapy on final and near-final height in 26 children with true precocious puberty treated at a median age of less than 5 years. J Clin Endocrinol Metab 1995;80:546–551.
86. Leiper AD, Stanhope R, Preece MA, Grant DB, Chessels JM. Precocious or early puberty and growth failure in girls treated for acute lymphoblastic leukaemia. Horm Res 1988;30:72–76.
87. Thomas BC, Stanhope R, Leiper AD. Gonadotropin releasing hormone analogue and growth hormone therapy in precocious and premature puberty following cranial irradiation for acute lymphoblastic leukaemia. Horm Res 1993;39:25–29.
88. Neely EK, Wilson DM, Lee PA, Stene M, Hintz RL. Spontaneous serum gonadotropin concentrations in the evaluation of precocious puberty. J Pediatr 1995;127:47–52.
89. Fass B. Glucocorticoid therapy for nonendocrine disorders: withdrawal and "coverage." Pediatr Clin North Am 1979;26:251–256.
90. Grinspoon SK, Biller BMK. Laboratory assessment of adrenal insufficiency. J Clin Endocrinol Metab 1994;79:923–931.
91. Oelkers W. Adrenal insufficiency. N Engl J Med 1996;335:1206–1212.
92. Thornton PS, Alter CA, Katz LE, Gruccio DA, Winyard PJ, Moshang T Jr. The new highly sensitive adrenocorticotropin assay improves detection of patients with partial adrenocorticotropin deficiency in a short-term metyrapone test. J Pediatr Endocrinol Metab 1994;7:317–324.
93. Tordjman K, Jaffe A Grazas N, Apter C, Stern N. The role of the low-dose (1 µg) adrenocorticotropin test in the evaluation of patients with pituitary disease. J Clin Endocrinol Metab 1995;80:1301–1305.
94. Broide J, Soferman R, Kivity S, et al. Low-dose adrenocorticotropin test reveals impaired adrenal function in patients taking inhaled corticosteroids. J Clin Endocrinol Metab 1995;80:1243–1246.
95. Schlagecke R, Kornely E, Santen RT, Ridderskamp P. The effect of long-term glucocorticoid therapy on pituitary-adrenal responses to exogenous corticotropin-releasing hormone. N Engl J Med 326;226–230.
96. Linder BL, Esteban NV, Yergey AL, Winterer JC, Loriaux DL, Cassorla F. Cortisol production rate in childhood and adolescence. J Pediatr 1990;117:892–896.
97. Perheentupa J, Czernichow P. Water regulation and its disorders. In: Kappy MS, Blizzard RM, Migeon CJ, eds. Wilkins Diagnosis and Treatment of Endocrine Disorders in Childhood and Adolescence, 4th ed. 1994, pp. 1139–1140.
98. Blevins LS, Wand GS. Diabetes insipidus. Crit Care Med 1992;20:69–79.
99. Ganong CA, Kappy MS. Cerebral salt wasting in children: the need for recognition and treatment. Am J Dis Child 1993;147:167–169.
100. Kappy MS, Ganong CA. Cerebral salt wasting in children: the role of atrial natriuretic hormone. Adv Pediatr 1996;43:271–308.
101. Ferry Jr RJ, Katz LEL, Weinzimer SA, and Moshang Jr T. Co-existent central diabetes insipidus and salt wasting in a child. National Cooperative Growth Study, Thirteenth Annual Investigators Meeting, 1999, Charleston, SC.

11 Endocrinologic Sequelae of Anorexia Nervosa

Catherine M. Gordon, MD, MSc and Estherann Grace, MD

CONTENTS

  INTRODUCTION
  HYPOTHALAMIC-PITUITARY-ADRENAL AXIS IN AN
  LEPTIN AND INSULIN ABNORMALITIES
  GROWTH HORMONE ABNORMALITIES
  THYROID HORMONE ABNORMALITIES
  HYPOTHALAMIC-PITUITARY-OVARIAN AXIS ABNORMALITIES
  PROLACTIN
  VASOPRESSIN
  OSTEOPENIA AND ABNORMALITIES IN SKELETAL DYNAMICS IN AN
  PATIENT EVALUATION
  MANAGEMENT
  CONCLUSION
  REFERENCES

INTRODUCTION

Anorexia nervosa (AN) is a severe psychiatric and medical condition once described as the "relentless pursuit of thinness" *(1)*. The disorder affects 0.48% of adolescent females in the US *(2)*, and represents the third most common chronic disease among American females. The disorder is most commonly seen among adolescent girls, with estimates of male-female prevalence ratio ranging from 1:6 to 1:10. However, 19–30% of younger patients with AN are male, and the overall prevalence of this disorder among adolescent boys appears to be increasing *(3–5)*. 85% of these patients present between the age of 13–20 yr-of-age during a critical period for growth, pubertal development, and the maximal bone accretion that culminates in peak bone mass. The disorder can result in a compromise in each of these important endocrinologic events. Patients with AN also have a characteristic clinical picture of endocrine dysfunction, including amenorrhea,

From: *Contemporary Endocrinology: Pediatric Endocrinology: A Practical Clinical Guide*
Edited by: S. Radovick and M. H. MacGillivray © Humana Press Inc., Totowa, NJ

Table 1
DSM-IV Criteria for Anorexia Nervosa

1. An intense fear of gaining weight or becoming fat, even though underweight
2. A disturbance in body image such that the patient feels fat even when emaciated
3. Refusal to maintain body weight over a minimal normal weight (weight loss leading to maintenance of body weight 15% below that expected for height)
4. Amenorrhea for three or more cycles

abnormal temperature regulation, elevated growth hormone (GH) levels, and abnormal eating suggestive of hypothalamic or pituitary dysfunction. Therefore, endocrine function has been studied extensively in these patients. The multiple endocrine abnormalities seen appear to represent an adaptation to the starvation state.

The primary clinical features of AN by Diagnostic and Statistical Manual of Mental Disorders, 4th Edition (DSM-IV) criteria are shown in Table 1. Of note, pubertal adolescent girls may fail to make normal weight gains and may gradually fall below the 85th percentile of expected weight for height, or lose the equivalent of 15% of expected body weight for height. Linear growth failure may also result from inadequate caloric intake at a critical stage of puberty, while small amounts of gonadal steroids may continue to be secreted, advancing bone age and resulting in the loss of final adult stature.

HYPOTHALAMIC-PITUITARY-ADRENAL AXIS IN AN

Patients with AN exhibit hyperactivity of their hypothalamic-pituitary-adrenal (HPA) axis.6,7 These patients typically have elevated serum cortisol levels, accompanied by increased corticotropin-releasing hormone (CRH) secretion and normal circulating levels of adrenocorticotropic hormone (ACTH). The elevation in cortisol could be secondary to increased cortisol production, decreased clearance, or a combination of both factors *(7)*. Boyar and colleagues *(8)* were the first to report decreased cortisol metabolism in AN, subsequently confirmed by other groups. Walsh and colleagues *(9)* noted that when body size was taken into account (cortisol production/kg), cortisol secretion was significantly increased.

Overactivity of the HPA axis appears to be largely secondary to increased CRH production, but with circadian rhythmicity maintained. These patients may also exhibit inadequate suppression of cortisol after an overnight oral dexamethasone challenge *(10–12)* Estour and colleagues *(13)* administered dexamethasone intravenously to 15 patients with AN and observed nonsuppression in 93%. Results of those studies suggest that hypercortisolism exists in AN that is not suppressible by exogenous glucocorticoid during the most acute phase of illness. These findings appear to reverse on refeeding and weight gain. Gold and colleagues *(6)* found increased cortisol response to CRH, while Hotta and colleagues *(14)* showed a decreased response. Both groups interpret their findings as an indication that there is increased HPA axis activity due to increased CRH secretion in AN.

LEPTIN AND INSULIN ABNORMALITIES

Studies examining the question of insulin dynamics in AN have yielded contradictory results *(15)*. Both insulin resistance and insulin deficiency have been documented previously in these patients. Low fasting glucose and insulin levels have been reported in AN *(15)*, as well as both normal *(16)* and increased insulin sensitivity *(17)*. Our group reported low baseline insulin levels, as well as subnormal insulin rises after oral glucose in patients with AN compared to healthy, normal-weight controls *(18)*. We concluded that these results represent either an isolated resistance to glucocorticoid on a pancreatic level or compromised pancreatic function after months of starvation, with less ability to respond to a high-glucose challenge.

Subnormal plasma leptin levels are seen in AN *(19)*, and likely reflect the decreased fat mass in these subjects. The low leptin in these patients may play a role in modulating the HPA axis. In the animal model, administration of leptin to calorically-deprived rats blunts the starvation-induced rises in cortisol and ACTH *(20)*. Overactivation of the HPA axis in patients with AN may thus be secondary to a leptin-deficient state. Subnormal leptin levels in these amenorrheic patients support previous suggestions that this hormone may serve as a metabolic signal to the reproductive axis *(20–22)*

GROWTH HORMONE ABNORMALITIES

Elevated serum growth hormone (GH) levels are found in at least one-half of emaciated anorexic patients *(23,24)* and return to normal with treatment and weight gain *(25)*. Whereas increased basal levels of GH are a reasonably constant finding in emaciated patients with AN, GH responses to provocative tests have been less consistent *(26)*. Patients with AN exhibit impaired GH responses to L-Dopa and apomorphine administration, and two reports have demonstrated that these findings persist even after nutritional rehabilitation *(27,28)*. The GH response to arginine has been reported as normal in one study *(29)*. A paradoxical increase in GH secretion following a glucose load has been reported by some investigators *(30,31)*. Thyrotropin-releasing hormone administration also parodoxically stimulates GH secretion in both underweight and weight-restored patients with AN *(32,33)*. Serum levels of insulin-like growth factor-I (IGF-I) are suppressed, which normalize with nutritional therapy *(26)*. These findings have been attributed to consequences of starvation, but conflicting data exist as to the relative contributions of severity of weight loss and caloric deprivation.

THYROID HORMONE ABNORMALITIES

Thyroid function tests are abnormal in many patients with AN and likely reflect an adaptive response to permit conservation of energy. Serum levels of T4 and T3 in these patients are significantly lower than in normal individuals. In AN, as in starvation, peripheral deiodination of T4 is diverted from formation of active T3 to production of reverse T3 (rT3), an inactive metabolite *(34)*. Levels of T3 correlate linearly with body weight, expressed as a percentage of ideal *(35)*, and normalize with weight gain *(36)*. Higher levels of rT3, the less active form of the hormone, may explain the occurrence of hypothyroid symptoms, such as fatigue, constipation, and hypothermia that occur commonly in these patients despite the normal to slightly subnormal T4 levels seen. Levels of thyroid-stimulating hormone (TSH) are within normal limits *(36,37)* and are not related to body weight *(36)*. However, peak TSH response to thyroid-releasing hormone (TRH) stimulation appears to be delayed (e.g., to 120 min) *(38)* and may be augmented *(35)*, suggestive of a hypothalamic defect.

HYPOTHALAMIC-PITUITARY-OVARIAN AXIS ABNORMALITIES

Amenorrhea is one of the cardinal features of AN and is due to hypogonadotropic hypogonadism. Studies in markedly underweight patients with AN show low plasma gonadotropin levels *(39)*. A positive relationship between resting luteinizing hormone (LH) levels and body weight has been shown, and LH levels normalize with weight gain *(40)*. Studies of 24-h secretory patterns of gonadotropins demonstrate that significant weight loss induces a pattern of follicle stimulating hormone (FSH) and LH secretion resembling that of prepubertal girls *(41)*. The pattern is characterized by either low LH levels throughout the day or decreased LH secretory episodes during waking hours. The LH response to gonadotropin releasing hormone (GnRH) may also be significantly reduced in these patients. This response is correlated with body weight, so that patients with the greatest weight loss have the smallest rise in LH in response to GnRH *(40)*.

Weight loss itself does not appear to explain the relationship between nutritional deprivation and disturbances in menstrual function, as amenorrhea precedes significant weight loss in half to two-thirds of patients *(39)* and may persist despite weight restoration *(42)*. Return of menstruation in patients with AN correlates with regaining weight, although not all patients recover menses *(43)*. A number of investigators have identified mean thresholds associated with reestablishment of menses in girls with AN based on estimates of percentages of body fat using height and weight measurements *(44)*, percentage of ideal body weight *(45)*, and body mass index (BMI) *(46)*. However, it has been shown that return of menses does not show a simple relationship to weight or fatness *(47)*. The majority of patients resume menstruation when weight has returned to at least 90% of ideal *(25)*. These findings are in accord with the work of Frisch and colleagues *(48)* indicating that the onset and continuation of regular menstrual function in women are dependent on the maintenance of a minimal weight for height. This threshold has been proposed to represent a critical level of percentage body fat *(44)* and implies that body composition may be an important determinant of reproductive fitness in the human female *(48)*. Following weight restoration and resumption of menses, patients with AN appear to have normal fertility *(43)*, although this has not been well-studied.

PROLACTIN

Fasting morning levels of prolactin are normal *(49,50)* and there is no relationship between basal prolactin and body weight, estradiol, or gonadotropins *(50)*. Prolactin responses to L-Dopa and chlorpromazine are also normal. The prolactin response to TRH is normal in magnitude, but delayed *(51)*. Nighttime prolactin levels are reduced *(52)*, possibly secondary to dietary factors as nocturnal prolactin is reduced by a vegetarian diet in healthy, normal-weight subjects *(53)*.

VASOPRESSIN

Partial diabetes insipidus has been reported in AN *(49,51)*. Increased CSF arginine vasopressin (AVP) levels and an increased cerebrospinal fluid (CSF) to plasma ratio of AVP have been reported in AN with a further increase noted immediately following weight restoration *(54)*. These findings appear to reverse with weight gain.

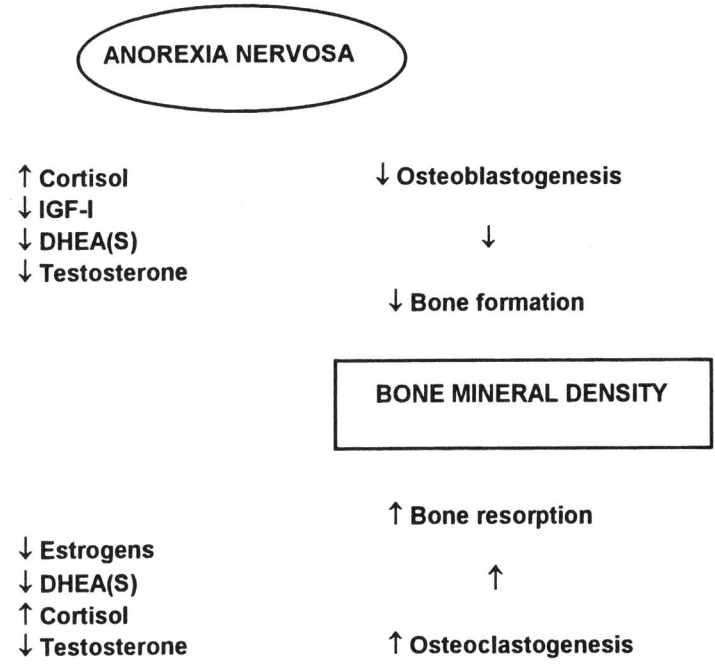

Fig. 1. Multifactorial etiology of bone loss in AN. Mechanisms behind the bone loss of anorexia nervosa are outlined.

OSTEOPENIA AND ABNORMALITIES IN SKELETAL DYNAMICS IN AN

The amenorrhea that accompanies AN in adolescence and young adulthood appears to have permanent effects on bone density, since rapid bone accretion occurs during puberty *(55–57)*. A serious complication of AN is profound osteopenia of both trabecular and cortical bone compartments *(58–62)* with spinal bone density reported to be greater than 2 SD below normal in 50% of young women with this disease *(59)*. The osteopenia is so severe that clinical fractures at multiple sites have been documented in women during late adolescence and young adulthood *(60,61,63)*.

The mechanisms of the bone loss in AN appear to be multi-factorial. Although estrogen deficiency is characteristic, estrogen therapy alone does not result in significant increases in bone density *(64)*. Klibanski and colleagues reported a positive effect of estrogen/progestin therapy on bone density only in young women who were <70% of ideal body weight *(64)*. There also appear to be direct effects of undernutrition on bone, as IGF-I levels are subnormal and correlate with markers of bone formation *(65,66)*. Grinspoon and colleagues have studied parenteral IGF-I therapy for its potential effect on bone density *(65)*. Deficiencies of androgens, most notably dehydroepiandrosteredione (DHEA), have also been noted *(67,68)* which may be significant as DHEA appears to have both anabolic and antiosteolytic effects on bone *(66,69)*. Gordon and colleagues have shown that short-term oral DHEA has promising effects on bone turnover markers *(66)*. Its long-term effects on BMD are currently under study.

PATIENT EVALUATION

Patients in whom AN is suspected should undergo a careful patient and family history, physical examination, laboratory tests, and mental health and nutritional assessment. The patient history should focus on weight changes, self-perception of weight and desired weight, a history of bingeing and out of control cycles of eating and purging, and use of laxatives, ipecac, and diet pills. Purging can include hyperexercising. Triggers for the weight loss should also be investigated, such as teasing at school or comments about weight that occurred either in the home or school setting. A careful history around the issues of growth, pubertal progression or delay, and a menstrual history is critical as girls with AN may have delayed puberty, impaired growth, delayed menarche, amenorrhea, or oligomenorrhea. A family history should include information about eating disorders, obesity, thyroid disease, depression, alcoholism, substance use, or other evidence of mental illness.

A review of systems should include questions about abdominal pain, bloating, constipation, esophagitis associated with bulimia, hair loss or texture change associated with AN, cold intolerance, fatigue, weakness, fainting, substance use, and depression. The level of athletic participation and hours per day of physical exercise should be obtained. Special note should be made of previous stress fractures that may allude to osteopenia. One should consider that it is often difficult to distinguish classic AN from the "female athlete triad" which includes osteoporosis, amenorrhea, and eating disorders *(70)*. Adolescent girls with this triad are at increased risk for developing stress fractures not only because of the osteopenia, but also because of an altered pain threshold, including an inability to stop exercising and rest with the onset of pain.

A dietary history should include a 24-h recall of intake. The amounts may be inaccurate because teenagers with AN often overreport their intake. Triggers of bingeing such as stress are important to address. The calcium intake should be estimated by determining the number of servings of dairy products per day or the use of calcium supplements. This assessment is helpful in planning treatment interventions to assure adequate calcium and vitamin D intake because of the increased risk of osteoporosis in patients with AN. It is also important to ask about consumption of caffeine-containing beverages which may decrease a patient's appetite and increase heartrate at the time of medical evaluations. Documentation of soda consumption is also important as recent reports have suggested an association between consumption of these beverages and fractures in healthy adolescent girls *(71–73)*.

The physical examination should include vital signs to assess bradycardia, hypotension, orthostasis, and hypothermia. The weight and height should be recorded in a gown, after urination, so that measurements are consistent between visits. Heights and weights should be plotted on age-appropriate growth charts to determine the patient's weight for height. The urine specific gravity should be measured since these patients often water load, and abnormalities of vasopressin (e.g., partial diabetes insipidus) have been reported *(49,51)*. During the skin examination, the clinician should assess for lanugo hair, dry skin, hypercarotenemia, hair changes, and calluses on the dorsum of the hand (the latter indicative of bulimic behaviors). On the abdominal exam, the abdomen is typically scaffoid with palpable stool. Other findings include breast atrophy, hypoestrogenic vaginal mucosa, and cool and wasted extremities. The cardiac examination should include an assessment for bradycardia, arrhythmias, and mitral valve prolapse. From chronic vomiting, there may be dental caries or acid erosion of the anterior teeth, and parotid hypertrophy.

In assessing the history and physical examination of an adolescent with suspected AN, the possibility of other diagnoses must be entertained: malignancy, central nervous system tumor, inflammatory bowel disease, celiac disease and other causes of malabsorption, diabetes mellitus, hypothyroidism, hypopituitarism, primary adrenal insufficiency, primary depression (with secondary anorexia), and human immunodeficiency virus (HIV) infection, among others. The typical laboratory evaluation obtained at the initial visit includes: complete blood count, differential, sedimentation rate, urinalysis, electrolytes, glucose, calcium, magnesium, phosphorus, blood urea nitrogen (BUN), creatinine, and thyroid function tests. If persistent or unexplained amenorrhea is present, serum levels of FSH and prolactin are obtained before initiation of hormonal replacement therapy. If a patient is sexually active, a urine pregnancy test is obtained. An electrocardiogram is also obtained if the patient is bradycardic or will be using medication with cardiac effects. CNS imaging should be considered in a patient with an early or unusual presentation of an eating disorder, growth failure, pubertal arrest, or neurological signs and symptoms. Other tests, including endocrinologic assessments, may be considered depending on the patient's presentation.

MANAGEMENT

The treatment of an adolescent with AN requires a multidisciplinary team approach. A physician typically assumes the role as manager of the team, performing vital sign and weight checks and coordinating the overall communication with the family. An endocrinologist can either assume the role of manager or can help to address specific endocrinologic issues, such as the amenorrhea and bone loss commonly seen in these patients. A nutritionist works with the adolescent and family around meal planning and recommendations for caloric requirements and calcium intake. A psychotherapist provides individual and/or family therapy.

The indications for hospitalization include unstable vital signs, hypotension, orthostasis, bradycardia, severe malnutrition (75–80% of ideal body weight), dehydration, abnormal electrolytes, arrythmias, acute food refusal, uncontrollable bingeing and purging, suicidality, and failure of outpatient therapy. Treatment options include medical hospitalization, psychiatric hospitalization, and day treatment psychiatric programs.

Osteoporosis is a significant health risk for adolescents with AN and often becomes a longterm follow-up issue for an endocrinologist. The bone loss and resulting low bone density are often irreversible and may be a source of both short- and long-term morbidity. The degree of osteoporosis has been associated with duration of both disease and amenorrhea. As short a period as 6 mo of estrogen deficiency may have a negative impact on bone density. Other factors to consider include inadequate calcium and vitamin D intake, hypercortisolism, and adrenal androgen deficiency. The most important approach to the prevention and treatment of low bone mass in AN is the restoration of a normal body weight. Hotta and colleagues *(46)* found that a BMI >16.4 ± 0.3 kg/m^2 was associated with an improvement in bone density. Shomento and Kreipe *(45)* have found that a mean of >92 ± 7% of ideal body weight was associated with the return of menses. Golden and colleagues have noted that even with restoration of normal body weight, persistent amenorrhea has been associated with low leptin levels *(74)*. Return of menses is an important milestone implying the provision of normal estrogen levels to all tissues, including the potential to improve bone mass. Hormonal therapies have been tested with mixed results. Estrogen/progestin replacement has been subjected to only a few trials. Replacement therapy with estrogen/progestin, DHEA and IGF-I are presently under study. Calcium and vitamin D supplements are important during the critical period for bone accretion. These patients should receive 1300–1500 mg of elemental calcium and 400 international units of vitamin D daily. Physical activity is associated with increased bone formation *(75)*. Exercise regimens should be tailored individually for a given patient that take into account hemodynamic stability, level of fitness and extent of bone loss.

CONCLUSION

Clinical investigators who study patients with AN are faced with multiple endocrinologic abnormalities. Most of the abnormalities noted are an adaptive response to starvation and reverse with weight restoration. Bone loss with potential osteoporosis appears to be the only irreversible endocrinologic abnormality cited to date. Research is clearly needed to understand the multifactorial etiology of disordered eating in adolescents and to develop strategies to promote healthy eating patterns in young people. In addition, given that the bone loss seen is often irreversible, future research will hopefully elucidate mechanisms behind this complication and provide guidance as to new treatment strategies.

REFERENCES

1. Bruch H. Thin, fat people. J Am Med Womens Assoc 1973;28:187–188.
2. Fisher M, Golden NH, Katzman DK, et al. Eating disorders in adolescents: A background paper. J Adolescen Health 1995;16:420–437.
3. Fosson A, Knibbs J, Bryant-Waugh R, Lask B. Early onset of anorexia nervosa. Arch Dis Childhood 1987;62:114–118.
4. Higgs JF, Goodyer IN, Birch J. Anorexia nervosa and food avoidance emotional disorder. Arch Dis Childhood 1989;64:346–351.
5. Lucas AR, Beard CM, O'Fallon WM, Kurland LT. 50-year trends in the incidence of anorexia nervosa in Rochester, Minnesota; A population-based study. Am J Psychiatry 1991;148:917–922.
6. Gold PW, Gwirtsman H, Averginoa PC, et al. Abnormal hypothalamic-pituitary-adrenal function in anorexia nervosa: Pathophysiologic mechanisms in underweight and weight-corrected patients. N Engl J Med 1986;314:1335–1342.
7. Licinio J, Wong M-L, Gold PW. The hypothlaamic-pituitary-adrenal axis in anorexia nervosa. Psychiatric Res 1996;62:75–83.
8. Boyar RM, Hellman LD, Roffwarg H, et al. Cortisol secretion and metabolism in anorexia nervosa. N Engl J Med 1977;296:190–193.
9. Walsh BT, Katz JL, Levin J, et al. Adrenal activity in anorexia nervosa. Psychosom Med 1978;40:499–506.
10. Doerr, P, Fichter, M, Pirke, KM., Lund, R.: Relationship between weight gain and hypothalamic pituitary adrenal function in patients with anorexia nervosa. J Steroid Biochem 1985;13:529–573.
11. Walsh BT, Roose SP, Katz JL, et al. Hypothalamic-pituitary-adrenocortical activity in anorexia nervosa and bulimia. Psychoneuroendocrinology 1987;12:131–140.
12. Schweitzer I, Szmukler GI, Maguire KP, Harrison LC, Tuckwell V, Davies BM. The dexamethasone suppression test in anorexia nervosa: The influence of weight, depression, adrenocorticotropic hormone and dexamethasone. Br J Psychiatry 1990;157:713–717.
13. Estour B, Pugeat M, Lang F, LeJeune H, Broutin F, Pellet J, Rouseet H, Tourniaire J. Rapid escape of cortisol from suppression in response to iv dexamethasone in anorexia nervosa. Clin Endocrinol 1990;33:45–52.

14. Hotta M, Shibasaki T, Masuda A, et al. The responses of plasma adrenocorticotropin and cortisol to corticotropin-releasing hormone (CRH) and cerebrospinal fluid immunoreactive CRH in anorexia nervosa patients. J Clin Endocrinol Metab 1986;62:319–324.
15. Nozaki T, Tamai H, Matsubayashi S, Komaki G, Kobayashi N, Nakagawa T. Insulin response to intravenous glucose in patients with anorexia nervosa showing low insulin response to oral glucose. J Clin Endocrinol Metab 1994;79:311–314.
16. Castillo M, Scheen A, Lefebvre PJ, Luyckx AS. Insulin-stimulated glucose disposal is not increased in anorexia nervosa. J Clin Endocrinol Metab 1985;60:311–314.
17. Zuniga-Guajardo S, Garfinkle PE, Zinman B. Changes in insulin sensitivity and clearance in anorexia nervosa. Metabolism 1986;85:1096–1100.
18. Gordon CM, Emans SJ, DuRant RH, et al. Endocrinologic and psychological effects of short-term dexamethasone in anorexia nervosa. Eat Weight Disord 2000;5(3):175–182.
19. Grinspoon S, Gulick T, Askari H, et al. Serum leptin levels in women with anorexia nervosa. J Clin Endocrinol Metab 1996;81:3861–3863.
20. Ahima RS, Prabakaran D, Mantzoros C, et al. Role of leptin in the neuroendocrine response to fasting. Nature 1996;382:250–252.
21. Audi L, Mantzoros CS, Vidal-Puig A, Vargas D, Guissinye M, Carrascosa A. Leptin in relation to resumption of menses in women with anorexia nervosa. Mol Psychol 1998;3:544–547.
22. Barash IA, Cheung CC, Weigle DS, et al. Leptin is a metabolic signal to the reproductive system. Endocrinol 1996;137:3144–3147.
23. Hurd HP, Palumbo PJ, Gharib H. Hypothalamic-endocrine dysfunction in anorexia nervosa. Mayo Clin Proc 1977;52:711.
24. Landon J, Greenwood FC, Stamp TCB, Wynn V. The plasma sugar, free fatty acid, cortisol and growth hormone response to insulin, and the comparison of this procedure with other tests of pituitary and adrenal function. II. In patients with hypothalamic or pituitary dysfunction or anorexia nervosa. J Clin Invest 1966;45:437–449.
25. Garfinkel PE, Brown GM, Stancer HC, Moldofsky H. Hypothalamic pituitary function in anorexia nervosa. Arch Gen Psychiatry 1975;32:739–744.
26. Newman MM, Halmi KA. The endocrinology of anorexia nervosa and bulimia nervosa. Endocrinol Metab Clin North Am 1988;17:195–213.
27. Casper RC, Davis JM, Pandley GN. The effect of the nutritional status and weight changes on hypothalamic function test in anorexia nersvoa. In: *Anorexia Nervosa* (Vigersky RA, ed.) Raven Press, New York. 1977, pp. 137–148.
28. Sherman BM, Halmi KA. Effect of nutritional rehabilitation on hypothalamic-pituitary function in anorexia nervosa. In: *Anorexia Nervosa* (Vigersky RA, ed.) Raven Press, New York. 1977, pp. 137–148.
29. Sizonenko PC, Rabinovitch A, Schneider P, Paunier L, Wollheim CB, Zahnd G. Plasma growth hormone, insulin and glucagon responses to arginine infusuion in children and adolescents with idiopathic short stature, isolated growth hormone deficiency, panhypopituitarism and anorexia nervosa. Pediatr Res 1975;9:733–738.
30. Blickle JF, Reville P, Stephan F, et al. The role of insulin, glucagon, and growth hormone in the regulation of plasma glucose and free fatty acids levels in anorexia nervosa. Horm Metab Res 1984;16:336.
31. Vander Laan WP, Parker DC, Rossman, LG, et al. Implications of growth hormone release in sleep. Metabolism 1978;19:891.
32. Macaron C, Wilbert J, Green O, et al. Studies of growth hormone, thyrotropin and prolactin secretion in anorexia nervosa. Psychoneuroendocrinology 1978;3:181.
33. Casper RC, Frohman L. Delayed TSH release in anorexia nervosa following injection of thyrotropin-releasing homrone (TRH). Psychoneuroendocrinology 1982;7:59.
34. Moshang T Jr, Parks JS, Bader L, et al. Low serum triiodothyronine in patients with anorexia nervosa. J Clin Endocrinol Metab 1975;40:470–473.
35. Leslie RD, Isaacs AJ, Gomez J, Raggart PR, Bayliss R. Hypothalamo-pituiatry-thryoid function in anorexia nervosa: Influence of weight gain. Br Med J 1978;2:526–528.
36. Wakeling A, DeSouza VFA, Gore MBR, Sabur M, Kingstone D, Boss AMB. Amenorrhea, body weight and serum hormone concentrations, with particular reference to prolactin and thyroid hormones in anorexia nervosa. Psychol Med 1979;9:265–272.
37. Moshang T, Jr, Utiger RD. Low triiodothyronine euthryoidism in anorexia nervsoa. In: *Anorexia Nervosa* (Vigersky RA, ed.) Raven Press, New York. 1977, pp. 137–148.

38. Vigersky RA, Loriaux DL, Andersen AE, Mecklenberg RS, Vaitukaitus JL. Delayed pituitary hormone response LRF and TRF in patients with anorexia nervosa and with secondary amenorrhea associated with simple weight loss. J Clin Endocrinol Metab 1976;43:893–900.
39. Hurd HP, Palumbo PJ, Gharid H. Hypothalamic-endocrine dysfunction in anorexia nersvoa. Mayo Clin Proc 1977;52:711–716.
40. Jeuniewic N, Brown GM, Garfinkel PE, Moldofsky H. Hypothalamic function as related to body weight and body fat in anorexia nersvoa. Psychosom Med 1978;40:187–198.
41. Boyar RM, Katz J, Finkelstein JW, et al. Anorexia nervosa: Immaturity of the 24-hour luteinizing hormone secretory pattern. N Engl J Med 1974;291:861–865.
42. Falk JR, Halmi KA. Amenorrhea in anorexia nervosa: Examination of the critical body weight hypothesis. Biol Psychiatry 1982;17:799.
43. Knuth UA, Hull MG, Jacobs HS. Amenorrhea and loss of weight. Br J Obstet Gynaecol 1977;84:801–807.
44. Frisch RE, McArthur JW. Menstrual cycles: Fatness as determinant of minimum weight for height necessary for their maintenance or onset. Science 1974;185:949–950.
45. Shomento SH and Kreipe RE. Menstruation and fertility following anorexia nervosa. Adolesc Pediatr Gynecol 1994;7:142–146.
46. Hotta M, Shibasaski T, Sato K, Demura H. The importance of body weight history in the occurrence and recovery of osteoporosis in patients with anorexia nervosa: Evaluation by dual x-ray absorptiometry and bone metabolic markers. Eur J Endocrinol 1998;139:276–283.
47. Katz JL, Boyar R, Roffwarg H, Hellman L, Weiner H. Weight and circadian luteinizing hormone secretory pattern in anorexia nervosa. Psychosom Med 1978;40:549–567.
48. Frisch RE. Food Intake, Fatness, and Reproductive Ability. In: *Anorexia Nervosa* (Vigersky RA, ed.) Raven Press, New York. 1977, pp. 137–148.
49. Mecklenberg RS, Loriaux DL, Thompson, RH, Andersen AE, Lipsett MB. Hypothalamic dysfunction in patients with anorexia nervosa. Medicine 1974;53:147–159.
50. Wakeling A, DeSouza VFA, Gore MBR, Sabur M, Kingstone D, Boss AMB. Amenorrhea, body weight and serum hormone concentrations with particular reference to prolactin and thyroid hormones in anorexia nervosa. Psychol Med 1979;9:265–272.
51. Vigersky RA, Loriaux DL. Anorexia nervosa as a model of hypothalamic dysfunction. In: *Anorexia Nervosa* (Vigersky RA, ed.) Raven Press, New York. 1977, pp. 137–148.
52. Tolis G, Woods I, Guyda H. Absence of hyperprolactinemia during sleep in anorexia nervosa. Meeting of Royal College of Physicians and Surgeons of Canada 1979, (Abstract) p. 40.
53. Hill P, Wynder F. Diet and prolactin release. Lancet 1976;2:806–807.
54. Kaye WH, Ebert MH, Lake CR. Central nervous system amine metabolism in anorexia nervosa (Abstract). Sci Proc Amer Psychiatr Assoc 1980, p. 126.
55. Bonjour JP, Theintz G, Buchs B, Slosman D, Rizzoli R. Critical years and stages of puberty for spinal and femoral bone mass accumulation during adolescence. J Clin Endocrinol Metab 1991;73:555–563.
56. Gilsanz V, Roe TF, Mora S, Costin G, Goodman WG. Changes in vertebral bone density in black girls and white girls during childhood and puberty. N Engl J Med 1991;325:1597–1600.
57. Theintz G, Buchs B, Rizzoli R, et al. Longitudinal monitoring of bone mass accumulation in healthy adolescents: Evidence for a marked reduction after 16 yr-of-age at the levels of lumbar spine and femoral neck in female subjects. J Clin Endocrinol Metab 1992;75:1060–1065.
58. Davies KM, Pearson PH, Huseman CA, Greger NG, Kimmerl DK, Recker RR. Reduced bone mineral in pateints with eaing disorders. Bone 1990;11:143–147.
59. Biller BMK, Saxe V, Herzog DB, Rosenthal DI, Holzman S, Klibanski A. Mechanisms of osteoporosis in adult and adolescent women with anorexia nervosa. J Clin Endocrinol Metab 1989;68:548–554.
60. Rigotti NA, Nussbaum SR, Herzog DB, Neer RM. Osteoporosis in women with anorexia nervosa. N Engl J Med 1984;311:1601–1606.
61. Kaplan FS, Pertschuck M, Fallon M, Haddad J. Osteoporosis and hip fracture in a young woman with anorexia nervosa. Clin Orthop Rel Res 1985;212:250–254.
62. Bachrach LK, Guido D, Katzman D, Litt IF, Marcus R. Decreased bone density in adolescent girls with anorexia nervosa. Pediatrics 1990;86:440–447.
63. Brotman AW, Stern TA. Osteoporosis and pathologic fractures in anorexia nervosa. Am J Psychiatry 1985;142:495–496.
64. Klibanski A, Biller BMK, Schoenfeld DA, et al. The effects of estrogen administration on trabecular bone loss in young women with anorexia nervosa. J Clin Endocrinol Metab 1995;80:898–904.

65. Grinspoon S, Baum H, Lee K, et al. Effects of short-term recombinant human insulin-like growth factor I administration on bone turnover in osteopenic women with anorexia nervosa. J Clin Endocrinol Metab 1996;81:3864–3870.
66. Gordon CM, Grace E, Emans SJ, Goodman E, Crawford MH, LeBoff MS. Changes in bone turnover markers and menstrual function after short-term oral DHEA in young women with anorexia nervosa. J Bone Miner Res 1999;14:136–145.
67. Zumoff B, Walsh BT, Katz JL, et al. Subnormal plasma dehydroepiandrosterone to cortisol ratio in anorexia nervosa: A second hormonal parameter of ontogenic regression. J Clin Endocrinol Metab 1983;56:668–671.
68. Devesa J, Perez-Fernandez R, Bokser L, Gaudeiero GJ, Lima L, Casanueva FF. Adrenal androgen secretion and dopaminergic activity in anorexia nervosa. Horm Metab Res 1987;20:57–60.
69. Gordon CM, Glowacki J, LeBoff MS. DHEA and the skeleton: Through the ages. Endocrine 1999;11:1–11.
70. Putukian M. The female athlete triad - eating disorders, amenorrhea, and osteoporosis. Med Clin North Am 1994;78:345–356.
71. Wyshak G. Teenaged girls, carbonated beverage consumption and bone fractures. Arch Pediatr Adolesc Med 2000;154:610–613.
72. Wyshak G, Frisch RE, Albright TE, Schiff I, Witschi J. Nonalcoholic carbonated beverage consumption and bone fractures among women former college athletes. J Orthop Res 1989;7:91–99.
73. Wyshak G, Frisch RE. Carbonated beverages, dietary calcium, the dietary calcium/phosphorus ratio and bone fractures in girls and boys. J Adolesc Health 1994;15:210–215.
74. Golden NH, Kretizer PM, Yoon DJ, et al. Leptin, resumption of menses, and anorexia nervosa. (Abstract) Eighth New York International Conference on Dating Disorders 1998, New York, NY.
75. Rubin CT, Lanyon LE. Regulation of bone formation by applied dynamic loads. J Bone Joint Surg Am 1984;66:397–402.

III ADRENAL DISORDERS

12 Adrenal Insufficiency

*Kathleen E. Bethin, MD, PhD
and Louis J. Muglia, MD, PhD*

CONTENTS

    INTRODUCTION
    ETIOLOGIES OF ADRENAL INSUFFIENCY
    CLINICAL PRESENTATION
    DIAGNOSIS
    THERAPY
    PSYCHOSOCIAL/QUALITY OF LIFE
    REFERENCES

INTRODUCTION

Disorders of adrenal function have long been known to cause clinically significant, often fatal, human disease. The initial description of anatomical abnormality of the adrenals in patients succumbing to a process manifest by progressive weakness, pallor, and overall physical decline was provided in 1849 by Thomas Addison *(1)*. While these initial cases may not have discerned the coincident sequelae of pernicious anemia and primary adrenal failure *(2)*, Addison's continued efforts clarified the association between abnormal adrenals and systemic pathology *(3)*. The first experimental verification of the importance of the adrenals in animal systems was provided shortly thereafter by Brown-Sequard *(4)*. Despite recognition of the importance of the adrenal and adrenal hormones in human health and disease during the 19th century, the prognosis for patients diagnosed with primary adrenal insufficiency remained very poor until scientists and physicians developed the capacity to chemically synthesize and replace these hormones in the 1940s. The experience of Dunlop, who detailed the outcome of 86 individuals diagnosed with adrenal insufficiency over the period 1929–1958, is particularly instructive *(5)*. He found that the average life expectancy following diagnosis in 1929–1938, a time during which only salt supplementation and crude adrenal extracts were available, was approx 1 yr. With the ability to administer deoxycorticosterone, a mineralocorticoid, during the interval 1939–1948, the life expectancy for patients with primary adrenal insufficiency

From: *Contemporary Endocrinology: Pediatric Endocrinology: A Practical Clinical Guide*
Edited by: S. Radovick and M. H. MacGillivray © Humana Press Inc., Totowa, NJ

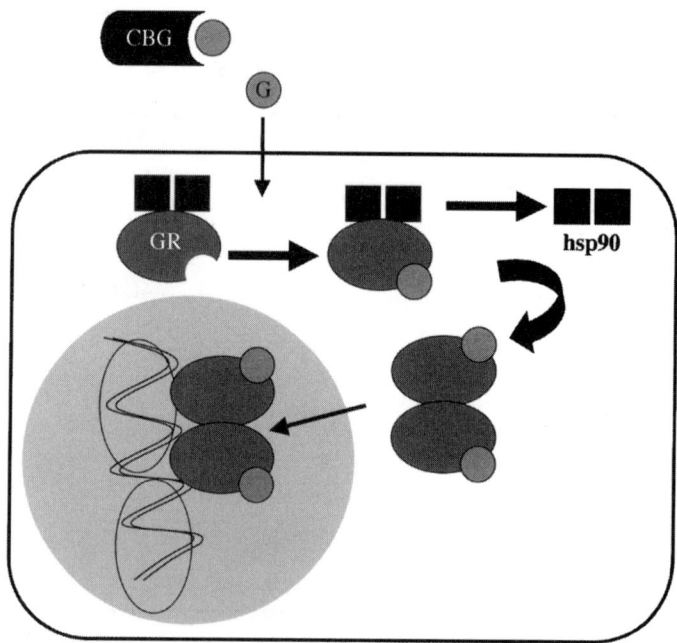

Fig. 1. Mechanism of glucocorticoid action. Glucocorticoids (G; small circles) circulate in the bloodstream primarily bound to corticosteroid binding globulin (CBG). Glucocorticoid dissociates from CBG, diffuses across cellular membranes, and binds the cytosolic, heat shock protein (hsp)-complexed, glucocorticoid receptor (GR; ovals). Upon ligand binding, the GR undergoes a conformational change resulting in dissociation from its molecular chaperones, such as hsp90 (black squares), dimerization, and exposure of nuclear targeting sequences. The dimerized GR enters the nucleus (large circle) to alter transcription of chromatin-packaged genes by direct binding of glucocorticoid response elements, recruitment of co-activators, or heterodimerization with other transcription factor partners.

improved marginally to approx 3 yr following diagnosis. Not until the ability to specifically replace glucocorticoids in the 1950s did the prognosis for those individuals with primary adrenal failure considerably improve, such that the average life expectancy exceeded 10 yr.

Primary adrenal insufficiency often combines defects in mineralocorticoid and glucocorticoid production. Glucocorticoid deficiency alone, however, can produce serious health risks as well. Patients treated with prolonged supraphysiological glucocorticoid doses for management of rheumatological disease were found to be at risk for sudden death during surgical stress if glucocorticoids had been recently terminated (6,7). Functions such as regulation of carbohydrate metabolism (8,9), free water excretion (10–13), vascular tone (14), and the inflammatory response (15) have been ascribed to glucocorticoids. The truly essential aspect(s) of glucocorticoid action, however, remain uncertain.

Cortisol, the primary glucocorticoid in humans, exerts its effects by diffusion from the blood stream across cell membranes where it binds high affinity glucocorticoid receptors (GRs) in the cytoplasm (Fig. 1). Two distinct gene products exhibit high-affinity glucocorticoid (GC) binding, the mineralocorticoid (type I) receptor and the glucocorticoid (type II) receptor. Similar to some other members of the nuclear hormone superfamily of receptors, in the non-ligand-bound state, GR exists in a cytoplasmic complex with heat shock proteins and immunophilins *(16,17)*. These GR "chaperones" serve to mask the GR nuclear translocation sequence, abrogating modulation of gene transcription by preventing access of GR to glucocorticoid response elements (GREs) or heterodimer partners. When ligand is bound, GR undergoes a conformational change such that the heat shock proteins dissociate, the nuclear translocation sequence is exposed, and GR dimers enter the nucleus where specific genes are either activated or repressed. GR-mediated changes in gene transcription occur by many mechanisms, some only beginning to be elucidated. One mechanism, for example, is that upon GR binding of GREs in nucleosome-packaged chromatin, co-activators (such as SRC-1/ NcoA-1, TIF2/GRIP1, or p300/CBP) are recruited *(18)*. These GR-co-activator complexes are histone acetylases, serving to "open" DNA-histone complexes for more efficient transcription by the basal transcription machinery, in addition to exposing sites for other transcription activators to bind. Conversely, while not yet demonstrated for GR, other members of the nuclear hormone receptor superfamily can also recruit co-repressors (such as SMRT and TIF1) with histone deacetylase activity that serve to "close" chromatin conformation and impede access of the basal transcription machinery *(19,20)*. Alternatively, GR actions at composite GREs, consisting of a low affinity GRE and a binding site for another type of transcription factor can differentially modulate transcription depending upon the relative abundance of each monomeric component *(21)*. Finally, GR can modulate transcription of genes which do not contain GREs. For instance, GR has the capacity to directly interact with the p65 subunit of transcription factor nuclear factor κB (NFκB) to block NFκB-mediated gene induction *(22,23)*. GR also induces transcription of a functional inhibitor of NFκB, IκBα, which then may serve to block NFκB-mediated gene activation *(24,25)*.

Considerable insight into the regulation of the hypothalamic-pituitary-adrenal (HPA) axis and the control of glucocorticoid release has been obtained through both human and animal studies (Fig. 2). Stress and circadian stimuli induce the release of hypothalamic neuropeptides, the most important of which are corticotropin-releasing hormone (CRH) and arginine vasopressin, into the hypophysial portal circulation *(26–29)*. These neuropeptides then stimulate release of adrenocorticotropin (ACTH) from anterior pituitary corticotrophs. ACTH released into the systemic circulation augments adrenocortical release of cortisol by acting upon specific G-protein coupled receptors on steroidogenic cells of the zona fasciculata and zona reticularis (Fig. 3) *(30,31)*. Cortisol then acts in a negative feedback manner at central nervous system and pituitary sites to decrease excessive release of hypothalamic neuropeptides and ACTH. Conversely, when insufficient glucocorticoid is present in the circulation, neuropeptide and ACTH release are augmented. In contrast, the control of mineralocorticoid (aldosterone) release by the zona glomerulosa of the adrenal is primarily determined by the renin-angiotensin system, with a smaller contribution from short-term changes in ACTH *(32,33)*. Changes in vascular volume sensed by the renal juxtaglomelar apparatus result in increased secretion of renin, a proteolytic enzyme that cleaves angiotensinogen to angiotensin I. Angiotensin I is then activated through further cleavage by angiotensin-converting enzyme to angiotensin II in the lung and other peripheral sites. Angiotensin II and its metabolite angiotensin III demonstrate vasopressor and potent aldosterone secretory activity.

Adrenal insufficiency can result from impaired function at each level of the HPA axis. Direct involvement of the pathologic process at the level of the adrenal, or primary

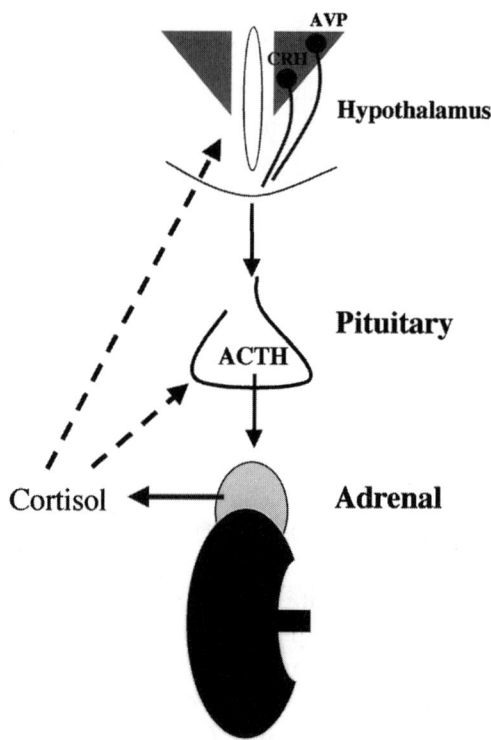

Fig. 2. Hypothalamic-pituitary-adrenal axis regulation. Stress, circadian stimuli, and glucocorticoid withdrawal stimulate cortical, hippocampal, and other higher neural centers to activate corticotropin-releasing hormone (CRH) and vasopressin (AVP) parvocellular neurons in the hypothalamic paraventricular nucleus (shaded triangles). These parvocellular neurons release CRH and AVP into the hypophysial portal circulation, augmenting release of ACTH from anterior pituitary corticotroph cells. ACTH directly stimulates adrenal cortisol release. Cortisol acts in a classical negative feedback manner (dotted arrows) to down-regulate excessive release of hypothalamic and pituitary mediators.

adrenal insufficiency, often causes both mineralocorticoid and glucocorticoid insufficiency by destruction of both glomerulosa and fasciculata/reticularis cells, repectively. Pituitary or hypothalamic defects result in secondary or tertiary adrenal insufficiency, respectively, manifest as isolated glucocorticoid insufficiency.

ETIOLOGIES OF ADRENAL INSUFFICIENCY

Primary Adrenal Insufficiency

The most common cause of primary adrenal insufficiency, or Addison's disease, is autoimmune adrenalitis (Table 1). Antibodies that react to all 3 zones of the adrenal cortex can be found in 60–75% of patients with autoimmune adrenal insufficiency *(34–37)*. After the onset of adrenal insufficiency, the titers decrease and sometimes completely disappear. Autoimmune adrenal insufficiency may occur as an isolated endocrinopathy or in association with other endocrinopathies *(36,37)*. Addison's disease in association with other endocrinopathies can be subdivided into two groups; polyglandular autoimmune disease type I and type II *(38)*. Polyglandular autoimmune disease III is diagnosed when autoimmune thyroid disease is present with another autoimmune

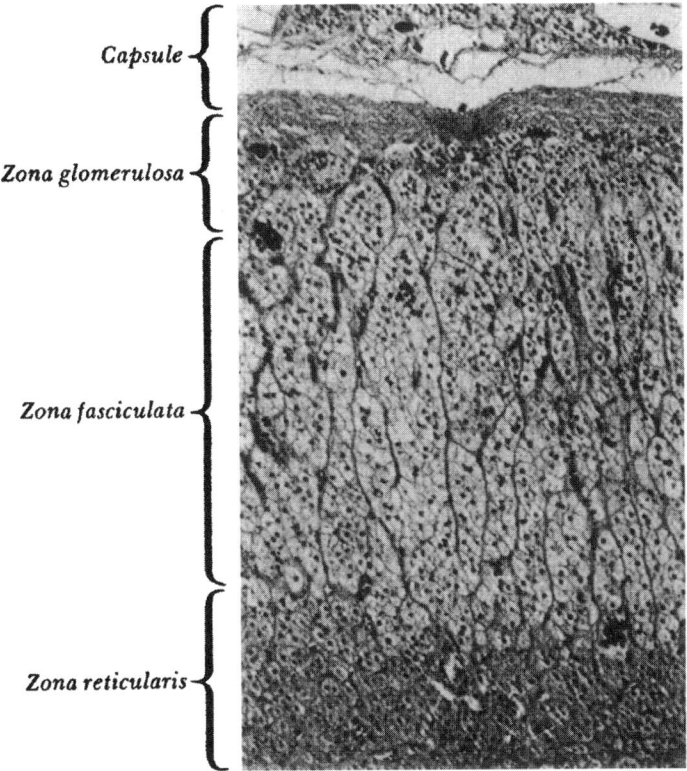

Fig. 3. Adrenal histology. Shown is a hematoxylin and eosin-stained section of a normal human adrenal. Relative sizes and positions of the zona glomerulosa, fasciculata, and reticularis are indicated (X40 magnification). Reproduced with permission from ref. *162*.

endocrinopathy without adrenal disease. The presence of adrenal antibodies in patients with other autoimmune diseases may precede the development of adrenal insufficiency by several years *(39,40)*.

Polyglandular autoimmune disease type I or autoimmune polyendocrinopathy candidiasis ectodermal dystrophy (APECED) is a rare autosomal recessive syndrome that usually presents in early childhood *(41)*. APECED is diagnosed when 2 of the following 3 diseases are present for at least 3 mo: hypoparathyroidism, chronic mucocutaneous candidiasis, and Addison's disease. Gonadal failure, enamel hypoplasia, and nail dystrophy are other common manifestations of this syndrome. Associated conditions include malabsorption syndromes, alopecia totalis or areata, pernicious anemia, autoimmune thyroid disease, chronic active hepatitis, vitiligo, type I diabetes mellitus, anterior hypophysitis, and diabetes insipidus *(41–43)*. Recently, the gene responsible for APECED has been characterized *(44)*. This gene encodes the autoimmune regulator protein (AIRE), a zinc finger protein with possible transcription factor function.

Polyglandular autoimmune disease type II is much more common than type I and usually presents in adulthood or late childhood. Polyglandular autoimmune disease II is diagnosed when adrenal failure and autoimmune thyroid disease or type I diabetes mellitus are present without hypoparathyroidism or candidiasis. Other diseases associated with this disorder include: gonadal failure, vitiligo, diabetes insipidus, alopecia,

Table 1
Causes of Adrenal Insufficiency

Primary adrenal insufficiency

Autoimmune	**Adrenal Hemorrhage**
Isolated Adrenal Insufficiency	Birth Trauma
Polyglandular Autoimmune Diseases I and II	Sepsis (Waterhouse-Friderichsen Syndrome)
	Shock
Inborn Errors of Metabolism	Coagulopathy
Congenital Adrenal Hypoplasia	Ischemia
StAR Deficiency	
Smith-Lemli-Opitz Syndrome	**Infection**
X-linked Adrenoleukodystrophy	Tuberculosis
DAX-1 Mutation (adrenal hypoplasia)	Amyloidosis
Familial Glucocorticoid Deficiency	Hemochromatosis
Wolman's Disease	Sarcoid
SF-1 Mutation	HIV/AIDS
	Hisotplasmosis
Drugs	Blastomycosis
Aminoglutethimide	Crypotcoccus
Etomidate	Coccidomycosis
Ketoconazole	
Metyrapone	
Suramin	
Phenytoin	
Barbituates	
Rifampicin	
Mitotane	

Secondary adrenal insufficiency

CNS Lesions	**Abnormalities in Neuropeptides**
Hypothalamic/Pituitary/Suprasellar Tumors	POMC
Trauma/hemorrhage	CRH
Hemochromatosis	
Sarcoidosis, Tuberculosis, Fungal Infection	**Abnormalities in Pituitary Development**
Empty Sella Syndrome	de Morsier Syndrome
	Hydrancephaly/Anencephaly
Cushing's Syndrome	Pituitary Aplasia/Hypoplasia
	Iatrogenic
	(supraphysiologic glucocorticoids)

pernicious anemia, myasthenia gravis, immune thrombocytopenia purpura, Sjögren's syndrome, rheumatoid arthritis, and celiac disease *(37,42,43)*.

Inborn errors of steroid metabolism provide another common cause of adrenal insufficiency. Congenital adrenal hyperplasia (CAH) is an inborn error of steroid metabolism resulting from defects in enzymes involved in the biosynthesis of cortisol from cholesterol (Fig. 4). Patients with congenital adrenal hyperplasia are cortisol deficient. Depending on the nature of enzyme deficiency, they may also be aldosterone deficient and require mineralocorticoid replacement and salt supplementation. The most common enzyme defects, 21-hydroxylase, 11β-hydroxylase or 3β-hydroxysteroid dehydrogenase lead to increased levels of the adrenal androgens androstenedione and/or dihydroepiandrosteredione (DHEA) *(45)*. These increases in adrenal androgens cause virilization of females, one of the primary clinical symptoms of congenital adrenal hyperplasia. Males with 21-hydroxylase or 11β-hydroxylase deficiency do not manifest genital ambiguity, while those with 3β-hydroxysteroid dehydrogenase deficiency demonstrate under-virilization since testosterone production is diminished.

Congenital lipoid adrenal hyperplasia (StAR, or steroidogenic acute regulatory protein deficiency) is a rare autosomal recessive condition that results in deficiency of all adrenal and gonadal steroid hormones *(46)*. Males with this condition usually have female external genitalia. The defective gene is on chromosome 8 and encodes the StAR protein. The StAR protein mediates cholesterol transport from the outer to inner mitochondrial membrane *(47)*.

Smith-Lemli-Opitz syndrome results from a deficiency of 7-dehydrocholesterol C-7 reductase. Individuals with this syndrome have low cholesterol and high 7-dehydrocholesterol *(48)* which may result in adrenal insufficiency and 46, XY gonadal dysgenesis *(49)*. Associated symptoms of this disorder include moderate to severe mental retardation, failure-to-thrive, altered muscle tone, microcephaly, dysmorphic facies, genitourinary anomalies, and limb anomalies *(50)*.

X-linked adrenoleukodystrophy (X-ALD) is a sex-linked, recessively inherited defect in a peroxisomal membrane protein, the adrenoleukodystrophy protein (ALDP), which belongs to the ATP-binding cassette superfamily of transmembrane transporters *(51,52)*. Defective ALDP function results in accumulation of very long chain fatty acids (VLCFA), demyelination in cerebral white matter, and destruction of the adrenal cortex *(53)*. Approximately 25% of patients with X-ALD develop adrenal insufficiency. Any male who presents with primary adrenal insufficiency should be screened for X-ALD by measuring serum VLCFA levels.

Genes affecting adrenal development in addition to those encoding steroid metabolic enzymes have also been found to cause congenital adrenal failure. X-linked adrenal hypoplasia congenita (AHC) with hypogonadotropic hypogonadism is a rare X-linked recessive disorder due to a deletion or mutation of the *AHC* (or *DAX-1* [dosage-sensitive sex reversal-adrenal hypoplasia congenita gene on the X-chromosome-1]) gene. Patients with this disorder have severe glucocorticoid, mineralocorticoid, and androgen deficiency *(54–56)*. In this disorder, the adrenal cortex resembles the fetal adrenal with large vacuolated cells. The miniature form of adrenal hypoplasia is a sporadic form associated with pituitary hypoplasia. More recently, heterozygous mutation of the autosomal steroidogenic factor-1 *(SF-1)* gene has been found to result in adrenal failure and 46, XY sex reversal in humans *(57)*. Homozygous SF-1 deficiency has not been found in humans, though completely SF-1 deficient mice demonstrate agenesis of the adrenal cortex, testes, and ovaries *(58)*.

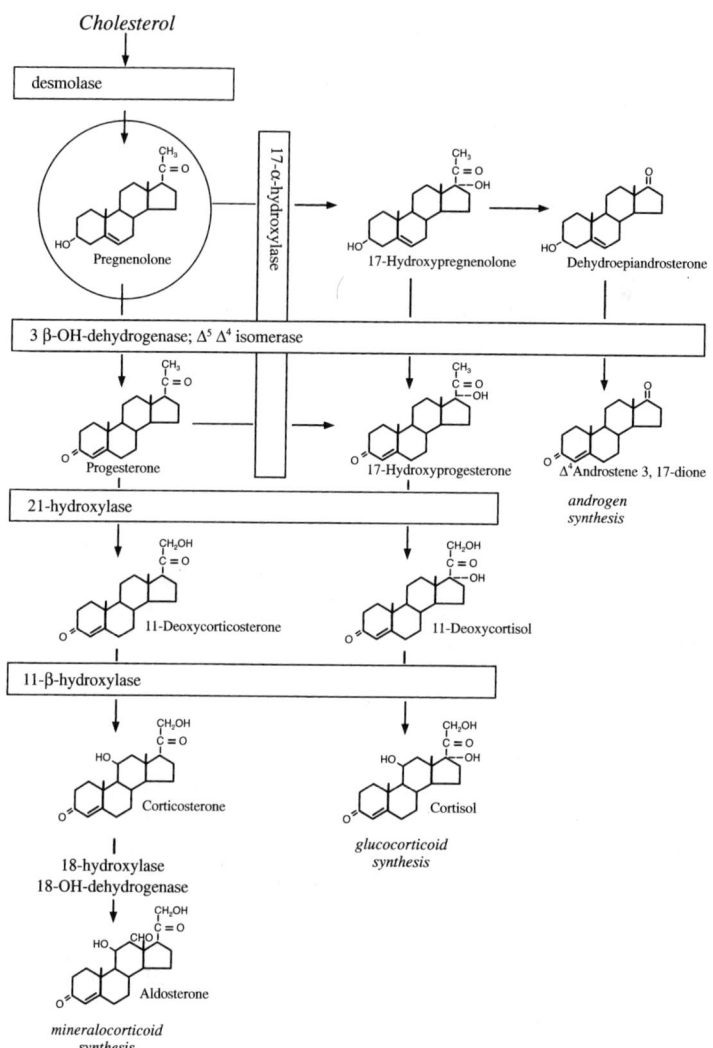

Fig. 4. Cortisol biosynthetic pathway. The enzymatic steps leading to mineralocorticoid, glucocorticoid, and adrenal androgen production are shown. Reproduced with permission from ref. *162*.

Familial glucocorticoid deficiency is a rare autosomal recessive disorder. Patients with this disorder present in childhood with hyperpigmentation, muscle weakness, hypoglycemia, and seizures because of low cortisol and elevated ACTH levels. Some families have been shown to have a defect in the ACTH receptor, while other families are thought to have a post-receptor defect *(59–61)*. Patients that also have achalasia and alacrima are classified as having Allgrove's or Triple-A syndrome.

Wolman's disease, a rare autosomal recessive disease that results from complete deficiency of lysosomal esterase, is usually fatal in the first year of life *(62)*. Features of this disease include mild mental retardation, hepatosplenomegaly, vomiting, diarrhea, growth failure, and adrenal calcifications. Calcifications that delineate the outline of both adrenals are pathognomonic for this disease and the less severe form of this disease, cholesterol ester storage disease *(63)*.

Birth trauma may cause adrenal hemorrhage and should be considered in a newborn presenting with signs and symptoms of adrenal insufficiency. Adrenal hemorrhage has also been reported as a sequelae of sepsis, traumatic shock, coagulopathies, or ischemic disorders. Adrenal hemorrhage in association with fulminant septicemia caused by *Neisseria meningitides* is known as the Waterhouse-Friderichsen syndrome.

Infiltrative disease of the adrenal due to tuberculosis had been a frequent cause of adrenal failure when Addison first described adrenal insufficiency. Today, tuberculosis is a rare cause of adrenal insufficiency, especially in children. Amyloidosis, hemochromatosis, and sarcoidosis have all been reported to cause primary adrenal insufficiency by invasion of the adrenal gland.

Patients with acquired immunodeficiency syndrome (AIDS) or who are human immunodeficiency virus (HIV) positive may acquire adrenal insufficiency. In patients with HIV, cytomegalovirus infection can cause necrotizing adrenalitis. Infection with *Mycobacterium avium-intracellulare*, or cryptococcus, or involvement of the adrenal gland by Kaposi's sarcoma also are significant causes of primary adrenal insufficiency in HIV positive patients *(64)*. In addition, most patients with AIDS have decreased adrenal reserves as measured by prolonged ACTH stimulation *(65)*.

Fungal disease has also been shown to cause primary adrenal insufficiency. Disseminated infection with histoplasmosis or blastomycosis may invade and destroy the adrenal glands *(66,67)*. Cryptococcus and coccidomycosis are rarer causes of adrenal insufficiency *(68,69)*.

Several drugs have been associated with the induction of adrenal insufficiency. Aminoglutethimide *(70)*, etomidate *(71)*, ketoconazole *(72)*, metyrapone *(73)*, and suramin *(74)* are drugs that may cause adrenal insufficiency by inhibiting cortisol synthesis. In most patients, an increase in ACTH will over-ride the enzyme block, but in patients with limited reserve, adrenal insufficiency may ensue. Drugs that accelerate metabolism of cortisol and synthetic steroids such as phenytoin *(75,76)*, barbiturates, and rifampicin *(76)* also may cause adrenal insufficiency in patients with limited reserve. Mitotane accelerates the metabolism of halogenated synthetic steroids (dexamethasone and fludrocortisone (Florinef)) and may precipitate an adrenal crisis in patients taking both drugs *(77)*.

Secondary and Tertiary Adrenal Insufficiency

With the widespread use of supraphysiological doses of glucocorticoids for the treatment of atopic, autoimmune, inflammatory, and neoplastic diseases, iatrogenic suppression of corticotroph ACTH release with secondary adrenocortical atrophy is a frequent, often unrecognized precipitant of adrenal insufficiency. Prolonged (greater than 7–10 d) supraphysiological glucocorticoid replacement places children and adults at risk for consequences of secondary/tertiary adrenal insufficiency *(78)*. Similarly, sustained, excessive glucocorticoid production in Cushing syndrome suppresses normal corticotroph responses. The duration of recovery of corticotroph function from iatrogenic adrenal suppression once pharmacological administration of glucocorticoids is discontinued, or Cushing syndrome after tumor resection, is quite variable, with evidence of suppression of the HPA axis evident in some patients for more than one year *(79)*.

Several acquired and congenital lesions of the hypothalamus and pituitary are also causes of secondary/tertiary adrenal insufficiency (Table 1). Disruption of corticotroph function commonly occurs by hypothalamic and pituitary tumors, or as a result of treatment of these tumors. In children, the most common tumors include craniopharyngiomas, dysgerminomas, and pituitary adenomas. Trauma to the hypothalamus, pituitary, or hypophysial portal circulation from significant head injury, cerebrovascular accident, Sheehan syndrome, or hydrocephalus/increased intracranial pressure provide additional etiologies of central adrenal insufficiency. Infiltrative diseases of the hypothalamus and pituitary such as autoimmune hypophysitis, sarcoidosis, tuberculosis, leukemia, and fungal infections also may result in adrenal insufficiency, often in the context of panhypopituitarism. Abnormalities in development of the hypothalamus and pituitary associated with adrenal insufficiency include de Morsier syndrome (septo-optic dysplasia) *(80,81)*, hydrancephaly/anencephaly, and pituitary hypoplasia/aplasia. Secondary adrenal insufficiency together with diabetes insipidus is particularly ominous in these patients, as sudden death during childhood has been found *(82)*.

Least commonly, inherited abnormalities of neuropeptides involved in HPA axis regulation have recently been reported. Deficiency of proopiomelanocortin results in adrenal insufficiency, pigmentary abnormalities, and obesity *(83,84)*. One kindred with suspected CRH deficiency and Arnold-Chiari type I malformation has been described *(85)*. While the mutation in this kindred is linked to the CRH locus, a specific mutation in CRH gene has not yet been defined.

CLINICAL PRESENTATION

Primary Adrenal Failure

Primary adrenal failure may present as acute, rapidly progressive deterioration or an insidious, chronic process. In infants with congenital adrenal hyperplasia, the first suspicion of adrenal insufficiency may be imparted by the observation of ambiguous genitalia in the delivery room. In caucasian infants, physical examination may additionally reveal hyperpigmentation of the labioscrotal folds, areolae, and buccal mucosa due to excessive propiomelanocortin synthesis and processing to ACTH and melanocyte-stimulating hormone (MSH). If of a salt-wasting variety, untreated CAH commonly causes hyponatremia, hyperkalemia, acidosis, and shock at 7–14 d-of-age. Infants with the rarer adrenal hypoplasia congenita do not manifest genital ambiguity, but may present with a similar adrenal crisis *(86)*.

Children and adults with primary adrenal insufficiency demonstrate a similar spectrum of signs and symptoms, whether of a gradual or sudden onset. The most common symptoms such as weakness, fatiguability, anorexia, vomiting, constipation or diarrhea, and depression are non-specific and do not immediately implicate adrenal insufficiency *(35)*. While salt-craving is highly suggestive of adrenal insufficiency, this symptom may not be elicited at presentation. Weight loss is another very common finding with adrenal insufficiency, though again does not strongly indicate the diagnosis. More specific signs such as hyperpigmentation of skin folds, gingiva, and non-sun exposed areas, hyponatremia with hyperkalemia, hypoglycemia, and hypotension often points toward the correct diagnosis. Hypercalcemia is sometimes found at presentation due to volume depletion and associated increased intravascular protein concentration *(87)*. In children with polyglandular autoimmune syndrome type I, mucocutaneous candidiasis and hypoparathyroidism ususally precede the appearance of adrenal insufficiency *(41)*. In X-linked adrenoleukodystrophy, neurological manifestations may either precede or follow the evolution of adrenal insufficiency *(88,89)*.

Secondary Adrenal Failure

The findings of secondary adrenal failure in large part recapitulate the consequences of isolated glucocorticoid deficiency in primary adrenal insufficiency, such as weakness, fatiguability, and an increased tendency toward hypoglycemia. Of note, salt-wasting does not occur because the renin-angiotensin-aldosterone system remains intact. Because glucocorticoids are required for appropriate renal free water clearance *(13)*, secondary adrenal insufficiency is associated with hyponatremia without hyperkalemia or volume depletion. Additionally, since ACTH production and secretion are the primary defects in secondary disease, skin hyperpigmentation does not occur unless as a manifestation of recently treated Cushing's Disease. Signs and symptoms of a central nervous system tumor such as headaches, vomiting, or visual disturbances, should be sought. Infants with congenital central nervous system malformations, physical evidence for possible hypopituitarism such as midline facial defects or microphallus, or optic nerve atrophy should be evaluated for adrenal deficiency. Individuals at risk for iatrogenic adrenal insufficiency will often appear Cushingoid on examination, with round facies, thinned skin, striae, and a buffalo hump due to prior glucocorticoid therapy.

DIAGNOSIS

Baseline Hormone Measurements

To verify suspected primary adrenal insufficiency in the patient presenting with classic signs and symptoms of Addison's disease, often little more is necessary than measurement of plasma ACTH, cortisol, renin activity, and aldosterone. Elevated ACTH and plasma renin activity together with low plasma cortisol and/or aldosterone confirms primary adrenal failure. In patients more than 6 mo-of-age, the age at which the circadian pattern of glucocorticoid production has been established *(90)*, not presenting in fulminant adrenal crisis, morning (approx 8 AM) ACTH and cortisol levels, along with electrolytes, plasma renin activity, and aldosterone, may establish the diagnosis. A morning cortisol of less than 3 µg/dL is indicative of adrenal insufficiency, while concentrations exceeding 20 µg/dL make adrenal failure quite unlikely *(91)*. Those with early adrenal failure, or secondary disease, will often require additional provocative testing as described below. Adrenal autoantibodies can be used to further establish the etiology of adrenal insufficiency as autoimmune *(34,36)*. All males diagnosed with primary adrenal failure without evidence of other autoimmune pathology should have plasma very long chain fatty acids measured to exclude X-linked adrenoleukodystrophy.

In newborns with ambiguous genitalia or a salt-wasting crisis where CAH is being considered, random measurement of cortisol precursors and precursor by products usually establishes or excludes the diagnosis. For a virilized female, where 21-hydroxylase, 11β-hydroxylase, or 3β-hydroxysteroid dehydrogenase deficiencies are possible, a typical hormone profile consists of measuring 17-hydroxypregnenolone, 17-hydroxyprogestone, dehydroepiandrosterone, androstenedione, testosterone, cortisol, plasma renin activity, and aldosterone. Males with under-virilization should be evaluated for 3β-hydroxysteroid dehydrogenase, 17-hydroxylase, or StAR deficiency, as well as non-adrenal etiologies of genital ambiguity, while normally virilized males with salt-wasting should be evaluated for 21-hydroxylase deficiency and aldosterone biosynthetic defects. In 11β-hydroxylase deficiency, hypertension, hypokalemia, and/or a suppressed plasma renin are found in normally virilized males, or virilized females. Since salt-wasting due to CAH does not typically occur within the first 3 d after birth, and adrenal hormone levels change dramatically in normal infants within this period *(92–94)*, random adrenal hormone measurements should be obtained on d of life 2 to 3. Additionally, the normal range of adrenal hormones differs for term and preterm infants and should be accounted for in interpretation of results *(95–97)*. Late-onset forms of CAH, and proximal lesions in the cortisol biosynthetic pathway, such as StAR deficiency or adrenal hypoplasia, often require cosyntropin stimulation testing, as described below, with cortisol precursors measured in addition to cortisol.

Cosyntropin Stimulation Test

Direct stimulation of adrenal cortisol release by admininstration of cosyntropin (1–24 ACTH; Cortrosyn) is the most commonly used diagnostic tool in evaluation of adrenal function *(91,98)*. In the standard cosyntropin test, baseline ACTH and cortisol samples are obtained and then 250 µg of cosyntropin is administered intravenously. If mineralocorticoid deficiency is also suspected, plasma renin activity, aldosterone, and electrolytes should be obtained with the baseline laboratories. 30 and/or 60 min following cosyntropin administration, a second plasma sample is obtained for cortisol determination. Plasma cortisol concentration ≥20 µg/dL, along with a normal baseline ACTH level rules out primary adrenal insufficiency. In addition, a normal response to this standard stimulation test also rules out long standing, severe secondary adrenal insufficiency. To evaluate recent onset, secondary adrenal insufficiency or milder forms of secondary adrenal insufficiency, a more sensitive stimulation test employing a lower dose of cosyntropin has been devised *(99–102)*. In this case, 1 µg, or 0.5 µg/m^2 of body surface area, of cosyntropin is administered intravenously, with cortisol measured at baseline and 20–60 min after administration. Plasma cortisol concentration above 18 µg/dL is considered a normal response.

Insulin-Induced Hypoglycemia

The response to hypoglycemia (blood glucose <40 mg/dL) requires the integrity of the entire HPA axis. After an overnight fast, 0.10–0.15 U/kg of regular insulin is administered intravenously. Blood glucose and cortisol are measured prior to, then 15, 30, 45, 60, 75, 90, and 120 min following insulin injection. Patients will experience some degree of discomfort during the hypoglycemic phase of this test due to neuroglycopenia and the consequences of catecholamine release, such as tachycardia, diaphoresis, anxiety, and tremulousness. A plasma cortisol of above 20 µg/dL is considered a normal response *(91,103)*. This test should be avoided in patients with a history of seizures or significant cardiovascular disease, and dextrose for intravenous rescue should be immediately accessible in the event of sustained severe hypoglycemia or a seizure.

Corticotropin-Releasing Hormone Stimulation Test

To directly assess corticotroph function, ovine corticotropin-releasing hormone can be administered intravenously at a dose of 1 µg/kg or 100 µg, followed by measurement of plasma ACTH and cortisol levels over the next 2 h *(104–106)*. Flushing occurs in some patients after administration. Peripheral CRH administration provides a less robust stimulus for ACTH release than hypoglycemia, and the normal range is less well established. However, studies directly comparing the responses to CRH and insulin-induced hypoglycemia have demonstrated good concordance in definition of adrenal status. In normal subjects, plasma ACTH peaks rapidly (15–30 min) following administration and remains at an elevated level. Cortisol peaks slightly later, at 30–60 min following injection, and also persists at an elevated level for 2 h. In patients with hypothalamic lesions, an exaggerated ACTH response is often obtained with an even longer prolongation in the duration of elevation. In contrast, patients with pituitary lesions do not respond to CRH administration with increases in either ACTH or cortisol.

Glucagon Stimulation Test

The glucagon stimulation test provides an alternative to insulin-induced hypoglycemia in evaluating central adrenal insufficiency as it requires endogenous ACTH secretion to cause cortisol release *(107,108)*. While glucagon doses of 0.03 mg/kg have been routinely used as a provocative test for growth hormone assessment, studies evaluating adrenal function have employed somewhat higher doses (0.1 mg/kg im; maximum 1.0 mg in children; in adult studies 1.0 mg if <90 kg and 1.5 mg if >90 kg) *(109–111)*. After an overnight fast, plasma is obtained at baseline, then 30, 60, 90, 120, 150, and 180 min following injection. A normal response is achieved if peak cortisol exceeds 20 µg/dL.

Metyrapone Test

Metyrapone inhibits the activity of the enzyme 11-β-hydroxylase, blocking the conversion of 11-deoxycortisol to cortisol. Thus, cortisol is unable to provide negative feedback at central nervous system and pituitary sites, increasing ACTH secretion. The increased plasma ACTH concentration stimulates increased production of 11-deoxycortisol and its urinary metabolites. Two general forms of the metyrapone test have been standardized: an overnight, single dose test *(112)*, and a multiple dose form *(113)*. Because of convenience, the single dose test is the more commonly performed. For the single dose test, 30 mg/kg to a maximum of 3.0 g is given at midnight with a snack to decrease the nausea associated with metyrapone ingestion. Cortisol, 11-deoxycortisol, and ACTH are measured at 8 AM following the dose. A normal response is the increase in plasma 11-deoxycortisol to more the 7 µg/dL *(114)*. Cortisol levels above 5 µg/dL imply inadequate suppression of enzyme activity such that low 11-deoxycortisol levels can not be taken as an index of inadequate hypothalamic or pituitary function.

Radiological Tests

In general, imaging studies should be utilized after the diagnosis of adrenal insufficiency is established by biochemical methods. The obvious exception to this rule is the patient presenting with symptoms suggesting an intracranial mass lesion. The resolution of magnetic resonance imaging (MRI) of the hypothalamus and pituitary in general exceeds that of computed tomography (CT) *(115)*, and is the initial imaging study of choice for evaluation of documented central adrenal insufficiency. If a mass is found, computed tomography may be performed to establish whether the tumor has calcifications characteristic of a craniopharyngioma.

In patients with primary adrenal insufficiency with positive adrenal autoantibodies or elevated VLCFA, establishing autoimmune adrenalitis or X-ALD as the etiology, respectively, adrenal imaging is not required. If these entities are not established as the diagnosis, CT or MRI of the adrenal should be performed *(116–119)*. Observation of calcifications in an older child is suggestive of tuberculous or other granulomatous disease, while in an infant, the diagnosis of Wolman disease should also be entertained. In a limited number of cases, CT-assisted needle biopsy for pathological diagnosis may be required.

THERAPY

Primary Adrenal Failure

CHRONIC REPLACEMENT

The daily cortisol production rate in man is 5.7–7 mg/m^2/d *(120–122)*. Since the bioavailability of oral steroids is approx 50% (but varies from individual to individual), the recommended dose for replacement hydrocortisone therapy is 10–15 mg/m^2/d divided 2–3× per day *(123,124)* (Table 2). It has been shown that twice-daily hydrocortisone produces a non-physiological low cortisol level 2–4 h prior to the next dose *(125,126)*. Therefore, younger children, who are more prone to hypoglycemia when cortisol levels are low, or children with CAH, where efficient suppression of adrenal androgens is required, should receive hydrocortisone divided 3× per day. Although steroids other than hydrocortisone may be used, hydrocortisone is preferred in children since it has less growth suppressive effects than synthetic steroids *(127–129)*.

Patients with primary adrenal insufficiency often do not produce adequate aldosterone. Although hydrocortisone has some mineralocorticoid activity, physiologic doses do not usually provide enough mineralocorticoid activity to prevent salt-wasting in children with primary adrenal insufficiency. Thus, children with mineralocorticoid deficiency are also treated with 0.05–0.2 mg/d of Florinef. Since the aldosterone secretion rate after the first week of life does not increase from infancy to adulthood, mineralocorticoid doses do not vary significantly with body size *(130)*. Because infant formulas are low in salt, infants are treated with 1–4g/d of NaCl supplementation *(131)*. Older children and adults usually have enough salt in their diet without additional salt supplementation to maintain normal electrolytes with the use of Florinef.

It is important that treatment adequacy be monitored on a regular basis. Growth velocity, weight gain, blood pressure, serum electrolytes, and plasma renin activity are the most useful tests every 3–6 mo. Hyperpigmentation in non-sun exposed areas is also an important sign that indicates inadequate therapy. Some physicians also like to monitor ACTH levels and maintain these in the high normal to mildly elevated range. Special considerations for children with CAH are discussed below.

Stress Replacement

In normal individuals, plasma ACTH and cortisol levels increase in response to surgery, trauma, and critical illness. Many researchers have measured plasma or urinary-free cortisol in healthy adults undergoing surgery or in acutely ill individuals and have found that the daily secretion rate of cortisol is proportional to the degree of stress *(132–137)*. Estimates of the daily cortisol secretory rate in adults after surgery range from 60–167 mg/24 h. Based on repeated cortisol measurements, it has been estimated that adults undergoing minor surgery secrete 50 mg/d of cortisol *(138,139)* and 75–150 mg/d after major surgery *(132)*. One comprehensive review of the literature *(140)* recommends that adults receive 25 mg for minor stress, 50–75 mg for minor surgery and 100–150 mg hydrocortisone per day for major surgery for 1–3 d.

Table 2
Management of Adrenal Insufficiency

Management of adrenal crisis

Obtain Blood for:
    Electrolytes
    Cortisol
    ACTH
Intravenous Fluid Administration
    500 mL/m^2 of D5NS over first 30–60 min to restore cardiovascular stability
    Correct sodium at a maximal rate of 0.5 mEq/L to prevent central pontine myelinolysis
Stress Dose Steroid
    Intravenous 100 mg/m^2 hydrocortisone, or if a new presentation, use 2.5 mg/m^2 of dexamethasone until ACTH stimulation test is done
    Continue 100 mg/m^2/d hydrocortisone divided q 6–8 h (or 2.5 mg/m^2/d dexamethasone) until stable for 24 h
If a new presentation, perform ACTH stimulation test
Frequent assessment of electrolytes, blood glucose, and vital signs

Chronic replacement

Glucocorticoid Replacement
    10–15 mg/m^2/d of hydrocortisone divided BID-TID
    Monitor clinical symptoms and morning plasma ACTH (Addison' disease)
        or adrenal androgens/cortisol precursors (congenital adrenal hyperplasia)
Mineralocorticoid Replacement
    Florinef 0.5–2.0 mg QD
    Infants need 1–4 g NaCl added to their formula divided QID
    Monitor blood pressure, plasma renin activity, and electrolytes
Treatment of Minor Febrile Illness or Stress
    Increase steroid dose to 30–100 mg/m^2/d until 24 hours after symptoms resolve
    Do not alter Florinef dose
    If unable to tolerate oral intake, administer 30–100 mg/m^2 of hydrocortisone acetate or 1–2.5 mg/m^2 of dexamethasone IM
Obtain Medical Alert Bracelet

Based on data from adults, children should receive 30–100 mg/m^2/d of hydrocortisone with the onset of fever, gastrointestinal, or other significant illness and continued for 24 h after symptoms resolve *(45,141,142)* (Table 2). If the child has emesis within 1 h of the dose, it should be repeated and if emesis occurs again, an intramuscular injection of 30–100 mg/m^2/d hydrocortisone or its equivalent should be given. The night prior to surgery, children should be given triple their normal dose of hydrocortisone. On the day of surgery, on-call to the operating room prior to anesthesia administration, they should be given an intravenous dose of 30–100 mg/m^2 of hydrocortisone, then continued on 30–100 mg/m^2/d divided every 6–8 h for the next 24–48 h post-operatively. There is no need to give extra Florinef for stress. However, salt intake must be maintained to prevent electrolyte imbalance.

During a suspected adrenal crisis, electrolytes, cortisol and ACTH levels should be drawn and treatment begun before lab values are available. Normal saline with 5% dextrose at a volume of 500 mL/m^2 should be infused over the first hour. Initially

100 mg/m^2 of hydrocortisone can be given intravenously and then 100 mg/m^2/d divided every 6–8 h. In order to confirm a suspected diagnosis of adrenal insufficiency, equivalent doses of dexamethasone (2.5 mg/m^2/d) should be given instead of hydrocortisone. Dexamethasone does not cross-react in standard cortisol assays, and allows cosyntropin stimulation testing to be performed shortly after the initiation of therapy. Once a cosyntropin stimulation test has been performed, children should be changed to the less growth-suppressive hydrocortisone. After re-expansion of vascular volume with normal saline to restore cardiovascular stability, hyponatremia should be corrected at a maximal rate of 0.5 mEq/L/h to minimize the risk for central pontine myelinolysis. Additionally, a glucose infusion should be continued during re-hydration to avoid hypoglycemia.

Central Adrenal Failure

ACTH or CRH deficiency is treated in much the same as primary adrenal insufficiency. The major difference is that while these patients do not require mineralocorticoid replacement, they do require evaluation for deficiency of other pituitary hormones. In addition, when first diagnosed, a head MRI, with special attention to views of the pituitary and hypothalamus, should be performed to look for a tumor or other anomalies.

Special Considerations for Virilizing Forms of CAH

STANDARD THERAPY

Treatment of all forms of CAH consists of replacement and, when indicated, stress doses of cortisol. Treatment of virilizing forms of CAH requires more than replacement doses of hydrocortisone to prevent further virilization and rapid fusion of the growth plates. The dose required varies from individual to individual but averages 10–20 mg/m^2/d in 2–3 divided doses *(45,143,144)*.

Patients with CAH, with or without salt-wasting, may benefit from mineralocorticoid therapy. In the salt-losing forms of CAH with elevation in plasma renin activity, the addition of Florinef at 0.05–0.2 mg/d is required. In patients with mildly elevated plasma renin activity without overt salt wasting, the addition of Florinef often helps to suppress excess adrenal androgen production. Depending on the degree of enzyme deficiency, children with CAH may also have aldosterone deficiency or increased levels of antagonists of aldosterone action *(145,146)*. Aldosterone deficiency causes hyperkalemia, hyponatremia, and volume depletion. Hyponatremia and volume depletion lead to increased renin and angiotensin II. Angiotensin II not only stimulates aldosterone secretion directly at the level of the adrenal cortex, it also stimulates ACTH secretion *(147–149)*. Therefore, by suppressing plasma renin activity with the use of Florinef, patients may require a lower dose of glucocorticoid. Infants with CAH also require approx 1–4 g/d of salt added to their formula or as supplementation to breast feeding *(131)*.

Follow-up evaluation should occur every 2–4 mo to monitor electrolytes, plasma renin activity, growth velocity, 17-hydroxyprogesterone and androstenedione. Suppression of 17-hydroxyprogesterone and androstenedione into the normal range may compromise growth *(150,151)*. In any patient where normal levels of these precursors suppress growth, steroid doses should be reduced to maintain levels in the slightly elevated range. A bone age should be monitored yearly to ensure that skeletal maturation is not advancing faster than the chronological age.

Newer Therapies: CAH

A major shortcoming in the therapy of CAH is compromised final adult height *(152–155)*. Inadequate suppression of 17-hydroxyprogesterone leads to relative advancement of bone age and ultimately short stature. Too much glucocorticoid also results in suppression of growth. One ongoing study is using 10 mg/kg/d of flutamide divided twice daily and 40 mg/kg/d testolactone divided three times daily to reduce the dose of glucocorticoid needed to prevent rapid advancement of the bone age *(156–158)*. The daily hydrocortisone dose for children in this study has been reduced to 8.6 ± 0.6 mg/m^2/d with maintenance of normal growth velocity and bone maturation.

X-linked Leukodystrophy

Conventional therapy consists of replacement and stress doses of cortisol, if indicated. Restriction of VLCFA intake and supplementation with glycerol trioleate and glycerol trierucate (Lorenzo's oil) has very little benefit *(159)*. In animal studies, 4-phenylbutyrate promotes the expression of a peroxisomal protein that corrects the metabolism of VLCFA and prevents the accumulation in the brain and adrenal glands *(53)*. Bone marrow transplantation has shown some success when performed before significant cognitive changes have occurred *(160,161)*. However, bone marrow transplantation does not reverse damage that has already occurred.

PSYCHOSOCIAL/QUALITY OF LIFE

Children with adrenal insufficiency generally lead normal lives. However, glucocorticoid deficiency places them at increased risk for usual illnesses becoming life-threatening. If appropriate stress steroid coverage is not given during an illness, these children have the potential of dying. Therefore, for both the child and the entire family, reinforcement of stress steroid administration during illness is essential. If oral intake of medications and salt is not possible due to gastrointestinal disease or mental status changes, further instruction for emergency assistance is important. All children with adrenal insufficiency should be provided with a medical alert bracelet stating their diagnosis to facilitate urgent therapy if required. Other factors affecting quality of life are determined by the etiology of adrenal failure.

Polyglandular Autoimmune Syndromes

Children with adrenal insufficiency in the context of one of the polyglandular autoimmune syndromes must contend with other endocrinopathies, or the anticipation of developing other endocrinopathies. Often, complicated, multi-drug therapeutic regimens develop with significant financial and emotional cost to the families. The development of type 1 diabetes mellitus, especially, places added demands on daily life. Additionally, enamel hypoplasia, nail dystrophy, vitiligo, and alopecia may be considered disfiguring by the patients with these disorders.

Central Adrenal Insufficiency

Secondary or tertiary adrenal insufficiency may be associated with insufficiency of other pituitary hormones. Similar to patients with polyglandular autoimmunes syndromes, multi-hormone deficiency states are common and require frequent medication administration and dosage adjustment. Long-term issues with decreased fertility and excessive weight gain due to hypothalamic damage pose the most challenging concerns.

Congenital Adrenal Hyperplasia

Determining the etiology of ambiguous genitalia is an endocrine emergency. Sex assignment of a newborn has obvious long-term implications, with optimization of adult sexual and emotional function being the primary goal. Recently, there has been controversy regarding the timing for sex assignment and reconstructive surgery. Members of the Intersex Society of North America (ISNA) propose that no reconstructive genital surgery should be performed on children before they are old enough to consent. In general though, 46,XX patients with CAH, if treated adequately, may be fertile as adult females. Therefore, the recommendation that 46,XX patients with CAH be raised as females, with prompt reconstructive surgery if needed, has been the standard of care. Management of all forms of genital ambiguity benefit from a multi-disciplinary approach with input from endocrinologists, surgeons, geneticists, and psychologists, allowing formulation of a consistent long-term plan for the child and family.

Adrenoleukodystrophy

The phenotype of X-ALD is variable with at least 7 clinical subtypes: childhood cerebral ALD, adolescent ALD, adult cerebral ALD, adrenomyeloneuropathy, Addison's disease only, asymptomatic, and heterozygote women. All of these subtypes can be present within the same family *(89)*. In 6–8% of cases, Addison's disease is the only manifestation of ALD. Any male sibling of an affected patient has a 50% chance of also being affected. Therefore, all male siblings should be screened and if positive, evaluated for adrenal insufficiency. Any female sibling of a patient has a 50% chance of being a carrier. Screening should be offered to any female siblings to evaluate the risk of disease to their children. The major psychosocial consideration in this disease is the anticipation of progressive neurological deterioration, with limited interventions of proven efficacy.

REFERENCES

1. Addison, T. Anemia - disease of the supra-renal capsules. London Medical Gazette 1849;43:517–518.
2. Graner, J.L. Disease discovery as process: the example of Addison's disease. Pharos 1987;50:13–16.
3. Addison T. 1855. On the Constitutional and Local Effects of Disease of the Supra-renal Capsules. Samuel Highley, London.
4. Brown-Sequard CE. Recherches experimentales sur la physiologie et al pathologie des capsules surrenales. CR Seances Acad Sci 1856;43:422–425,542–426.
5. Dunlop D. Eighty-six cases of Addison's disease. Brit Med J 1963;2:887–891.
6. Fraser CG, Preuss FS, Bigford WD. Adrenal atrophy and irreversible shock associated with cortisone therapy. JAMA 1952;149:1542–1543.
7. Lewis L, Robinson RF, Yee J, Hacker LA, Eisen G. Fatal adrenal cortical insufficiency precipitated by surgery during prolonged continuous cortisone treatment. Ann Int Med 1953;39:116–125.
8. Orth DN, Kovacs WJ, Debold CR. The adrenal cortex. In: Williams Textbook of Endocrinology (Wilson JD, Foster DW, eds.) WB Saunders Co., Philadelphia. 1992, pp. 489–619.
9. Van Cauter E, Shapiro ET, Tillil H, Polonsky KS. Circadian modulation of glucose and insulin responses to meals: relationship to cortisol rhythm. Am J Physiol 1992;262:E467–E475.
10. Ahmed AB, George BC, Gonzalez-Auvert C, Dingman JF. Increased plasma arginine vasopressin in clinical adrenocortical insufficiency and its inhibition by glucosteroids. J Clin Invest 1967;46:111–123.
11. Iwasaki Y, Kondo K, Hasegawa H, Oiso Y. Osmoregulation of plasma vasopressin in three cases with adrenal insufficiency of diverse etiologies. Horm Res 1997;47:38–44.

12. Kleeman CR, Czaczkes JW, Cutler R. Mechanisms of impaired water excretion in adrenal and pituitary insufficiency. IV. Antidiuretic hormone in primary and secondary adrenal insufficiency. J Clin Invest 1964;43:1641–1648.
13. Green HH, Harrington AR, Valtin H. On the role of antidiuretic hormone in the inhibition of acute water diuresis in adrenal insufficiency and the effects of gluco- and mineralocorticoids in reversing inhibition. J Clin Invest 1970;49:1724–1736.
14. Munck A, Guyre PM. Glucocorticoid physiology, pharmacology, stress. Adv Exp Med Biol 1984;196:81–96.
15. Chrousos GP. The hypothalamic-pituitary-adrenal axis and immune-mediated inflammation. N Engl J Med 1995;332:1351–1362.
16. Truss M, Beato M. Steroid hormone receptors: interaction with deoxyribonucleic acid and transcription factors. Endo Rev 1993;14:459–479.
17. Barnes PJ. Anti-inflammatory actions of glucocorticoids: molecular mechanisms. Clin Sci 1998;94:557–572.
18. Collingwood TN, Urnov FD, Wolffe AP. Nuclear receptors: coactivators, corepressors and chromatin remodeling in the control of transcription. J Mol Endocrinol 1999;23:255–275.
19. Chen JD, Evans RM. A transcriptional co-repressor that interacts with nuclear hormone receptor. Nature 1995;377:454–457.
20. Le Douarin B, Nielsen AL, Garnier JM, et al. The involvement of TIF1 alpha and TIF1 beta in the epigenetic control of transcription by nuclear receptors. EMBO J 1996;14:2020–2033.
21. Miner JN, Yamamoto KR. Regulatory crosstalk at composite response elements. Trends Biochem Sci. 1991;16:423–426.
22. McKay LI, Cidlowski JA. Cross-talk between nuclear factor-kappa B and the steroid hormone receptors: mechanisms of mutual antagonism. Mol Endocrinol 1998;12:45–56.
23. McKay LI, Cidlowski JA. Molecular control of immune/inflammatory responses: interactions between nuclear factor-kappa B and steroid receptor-signaling pathways. Endocr Rev 1999;20:435–459.
24. Auphan N, DiDonato JA, Rosette C, Helmberg A, Karin M. Immunosuppression by glucocorticoids: inhibition of NF-kB activity through induction of IkB synthesis. Science 1995;270:286–290.
25. Scheinman RI, Cogswell PC, Lofquist AK, Baldwin ASJ. Role of transcriptional activation of IkBα in mediation of immunosuppression by glucocorticoids. Science 1995;270:283–286.
26. Aguilera G. Regulation of pituitary ACTH secretion during chronic stress. Front Neuroendocrinol 1994;15:312–350.
27. Dallman MF, Akana SF, Cascio CS, Darlington DN, Jacobson L, Levin N. Regulation of ACTH secretion: variations on a theme of B. Recent Prog Horm Res 1987;43:113–173.
28. Dallman MF, Strack AM, Akana SF, et al. Feast and Famine: critical role of glucocorticoids with insulin in daily energy flow. Front Neuroendocrinol 1993;14:303–347.
29. Plotsky P, Bruhn T, Vale W. Hypophysiotropic response of adrenocorticotropin in response to insulin induced hypoglycemia. Endocrinology 1985;117:323–329.
30. Clark AJ, Cammas FM. The ACTH receptor. Baillieres Clin Endocrinol Metab 1996;10:29–47.
31. Allolio B, Reincke M. Adrenocorticotropin receptor and adrenal disorders. Horm Res 1997;47:273–278.
32. Gibbons GH, Dzau VJ, Farhi ER, Barger AC. Interaction of signals influencing renin release. Ann Rev Physiol 1984;46:291–308.
33. Dzau VJ. Molecular and physiological aspects of tissue renin-angiotensin system: emphasis on cardiovascular control. J Hypertens Suppl 1988;6:S7–S12.
34. Blizzard RM, Chee D, Davis W. The incidence of adrenal and other antibodies in the sera of patients with idiopathic adrenal insufficiency (Addison's disease). Clin Exp Immunol 1967;2:19–30.
35. Nerup J. Addison's disease clinical studies. A report for 108 cases. Acta Endocrinol (Copenh) 1974;76:127–141.
36. Falorni A, Nikoshkov A, Laureti S, et al. High diagnostic accuracy for idiopathic Addison's disease with a sensitive radiobinding assay for autoantibodies against recombinant human 21-hydroxylase. J Clin Endocrinol Metab 1995;80:2752–2755.
37. Barnes WIAE. Adrenocortical Insufficiency. Clin Endocrinol Metab 1972;1:549–594.
38. Riley PBAW. Autoimmune Polyglandular Syndrome. In: Pediatric Endocrinology (Sperling MA, ed.) WB Saunders, Philadelphia. 1996, pp. 509–522.

39. Ahonen P, Miettinen A, Perheentupa J. Adrenal and steroidal cell antibodies in patients with autoimmune polyglandular disease type I and risk of adrenocortical and ovarian failure. J Clin Endocrinol Metab 1987;64:494–500.
40. Boscaro M, Betterle C, Sonino N, Volpato M, Paoletta A, Fallo F. Early adrenal hypofunction in patients with organ-specific autoantibodies and no clinical adrenal insufficiency. J Clin Endocrinol Metab 1994;79:452–455.
41. Ahonen P, Myllarniemi S, Sipila I, Perheentupa J. Clinical variation of autoimmune polyendocrinopathy-candidiasis-ectodermal dystrophy (APECED) in a series of 68 patients. N Engl J Med 1990;322:1829–1836.
42. Neufeld M, Maclaren NK, Blizzard RM. Two types of autoimmune Addison's disease associated with different polyglandular autoimmune (PGA) syndromes. Med 1981;60:355–362.
43. Leshin M. Polyglandular autoimmune syndromes. Am J Med Sci 1985;290:77–88.
44. Nagamine K, Peterson P, Scott HS, et al. Positional cloning of the APECED gene. Nat Genet 1997;17:393–398.
45. New MI. Congenital Adrenal Hyperplasia. In: Endocrinology (DeGroot LJ, ed.) WB Saunders, Philadelphia. 1995, pp. 1813–1835.
46. Hauffa BP, Miller WL, Grumbach MM, Conte FA, Kaplan SL. Congenital adrenal hyperplasia due to deficient cholesterol side-chain cleavage activity (20, 22-desmolase) in a patient treated for 18 years. Clin Endocrinol 1985;23:481–493.
47. Lin D, Sugawara T, Strauss 3rd JF, et al. Role of steroidogenic acute regulatory protein in adrenal and gonadal steroidogenesis. Science 1995;267:1828–1831.
48. Tint GS, Salen G, Batta AK, et al. Correlation of severity and outcome with plasma sterol levels in variants of the Smith-Lemli-Opitz syndrome. J Pediatr 1995;127:82–87.
49. Bialer MG, Penchaszadeh VB, Kahn E, Libes R, Krigsman G, Lesser ML. Female external genitalia and mullerian duct derivatives in a 46,XY infant with the Smith-Lemli-Opitz syndrome. Am J Med Genet 1987;28:723–731.
50. Jones KL. Smith-Lemli-Opitz Syndrome. In: Smith's Recognizable Patterns of Human Malformation. WB Saunders, Philadelphia. 1997, pp. 112–115.
51. Mosser J, Douar AM, Sarde CO, et al. Putative X-linked adrenoleukodystrophy gene shares unexpected homology with ABC transporters. Nature 1993;361:726–730.
52. Mosser J, Lutz Y, Stoeckel ME, et al. The gene responsible for adrenoleukodystrophy encodes a peroxisomal membrane protein. Hum Mol Genet 1994;3:265–271.
53. Kemp S, Wei HM, Lu JF, et al Gene redundancy and pharmacological gene therapy: implications for X-linked adrenoleukodystrophy. Nat Med 1998;4:1261–1268.
54. Zanaria E, Muscatelli F, Bardoni B, et al. An unusual member of the nuclear hormone receptor superfamily responsible for X-linked adrenal hypoplasia congenita. Nature 1994;372:635–641.
55. Muscatelli F, Strom TM, Walker AP, et al. Mutations in the DAX-1 gene give rise to both X-linked adrenal hypoplasia congenita and hypogonadotropic hypogonadism. Nature 1994;372:672–676.
56. Guo W, Burris TP, Zhang YH, et al. Genomic sequence of the DAX1 gene: an orphan nuclear receptor responsible for X-linked adrenal hypoplasia congenita and hypogonadotropic hypogonadism. J Clin Endocrinol Metab 1996;81:2481–2486.
57. Achermann JC, Ito M, Ito M, Hindmarsh PC, Jameson JL. A mutation in the gene encoding steroidogenic factor-1 causes XY sex reversal and adrenal failure in humans. Nat Genet1999;22:125–126.
58. Luo X, Ikeda Y, Parker KL. A cell-specific nuclear receptor is essential for adrenal and gonadal development and sexual differentiation. Cell 1994;77:481–490.
59. Weber A, Clark AJ. Mutations of the ACTH receptor gene are only one cause of familial glucocorticoid deficiency. Hum Mol Genet1994;3:585–588.
60. Yamaoka T, Kudo T, Takuwa Y, Kawakami Y, Itakura M, Yamashita K. Hereditary adrenocortical unresponsiveness to adrenocorticotropin with a postreceptor defect. J Clin Endocrinol Metab 1992;75:270–274.
61. Weber A, Toppari J, Harvey RD, et al. Adrenocorticotropin receptor gene mutations in familial glucocorticoid deficiency: relationships with clinical features in four families. J Clin Endocrinol Metab 1995;80:65–71.
62. Anderson RA, Byrum RS, Coates PM, Sando GN. Mutations at the lysosomal acid cholesteryl ester hydrolase gene locus in Wolman disease. Proc National Acad Sci USA 1994;91:2718–2722.
63. Wolman M. Wolman disease and its treatment. Clin Pediatr 1995;34:207–212.
64. Glasgow BJ, Steinsapir KD, Anders K, Layfield LJ. Adrenal pathology in the acquired immune deficiency syndrome. Am J Clin Pathol 1985;84:594–597.

65. Membreno L, Irony I, Dere W, Klein R, Biglieri EG, Cobb E. Adrenocortical function in acquired immunodeficiency syndrome. J Clin Endocrinol Metab 1987;65:482–487.
66. Sarosi GA, Voth DW, Dahl BA, Doto IL, Tosh FE. Disseminated histoplasmosis: results of long-term follow-up. A center for disease control cooperative mycoses study. Ann Intern Med 1971;75:511–516.
67. Moreira AC, Martinez R, Castro M, Elias LL. Adrenocortical dysfunction in paracoccidioidomycosis: comparison between plasma beta-lipotrophin/adrenocorticotrophin levels and adrenocortical tests. Clin Endocrinol 1992;36:545–551.
68. Maloney P. Addison's Disease due to Chronic Disseminated Coccidiomycosis. Arch Intern Med 1952;90:869–878.
69. Walker BF, Gunthel CJ, Bryan JA, Watts NB, Clark, RV. Disseminated cryptococcosis in an apparently normal host presenting as primary adrenal insufficiency: diagnosis by fine needle aspiration. Am J Med 1989;86:715–717.
70. Fishman LM, Liddle GW, Island DP, Fleischer N, Kuchel O. Effects of amino-glutethimide on adrenal function in man. J Clin Endocrinol Metabol 1967;27:481–490.
71. Wagner RL, White PF, Kan PB, Rosenthal MH, Feldman D. Inhibition of adrenal steroidogenesis by the anesthetic etomidate. N Engl J Med 1984;310:1415–1421.
72. Sonino N. The use of ketoconazole as an inhibitor of steroid production. N Engl J Med 1987;317: 812–818.
73. Liddle GW, Island D, Lance EM, et al. Alterations of adrenal steroid patterns in man resulting from treatment with a chemical inhibitor of 11β-hydroxylation. J Clin Endocrinol Metab 1958;18: 906–912.
74. Ashby H, DiMattina M, Linehan WM, Robertson CN, Queenan JT, Albertson BD. The inhibition of human adrenal steroidogenic enzyme activities by suramin. J Clin Endocrinol Metab 1989;68:505–508.
75. Keilholz U, Guthrie Jr GP. Adverse effect of phenytoin on mineralocorticoid replacement with fludrocortisone in adrenal insufficiency. Am J Med Sci 1986;291:280–283.
76. Elias AN, Gwinup G. Effects of some clinically encountered drugs on steroid synthesis and degradation. Metabolism 1980;29:582–595.
77. Robinson BG, Hales IB, Henniker AJ, et al. The effect of o,p'-DDD on adrenal steroid replacement therapy requirements. Clin Endocrinol 1987;27:437–444.
78. Axelrod L. Glucocorticoid therapy. Medicine 1976;55:39–65.
79. Livanou T, Ferriman D, James VHT. Recovery of hypothalamo-pituitary-adrenal function after corticosteroid therapy. Lancet 1967;2:856–859.
80. de Morsier G. Etudes sur les dysraphies cranioencephaliques. III. Agenesie du septum lucidum avec malformation du tractus optique. La dysplasie septo-optique. Schweiz Arch Neurol Neurochir Psychiatr 1956;77:267–292.
81. Willnow S, Kiess W, Butenandt O, et al. Endocrine disorders in septo-optic dysplasia (De Morsier syndrome)—evaluation and follow up of 18 patients. Eur J Pediatr 1996;155:179–184.
82. Brodsky MC, Conte FA, Taylor D, Hoyt CS, Mrak RE. Sudden death in septo-optic dysplasia. Report of 5 cases. Arch Ophthalmol 1997;115:66–70.
83. Krude H, Biebermann H, Luck W, Horn R, Brabant G, Gruters A. Severe early-onset obesity, adrenal insufficiency and red hair pigmentation caused by POMC mutations in humans. Nat Genet 1998;19:155–157.
84. Pernasetti F, Toledo SP, Vasilyev VV, et al. Impaired adrenocorticotropin-adrenal axis in combined pituitary hormone deficiency caused by a two-base pair deletion (301-302delAG) in the prophet of Pit-1 gene. J Clin Endocrinol Metab 2000;85:390–397.
85. Kyllo JH, Collins MM, Vetter KL, Cuttler L, Rosenfield RL, Donohoue PA. Linkage of congenital isolated adrenocorticotropic hormone deficiency to the corticotropin releasing hormone locus using simple sequence repeat polymorphisms. Am J Med Genet 1996;62:262–267.
86. Guo W, Mason JS, Stone CG, et al. Diagnosis of X-linked adrenal hypoplasia congenita by mutation analysis of the DAX1 gene. JAMA 1995;274:324–330.
87. Walser M, Robinson BHB, Duckett JWJ. The hypercalcemia of adrenal insufficiency. J Clin Invest 1963;42:456–465.
88. Moser HW, Moser AE, Singh I, O'Neill BP. Adrenoleukodystrophy: survey of 303 cases: biochemistry, diagnosis, and therapy. Ann Neurol 1984;16:628–641.

89. Laureti S, Casucci G, Santeusanio F, Angeletti G, Aubourg P, Brunetti P. X-linked adrenoleukodystrophy is a frequent cause of idiopathic Addison's disease in young adult male patients. J Clin Endocrinol Metab 1996;81:470–474.
90. Onishi S, Miyazawa G, Nishimura Y, et al. Postnatal development of circadian rhythm in serum cortisol levels in children. Pediatrics 1983;72:399–404.
91. Grinspoon SK, Biller BMK. Laboratory assessment of adrenal insufficiency. J Clin Endocrinol Metab 1994;79:923–931.
92. Sippel WG, Becker H, Versmold HT, Bidlingmaier F, Knorr D. Longitudinal studies of plasma aldosterone, corticosterone, deoxycorticosterone, progesterone, 17-hydroxyprogesterone, cortisol, and cortisone determined simultaneously in mother and child at birth and during the early neonatal period. I. Spontaneous delivery. J Clin Endocrinol Metab 1978;46:971–985.
93. de Peretti E, Forest MG. Unconjugated dehydroepiandrosterone plasma levels in normal subjects from birth to adolesence in human: the use of a sensitive radioimmunoassay. J Clin Endocrinol Metab 1976;43:982–991.
94. Doerr HG, Sippell WG, Versmold HT, Bidlingmaier F, Knorr D. Plasma aldosterone and 11-deoxycortisol in newborn infants: a reevaluation. J Clin Endocrinol Metab 1987;65:208–210.
95. Lee MM, Rajagopalan L, Berg GJ, Moshang TJ. Serum adrenal steroid concentrations in premature infants. J Clin Endocrinol Metab 1989;69:1133–1136.
96. Thomas S, Murphy JF, Dyas J, Ryallis M, Hughes, IA. Response to ACTH in the newborn. Arch Dis Child 1986;61:57–60.
97. Doerr HG, Sippell WG, Versmold HT, Bidlingmaier F, Knorr D. Plasma mineralocorticoids, glucocorticoids, and progestins in premature infants: longitudinal study during the first week of life. Pediatr Res 1988;23:525–529.
98. Oelkers W, Diederich S, Bahr V. Diagnosis and therapy surveillance in Addison's disease: rapid adrenocorticotropin (ACTH) test and measurement of plasma ACTH, renin activity, and aldosterone. J Clin Endocrinol Metabol 1992;75:259–264.
99. Dickstein G, Shechner C, Nicholson WE, et al. Adrenocortropin stimulation test: effects of basal cortisol level, time of day, suggested new sensitive low dose test. J Clin Endocrinol Metab 1991;72:773–778.
100. Tordjman K, Jaffe A, Grazas N, Apter C, Stern N. The role of the low dose (1 microgram) adrenocorticotropin test in the evaluation of patients with pituitary diseases. J Clin Endocrinol Metab 1995;80:1301–1305.
101. Tordjman K, Jaffe A, Trostanetsky Y, Greenman Y, Limor R, Stern N. Low-dose (1 microgram) adrenocorticotrophin (ACTH) stimulation as a screening test for impaired hypothalamo-pituitary-adrenal axis function: sensitivity, specificity and accuracy in comparison with the high-dose (250 microgram) test. Clin Endocrinol 2000;52:633–640.
102. Merry WH, Caplan RH, Wickus GG, et al. Postoperative acute adrenal failure caused by transient corticotropin deficiency. Surgery 1994;116:1095–1100.
103. Pavord SR, Girach A, Price DE, Absalom SR, Falconer-Smith J, Howlett TA. A retrospective audit of the combined pituitary function test, using the insulin stress test, TRH and GnRH in a district laboratory. Clin Endocrinol 1992;36:135–139.
104. Schulte HM, Chrousos GP, Avgerinos P, et al. The corticotropin-releasing hormone stimulation test: a possible aid in the evaluation of patients with adrenal insufficiency. J Clin Endocrinol Metab 1984;58:1064–1067.
105. Schulte HM, Chrousos GP, Oldfield EH, Gold PW, Cutler GB, Loriaux DL. Ovine corticotropin-releasing factor administration in normal men. Pituitary and adrenal responses in the morning and evening. Horm Res 1985;21:69–74.
106. Schlaghecke R, Kornely E, Santen RT, Ridderskamp P. The effect of long-term glucocorticoid therapy on pituitary-adrenal responses to exogenous corticotropin-releasing hormone. N Engl J Med 1992;326:226–230.
107. Littley MD, Gibson S, White A, Shalet SM. Comparison of the ACTH and cortisol responses to provocative testing with glucagon and insulin hypoglycaemia in normal subjects. Clin Endocrinol 1989;31:527–533.
108. Spathis GS, Bloom SR, Jeffcoate WJ, et al. Subcutaneous glucagon as a test of the ability fo the pituitary to secrete GH and ACTH. Clin Endocrinol 1974;3:175–186.
109. Vanderschueren-Lodeweyckx M, Wolter R, Malvaux P, Eggermont E, Eeckels R. The glucagon stimulation test: effect on plasma growth hormone and on immunoreactive insulin, cortisol, and glucose in children. J Pediatr 1974;85:182–187.

110. Chanoine JP, Rebuffat E, Kahn A, Bergmann P, Van Vliet G. Glucose, growth hormone, cortisol, and insulin responses to glucagon injection in normal infants, aged 0.5-12 months. J Clin Endocrinol Metab 1995;80:3032–3035.
111. Orme SM, Peacey SR, Barth JH, Belchetz PE. Comparison of test of stress-related cortisol secretion in pituitary disease. Clin Endocrinol 1996;45:135–140.
112. Spiger M, Jubiz W, Meikle W, West CD, Tylor FH. Single dose metyrapone test. Arch Intern Med 1975;135:698–700.
113. Liddle GW, Estep HL, Kendall JW, Williams WC, Townes AW. Clinical application of a new test of pituitary reserve. J Clin Endocrinol Metab 1959;19:875–894.
114. Fiad TM, Kirby JM, Cunningham SK, McKenna TJ. The overnight single-dose metyrapone test is a simple and reliable index of the hypothalamic-pituitary-adrenal axis. Clin Endocrinol 1994;40:603–609.
115. Kulkarni MV, Lee KF, McArdle CB, Yeakley JW, Haar FL. 1.5-T MR imaging of pituitary microadenomas: technical considerations and CT correlation. Am J Neuroradiol 1988;9:5–11.
116. Lee MJ, Mayo-Smith WW, Hahn PF, et al. State-of-the-art MR imaging of the adrenal gland. Radiographics 1994;14:1015–1029.
117. Krebs TL, Wagner BJ. The adrenal gland: radiologic-pathologic correlation. Mag Reson Imaging Clin N Am 1997;5:127–146.
118. Sosa JA, Udelsman R. Imaging of the adrenal gland. Surg Oncol Clin N Am 1999;8:109–127.
119. Weishaupt D, Debatin JF. Magnetic resonance: evaluation of adrenal lesions. Curr Opin Urol 1999;9:153–163.
120. Esteban NV, Loughlin T, Yergey AL, et al. Daily cortisol production rate in man determined by stable isotope dilution/mass spectrometry. J Clin Endocrinol Metab 1991;72:39–45.
121. Kerrigan JR, Veldhuis JD, Leyo SA, Iranmanesh A, Rogol AD. Estimation of daily cortisol production and clearance rates in normal pubertal males by deconvolution analysis. J Clin Endocrinol Metab 1993;76:1505–1510.
122. Linder BL, Esteban NV, Yergey AL, Winterer JC, Loriaux DL, Cassorla F. Cortisol production rate in childhood and adolescence. J Pediatr 1990;117:892–896.
123. Heazelwood VJ, Galligan JP, Cannell GR, Bochner F, Mortimer RH. Plasma cortisol delivery from oral cortisol and cortisone acetate: relative bioavailability. Br J Clin Pharmacol 1984;17:55–59.
124. Keenan BS, Eberle AE, Lin TH, Clayton GW. Inappropriate adrenal androgen secretion with once-a-day corticosteroid therapy for congenital adrenal hyperplasia. J Pediatr 1990;116:133–136.
125. DeVile CJ, Stanhope R. Hydrocortisone replacement therapy in children and adolescents with hypopituitarism. Clin Endocrinol 1997;47:37–41.
126. Groves RW, Toms GC, Houghton BJ, Monson JP. Corticosteroid replacement therapy: twice or thrice daily? J R Soc Med 1988;81:514–516.
127. Van Metre, TEJ, Niemann WA, Rosen LJ. A comparison of the growth suppressive effect of cortisone, prednisone and other adrenal cortical hormones. J Allergy 1960;31:531.
128. Stempfel RS Jr, Sheikholislam BM, Lebovitz HE, Allen E, Franks RC. Pituitary growth hormone suppression with low-dosage, long-acting corticoid administration. J Pediatr 1968;73:767–773.
129. Laron Z, Pertzelan A. The comparative effect of 6 alpha-fluoroprednisolone, 6 alpha-methylprednisolone, and hydrocortisone on linear growth of children with congenital adrenal virilism and Addison's disease. J Pediatr 1968;73:774–782.
130. Weldon VV, Kowarski A, Migeon CJ. Aldosterone secretion rates in normal subjects from infancy to adulthood. Pediatrics 1967;39:713–723.
131. Mullis PE, Hindmarsh PC, Brook CG. Sodium chloride supplement at diagnosis and during infancy in children with salt-losing 21-hydroxylase deficiency. Eur J Pediatr 1990;150:22–25.
132. Kehlet H, Binder C. Value of an ACTH test in assessing hypothalamic-pituitary-adrenocortical function in glucocorticoid-treated patients. Br Med J 1973;2:147–149.
133. Espiner E. Urinary Cortisol Excretion in Stress Situations and in Patients with Cushing's Syndrome. J Endocrinol 1966;35:29–44.
134. Chernow B, Alexander HR, Smallridge RC, et al. 1987. Hormonal responses to graded surgical stress. Arch Intern Med 147:1273–1278.
135. Wise L, Margraf HW, Ballinger WF. A new concept on the pre- and postoperative regulation of cortisol secretion. Surgery 1972;72:290–299.
136. Hume DM, Bell CC, Bartter F. Direct measurement of adrenal secretion during operative trauma and convalescence. Surgery 1962;52:174–187.

137. Ichikawa Y. Metabolism of cortisol-4-C14 in patients with infections and collagen diseases. Metabolism 1966;15:613–625.
138. Kehlet H, Binder C. Adrenocortical function and clinical course during and after surgery in unsupplemented glucocorticoid-treated patients. Br J Anaesth 1973;45:1043–1048.
139. Kehlet H. A rational approach to dosage and preparation of parenteral glucocorticoid substitution therapy during surgical procedures. A short review. Acta Anaesthesiol Scand 1975;19:260–264.
140. Salem M, Tainsh Jr RE, Bromberg J, Loriaux DL, Chernow B. Perioperative glucocorticoid coverage. A reassessment 42 years after emergence of a problem. Ann Surg 1994;219:416–425.
141. Nickels DA, Moore DC. Serum cortisol responses in febrile children. Pediatr Infect Dis J 1989;8:16–20.
142. Miller WL. Congenital adrenal hyperplasias. Endocrinol Metab Clin N Am 1991;20:721–749.
143. Girgis R, Winter JS. The effects of glucocorticoid replacement therapy on growth, bone mineral density, and bone turnover markers in children with congenital adrenal hyperplasia. J Clin Endocrinol Metab 1997;82:3926–3929.
144. Winter JS, Couch RM. Modern medical therapy of congenital adrenal hyperplasia. A decade of experience. Ann NY Acad Sci 1985;458:165–173.
145. Ulick S, Eberlein WR, Bliffeld AR, Chu MD, Bongiovanni AM. Evidence for an aldosterone biosynthetic defect in congenital adrenal hyperplasia. J Clin Endocrinol Metab 1980;51:1346–1353.
146. Horner JM, Hintz RL, Luetscher JA. The role of renin and angiotensin in salt-losing, 21-hydroxylase-deficient congenital adrenal hyperplasia. J Clin Endocrinol Metab 1979;48:776–783.
147. Ames RP, Borkowski AJ, Sicinski AM, Laragh JH. Prolonged infusions of angiotensin II and norepinephrine and blood pressure, electrolyte balance, and aldosterone and cortisol secretion in normal man and in cirrhosis with ascites. J Clin Invest 1965;44:1171–1186.
148. Rayyis SS, Horton R. Effect of angiotensin II on adrenal and pituitary function in man. J Clin Endocrinol Metab 1971;32:539.
149. Rosler A, Levine LS, Schneider B, Novogroder M, New MI. The interrelationship of sodium balance, plasma renin activity, and ACTH in congenital adrenal hyperplasi. J Clin Endocrinol Metab 1977;45:500.
150. Brook CG, Zachmann M, Prader A, Murset G. Experience with long-term therapy in congenital adrenal hyperplasia. J Pediatr 1974;85:12–19.
151. Silva IN, Kater CE, Cunha CF, Viana MB. Randomised controlled trial of growth effect of hydrocortisone in congenital adrenal hyperplasia. Arch Dis Child 1997;77:214–218.
152. DiMartino-Nardi J, Stoner E, O'Connell A, New MI. The effect of treatment of final height in classical congenital adrenal hyperplasia (CAH). Acta Endocrinol Suppl 1986;279:305–314.
153. Jaaskelainen J, Voutilainen R Growth of patients with 21-hydroxylase deficiency: an analysis of the factors influencing adult height. Pediatr Res 1997;41:30–33.
154. New MI, Gertner JM, Speiser PW, Del Balzo P. Growth and final height in classical and nonclassical 21-hydroxylase deficiency. J Endocrinol Invest 1989;12:91–95.
155. Urban MD, Lee PA, Migeon CJ. Adult height and fertility in men with congenital virilizing adrenal hyperplasia. N Engl J Med 1978;299:1392–1396.
156. Merke DP, Cutler Jr GB. New approaches to the treatment of congenital adrenal hyperplasia. JAMA 1997;277:1073–1076.
157. Laue L, Merke DP, Jones JV, Barnes KM, Hill S, Cutler Jr GB. A preliminary study of flutamide, testolactone, and reduced hydrocortisone dose in the treatment of congenital adrenal hyperplasia. J Clin Endocrinol Metab 1996;81:3535–3539.
158. Merke DP, Keil MF, Jones JV, Fields J, Hill S, Cutler Jr GB. Flutamide, testolactone, and reduced hydrocortisone dose maintain normal growth velocity and bone maturation despite elevated androgen levels in children with congenital adrenal hyperplasia. J Clin Endocrinol Metab 2000;85:1114–1120.
159. Zinkham WH, Kickler T, Borel J, Moser HW. Lorenzo's oil and thrombocytopenia in patients with adrenoleukodystrophy. N Engl J Med 1993;328:1126–1127.
160. Krivit W, Lockman LA, Watkins PA, Hirsch J, Shapiro EG. The future for treatment by bone marrow transplantation for adrenoleukodystrophy, metachromatic leukodystrophy, globoid cell leukodystrophy and Hurler syndrome. J Inherit Metab Dis 1995;18:398–412.
161. Aubourg P, Blanche S, Jambaque I, et al. Reversal of early neurologic and neuroradiologic manifestations of X-linked adrenoleukodystrophy by bone marrow transplantation. N Engl J Med 1990;322:1860–1866.
162. Bethune JE. 1975. The Adrenal Cortex. The Upjohn Company, Kalamazoo.

13 Congenital Adrenal Hyperplasia

Lenore S. Levine, MD
and Sharon E. Oberfield, MD

Contents

Introduction
Lipoid Adrenal Hyperplasia
3β Hydroxysteroid (3β HSD)/Δ4,5-Isomerase Deficiency
17-Hydroxylase/17,20 Lyase Deficiency
21-Hydroxylase Deficiency
11β-Hydroxylase Deficiency
Therapy, Monitoring, and Outcome
Prenatal Diagnosis and Treatment of CAH
Newborn Screening for CAH
Conclusion
References

INTRODUCTION

Congenital adrenal hyperplasia (CAH) is a family of autosomal recessive disorders in which there is a deficiency of one of the enzymes necessary for cortisol synthesis *(1)* (*see* Fig. 1). An abnormality in each of the enzymatic activities required for cortisol synthesis has been described. As a result of the disordered enzymatic step, there is decreased cortisol synthesis, increased ACTH via the negative feedback system, overproduction of the hormones prior to the enzymatic step or not requiring the deficient enzyme, and deficiency of the hormones distal to the disordered enzymatic step. Since certain of the enzymatic steps are required for sex hormone synthesis by the gonad, a disordered enzymatic step in the gonad, resulting in gonadal steroid hormone deficiency, may also be present *(2)*.

The symptoms of the disorder depend upon which hormones are overproduced and which are deficient. As a result, CAH may present with virilization of the affected female infant and subsequent signs of androgen excess in both males and females, incomplete virilization of the male and signs of sex hormone deficiency at puberty in both males and females, salt-wasting crisis secondary to aldosterone deficiency, or hormonal hyperten-

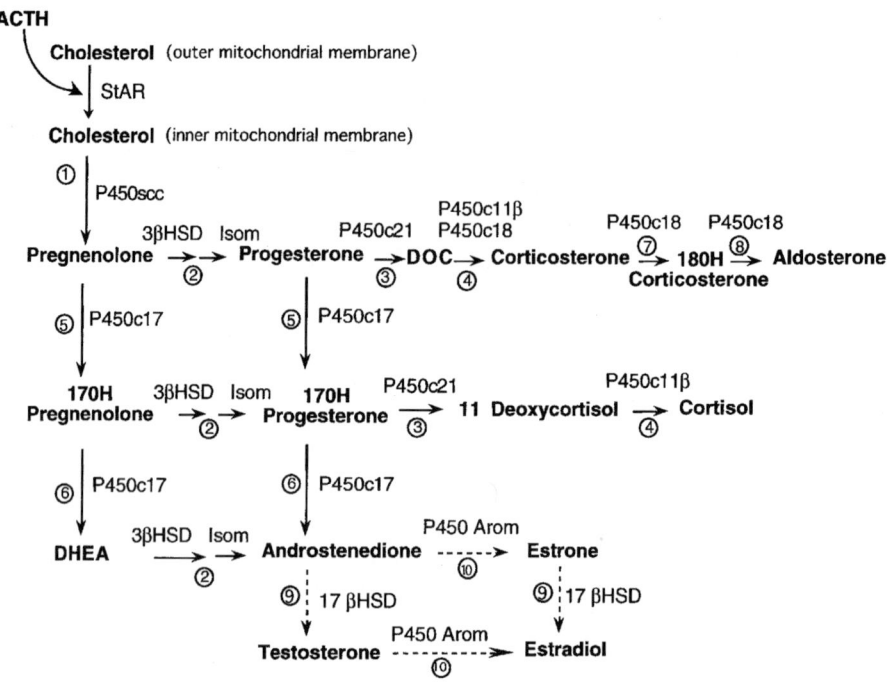

Fig. 1. Simplified scheme of adrenal steroidogenesis. Two reactions (dotted arrows) occur primarily in gonads, not in adrenal gland. Chemical names for enzymes shown above or to right of arrows; circled numbers refer to traditional names: 1) 20,22-desmolase; 2) 3β–hydroxysteroid dehydrogenase/isomerase; 3) 21-hydroxylase; 4) 11β–hydroxylase; 5) 17α-hydroxylase; 6) 17,20-lyase; 7) 18-hydroxylase; 8) 18-oxidase; 9) 17β–hydroxysteroid dehydrogenase; 10) aromatase; StAR = steroidogenic acute regulatory protein; DOC = 11-deoxycorticosterone.

sion secondary to increased deoxycorticosterone (DOC), a mineralocorticoid *(1–6)*. The enzymes of adrenal steroidogenesis, their cellular location, the genes encoding the enzymes, and their chromosomal locations are presented in Table 1. The clinical presentations of this family of disorders is presented in Table 2. This chapter will present an overview of all of the enzymatic deficiencies resulting in CAH with the most extensive review of 21-hydroxylase deficiency, the most common, first described, and the most intensively studied of the enzymatic disorders.

LIPOID ADRENAL HYPERPLASIA

Lipoid adrenal hyperplasia is due to a deficiency of cholesterol desmolase activity. As a result, there is a deficiency in all of the adrenal hormones: glucocorticoids (cortisol), mineralocorticoids (aldosterone), and the sex steroids (Fig. 1). In addition, since this enzymatic activity is necessary for sex hormone synthesis in the gonad, there is also deficiency of gonadal steroids. Affected infants usually present early in life with salt-wasting crisis manifested by cardiovascular collapse, hyponatremia, and hyperkalemia. Males have phenotypically female external genitalia. Females exhibit no genital abnormalities. Increased pigmentation, secondary to increased ACTH, may be of such a degree as to produce "bronzing" in the newborn. Occasionally, infants have been reported to

Table 1
Enzymes and Genes of Adrenal Steroidogenesis[a]

Enzymatic Activity	Enzyme	Cellular Location	Gene	Chromosomal Location
Cholesterol Desmolase (side chain cleavage)	P450scc (CYP11A1)	mitochondrion	CYP11A1	15q23–q24
3β-Hydroxysteroid Dehydrogenase	3βHSD (3βHSDII)	endoplasmic reticulum	HSD3B2	1p13.1
17α-Hydroxylase/17,20 lyase	P450c17 (CYP17)	endoplasmic reticulum	CYP17	10q24.3
21α-Hydroxylase	P450c21 (CYP21A2)	endoplasmic reticulum	CYP21A2	6p21.3
11β-Hydroxylase	P450c11 (CYP11B1)	mitochondrion	CYP11B1	8q21–22
Aldosterone synthase (corticosterone 18-methylcorticosterone oxidase/lyase)	P450c18 (CYP11B2)	mitochondrion	CYP11B2	8q21–22

[a]Adapted with permission from ref. *(1)*.

present with salt-wasting crisis beyond the newborn period. Because of the gonadal sex steroid deficiency, males are unable to produce gonadal steroids at the time of puberty. Affected females may have sufficient gonadal function remaining at puberty to begin feminization and progress to menarche, but gonadal failure ultimately ensues (Table 2). Laboratory evaluation in patients with lipoid adrenal hyperplasia reveals low levels of all steroid hormones, with no response to ACTH or human chorionic gonadotropin (HCG) administration. ACTH and plasma renin activity (PRA) are very elevated. Imaging studies of the adrenal gland will reveal marked enlargement of the adrenals secondary to the accumulation of lipoid droplets. Females with this disorder have normal internal and external genitalia.

Males, as noted above, are phenotypically female. Males incorrectly diagnosed as females with adrenal insufficiency have been noted subsequently to have inguinal gonads, which has led to the correct diagnosis.

Lipoid adrenal hyperplasia is rare. It has been reported in approx 100 patients, the majority of whom are Japanese. In this disorder, the gene coding for P450 SCC, a mitochondrial enzyme, has been normal in almost all cases studied (Table 1). It has now been established that congenital lipoid adrenal hyperplasia is most often due to a mutation in the gene for steroidogenic acute regulatory protein (StAR). The StAR gene is located on chromosome 8p11.2 and is expressed in adrenals and gonads. StAR is a mitochondrial protein that promotes the movement of cholesterol from the outer to the inner mitochondrial membrane. Recently, mutations in the P450scc gene were described in two patients with lipoid adrenal hyperplasia: a 46XY patient with a heterozygous mutation, and a 46XX patient with compound heterozygous mutations. Thus, lipoid adrenal hyperplasia is the only form of CAH which is not usually caused by a mutation in a gene coding for a steroidogenic enzyme *(7–10)*.

Table 2
Clinical and Hormonal Data

Enzymatic deficiency	Signs and symptoms	Laboratory findings	Therapeutic measures
Lipoid CAH (Cholesterol desmolase deficiency)	Salt-wasting crisis Male pseudohermaphoditism	Low levels of all steroid hormones, with decreased/absent response to ACTH Decreased/absent response to HCG in male pseudohermaphroditism ↑ACTH ↑PRA	Glucocorticoid and mineralocorticoid administration Sodium chloride supplementation Gonadectomy of male pseudohermaphrodite Sex hormone replacement consonant with sex of rearing
3β-HSD deficiency	Classic form: Salt-wasting crisis Male and female pseudohermaphroditism Precocious pubarche Disordered puberty	↑↑Baseline and ACTH-stimulated Δ5 steroids (pregnenolone, 17-OH pregnenolone, DHEA, and their urinary metabolites) ↑↑Δ5/Δ4 serum and urinary steroids ↑ACTH ↑PRA Suppression of elevated adrenal steroids after glucocorticoid administration	Glucocorticoid and mineralocorticoid administration Sodium chloride supplementation Surgical correction of genitalia and sex hormone replacement as necessary consonant with sex of rearing
3β-HSD deficiency	Nonclassic form: Precocious pubarche, disordered puberty, menstrual irregularity, hirsutism, acne, infertility	↑Baseline and ACTH-stimulated Δ5 steroids (pregnenolone, 17-OH pregnenolone, DHEA, and their urinary metabolites) ↑Δ5/Δ4 serum and urinary steroids Suppression of elevated adrenal steroids after glucocorticoid administration	Glucocorticoid administration

21-OH deficiency	Classic form: Salt-wasting crisis Female pseudohermaphroditism Postnatal virilization	↑↑Baseline and ACTH-stimulated 17-OH progesterone and pregnanetriol ↑↑Serum androgens and urinary metabolites ↑ACTH ↑PRA Suppression of elevated adrenal steroids after glucocorticoid administration	Glucocorticoid and mineralocorticoid replacement Sodium chloride supplementation Vaginoplasty and clitoral recession in female pseudohermaphroditism
21-OH deficiency	Nonclassic form: Precocious pubarche, disordered puberty, menstrual irregularity, hirsutism, acne, infertility	↑↑Baseline and ACTH-stimulated 17-OH progesterone and pregnanetriol ↑↑Serum androgens and urinary metabolites Suppression of elevated adrenal steroids after glucocorticoid administration	Glucocorticoid administration
11β-Hydroxylase deficiency	Classic Form: Female pseudohermaphroditism Postnatal virilization in males and females Hypertension	↑↑Baseline and ACTH-stimulated compound S and DOC and their urinary metabolites ↑↑Serum androgens and their urinary metabolites ↑ACTH ↓PRA Hypokalemia Suppression of elevated steroids after glucocorticoid administration	Glucocorticoid administration Vaginoplasty and clitoral recession in female pseudo-hermaphroditism

(continued)

Table 2 (continued)
Clinical and Hormonal Data

Enzymatic deficiency	Signs and symptoms	Laboratory findings	Therapeutic measures
17α-OH/17,20 lyase deficiency	Male pseudohermaphroditism Sexual infantilism Hypertension	↑↑DOC, 18-OH DOC, corticosterone 18-hydroxycorticosterone Low 17α-hydroxylated steroids and poor response to ACTH Poor response to HCG in male pseudohermaphroditism ↓PRA ↑ACTH Hypokalemia Suppression of elevated adrenal steroids after glucocorticoid administration	Glucocorticoid administration Surgical correction of genitalia and sex hormone replacement in male pseudohermaphroditism consonant with sex or rearing Sex hormone replacement in female

Adapted with permission from ref. (83).

3β HYDROXYSTEROID (3β HSD)/Δ4,5-ISOMERASE DEFICIENCY

3β HSD/Δ4,5-Isomerase deficiency is also a rare form of CAH occurring in fewer than 5% of patients. As can be seen in Figure 1, 3β HSD/Δ4,5-Isomerase is necessary for the conversion of pregnenolone to progesterone, 17-hydroxypregnenelone to 17-hydroxyprogesterone, and dehydroepiandrosterone (DHEA) to Δ4-androstenedione. Decreased ability to convert these Δ5 steroids to Δ4 steroids results in decreased synthesis of cortisol, aldosterone, and androstenedione. In the testes, it results in decreased ability to form testosterone. The deficiency of cortisol results in increased ACTH with overproduction of Δ5 steroids, including DHEA. The increased level of DHEA is sufficient to result in some virilization of the external genitalia in affected females, although the virilization is not as marked as in the other forms of virilizing CAH, 21-hydroxylase deficiency and 11-hydroxylase deficiency. Female infants with 3β HSD/Δ4,5-Isomerase deficiency may have clitoromegaly and partial fusion of the labial folds. Males with this disorder manifest a deficiency of prenatal testosterone and are born with varying degrees of ambiguity of the external genitalia ranging from hypospadius to more significant degrees of incomplete virilization with partial fusion of the scrotal folds. Most infants with 3β HSD/Δ4,5-Isomerase deficiency have aldosterone deficiency and present in the newborn period with salt-wasting crisis. Postnatally there is continued excessive DHEA secretion with growth acceleration and the early onset of pubic and/or axillary hair. Symptoms of ongoing excessive adrenal androgens include hirsutism, acne, menstrual irregularity or amenorrhea, and infertility. Increased pigmentation of skin creases occurs secondary to increased ACTH. Laboratory evaluation reveals elevation of the Δ5 steroids, specifically the diagnostic hormone 17-hydroxypregnenolone, and DHEA, with a further rise following ACTH stimulation, to levels of 10,000–60,000 ng/dL and 3000–12,000 ng/dL, respectively. The ratios of Δ5 to Δ4 steroids (17-hydroxypregnenolone/17-hydroxyprogesterone and DHEA/androstenedione) post ACTH stimulation have been reported to reach 18–25 and 18–30, respectively. Males with this disorder have been reported to undergo normal male puberty. However, this occurs with marked elevation of the Δ5 steroids sufficient to produce adequate levels of testosterone. ACTH levels are increased, and in those with aldosterone deficiency, plasma renin activity is markedly elevated as well. Glucocorticoid administration results in a decrease in ACTH followed by a decrease in the overproduced adrenal androgens (Table 2).

The 3β HSD enzyme, located in the endoplasmic reticulum, mediates both 3β HSD and isomerase activities. (Table 1) 3β HSD/Δ4,5-Isomerase deficiency is due to a mutation in the HSD3β2 gene, located on chromosome 1. A number of mutations in this gene have been described. In the past, signs of mild androgen excess in children and adults (precocious pubarche, acne, hirsutism, menstrual problems) have been attributed to a non-classic form of 3β HSD deficiency in which a less severe enzymatic deficiency results in lesser elevations of the Δ5 steroids and Δ5/Δ4 ratios. Although mutations in the 3β HSD gene have been described in premature pubarche, a number of children and adults thought to have non-classic 3β HSD deficiency have been demonstrated to have normal 3β HSD genes, bringing into question the diagnosis and suggesting that hormonal criteria remain to be established for the diagnosis of the non-classic or mild form of the disease *(11–16)*.

17-HYDROXYLASE/17,20 LYASE DEFICIENCY

17-hydroxylase/17,20 lyase deficiency is another relatively rare form of CAH, described in 125 to 150 patients. In this disorder, there is a deficiency of 17-hydroxylation by which pregnenolone and progesterone are converted to 17-hydroxypregnenolone and 17-hydroxyprogesterone, and deficiency as well in the 17,20 lyase reaction resulting in the conversion of 17-hydroxypregnenolone and 17-hydroxyprogesterone to DHEA and $\Delta 4$-androstenedione, respectively (Fig. 1). Similar to other forms of CAH, the deficiency in cortisol results in increased ACTH. Overproduction of DOC, a mineralocorticoid, ensues, producing hypertension and hypokalemia that may be the presenting symptoms. Because this enzymatic deficiency is present also in the gonad, there is a deficiency of sex steroids as well, so that affected males are incompletely virilized and are phenotypically female or ambiguous. These males are unable to undergo normal male puberty due to testosterone deficiency. Affected females have normal female external genitalia and may present with failure of sexual development at adolescence (Table 2). Rarely, patients have been described with isolated 17,20 lyase deficiency. 17-hydroxylase/17,20 lyase deficiency is diagnosed by the presence of low levels of all 17-hydroxylated steroids, with a poor response to ACTH and HCG administration. Levels of DOC (10–40×), 18-OH DOC (30–60×), corticosterone (B) (30–100×) and 18-OHB (10×) are markedly elevated and PRA and aldosterone are suppressed. Glucocorticoid administration results in suppression of the overproduced hormones. As DOC is suppressed, there is resolution of the volume expansion and PRA increases, thus stimulating aldosterone secretion.

P450c17, found in the endoplasmic reticulum, is responsible for catalyzing steroid 17-hydroxylation and 17,20 lyase reactions. It is coded for by a gene located on chromosome 10 expressed both in the adrenal cortex and in the gonads (Table 1). Approximately 20 different genetic lesions have been documented in these patients. The molecular basis for isolated 17,20 lyase deficiency has been elucidated *(17–19)*.

21-HYDROXYLASE DEFICIENCY

21-hydroxylase deficiency is the most common form of CAH, affecting approx 90% of individuals with CAH. It occurs with a world-wide frequency of approx 1:15,000 newborns, with increased frequency among certain ethnic groups (Yupik Eskimos; LaReunion, France). In this disorder, there is decreased ability to 21-hydroxylate progesterone and 17-hydroxyprogesterone to DOC and 11-deoxycortisol (S), respectively (Fig. 1). As a result, there is decreased cortisol secretion, increased ACTH, adrenal hyperplasia, and overproduction of the steroids prior to 21-hydroxylation. 17-hydroxyprogesterone is the most elevated and is the diagnostic hormone in this disorder. There is overproduction of the adrenal androgens, especially $\Delta 4$-androstenedione, and by peripheral conversion, testosterone, resulting in virilization, the hallmark of this disorder.

In addition, approx 2/3 of these patients will have aldosterone deficiency presenting with salt-wasting crisis in the newborn period, most often between 1 wk and 1 mo of-age. Salt-wasting may become manifest later in infancy and occasionally beyond the time of infancy, often in the setting of an intercurrent illness. Because this disorder begins *in utero*, the female fetus is exposed to excessive adrenal androgens resulting in virilization of the external genitalia ranging from clitoromegaly, with or without mild degrees of labial fusion, to marked virilization of the external genitalia such that the female infant appears to be a male infant with hypospadius (occasionally with the appearance of a penile urethra) and undescended testes. There is a urogenital sinus with one outflow track to the perineum. As with all forms of CAH, a female infant will have normal ovaries, fallopian tubes, uterus, and proximal vagina.

Post-natally, there is continued virilization with progressive clitoromegaly and penile enlargement, rapid growth, and premature development of pubic and/or axillary hair. Additionally, signs of androgen excess secondary to late or inadequate treatment include acne, delayed menarche or primary amenorrhea, menstrual irregularity, hirsutism, and infertility. Although rapid growth and tall stature are present in early childhood, bone age advancement is greater than height advancement, resulting in short final height in late or poorly treated patients. True precocious puberty may occur with bone age advancement to 10 yr or older, contributing to short final height. Increased ACTH secretion results in increased pigmentation of skin creases, nipples, and genitalia. Unilateral testicular enlargement may occur secondary to stimulation of adrenal rest tissue and formation of adrenal rest tumors (Table 2).

A milder non-classic form of 21-hydroxylase deficiency is well recognized. It occurs most commonly in Ashkenazi Jews with an estimated frequency of 0.1%. There is no salt-wasting in the non-classic disorder and female genitalia are normal at birth. Signs of androgen excess may appear in childhood; premature pubarche, acne, hirsutism, menstrual irregularity, and infertility may be presenting symptoms. Males with this disorder may also present with unilateral testicular enlargement similar to males with the classical disorder (Table 2).

The diagnostic hormone in 21-hydroxylase deficiency is 17-OH progesterone. Levels in the classic form are markedly elevated throughout the day in the range of 10,000–100,000 ng/dL and rise to levels of 25,000–100,000 ng/dL or greater following ACTH stimulation. Androstenedione levels are also elevated and may be in the range of 250 ng/dL to greater than 1000 ng/dL. Testosterone levels are elevated to a variable degree and range from an early male pubertal level to levels in the adult male range (350–1000 ng/dL). The 24-h urinary excretion of pregnanetriol and 17-ketosteroids, the metabolic products of 17-hydroxyprogesterone and androgens, respectively, are also elevated. The elevated serum and urinary hormones promptly decrease following glucocorticoid administration. ACTH levels are increased throughout the day in classic 21-OH deficiency and PRA and PRA/aldosterone are increased in overt or subtle salt-wasting. Salt-wasting crisis presents with hyponatremia, hyperkalemia, acidosis, and azotemia. Hypoglycemia may also be present. Cortisol levels may be decreased or in the normal range but usually do not increase with ACTH, indicating that the adrenal gland has maximally compensated for the enzymatic deficiency. Laboratory findings are less marked in the non-classic form. 17-hydroxyprogesterone may be only mildly elevated particularly if drawn in late morning or afternoon, paralleling the diurnal pattern of ACTH. Following ACTH administration, 17-hydroxyprogesterone rises to levels of 2000-10,000 ng/dL. Serum androgens are also less elevated compared to the classic form. Glucocorticoid administration results in a prompt decrease in the elevated hormones. Basal cortisol levels are normal and usually increase normally in response to ACTH administration (Table 2).

21-hydroxylation is mediated by P450c21, found in the endoplasmic reticulum (Table 1). The gene for P450c21 was initially mapped to within the HLA complex on the short arm of chromosome 6 between the genes for HLA-B and DR, by HLA studies of families with classic CAH. In these studies, it was demonstrated that within a family, all affected siblings were HLA-B identical and different from their unaffected siblings. Family members sharing one HLA-B antigen with the affected index case were predicted to be heterozygote carriers of the *CAH* gene and family members sharing no HLA-B antigen with the affected index case were predicted to be homozygous normal. Subsequently, molecular genetic analysis demonstrated that there are two highly homologous human *P450c21* genes - one active (*CYP21B, CYP 21A2*) and one inactive (*CYP21P, CYP21A*). The two genes are located in tandem with two highly homologous genes for the fourth component of complement (*C4A, C4B*). A number of other genes of known and unknown function are also located in this cluster.

The genetic mutations in patients with 21-OH deficiency have been extensively studied. Most patients are compound heterozygotes, having a different mutation on each allele. The severity of the disease is determined by the less severely affected allele. Approximately 75% of mutations are recombinations between the inactive CYP21A gene and the active CYP21A2 gene, resulting in microconversions. Large gene conversions and gene deletions also occur.

The classic form of the disorder results from the combination of two severe deficiency genes, while the non-classic form of the disease results from a combination of a severe *CYP21A2* deficiency gene (found in the classic form of the disease) and a mild *CYP21A2* deficiency gene or a combination of two mild deficiency genes. Point mutations, gene conversions, and gene duplications have been found in the mild *CYP21A2* deficiency genes. A valine to leucine substitution in codon 281 is a frequently found point mutation and is highly associated with HLA-B14DR1 *(1–6)*.

11β-HYDROXYLASE DEFICIENCY

CAH due to 11β-hydroxylase deficiency accounts for approx 5% of reported cases of CAH. It occurs in approximately 1:100,000 births in a diverse Caucasian population but is more common in Jews of North African origin. In this disorder, the enzymatic deficiency results in a block in 11-hydroxylation of 11-deoxycortisol (compound S) to cortisol and 11-deoxycorticosterone (DOC) to corticosterone (B). Decreased cortisol results in increased ACTH and adrenal hyperplasia and overproduction of 11-deoxycortisol and DOC. As in 21-hydroxylase deficiency, there is shunting into the androgen pathway with overproduction of adrenal androgens, especially androstenedione, and by peripheral conversion, testosterone (Fig. 1).

This results in virilization, similar to 21-hydroxylase deficiency, with prenatal virilization of the female fetus, and postnatal virilization of affected males and females. The excessive DOC secretion results in sodium and water retention and plasma volume expansion. Hypertension and hypokalemia may ensue.

The diagnosis of 11β-hydroxylase deficiency is based upon marked elevation of serum 11-deoxycortisol (1400–4300 ng/dL) and DOC (183–2050 ng/dL). Increased excretion of their metabolites tetrahydro-11-deoxycortisol (THS) and tetrahydro-11-deoxycorticosterone (TH-DOC)in a 24-h urine can confirm the diagnosis. Serum androstenedione and testosterone and urinary ketosteroids are also elevated. PRA and aldosterone are suppressed secondary to the volume expansion mediated by the excessive DOC, and hypokalemia may also be present. Glucocorticoid therapy results in suppression of the excessive S, DOC, and androgens. As DOC is suppressed, there is remission of the volume expansion, PRA and aldosterone rise and hypokalemia reverses. A milder form of 11-hydroxylase deficiency has also been reported, presenting in later childhood, adolescence, or adulthood with signs of androgen excess: premature pubarche, acne, hirsutism, menstrual irregularity, and infertility (Table 2).

P450c11β, a mitochondrial enzyme, is coded for by *CYP11B1*. It mediates 11β-hydroxylation in the zona fasciculata leading to cortisol synthesis. P450c18, also located in the mitochondria and coded for by CYP11B2, mediates 11β-hydroxylase, 18-hydroxylase, and 18-oxidase activities in the zona glomerulosa leading to aldosterone synthesis. These genes lie on chromosome 8q21–22 (Table 1). CAH due to 11β-hydroxylase deficiency results from a mutation in the *CYP11B1* gene. A number of mutations in this gene have been reported in patients with 11β-hydroxylase deficiency. Almost all Moroccan Jewish patients with this disorder have a point mutation in codon 448 in CYP11B1, resulting in an arginine→histidine substitution *(20–23)*.

THERAPY, MONITORING, AND OUTCOME

The principle of therapy of CAH is to replace the hormones that are deficient and to decrease the hormones that are overproduced. Glucocorticoids have been the mainstay of treatment for over 50 yr. As noted previously, administration of glucocorticoid reduces ACTH overproduction, reverses adrenal hyperplasia, and reduces the levels of hormones that are overproduced—androgens in the virilizing disorders (21-hydroxylase, 11-hydroxylase, 3β HSD/Δ4,5 Isomerase deficiencies) and DOC in the hypertensive disorders (11-hydroxylase, 17-hydroxylase). In the salt-wasting disorders (Lipoid Adrenal Hyperplasia, 3β HSD/Δ4,5 Isomerase, 21-Hydroxylase), mineralocorticoid and sodium supplementation are provided. In disorders with sex steroid deficiency (Lipoid Adrenal Hyperplasia, 17-Hydroxylase, 3βHSD/Δ4,5 Isomerase) sex hormone replacement consonant with the sex of assignment is necessary. Surgical correction of ambiguous genitalia may also be necessary.

The objective of therapy is to achieve normal growth and pubertal development, normal sexual function and normal reproductive function, in those disorders with potential fertility. Therapy must be individualized according to the clinical course and hormonal levels.

Glucocorticoid

Hydrocortisone is most commonly used in childhood. Because of the short half life, 3 daily divided doses are generally recommended. The dose of hydrocortisone is usually in the range of 10–20 mg/m^2/d. Lower doses can often be used in the non-classical disorders. Whether the dose should be equally divided or a higher dose given in the morning or in the evening is controversial. Some pediatric endocrinologists prefer cortisone acetate intramuscularly 15–20 mg every 3 d for the first 2 yr of life. Equivalent doses of longer acting steroids, such as prednisone or dexamethasone, may be used in the older adolescent/young adult, allowing for less frequent dosing. The longer acting steroids are used less frequently in the growing child because of concern in regard to overtreatment, although there are reports of successful treatment with the more potent steroids in childhood *(1–6,24)*.

Mineralocorticoid and Salt

In the presence of aldosterone deficiency, florinef, a synthetic mineralocorticoid is administered. The dose is usually between 0.1–0.3 mg daily. Sodium chloride supplementation, 1–3 g daily is necessary, especially in the infant and young child. As sodium chloride in the diet increases, it may be possible to decrease and ultimately discontinue sodium supplementation. Similarly, there may be a decreasing dose requirement for florinef.

Sex Steroids

In those conditions with sex steroid deficiency (Lipoid Adrenal Hyperplasia, 17-hydroxylase, 3β HSD/Δ4,5 Isomerase), sex hormone replacement therapy to induce or maintain normal secondary sexual characteristics may often be required. Therapy is begun at an age appropriate for puberty and the achievement of a satisfactory final height. Estrogen therapy to induce breast development is often begun with premarin. A progestational agent is added to induce menses in the genetic female, and therapy is often subsequently changed to an oral contraceptive agent. Testosterone enanthate is used to induce male pubertal changes. The newer testosterone patches may also be used. Menstrual irregularity or amenorrhea may occur in females with the virilizing disorders. Oral contraceptives may also be used in these patients.

Genitalia Surgery

In females with virilizing forms of CAH, surgical correction of the genitalia may be necessary depending on the degree of virilization. If significant clitoromegaly is present but not marked, clitoral recession may be possible. The clitoris is freed and repositioned beneath the pubis, with preservation of the glans, corporal components, and all neural and vascular elements. If there is marked clitoromegaly, the clitoris is reduced, with partial excision of the corporal bodies and preservation of the neurovascular bundle. Vaginoplasty and correction of the urogenital sinus is usually performed at the time of clitoral surgery. This initial surgery most often is performed within the first year of life; later revision may be necessary.

In conditions with gonadal sex hormone deficiency resulting in incomplete virilization of the external genitalia in the genetic male, surgical correction to conform with the sex of rearing is often necessary. Males with lipoid adrenal hyperplasia have phenotypically normal female genitalia and are raised as females. A gonadectomy is performed to avoid the risk of gonadal malignancy. The degree of genital ambiguity in males with 3β HSD/Δ4,5 Isomerase or 17-hydroxylase deficiencies is variable and ranges from phenotypically female to male with hypospadius. In those given a female sex assignment, gonadectomy and surgery to create normal female appearing external genitalia are performed. In incompletely virilized males given a male sex assignment, corrective surgery may include repair of hypospadius, orchiopexy, and phalloplasty.

Our present practices in regard to genital surgery in infants with intersex problems are currently undergoing intensive re-examination and re-evaluation. It has been suggested by some patient groups and professionals that surgery should not be performed until the child can participate in the decision. The need for better education of parents, more attention to psychosocial issues, and better communication between all the involved professionals, parents, and patients is clearly demonstrated in reports of problematic psychosocial outcome in intersex patients. Many groups are exploring methods to improve outcome but there is, at the present time, no clear consensus how this can be achieved *(25–28)*.

LHRH Agonists

Precocious puberty may occur in late diagnosed or poorly controlled children whose bone ages are advanced to 10 yr or more. Lutenizing hormone releasing hormone (LHRH) agonists have been used to delay puberty, retard bone age advancement, and prolong the time available for continued growth. The dose of Lupron Depot-Ped, commonly used in the US, is similar to that used in non-CAH children with precocious puberty, approx 0.3 mg/kg im every 28 d *(29)*.

Other Treatments

Use of a combination of an anti-androgen (to block androgen effect) and an aromatase inhibitor (to block conversion of androgen to estrogen) with reduced hydrocortisone dose has been reported in a 2-yr study. The preliminary report suggests this regimen is efficacious, resulting in normal growth and normal bone age advancement *(30,31)*.

There have been preliminary reports of growth hormone treatment, with or without LHRH agonists, in children with CAH. Initial data suggests improvement in predicted adult height but long-term results and final heights have not been reported *(32,33)*.

Adrenalectomy has been reported in children with salt-wasting 21-OH deficiency and 11-OH deficiency who could not be well controlled medically *(34–37)*.

Long-term studies of these new treatment regimens are required to determine if they result in better final outcome.

Monitoring

Therapy is evaluated by clinical course and appropriate hormonal levels. Normal gain in height and weight, normal onset and progress of puberty, absence of signs of androgen excess in virilizing disorders (rapid growth, acne, hirsutism, phallic enlargement), normotension in the hypertensive disorders and in patients on mineralocorticoid and/or salt replacement are goals of therapy. Glucocorticoid excess results in poor growth, excess weight gain and Cushingoid appearance. Inadequate sodium repletion may result in poor growth and worsening of hormonal control while inadequate androgen suppression results in rapid growth and bone age advancement. Hormonal monitoring includes measurement of adrenal androgens in the virilizing disorders, PRA in the salt-losing disorders, and PRA and DOC in the hypertensive disorders.

Measurement of the precursor hormones, such as 17-OH progesterone in 21-hydroxylase deficiency, compound S in 11-OH deficiency, and 17-OH pregnenolone in 3β HSD/Δ4,5 Isomerase deficiency should also be performed (Table 2).

The aim of therapy is to keep the precursor hormones in a range sufficiently low to maintain adrenal androgens in the normal range in the virilizing disorders. PRA should be in the high normal range in the salt-wasting disorders. PRA and DOC should be in the normal range in the hypertensive disorders.

The optimal time and relationship to dose for the hormonal measurements are not established. Early morning bloods before the morning glucocorticoid dose and random bloods drawn while on the usual therapeutic regimen are utilized. Measurement of 24-h excretion of urinary metabolites can provide an additional measure of control *(1–6)*.

Outcome

The outcome of treatment of CAH due to 21-hydroxylase deficiency has been the most extensively reported. Normal final height and normal pubertal development, sexual function, and fertility have been reported. However, there have been frequent reports of short stature, disordered puberty, menstrual irregularity, infertility, inadequate vaginal reconstruction, and lack of sexual function. Cross-gender development and gender change from female to male have occurred *(1–6,26,28,38–50)*. Recently, decreased bone mineral density in adult women with CAH has been reported *(51)*.

It is hoped that earlier diagnosis by newborn screening, the development of improved methods to monitor these patients, improved surgical techniques, and new therapies will result in better outcome.

The increased awareness of psychosocial issues and the need for extensive psychologic support for patients and families as well as the current re-examination and discussion of issues relating to genital surgery should contribute to the development of more successful therapy and better outcome.

PRENATAL DIAGNOSIS AND TREATMENT OF CAH

Prenatal Diagnosis of CAH

There have been numerous reports of the prenatal diagnosis and treatment of CAH due to 21-hydroxylase deficiency. Initially, the prenatal diagnosis of CAH due to 21-OH deficiency was based upon elevated levels of 17-hydroxyprogesterone and androstenedione (and testosterone in females) in amniotic fluid of a pregnancy at risk. The demonstration of genetic linkage between CAH due to 21-OH deficiency and HLA made possible the prenatal prediction of the disorder by HLA genotyping of cultured amniotic fluid cells and cultured chorionic villous cells. A fetus HLA identical to the affected index case would be predicted to be affected. The fetus that has one HLA haplotype in common with the index case would be predicted to be a heterozygous carrier, and the fetus in which both HLA haplotypes are different from the index case would be predicted to be homozygous normal. Molecular genetic analysis of DNA extracted from chorionic villous cells or amniocytes for *P450c21B, C4, HLA* class I and II genes has largely replaced hormonal evaluation and *HLA* genotyping in the prenatal diagnosis of CAH due to 21-hydroxylase deficiency. Causative mutations can now be identified in 95% of chromosomes by 21B gene analysis. A newly developed, rapid allele-specific polymerase chain reaction has recently been used for prenatal diagnosis. Determination of satellite markers may also be informative. Mutations not detected by this approach can be characterized by Southern blot analysis or direct sequencing of CYP21B genes. *De novo* mutations, found in patients with CAH but not in parents, are found in 1% of disease-causing CYP21B mutations *(1–6,52,53)*.

Prenatal diagnosis of 11β-hydroxylase deficiency has been made utilizing measurement of amniotic fluid 11-deoxycortisol and THS and DNA analysis of chorionic villus cells *(51,52)*. Lipoid adrenal hyperplasia has also been diagnosed prenatally using ultrasonography, amniotic fluid hormone levels and maternal plasma and urinary hormone measurements *(56,57)*. Theoretically, all forms of CAH can now be diagnosed prenatally by DNA analysis of chorionic villus cells.

Prenatal Treatment of CAH

Successful prenatal treatment of CAH due to 21-OH deficiency to prevent virilization of a female fetus was first reported in 1984. In a pregnancy at risk, dexamethasone 0.5 mg twice daily was administered to the mother from 5 wk of fetal age. The fetus was identified as an affected female by karyotyping and HLA genotyping of amniotic cells, and dexamethasone was continued to term. The infant had normal genitalia at birth and was confirmed to be affected. In a second pregnancy in this report, administration of hydrocortisone to the mother resulted in an affected female with minimally virilized genitalia *(58)*.

Since this initial report, there have been at least 88 CAH female infants treated prenatally. Dexamethasone, in doses as low as 0.5 mg to as high as 2 mg/d, has been administered in 1–4 divided doses. In some cases, treatment was interrupted for 5–7 d before amniocentesis, and in a few cases treatment was discontinued at 21–26 wk.

All newborns in whom treatment was initiated after 10 wk of fetal age or in whom treatment was discontinued by the end of the second trimester were severely virilized. In those treated from early in the first trimester to birth, treatment was considered successful and surgical correction unnecessary in 83% and not effective in 17%. Variability in maternal metabolic clearance and placental metabolism may contribute to the variability of results in addition to inadequate dosing and interruption or delay in treatment.

Spontaneous abortion, late pregnancy fetal demise, intrauterine growth retardation, liver steatosis, hydrocephalus, agenesis of the corpus callosum, and hypospadius with unilateral cryptochidism occasionally have occurred in short-term treated unaffected pregnancies or longer treated affected pregnancies. These events have not been considered to be related to the treatment. In long-term follow-up of most infants treated prenatally until midgestation or throughout the pregnancy, development seems to be normal, and growth has been consistent with the family pattern and the other affected siblings. However, the long-term follow-up is limited and most infants have been followed only for a brief period of time. Detailed neuropsychologic evaluations have not been reported. Rare adverse events including failure to thrive and psychomotor and psychosocial delay in development have been observed but cannot be definitively ascribed to the prenatal therapy *(52,53,59–62)*.

In a recent preliminary report, cognitive and behavioral development of young children aged 6 mo to 5 yr treated prenatally with dexamethasone (DEX) because of CAH risk was assessed by mother-completed standard questionnaires and compared with development of children from untreated CAH at risk pregnancies. No significant differences in cognitive abilities or behavior problems were identified. Dex-exposed children were reported to demonstrate more shyness, emotionality and avoidance, and less sociability than unexposed children *(63)*.

Successful prenatal treatment has also been reported in 11β-hydroxylase deficiency *(55)*.

Maternal Complications of Prenatal Treatment of CAH

There have been a number of reports of maternal adverse effects of prenatal dexamethasone treatment. The frequency of adverse effects has varied from approx 1/3 to 100% in mothers treated until delivery. The most common problem reported has been marked weight gain, found in 1/4 to 100% of mothers in various reports. Other side effects include edema, irritability, nervousness, mood swings, hypertension, glucose intolerance, epigastric pain, gastroenteritis, Cushingoid facial features, increased facial hair growth, and severe striae with permanent scarring. Studies of possible long term maternal adverse effects have not been reported *(60,62,64)*.

The maternal effects have prompted decreasing the dose or discontinuing the treatment. Non-compliance and unsatisfactory genital outcome may have resulted. Symptoms of glucocorticoid deficiency following tapering or discontinuing treatment have been rarely observed *(59)*.

Maternal anxiety about short and long term side effects of prenatal dexamethasone treatment on the fetus and child and on the mother has been documented *(65)*. In one report, 1/3 of all dexamethasone treated mothers stated they would not undergo prenatal treatment again *(62)*.

Protocol for Prenatal Treatment of CAH

Prenatal treatment of CAH due to 21-OH deficiency appears to be effective in ameliorating the virilization of the affected female fetus. However at present, the short and long-term complications to the fetus and mother are not fully defined. Therefore, parents seeking genetic counseling should be fully informed of the presently unknown long term side effects on treated mothers and prenatally treated children, the known possible maternal side effects, and the variable genital outcome *(66)*.

Treatment should be offered only to patients who have a clear understanding of the possible risks and benefits and who are able to comply with the need for very close monitoring throughout pregnancy and, postnatally, continued follow-up of the prenatally treated child. In the presence of maternal medical or mental conditions that may be worsened by dexamethasone treatment, such as hypertension, overt gestational diabetes, or toxemia, treatment should not be undertaken or undertaken only with extreme caution *(59)*.

Maternal monitoring for physical, hormonal, and metabolic changes should begin at the initiation of treatment and should be continued throughout the pregnancy. Treatment should be initiated in the 5th to 7th wk of gestation with dexamethasone, at a dose of approx 20–25 µg/kg/d, given in two–three divided doses. Chorionic villus sampling in the 9 wk for prenatal diagnosis should be performed with karyotyping and *HLA/21B/C4* gene analysis (HLA typing if gene analysis is not available) of chorionic villus cells. If chorionic villus sampling is performed in the 10th to 11th wk, a small amount of amniotic fluid can be obtained for hormonal analysis as well, to obtain some measure of fetal adrenal suppression. If the fetus is a male or an unaffected female, treatment is discontinued. If the fetus is an affected female, or if prenatal diagnosis by chorionic villus sampling is unsuccessful or not performed, treatment is continued. If necessary, amniocentesis is performed at 15 wk with genetic analysis of amniocytes and hormonal determination in amniotic fluid. If the fetus is an affected female, treatment is continued to term.

It is important to note that if the mother is receiving treatment with dexamethasone, hormonal analysis of amniotic fluid cannot be relied on for prenatal diagnosis.

Serum estriol level to evaluate adequacy of fetal adrenal suppression and fasting blood sugar should be determined monthly, and an oral glucose tolerance test should be performed during the second and third trimesters. Prompt intervention in the presence of excessive weight gain, increased blood pressure, and glucose intolerance or other side effects should be instituted. Consideration should be given to reducing the dose of dexamethasone during the second and third trimesters *(52,53,59)*.

NEWBORN SCREENING FOR CAH

The development in 1977 of the methodology to measure 17-hydroxyprogesterone in a heel stick capillary blood specimen on filter paper made possible newborn screening for CAH due to 21-OH deficiency *(67)*. Shortly thereafter, a pilot newborn screening program was developed in Alaska *(68)*. Screening programs have been developed worldwide in various countries including Brazil, Canada, France, Germany, Israel, Japan, New Zealand, Portugal, Saudi Arabia, Scotland, Spain, Sweden, and Switzerland. More than 20 states in the US include CAH due to 21-OH deficiency in their screening programs.

All CAH newborn screening programs employ the measurement of 17-OH progesterone in a filter paper blood spot sample obtained by the heel prick technique concurrently with samples collected for newborn screening of other disorders. Data on more than 17 million neonates screened is available. The disorder occurs in 1 of 21,000 newborns in Japan, 1 of 10,000-16,000 in Europe and North America, 1 in 5000 in La Reunion, France, and 1 of 300 in Yupik Eskimos of Alaska. About 75% of affected infants have the salt-losing form and 25% have the simple virilizing form of the disorder. The non-classic form is not reliably detected by newborn screening and its frequency remains to be established. Almost all of the screening programs use a single sample screening test, although a number of programs perform a second test on the initial sample in the presence of a borderline level on the initial screening, and a few programs utilize two sample screenings. Accurate measurement of serum 17-hydroxyprogesterone requires an assay with high specificity with an extraction step because of the many cross reacting steroids present. Cut-off levels of 17-OH progesterone have been established by each screening laboratory. The majority of false-positive results have occurred in low birth weight and premature births since 17-OH progesterone levels are generally higher in premature infants. Separate normative reference levels based on birth weight or gestational age have been developed, which have minimized the false positive rates among this population of newborns. The false negative rate for screening is very low *(67–82)*.

CONCLUSION

Our understanding of the pathophysiology of the disorders of adrenal steroidogenesis which result in Congenital Adrenal Hyperplasia expanded markedly in the second half of the twentieth century. The clinical spectrum of these disorders and their biochemical basis; the cellular locations, function, and abnormalities of the affected enzymes; and the genes encoding these enzymes and the molecular mutations resulting in CAH have been elucidated. Prenatal diagnosis and treatment and newborn screening are now possible. Despite 50 yr of treatment however, the optimal therapy eludes us and efforts must continue in the 21st century to develop better treatment protocols to achieve more successful outcomes in these disorders.

REFERENCES

1. Levine LS. Congenital adrenal hyperplasia. Pediatr Rev 2000;21:159–170.
2. Grumbach MM, Conte FA. Disorders of sex differentiation. In: Wilson JD, ed. Williams Textbook of Endocrinology, 9th ed. Saunders, Philadelphia, 1998, pp. 1361–1374.
3. Pang S. Congenital adrenal hyperplasia. Endocrinol Metab Clin North Am 1997;26:853–891.
4. Miller WL. Molecular biology of steroid hormone synthesis. Endocr Rev 1998;9:295–318.
5. White PC, Speiser PW. Congenital adrenal hyperplasia due to 21-hydroxylase deficiency. Endocr Rev 2000;21:245–291.
6. New MI. Diagnosis and management of congenital adrenal hyperplasia. Ann Rev Med 1998;49: 311–328.
7. Bose HS, Sugawara T, Strauss III JF, et al. The pathophysiology and genetics of congenital lipoid adrenal hyperplasia. N Engl J Med 1996;355:1870–1878.
8. Miller WL. Congenital lipoid adrenal hyperplasia: The human gene knockout for the steroidogenic acute regulatory protein. J Mol Endocrinol 1997;19:227–240.
9. Fujieda K, Tajima T, Nakae J, et al. Spontaneous puberty in 46,XX subjects with congenital lipoid adrenal hyperplasia. J Clin Invest 1997;99:1265–1271.
10. Bose HS, Sato S, Aisenberg J, et al. Mutations in the steroidogenic acute regulatory protein (StAR) in six patients with congenital lipoid adrenal hyperplasia. J Clin Endocrinol Metab 2000;85: 3636–3639.
10a. Tajima T, Fujieda K, Kouda N, et al. Heterozygous mutation in the cholesterol side chain cleavage enzyme (P450scc) gene in a patient with 46,XY sex reversal and adrenal insufficiency. J Clin Endocrinol Metab 2001;86:3820–3825.
10b. Katsumata N, Ohtake M, Hojo T, et al. Compound heterozygous mutations in the cholesterol side-chain cleavage enzyme gene (*CYP11A*) cause congenital adrenal insufficiency in humans. J Clin Endocrinol Metab 2002;87:3808–3813.
11. Simard J, Rhéaume E, Sanchez R, et al. Molecular basis of congenital adrenal hyperplasia due to 3β–hydroxysteroid deficiency. Mol Endocrinol 1993;7:716–728.
12. Mason JI. The 3β–hydroxysteroid dehydrogenase gene family of enzymes. Trends Endocrinol Metab 1993;6:199.
13. Chang YT, Zhang L, Alkaddour HS, et al. Absence of molecular defect in the Type II 3β–hydroxysteroid dehydrogenase (3β–HSD) gene in premature pubarche children and hirsute female patients with moderately decreased adrenal 3β-HSD activity. Pediatr Res 1995;37:820–824.
14. Pang S. Genetics of 3β–hydroxysteroid dehydrogenase deficiency disorder. Growth Genet Horm 1996;12:5–9.
15. Moison AM, Ricketts ML, Tardy V, et al. New insight into the molecular basis of 3β–hydroxysteroid dehydrogenase deficiency: Identification of eight mutations in the *HSD3B2* gene in eleven patients from seven new families and comparison of the functional properties of twenty-five mutant enzymes. J Clin Endocrinol Metab 1999;84:4410–4425.
16. Marui S, Castro M, Latronico AC, et al. Mutations in the type II 3β–hydroxysteroid dehydrogenase (HSD3B2) gene can cause premature pubarche in girls. Clin Endocrinol 2000;52:67–75.
17. Yanase T, Simpson ER, Waterman MR. 17α-hydroxylase/17,20-lyase deficiency: From clinical investigation to molecular definition. Endocr Rev 1991;12:91–108.
18. Zachmann M. Prismatic cases: 17,10-desmolase (17,20-lyase) deficiency. Clin Endocrinol 1996; 81:457–459.
19. Geller DH, Auchus RJ, Mendonca BB, et al. The genetic and functional basis of isolated 17,20-lyase deficiency. Nat Genet 1997;17:201–205.
20. Geley S, Kapelari K, Jöhrer K, et al. CYP11B1 mutations causing congenital adrenal hyperplasia due to 11β–hydroxylase deficiency. J Clin Endocrinol Metab 1996;81:2896–2901.
21. White PC, Curnow KC, Pascoe L. Disorders of steroid 11β–hydroxylase isozymes. Endocr Rev 1994;15:421–438.
22. Merke DP, Tajima T, Chhabra A, et al. Novel CYP11B1 mutations in congenital adrenal hyperplasia due to steroid 11β–hydroxylase deficiency. J Clin Endocrinol Metab 1998;83:270–273.
23. Zachmann M, Tassinari D, Prader A. Clinical and biochemical variability of congenital adrenal hyperplasia due 11β–hydroxylase deficiency: A study of 25 patients. J Clin Endocrinol Metab 1983;56:222–229.
24. Rivkees SA, Crawford JD. Dexamethasone treatment of virilizing congenital adrenal hyperplasia: The ability to achieve normal growth. Pediatrics 2000;106:767–773.

25. Schober JM. Feminizing genitoplasty for intersex. In: Stringer MD, Oldham KT, and Moriquand PDE, and Howard BR eds. Pediatric surgery and urology: Long term outcomes. Saunders, Philadelphia, 1998, pp. 549–558.
26. Meyer-Bahlburg HFL. What causes low rates of child-bearing in congenital adrenal hyperplasia? J Clin Endocrinol Metab 1999;84:1844–1847.
27. Alizai NK, Thomas DFM, Lilford TRJ, Batchelor AGG, Johnson N. Feminizing genitoplasty for congenital adrenal hyperplasia: What happens at puberty? J Urol 1999;161:1588–1591.
28. Krege S, Walz KH, Hauffa BP, et al. Long-term follow-up of female patients with congenital adrenal hyperplasia from 21-hydroxylase deficiency, with special emphasis on the results of vaginoplasty. BJU Int 2000;86:253–259.
29. Soliman AT, AlLamki M, AlSalmi I, et al. Congenital adrenal hyperplasia complicated by central precocious puberty: Linear growth during infancy and treatment with gonadotropin-releasing hormone analog. Metab, 1997;46:513–517.
30. Laue L, Merke SP, Jones JV, et al. A preliminary study of flutamide, testolactone, and reduced hydrocortisone dose in the treatment of congenital adrenal hyperplasia. J Clin Endocrinol Metab 1996;81:3535–3539.
31. Merke DP, Keil MF, Jones JV, et al. Flutamide, testolactone, and reduced hydrocortisone dose maintain normal growth velocity and bone maturation despite elevated androgen levels in children with congenital adrenal hyperplasia. J Clin Endocrinol Metab 2000;85:1114–1120.
32. Alvi S, Shaw NJ, Rayner PHW, et al. Growth hormone and goserelin in congenital adrenal hyperplasia. Horm Res 1997;48(Suppl 2):1–201.
33. Quintos JB, Vogiatzi MG, Harbison MD, et al. Growth hormone and depot leuprolide therapy for short stature in children with congenital adrenal hyperplasia. Annual Meeting Endocrine Society 1999. Program & Abstracts:110.
34. Van Wyk JJ, Gunther DF, Ritzen EM, et al. Therapeutic Controversies: The use of adrenalectomy as a treatment for congenital adrenal hyperplasia. J Clin Endocrinol Metab 1996;81:3180–3190.
35. Gunther DF, Bukowski TP, Titzen EM, et al. Prophylactic adrenalectomy of a three-year-old girl with congenital adrenal hyperplasia: Pre- and postoperative studies. J Clin Endocrinol Metab 1997;82:3324–3327.
36. Nasir J, Royston C, Walton C, et al. 11β–hydroxylase deficiency: Management of a difficult case by laparoscopic bilateral adrenalectomy. Clin Endocrinol 1996;45:225–228.
37. Chabre O, Portrat-Doyen S, Chaffanjon P, et al. Bilateral laparoscopic adrenalectomy for congenital adrenal hyperplasia with severe hypertension, resulting from two novel mutations in splice donor sites of CYP11B1. J Clin Endocrinol Metab 2000;85:4060–4068.
38. Lo JC, Schwitzgebel VM, Tyrrell JB, et al. Normal female infants born of mothers with classic congenital adrenal hyperplasia due to 21-hydroxylase deficiency. J Clin Endocrinol Metab 1999;84:930–936.
39. Lim YJ, Batch JA, Warne GL. Adrenal 21-hydroxylase deficiency in childhood: 25 years' experience. J Paediatr Child Health 1995;31:222–227.
40. Rasat R, Espiner EA, Abbott GD. Growth patterns and outcomes in congenital adrenal hyperplasia: Effect of chronic treatment regimes. NZ Med J 1995;108:311–314.
41. Yu ACM, Grant DB. Adult height in women with early-treated congenital adrenal hyperplasia (21-hydroxylase type): Relation to body mass index in earlier childhood. Acta Päediatr 1995;84:899–903.
42. Hauffa BP, Winter A, Stolecke H. Treatment and disease effects on short-term growth and adult height in children and adolescents with 21-hydroxylase deficiency. Klin Padiatr 1997;209:71–77.
43. Jaaskelainen J, Voutilainen R. Growth of patients with 21-hydroxylase deficiency: An analysis of the factors influencing adult height. Pediatr Res 1997;41:30–33.
44. Kandemir N, Yordam N. Congenital adrenal hyperplasia in Turkey: A review of 273 patients. Acta Paediatr 1997;86:22–25.
45. Kuhnle U, Bullinger M. Outcome of congenital adrenal hyperplasia. Pediatr Surg Int 1997;12:511–515.
46. Premawardhana LDKE, Hughes IA, Read GH, et al. Longer term outcome in females with congenital adrenal hyperplasia (CAH): The Cardiff experience. Clin Endocrinol 1997;46:327–332.
47. Eugster EA, DiMeglio LA, Wright JC, et al. Height outcome in congenital adrenal hyperplasia caused by 21-hydroxylase deficiency: A meta-analysis. J Pediatr 2001;138:26–32.
48. Schwartz RP. Back to basics: Early diagnosis and compliance improve final height outcome in congenital adrenal hyperplasia. J Pediatr 2001;138:3–5.
49. Diamond M. Prenatal predisposition and the clinical management of some pediatric conditions. J Sex Marital Ther 1996;22:139.

50. Diamond M, Sigmundson HK. Sex reassignment at birth. Arch Pediatr Adolesc 1997;151:298.
51. Hagenfeldt K, Ritzen EM, Ringertz H, et al. Bone mass and body composition of adult women with congenital virilizing 21-hydroxylase deficiency after glucocorticoid treatment since infancy. Eur J Endocrinol 2000;143:667–671.
52. Forest MG, Morel Y, David M. Prenatal treatment of congenital adrenal hyperplasia due to steroid 21-hydroxylase deficiency. Frontiers Endocrinol 1996;17:77–89.
53. Carlson AD, Obeid JS, Kanellopoulou N, et al. Congenital adrenal hyperplasia: Update on prenatal diagnosis and treatment. J Steroid Biochem Mol Biol 1999;69:19–29.
54. Rosler A, Weshler N, Leiberman E, et al. 11β–hydroxylase deficiency congenital adrenal hyperplasia: Update of prenatal diagnosis. J Clin Endocrinol Metab 1988;66:830–838.
55. Cerame BI, Newfield RS, Pascoe L, et al. Prenatal diagnosis and treatment of 11β–hydroxylase deficiency congenital adrenal hyperplasia resulting in normal female genitalia. J Clin Endocrinol Metab 1999;84:3129–3134.
56. Izumi H, Saito N, Ichiki S, et al. Prenatal diagnosis of congenital lipoid adrenal hyperplasia. Obstet Gynecol 1993;81:839–841.
57. Saenger P. New developments in congenital lipoid adrenal hyperplasia and steroidogenic acute regulatory protein. Pediatr Clin North Am 1997;44:397–421.
58. David M, Forest MG. Prenatal treatment of congenital adrenal hyperplasia resulting from 21-hydroxylase deficiency. J Pediatr 1984;105:799–803.
59. Levine LS, Pang S. Prenatal diagnosis and treatment of congenital adrenal hyperplasia. In: Milunsky A, ed. Genetic disorders and the fetus: Diagnosis, prevention and treatment. Fourth edition. The Johns Hopkins University Press, Baltimore, 1998, pp. 529–549.
60. Pang S, Clark AT, Freeman LC, et al. Maternal side effects of prenatal dexamethasone therapy for fetal congenital adrenal hyperplasia. J Clin Endocrinol Metab 1992;75:249–253.
61. Forest MG, Dorr HG. Prenatal treatment of congenital adrenal hyperplasia resulting from 21-hydroxylase deficiency: European experience in 253 pregnancies at risk. Clin Cour 1993;11:2–3.
62. Lajic S, Wedell A, Bui T, et al. Long-term somatic follow-up of prenatally treated children with congenital adrenal hyperplasia. J Clin Endocrinol Metab 1998;83:3872–3880.
63. Trautman PD, Meyer-Bahlburg HFL, Postelnek J, et al. Effects of early prenatal dexamethasone on the cognitive and behavioral development of young children: Results of a pilot study. Psychoneuroendocrinology 1995;20:439–449.
64. Forest MG, Morel Y, David M. Prenatal treatment of congenital adrenal hyperplasia. Trends Endocrinol Metab 1998;9:284–288.
65. Trautman PD, Meyer-Bahlburg HF, Postelnek J, et al. Mothers' reactions to prenatal diagnostic procedures and dexamethasone treatment of congenital adrenal hyperplasia. J Psychosom Obstet Gynaecol 1996;17:175–181.
66. Miller WL. Prenatal treatment of congenital adrenal hyperplasia: A promising experimental therapy of unproven safety. Trends Endocrinol Metab 1998;9:290–293.
67. Pang S, Hotchkiss J, Drash AL, et al. Microfilter paper method for 17α-hydroxyprogesterone radioimmunoassay; its application for rapid screening for congenital adrenal hyperplasia. J Clin Endocrinol Metab 1977;45:1003–1008.
68. Pang S, Murphey W, Levine LS, et al. A pilot newborn screening for congenital adrenal hyperplasia in Alaska. J Clin Endocrinol Metab 1982;55:413–420.
69. Pang S, Wallace MA, Hofman L, et al. Worldwide experience in newborn screening for classical congenital adrenal hyperplasia due to 21-hydroxylase deficiency. Pediatrics 1988;81:866–874.
70. Pang S, Clark A. Congenital adrenal hyperplasia due to 21-hydroxylase deficiency: Newborn screening and its relationship to the diagnosis and treatment of the disorder. Screening 1993;2:105–139.
71. Balsamo A, Cacciari E, Piazzi S, et al. Congenital adrenal hyperplasia: Neonatal mass screening compared with clinical diagnosis only in the Emilia-Romagna region of Italy. Pediatrics 1996;98:362–367.
72. Cutfield WS, Webster D. Newborn screening for congenital adrenal hyperplasia in New Zealand. J Pediatr 1995;126:118–121.
73. Dotti G, Pagliardini S, Vuolo A, et al. Congenital adrenal hyperplasia in the experience of the Piemonte and Valle d' Aosta regions program (1987–1995). In: Programs & Abstracts of the 3rd International Newborn Screening Meeting, Oct.22–23, 1996 Boston, MA USA. Abstract No.P-82.
74. Nordenstrom A, Thilen A, Hagenfeldt L, et al. Benefits of screening for congenital adrenal hyperplasia (CAH) in Sweden. In: Proceedings, Third Meeting of the International Society for Neonatal Screening, Levy HL, Hermos RJ, Grady GF, eds. Oct.22–23, 1996 Boston, MA USA. P:211–216.

75. Sack J, Front H, Kaiserman I, et al. Screening for 21-hydroxylase deficiency in Israel. In: Programs & Abstracts of the 3rd International Newborn Screening Meeting, Oct.22–23, 1996 Boston, MA USA. Abstract No. P-87.
76. Al-Nuaim AA. Newborn screening program (NSP) in Saudi Arabia (SA). In: Programs & Abstracts of the 3rd International Newborn Screening Meeting, Oct.22–23, 1996 Boston, MA USA. Abstract No.P-90.
77. Pang S, Shook M. Current status of neonatal screening for congenital adrenal hyperplasia. Curr Opin Pediatr 1997;9:419–423.
78. Tajima T, Fujieda K, Nakae J, et al. Molecular basis of nonclassical steroid 21-hydroxylase deficiency detected by neonatal mass screening in Japan. J Clin Endocrinol Metab 1997;82:2350–2356.
79. herrel BL Jr., Berenbaum SA, Manter-Kapanke V, et al. Results of screening 1.9 million Texas newborns for 21-hydroxylase-deficient congenital adrenal hyperplasia. Pediatrics 1998;101: 583–590.
80. Allen DB, Hoffman GL, Mahy SL, et al. Improved precision of newborn screening for congenital adrenal hyperplasia using weight adjusted criteria for 17-hydroxyprogesterone levels. J Pediatr 1997;130:120–133.
81. Brosnan PG, Brosnan CA, Kemp SF, et al. Effect of newborn screening for congenital adrenal hyperplasia. Arch Pediatr Adolesc Med 1999;153:1272–1278.
82. Kwon C, Farrell PM. The magnitude and challenge of false-positive newborn screening test results. Arch Pediatr Adolesc Med 2000;154:714–718.
83. Adapted from Miller WL, Levine LS. Molecular and clinical advances in congenital adrenal hyperplasia. J Pediatr 1987;111:1.

14 Cushing Syndrome in Childhood

Sandra Bonat, MD
and Constantine A. Stratakis, MD, D(MED)Sc

CONTENTS

> INTRODUCTION
> NORMAL HYPOTHALAMIC-PITUITARY-ADRENAL AXIS
> EPIDEMIOLOGY AND ETIOLOGY
> CLINICAL PRESENTATION
> DIAGNOSTIC GUIDELINES
> TREATMENT
> GLUCOCORTICOID REPLACEMENT
> PSYCHOSOCIAL IMPLICATIONS
> REFERENCES

INTRODUCTION

Although the initial description of the adrenal glands was made by Eustachio in 1563, it wasn't until 1912 that Harvey Cushing first described the classical Cushing syndrome. At that time, he thought that the syndrome that later bore his name could only result from tumors of the anterior pituitary or adrenal cortex. It was not until 1962 that the first case of ectopic Cushing syndrome was described. Over the last 3 decades, significant advances in the nosology and therapy of Cushing syndrome have been made.

Cushing syndrome is a multisystem disorder resulting from the body's prolonged exposure to excess production of glucocorticoids. It is characterized by truncal obesity, growth deceleration, characteristic skin changes, muscle weakness, and hypertension *(1)*. Most commonly, Cushing syndrome in childhood results from the exogenous administration of glucocorticoids. However, in this chapter, we will only analyze the causes and discuss the treatment of endogenous Cushing syndrome.

NORMAL HYPOTHALAMIC-PITUITARY-ADRENAL AXIS

Corticotropin releasing hormone (CRH) is synthesized in the hypothalamus and carried to the anterior pituitary in the portal system. CRH stimulates corticotropin (ACTH) release from the anterior pituitary, which in turn stimulates the adrenal cortex to secrete

From: *Contemporary Endocrinology: Pediatric Endocrinology: A Practical Clinical Guide*
Edited by: S. Radovick and M. H. MacGillivray © Humana Press Inc., Totowa, NJ

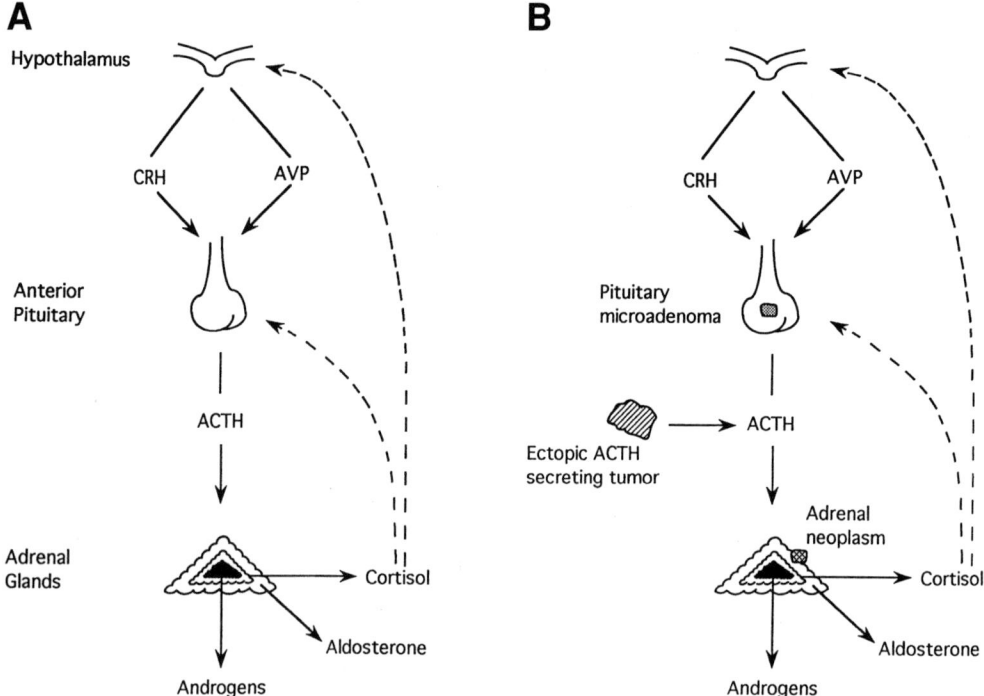

Fig. 1. (A) (Left panel) Physiologic regulation of cortisol secretion (Abbreviations : CRH = corticotropin-releasing hormone, AVP = arginine-vasopressin, ACTH = adrenocorticotropin). **(B)** (right panel) Causes of Cushing syndrome; adrenal neoplasms include PPNAD, benign tumors and adrenocortical carcinomas. Straight arrows represent stimulation, whereas dotted lines represent inhibition.

cortisol (hypothalamic-pituitary-adrenal or HPA axis) *(2,3)*. Cortisol inhibits the synthesis and secretion of both CRH and ACTH in a negative feedback regulation system (Fig. 1A). In Cushing syndrome, the HPA axis has lost its ability for self-regulation, because of excessive secretion of either ACTH or cortisol and the loss of the negative feedback function (Fig. 1B). Diagnostic tests, on the other hand, take advantage of the tight regulation of the HPA axis in the normal state and its disturbance in Cushing syndrome to guide therapy towards the primary cause of this disorder.

EPIDEMIOLOGY AND ETIOLOGY

Cushing syndrome is a rare entity, especially in children *(1)*. The overall incidence of Cushing syndrome is approx 2–5 new cases per million people per year. Only approx 10% of new cases each year occur in children. As in adult patients, there is a female to male predominance in children, that decreases with younger age; there may even be a male to female predominance in infants and young toddlers with Cushing syndrome *(1–3)*.

The most common cause of Cushing syndrome in children is exogenous or iatrogenic Cushing syndrome. This is the result of chronic administration of glucocorticoids or ACTH. Glucocorticoids are being used frequently for the treatment of many non-endocrine diseases including pulmonary, autoimmune, hematologic and neoplastic disorders. In addition, ACTH is being used for the treatment of certain seizure disorders.

The most common cause of endogenous Cushing syndrome in children is ACTH overproduction from the pituitary; this is called Cushing's disease. It is usually caused by an ACTH-secreting pituitary microadenoma or, rarely, a macroadenoma. ACTH secretion occurs in a semiautonomous manner, maintaining some of the feedback of the HPA axis. Cushing's disease accounts for approximately 75% of all cases of Cushing's syndrome in children over 7 yr. In children under 7 yr, Cushing disease is less frequent; adrenal causes of Cushing syndrome (adenoma, carcinoma, or bilateral hyperplasia) are the most common causes of the condition in infants and young toddlers. Ectopic ACTH production is almost unheard of in young children; it also accounts for less than 1% of the cases of Cushing syndrome in adolescents. Sources of ectopic ACTH include small cell carcinoma of the lungs; carcinoid tumors in the bronchus, pancreas, or thymus; medullary carcinomas of the thyroid; pheochromocytomas; and other neuroendocrine tumors.

Rarely, ACTH overproduction by the pituitary may be the result of CRH oversecretion by the hypothalamus or by an ectopic CRH source. However, this cause of Cushing syndrome has only been described in a small number of cases, and never in young children. Its significance lies in the fact that diagnostic tests usually used for the exclusion of ectopic sources of Cushing syndrome have frequently misleading results in the case of CRH-induced ACTH oversecretion.

Autonomous secretion of cortisol from the adrenal glands, or ACTH-independent Cushing syndrome, accounts for approx 15% of all the cases of Cushing syndrome in childhood. However, although adrenocortical tumors are rare in older children, in younger children they are more frequent.

Adrenocortical neoplasms account for 0.6% of all childhood tumors; Cushing syndrome is a manifestation of approximately one third of all adrenal tumors *(2–4)*. In children, most adrenal tumors presenting with Cushing's syndrome (70%) are malignant. The majority of patients present under age 5, contributing thus to the first peak of the known bimodal distribution of adrenal cancer across the life span. As in adults, there is a female to male predominance. The tumors usually occur unilaterally; however, in 2–10% of patients they occur bilaterally.

Bilateral nodular adrenal disease has been appreciated more recently as a rare cause of Cushing syndrome *(4)*. Primary pigmented adrenocortical nodular disease (PPNAD) is a genetic disorder with the majority of cases associated with Carney complex, a syndrome of multiple endocrine gland abnormalities in addition to lentigines and myxomas. The adrenal glands in PPNAD are most commonly normal or even small in size with multiple pigmented nodules surrounded by an atrophic cortex. The nodules are autonomously functioning resulting in the surrounding atrophy of the cortex. Children and adolescents with PPNAD frequently have periodic Cushing's syndrome.

Massive macronodular adrenal hyperplasia (MMAD) is another rare disease, which leads to Cushing's syndrome *(4)*. The adrenal glands are massively enlarged with multiple, huge nodules that are typical, yellow-to-brown cortisol-producing adenomas. Most cases of MMAD are sporadic, although few familial cases have been described; in those, the disease appears in children. In some patients with MMAD, cortisol levels appear to increase with food ingestion (food-dependent Cushing syndrome). These patients have an aberrant expression of the GIP receptor (GIPR) in the adrenal glands. In the majority of patients with MMAD, however, the disease does not appear to be GIPR-dependent; aberrant expression of other receptors might be responsible.

Table 1
Clinical Presentation of CS in Pediatric Patients[a]

Symptoms/signs	Frequency (Percent)
Weight gain	90
Growth retardation	83
Menstrual irregularities	81
Hirsutism	81
Obesity (Body Mass Index > 85 percentile)	73
Violaceous skin striae	63
Acne	52
Hypertension	51
Fatigue-weakness	45
Precocious puberty	41
Bruising	27
Mental changes	18
Delayed bone age	14
Hyperpigmentation	13
Muscle weakness	13
Acanthosis nigricans	10
Accelerated bone age	10
Sleep disturbances	7
Pubertal delay	7
Hypercalcemia	6
Alkalosis	6
Hypokalemia	2
Slipped femoral capital epiphysis	2

[a]National Institutes of Health series-modified from Ref. *1*.

Bilateral macronodular adrenal hyperplasia can also be seen in McCune Albright syndrome (MAS) *(5)*. In this syndrome there is a somatic mutation of the *GNAS1* gene leading to constitutive activation of the Gsα protein and continuous, non-ACTH-dependent stimulation of the adrenal cortex. Cushing syndrome in MAS is rare and usually presents in the infantile period (before 6 mo-of-age); interestingly, a few children have had spontaneous resolution of their Cushing syndrome.

CLINICAL PRESENTATION

In most children, the onset of Cushing's syndrome is rather insidious *(1–3,7)*. The most common presenting symptom of the syndrome is weight gain (Table 1). In childhood, a unique frequently encountered feature of Cushing syndrome is growth retardation. Other common problems reported in children include facial plethora, headaches, hypertension, hirsutism, amenorrhea, and delayed sexual development. Pubertal children may present with virilization. Skin manifestations, including acne, violaceous striae, and bruising and acanthosis nigricans are also common (Fig. 2). In comparison to adult patients with Cushing syndrome, symptoms that are less commonly seen in children include sleep disruption, weakness, and mental changes.

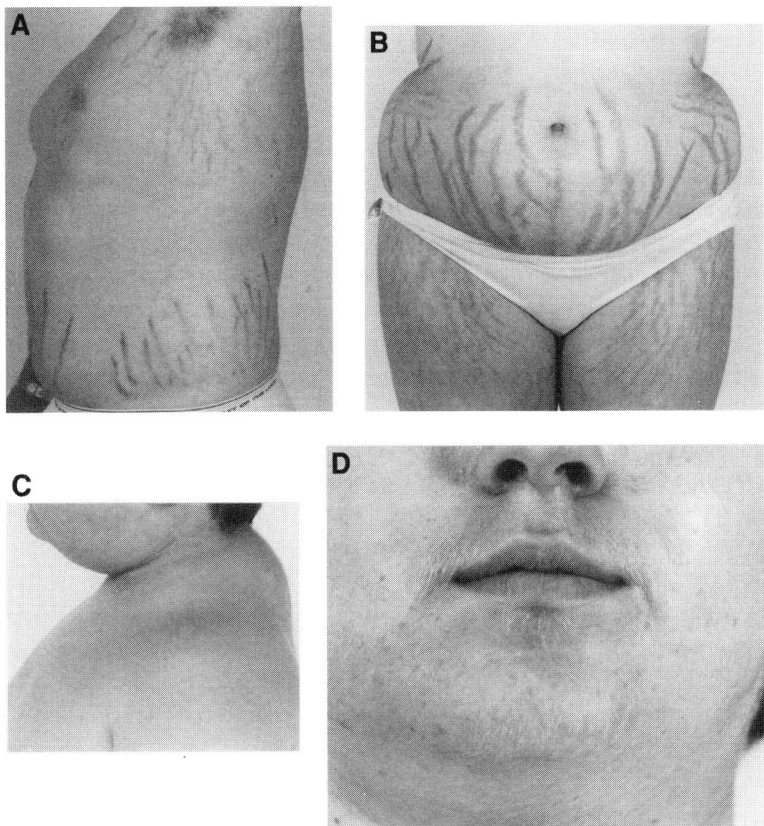

Fig. 2. Striae caused by endogenous Cushing syndrome in a 18-yr-old girl (**A** and **B**); acanthosis nigricans and ringworm (tinea corporis) lesions in a 9-yr-old; (**C**), and hypertrichosis in a teenager girl; (**D**) both patients had long-standing Cushing disease.

DIAGNOSTIC GUIDELINES

The appropriate therapeutic interventions in Cushing syndrome depend on accurate diagnosis and classification of the disease. The history and clinical evaluation, including growth charts, are important the initial diagnosis of Cushing syndrome. Upon suspicion of the syndrome, laboratory and imaging confirmations are necessary. An algorithm of the diagnostic process is presented in Fig. 3.

The first step in the diagnosis of Cushing syndrome is to document hypercortisolism *(6)*. This step is usually done in the outpatient setting. Because of the circadian nature of cortisol and ACTH, isolated cortisol and ACTH measurements are not of great value in diagnosis. One excellent screening test for hypercortisolism is a 24 h urinary free cortisol (UFC) excretion corrected for body surface area. A normal 24-h UFC value is <70 µg/m^2/d. A 24-h urine collection is often difficult for parents to perform with children and may be done incorrectly, especially in the outpatient setting. Falsely high UFC may be obtained because of physical and emotional stress, chronic and severe obesity, pregnancy, chronic exercise, depression, alcoholism, anorexia, narcotic withdrawal, anxiety,

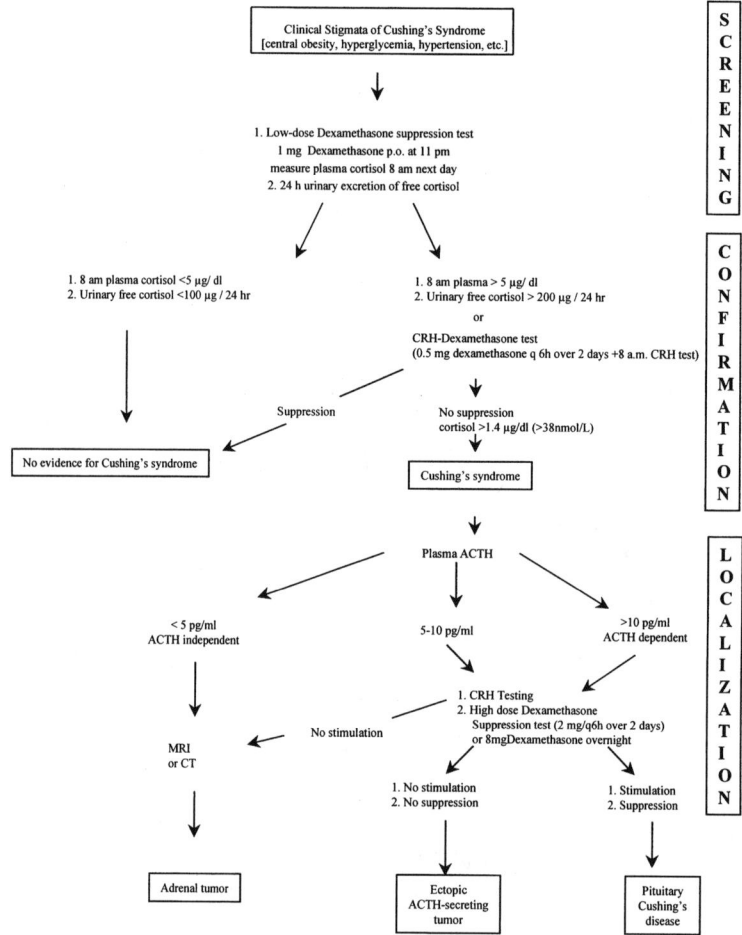

Fig. 3. Suggested diagnostic algorithm for the work up of suspected Cushing syndrome or hypercortisolemia. The details are discussed in the text; *see* also ref. *6*.

malnutrition, and high water intake. These conditions may cause sufficiently high UFC to cause what is known as pseudo-Cushing syndrome. On the other hand, falsely low UFC may be obtained mostly with inadequate collection.

Another baseline test for the establishment of the diagnosis of Cushing's syndrome is a low-dose dexamethasone suppression test. This test involves giving a 1 mg of Dexamethasone at 11 PM and measuring a serum cortisol level the following morning at 8 AM. The cortisol level should be <5 ug/dL. If it is greater than 5 µg/dL, further evaluation is necessary. This test has a low percentage of false normal suppression; however, the percentage of false positives is higher (approx 15–20%). It should be remembered that the 1-mg overnight test, like the 24-h UFC, does not distinguish between hypercortisolism from Cushing's syndrome and other hypercortisolemic states.

If the response to both the 1 mg dexamethasone overnight suppression test and the 24-h urinary free cortisol are both normal, a diagnosis of Cushing syndrome may be excluded with the following caveat: 5–10% of patients may have intermittent or periodic cortisol hypersecretion and may not manifest abnormal results to either test. If periodic or intermittent Cushing syndrome is suspected, continuous follow-up of the patients is recommended.

If one of the tests suggests Cushing syndrome or if there is any question about the diagnosis, tests that distinguish between pseudo-Cushing syndrome states and Cushing syndrome may be obtained. One such test is the combined dexamethasone-CRH test *(8)*. In this test, the patient is treated with low dose dexamethasone (0.5 mg adjusted for weight for children <70 kg) every 6 h for 8 doses prior to the administration of CRH (ovine CRH [oCRH]) the following morning. ACTH and cortisol levels are measured at baseline and every 15 min for 1 h after the administration of oCRH. The patient with pseudo-Cushing syndrome will exhibit low or undetectable basal plasma cortisol and ACTH, and have a diminished or no response to oCRH stimulation. Patients with Cushing syndrome will have higher basal cortisol and ACTH levels and will also have a greater peak value with oCRH stimulation. The criterion used for the diagnosis of Cushing's disease is a cortisol level of greater than 38 nmol/L 15 min after oCRH administration.

Once the diagnosis of Cushing's syndrome is confirmed, there are several tests to distinguish ACTH-dependent disease from the ACTH-independent syndrome. A spot plasma ACTH may be measured; if this measurement is <5ng/L it is indicative of ACTH-independent Cushing syndrome, although the sensitivity and specificity of this one ACTH measurement are not high because of the great variability in plasma ACTH levels and the instability of the molecule after sample collection. The standard high dose dexamethasone suppression test (Liddle's test) is used to differentiate Cushing disease from ectopic ACTH secretion and adrenal causes of Cushing syndrome. In the classic form of this test, a 2 mg dose of dexamethasone (adjusted per weight for children <70kg, 120 µg/kg/dose) is given every 6 h for 8 doses. Urinary free cortisol and 17-hydroxy-steroid excretion are measured at baseline and after dexamethasone administration. Approximately 85% of patients with Cushing disease will have suppression of cortisol and 17-hydroxysteroid values, whereas less than 10% of patients with ectopic ACTH secretion will have suppression. Urinary free cortisol values should suppress to 90% of baseline value and 17-hydroxysteroid excretion should suppress to less than 50% of baseline value. The Liddle test has been modified to giving a high dose of dexamethasone (8 mg, in children adjusted for weight <70 kg) at 11 PM and measuring the plasma cortisol level the following morning. This overnight, high-dose dexamethasone test has sensitivity and specificity values similar to those of the classic Liddle's test.

An oCRH stimulation test may also be obtained for the differentiation of Cushing disease from ectopic ACTH secretion *(9)*. In this test, 85% of patients with Cushing disease respond to oCRH with increased plasma ACTH and cortisol production. 95% of patients with ectopic ACTH production do not respond to administration of oCRH. The criterion for diagnosis of Cushing's disease is a mean increase of 20% above baseline for cortisol values at 30 and 45 min, and an increase in the mean corticotropin concentrations of at least 35% over basal value at 15 and 30 min after CRH administration. When the oCRH and high-dose dexamethasone (Liddle or overnight) tests are used together, diagnostic accuracy improves to 98%.

Another important tool in the localization and characterization of Cushing syndrome is diagnostic imaging. The most important initial imaging when Cushing disease is suspected is pituitary magnetic resonance imaging (MRI). The MRI should be done in thin sections with high resolution and always with contrast (gadolinium). The latter is important since only macroadenomas will be detectable without contrast; after contrast, an otherwise normal-looking pituitary MRI might show a hypoenhancing lesion, usually a microadenoma. More than 90% of ACTH-producing tumors are hypoenhancing, whereas only about 5% are hyperenhancing after contrast infusion. However, even with the use of contrast material, pituitary MRI may detect only up to approx 50% of ACTH-producing pituitary tumors.

Computed tomography (CT) (more preferable than MRI) of the adrenal glands is useful in the distinction between Cushing disease and adrenal causes of Cushing syndrome, mainly unilateral adrenal tumors. The distinction is harder in the presence of bilateral hyperplasia (MMAD or PPNAD) or bilateral adrenal carcinoma, which, however, are rare. Most patients with Cushing disease have ACTH-driven bilateral hyperplasia, and both adrenal glands will appear enlarged and nodular on CT or MRI. Most adrenocortical carcinomas are unilateral and quite large by the time they are detected. Adrenocortical adenomas are usually small, less than 5 cm in diameter and, like most carcinomas, they involve one adrenal gland. MMAD presents with massive enlargement of both adrenal glands, whereas PPNAD is more difficult to diagnose radiologically because it is usually associated with normal or small-sized adrenal glands, despite the histologic presence of hyperplasia.

Ultrasound may also be used to image the adrenal glands, but its sensitivity and accuracy is much less than CT or MRI. A CT or MRI scan of the neck, chest, abdomen, and pelvis may be used for the detection of an ectopic source of ACTH production. Labeled octreotide scanning and venous sampling may also help in the localization of an ectopic ACTH source.

Since up to 50% of pituitary ACTH secreting tumors and many ectopic ACTH tumors can not be detected on routine imaging, and often laboratory diagnosis is not completely clear, catheterization studies must be used to confirm the source of ACTH secretion in ACTH-dependent Cushing syndrome. Bilateral inferior petrosal sinus sampling (IPSS) is used for the confirmation of a pituitary microadenoma *(10)*. In brief, sampling from each inferior petrosal sinuses is taken for measurement of ACTH concentration simultaneously with peripheral venous sampling. ACTH is measured at baseline and at 3, 5, and 10 min after oCRH administration. Patients with ectopic ACTH secretion have no gradient between either sinus and the peripheral sample. On the other hand, patients with an ACTH-secreting pituitary adenoma have at least a 2-to-1 central-to-peripheral gradient at baseline or 3- to -1 after stimulation with oCRH. IPSS is an excellent test for the differential diagnosis between ACTH-dependent forms of Cushing syndrome with a diagnostic accuracy that approximates 100%, as long as it is performed in an experienced clinical center. IPSS, however, may not lead to the correct diagnosis, if obtained when the patient is not sufficiently hypercortisolemic or, if venous drainage of the pituitary gland does not follow the expected, normal anatomy.

TREATMENT

The treatment of choice for almost all patients with an ACTH-secreting pituitary adenoma (Cushing disease) is transsphenoidal surgery (TSS). In most specialized centers with experienced neurosurgeons the success rate of the first TSS is close to, or even higher than 90%. Treatment failures are most commonly the result of a macroadenoma or a small tumor invading the cavernous sinus. The success rate of repeat TSS is lower, closer to 60%. Post-operative complications include transient diabetes insipidus (DI) and, occasionally, syndrome of inappropriate antidiuretic hormone secretion (SIADH), central hypothyroidism, growth hormone deficiency, hypogonadism, bleeding, infection (meningitis), and pituitary apoplexy. The mortality rate is extremely low (<1%). Permanent pituitary dysfunction (partial or pan-hypopituitarism) and DI are rare, but more likely after repeat TSS or larger adenomas.

Pituitary irradiation is considered an appropriate treatment in patients with Cushing disease, following a failed TSS. Up to 80% of patients will have remission after irradiation of the pituitary gland. Hypopituitarism is the most common side effect and is more frequent when surgery precedes the radiotherapy. The recommended dosage is 4500/5000 cGy total, usually given over a period of 6 wk. Newer forms of stereotactic radiotherapy are now available as options for treatment of ACTH-secreting pituitary tumors. The photon knife (computer assisted linear accelerator) or the gamma knife (Cobalt-60) are now available; however, experience with these techniques is limited, especially in children. These modalities may be attractive because of the smaller amount of time required and the possibility for fewer side effects.

The treatment of choice for benign adrenal tumors is surgical resection. This procedure can be done by both transperitoneal and retroperitoneal approaches. In addition, laparoscopic adrenalectomy is also available at many institutions. Adrenal carcinomas may also be surgically resected, unless at later stages. Solitary metastases should also be removed, if possible. Therapy with mitotane, which is an adrenocytolytic agent, can be used as an adjuvant therapy or if the tumor is inoperable. Other chemotherapeutic options include cisplatin, 5-flurouracil, suramin, doxorubicin, and etoposide. Occasionally, glucocorticoid antagonists and steroid synthesis inhibitors are needed to correct the hypercortisolism. Radiotherapy can also be used in the case of metastases. The prognosis for adrenal carcinoma is poor, but usually children have a better prognosis than adults do.

Bilateral total adrenalectomy is usually the treatment of choice in bilateral micro- or macronodular adrenal disease, such as PPNAD and MMAD. In addition, adrenalectomy may be considered as a treatment for those patients with Cushing disease or ectopic ACTH-dependent Cushing syndrome who have either failed surgery or radiotherapy, or their tumor has not been localized, respectively. Nelson syndrome, which describes increased pigmentation, elevated ACTH levels, and a growing ACTH-producing pituitary tumor, may develop in up to 15% of patients with Cushing disease treated with bilateral adrenalectomy. It is possible that children with untreated Cushing disease are especially vulnerable to Nelson syndrome after bilateral adrenalectomy.

Pharmacotherapy is an option in the case of failure of surgery for Cushing's disease or in ectopic ACTH secretion where the source can not be identified. Mitotane is an inhibitor of the biosynthesis of corticosteroids by blocking the action of 11-β-hydroxylase and cholesterol side chain cleavage enzymes. It also acts by destroying adrenocortical cells that secrete cortisol. Other adrenal enzyme inhibitors, such as aminoglutethimide, metyrapone, trilostane, and ketoconazole may also be used alone or in combinations to control hypercortisolism. Aminoglutethimide blocks the conversion of cholesterol to pregnenolone in the adrenal cortex inhibiting the synthesis of cortisol, aldosterone, and androgens. Metyrapone acts by preventing the conversion of 11-deoxycortisol to cortisol. It can cause hypertension secondary to the accumulation of 11-deoxycorticosterone. Trilostane inhibits the conversion of pregnenolone to progesterone. Ketoconazole affects many pathway steps and is excellent in blocking adrenal steroidogenesis.

In ectopic ACTH production, if the source of ACTH secretion can be identified, the treatment of choice is surgical resection of the tumor. If surgical resection is impossible or if the source of ACTH can not be identified, pharmacotherapy is indicated as previously discussed. If the tumor can not be located, repeat searches for the tumor should be performed at least yearly. Bilateral adrenalectomy should be performed in the case of failure of pharmacotherapy or failure to locate the tumor after many years.

GLUCOCORTICOID REPLACEMENT

After the completion of successful TSS in Cushing disease or excision of an autonomously functioning adrenal adenoma, there will be a period of adrenal insufficiency while the hypothalamic pituitary adrenal axis is recovering. During this period, glucocorticoids should be replaced at the suggested physiologic replacement dose (12–15mg/m^2/d bid or tid). In the immediate post-operative period, stress doses of cortisol should be initiated. These should be weaned relatively rapidly to a physiologic replacement dose. The patient should be followed every few months, and the adrenocortical function should be periodically assessed with a 1 h ACTH test (normal response is a cortisol level over 18 µg/dL at 30 or 60 min after ACTH stimulation).

After bilateral adrenalectomy, patients require lifetime replacement with both glucocorticoids (as above) and mineralocorticoids (fludrocortisone 0.1–0.3 mg qday). These patients also need stress doses of glucocorticoids immediately postoperatively; they are weaned to physiologic replacement relatively quickly.

PSYCHOSOCIAL IMPLICATIONS

Cushing's syndrome has been associated with multiple psychiatric and psychological disturbances, most commonly depression and anxiety. Other abnormalities have included mania, panic disorder, suicidal ideation, schizophrenia, obsessive compulsive symptomatology, psychosis, impaired self-esteem, and distorted body image. Significant psychopathology can even remain after remission of hypercortisolism and even after recovery of the hypothalamic pituitary adrenal axis. Up to 70% of patients will have significant improvements in the psychiatric symptoms gradually after the correction of the hypercortisolism.

REFERENCES

1. Magiakou M, Mastorakos G, Oldfield EH, ET AL. Cushing's Syndrome in Children and Adolescents: Presentation, diagnosis and therapy. N Engl J Med 1994;331:629–636.
2. Tsigios C, Chrousos GP. Differential Diagnosis and Management of Cushing's Syndrome. Ann Rev Med 1996;47:443–461.
3. Orth DN. Cushing's Syndrome. N Engl J Med 1995;332:791–803.
4. Stratakis C, Kirschner LS. Clinical and Genetic Analysis of Primary Bilateral Adrenal Diseases (Micro- and Macronodular Disease) Leading to Cushing Syndrome. Horm Metab Res 1998;30:456–463.
5. Kirk JM, Brain CE, Carson DJ, Hyde JC, Grant DB. Cushing's Syndrome Caused by Nodular Adrenal Hyperplasia in Children with McCune-Albright Syndrome. J Pediatr 1999;134:789–792.
6. Bornstein SR, Stratakis C, Chrousos GP, Adrenocortical Tumors: Recent Advances in Basic Concepts and Clinical Management. Ann Intern Med 1999;130:759–771.
7. Stratakis C, Chrousos G. Adrenal Cancer. Endocrinol Metab Clin North Am 2000;29:15–25.

8. Yanovski JA, Cutler GB, Chrousos GP, Nieman LK. Corticotropin-releasing Hormone Stimulation Following Low-Dose Dexamethasone Administration: a new test to distinguish Cushing's syndrome from pseudo-Cushing's states. JAMA 1993;269:2232–2238.
9. Chrousos GP, Schulte HM, Oldfield EH, Gold PW, Cutler GB, Loriaux DL. The Corticotropin-Releasing Factor Stimulation Test: an aid in the evaluation of patients with Cushing's syndrome. N Engl J Med 1984;310:622–626.
10. Oldfield EH, Doppman JL, Nieman LK, et al. Petrosal Sinus Sampling with and without Corticotropin-Releasing Hormone for the Differential Diagnosis of Cushing's Syndrome. N Engl J Med 1991;325:897–905.

15 Mineralocorticoid Disorders

Christina E. Luedke, MD, PhD

CONTENTS

INTRODUCTION
DISORDERS OF DEFICIENT MINERALOCORTICOID
DISORDERS OF EXCESS MINERALOCORTICOID
REFERENCES

INTRODUCTION

Mineralocorticoids are steroid hormones produced by the adrenal cortex whose function is to control electrolyte and water balance. Disorders of either mineralocorticoid production or function can lead to severe alterations in the sodium, potassium, and water content of the body. Manifestations of decreased mineralocorticoid activity include hyponatremia, hyperkalemia, dehydration, hypotension, cardiac arrest, and death. Increased mineralocorticoid activity leads to hypervolemia, hypertension, and hypokalemia.

Under normal circumstances, aldosterone is the only functioning mineralocorticoid in humans. Aldosterone is synthesized from cholesterol in the zona glomerulosa of the adrenal cortex. Its synthesis is stimulated principally by angiotensin II (Fig. 1). Decreased renal blood flow, often an indicator of hypovolemia and hypotension, leads to secretion of renin by the juxtaglomerular apparatus of the afferent glomerular arterioles in the kidney. Renin, released into the blood, acts enzymatically to cleave circulating angiotensinogen into angiotensin I. Angiotensin converting enzyme, found ubiquitously on the endothelial surface of the vascular system, can then perform a second cleavage to create angiotensin II. Angiotensin II binds to receptors on the surface of glomerulosa cells and activates the aldosterone synthetic pathway. Aldosterone is secreted and acts on the distal and collecting tubules of the nephron to increase sodium retention by the kidneys. Water follows the osmotic gradient created by the sodium influx, and more water is retained. Euvolemia is reinstated and blood pressure normalized.

High plasma potassium levels act directly on the zona glomerulosa to stimulate aldosterone secretion, thereby starting the cascade of events in the kidney and elsewhere that will allow excretion of the excess potassium. In addition, adrenocorticotropic hormone (ACTH) has a transient stimulatory effect on aldosterone production by glomerulosa cells.

From: *Contemporary Endocrinology: Pediatric Endocrinology: A Practical Clinical Guide*
Edited by: S. Radovick and M. H. MacGillivray © Humana Press Inc., Totowa, NJ

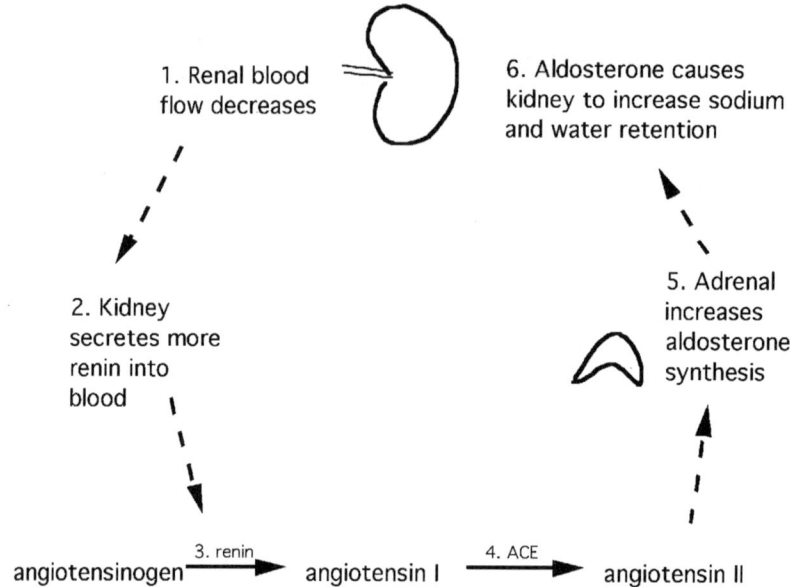

Fig. 1. Aldosterone production and action. A decrease in renal blood flow (**1**) leads to secretion of renin from the kidney (**2**). Plasma renin catalyzes the cleavage of angiotensin I from circulating angiotensinogen (**3**). Angiotensin I is then cleaved by endothelial angiotensin-converting enzyme (ACE) to form the active angiotensin II (**4**), which acts directly on the adrenal cortex to stimulate aldosterone synthesis and release (**5**). Aldosterone in turn acts on the kidney to increase blood volume (**6**).

Aldosterone's actions are mediated by binding to the mineralocorticoid receptor (MR) in target tissues, such as the kidney. The aldosterone-MR complex alters gene expression in the tubule cells to affect electrolyte flow (Fig. 2). Foremost is the insertion of increased numbers of the epithelial sodium channel protein into the luminal membrane of the tubule, allowing sodium to flow down the gradient from the lumen into the cell. In addition, the aldosterone-MR complex stimulates the expression and activity of the basal membrane sodium-potassium pump, allowing intracellular sodium to be transferred into the extracellular fluid in exchange for potassium. This creates an osmotic gradient that draws water from the lumen to the extracellular fluid and back into the bloodstream. Potassium and hydrogen flow in the opposite direction of sodium and are excreted into the urine. Other mineralocorticoid-target tissues, such as sweat glands and the colon, show similar flow of sodium and water into the blood and of potassium and hydrogen into the luminal fluids.

Other steroids that can bind with high affinity to MR include deoxycorticosterone (DOC), an intermediary in the synthetic pathway of aldosterone, and cortisol, the major glucocorticoid hormone. However, under normal conditions, their effects on water and electrolyte balance are negligible. DOC is secreted by the adrenal gland and circulates at similar concentrations as aldosterone, but most is protein-bound and not available to bind with MR. Only in certain diseases of excess DOC production will binding to MR be clinically significant. Cortisol, although present in 1000-fold higher concentration in the blood than aldosterone, is unable to gain access to MR in the kidney and other mineralocorticoid-target tissues because of local metabolism of cortisol to inactive cor-

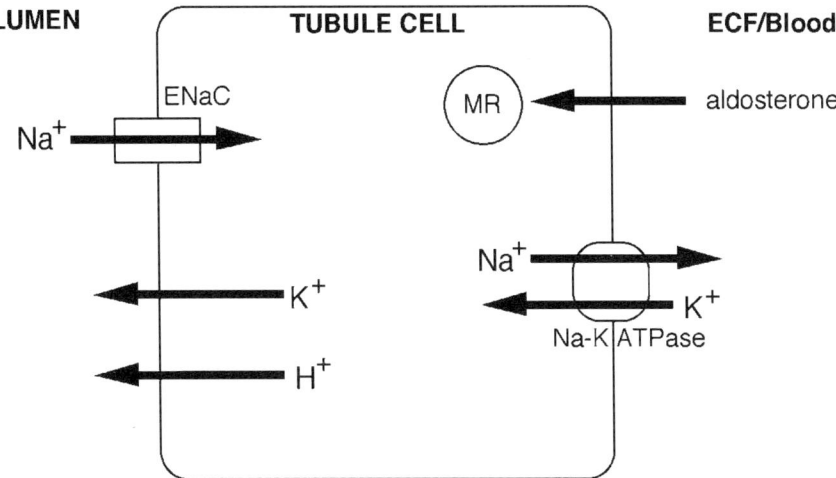

Fig. 2. Direction of ion flow in renal tubule cells in presence of aldosterone. ECF, extracellular fluid; ENaC, epithelial sodium channel; MR, mineralocorticoid receptor; Na-K ATPase, sodium potassium exchange pump.

tisone by the enzyme 11β-hydroxysteroid dehydrogenase type 2 (11β-HSD2). Thus, tissue specificity for aldosterone over cortisol by MR is achieved by local expression of this enzyme.

DISORDERS OF DEFICIENT MINERALOCORTICOID

Introduction

Mineralocorticoid deficiency is a typical concomitant of glucocorticoid deficiency in all causes of primary adrenal failure. Thus, aldosterone deficiency is common in adrenal aplasia, adrenal hypoplasia, most forms of congenital adrenal hyperplasia (the exceptions being 11β-hydroxylase and 17α-hydroxylase deficiencies), and in postnatally acquired adrenal failure, such as Addison's disease, adrenal hemorrhage and infection, and adrenoleukodystrophy. These conditions are discussed in detail in another chapter. Isolated aldosterone deficiency is much rarer and encompasses far fewer etiologic possibilities than complete adrenocortical insufficiency (Table 1). It results from defects in aldosterone synthase, an enzyme unique to the mineralocorticoid pathway that converts cholesterol to aldosterone. This enzyme is not involved in glucocorticoid synthesis by the zona fasciculata. It catalyzes three separate reactions: 11-hydroxylation, 18-hydroxylation, and 18-dehydrogenation of DOC (Fig. 3). Previously it was thought that these three reactions were catalyzed by three separate enzymes: 11β-hydroxylase (erroneously thought to be the same enzyme as that found in the fasciculata), corticosterone methyloxidase type I (CMO I), and CMO II. Now it is understood that mutations in different loci of the single aldosterone synthase gene lead to differential loss of enzymatic function.

The *CYP11B2* gene encodes aldosterone synthase and is closely related to *CYP11B1*, the gene for 11β-hydroxylase of the glucocorticoid synthetic pathway. *CYP11B2* is expressed only in the zona glomerulosa, while *CYP11B1* is expressed only in the fasciculata and reticularis of the adrenal gland.

Table 1
Disorders of Isolated Mineralocorticoid Deficiency

Aldosterone deficiency
   aldosterone synthase deficiency
     type 1 (CMO I deficiency)
     type 2 (CMO II deficiency)
   glomerulosa atrophy (transient deficiency)
   11β-hydroxylase deficiency
   17α-hydroxylase deficiency
Mineralocorticoid resistance = pseudohypoaldosteronism
   MR mutations
   post-MR mutations

Symptoms of mineralocorticoid deficiency can also result from the inability of target tissues to respond to aldosterone. This condition is called mineralocorticoid resistance or pseudohypoaldosteronism type I (Pseudohypoaldosteronism type II is an unrelated condition, not discussed in this chapter). Both MR defects and post-receptor defects have been identified.

Molecular Mechanisms

In CMO I deficiency, or more recently, type 1 aldosterone synthase deficiency, the 11-hydroxylase activity is present, the 18-hydroxylase activity diminished, and the 18-dehydrogenation generally not measurable. As a result, 18-hydroxycorticosterone and aldosterone levels are low, although 18-hydroxycorticosterone is measurable, and the 18-hydroxycorticosterone to aldosterone ratio is not significantly elevated above normal. Diminished mineralocorticoid activity leads to sodium loss ("salt-wasting") and hypovolemia, causing continuous activation of the renin angiotensin system. High angiotensin II levels drive the glomerulosa to synthesize precursors up to the enzymatic block. DOC produced by the glomerulosa still undergoes 11-hydroxylation, perhaps aided by the 11β-hydroxylase of the fasciculata, and corticosterone builds up.

In CMO II deficiency, or type 2 aldosterone synthase deficiency, the enzyme retains its ability to hydroxylate at the 11 and 18 positions, but is unable to carry out the final dehydrogenation step. Thus, 18-hydroxycorticosterone, the last intermediary before the enzymatic block, builds up, and the ratio of 18-hydroxycorticosterone to aldosterone is markedly elevated.

Both CMO I and II deficiencies are inherited as autosomal recessive. Genetic studies of individuals with both CMO I and II deficiency have shown point mutations in the *CYP11B2* gene in most cases *(1,2)*. Other genes that might be able to cause a similar biochemical and clinical syndrome have not yet been identified.

In mineralocorticoid resistance or pseudohypoaldosteronism type I, aldosterone production is normal, but the kidney is unable to respond to mineralocorticoid. An autosomal dominant form of pseudohypoaldosteronism, has been shown to result from mutations in the *MR* gene *(3)*. Others with autosomal dominant pseudohypoaldosteronism may have another defect, as MR mutations have not been found in all individuals with this phenotype *(3)*. Autosomal recessive pseudohypoaldosteronism has been shown to be caused by

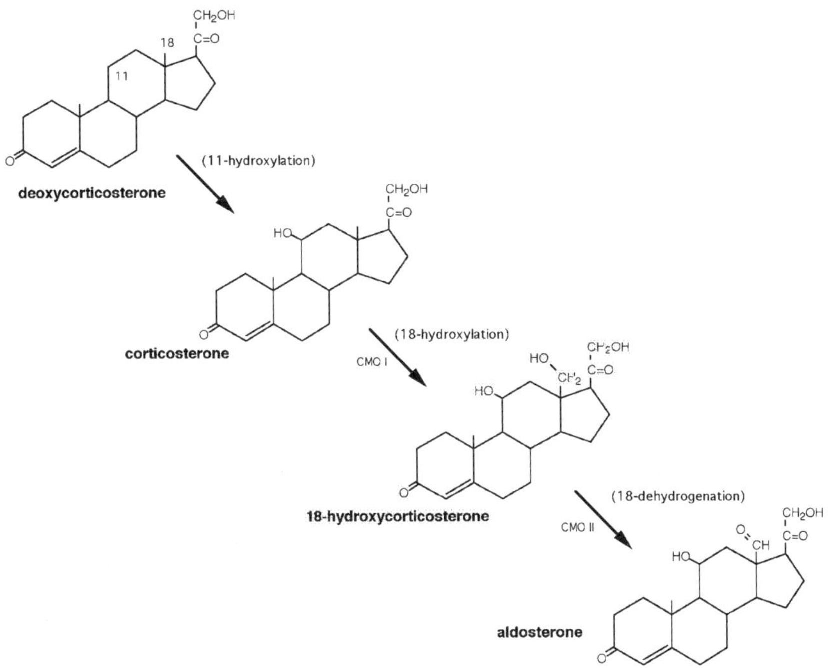

Fig. 3. The reactions catalyzed by aldosterone synthetase. CMO, corticosterone methyl oxidase.

inactivating mutations in the epithelial sodium channel, whose insertion into the luminal membrane is normally stimulated by binding of aldosterone to MR *(4,5)*.

Clinical Presentation

Isolated mineralocorticoid deficiency, either by inadequate production or by mineralocorticoid resistance, presents almost exclusively in infants. In its most severe form, the neonate presents within 1–2 wk of birth with dehydration, vomiting, and hypotension secondary to marked urinary sodium and water loss. Hyponatremia is present, but hyperkalemia and acidosis may or may not be present initially. If the electrolyte abnormality is not discovered and treated, life threatening hyperkalemia may occur. A history of multiple hospitalizations for recurrent vomiting and dehydration in the first year of life, treated successfully with intravenous saline, may also be elicited. If the deficiency is milder, the child may present at weeks to months of age with failure to thrive.

In general, defects in aldosterone production have milder presentations than aldosterone resistance, perhaps because some mineralocorticoid activity is present in CMO deficiency secondary to high levels of intermediates with weak MR-binding capacity. Furthermore, autosomal dominant pseudohypoaldosteronism typically is milder than the autosomal recessive forms, presumably because in the heterozygous state, there is still a significant response to aldosterone, although it is diminished.

Interestingly, children with mineralocorticoid deficiency or resistance may be mistakenly diagnosed with cystic fibrosis, which also presents with failure to thrive and leads to an elevated sodium level on sweat testing. In addition, children with autosomal recessive pseudohypoaldosteronism have more frequent lung infections, because of dysfunction of the sodium channel, also present in the lung *(6,7)*.

Diagnosis

The diagnosis of isolated mineralocorticoid deficiency should be entertained in infants presenting with hyponatremia and dehydration, once more common etiologies, such as adrenal insufficiency, have been ruled out. The classic laboratory findings include hyponatremia, hyperkalemia, metabolic acidosis, high urine sodium, and high plasma renin levels. CMO deficiency will present with a low or low-normal aldosterone level (normal aldosterone level in infancy, 20–120 ng/dL [8]), clearly inappropriate for the clinical situation with hyponatremia and dehydration. On the other hand, in pseudohypoaldosteronism, the aldosterone level is markedly and appropriately elevated. If the patient's hyponatremia and dehydration have resolved prior to the measurement of hormone levels, the renin level may be normal, in which case the aldosterone level may not be useful. The physiologic system must either be stressed by salt depletion or more safely by ACTH stimulation (9) to reassess hormone levels in this case. The differentiation between CMO deficiencies type I and II, based on low or high 18 hydroxycorticosterone levels, is of academic and research interest but does not alter management or outcome. Further confirmation of aldosterone deficiency is provided by positive response to treatment with mineralocorticoid agonist, while aldosterone resistance will fail to respond to this treatment.

Treatment and Outcome

Treatment in all cases of low aldosterone production includes an MR agonist and replacement of sodium. In the hospitalized child in the midst of a salt-wasting crisis, normal saline should be infused by bolus for hypotension and then at a steady rate until the body is replete of sodium. No intravenous selective MR agonist is available, and usually rigorous saline replacement will suffice to stabilize the infant. If enteral medication is not possible and saline not fully effective, mineralocorticoid activity can be obtained by using intravenous hydrocortisone at a dose of 50–100 mg/m^2/d. However, glucocorticoid effects will be a side-effect of this treatment.

As soon as enteral medication is possible, an oral MR agonist should be started. The MR agonist used is fludrocortisone, and its dose is uniform throughout all ages and sizes. For severe aldosterone deficiency, 100 µg/d is required. For optimal salt retention, such as at diagnosis, 50 µg every 12 h is preferable. However, this dosing scheme may eventually result in hypertension in some individuals, at which time switching to 100 µg once daily will usually work, by allowing a period of natriuresis before the next dose, in essence, an escape valve. For milder aldosterone deficiency, 50 µg once daily may be enough. There is no liquid form, so the tablet must be crushed and given in a small volume of milk or baby food for infants. Toddlers will usually chew the pill without difficulty.

For infants, who do not control their diet and therefore cannot respond to increased salt appetite, continued oral sodium supplementation is required in most cases. A good starting dose is 5 mEq/kg/d, given as NaCl and preferably divided into three doses. By the toddler age, the child will generally choose salty foods appropriately and self-regulate the sodium intake.

In pseudohypoaldosteronism, treatment relies entirely on sodium repletion, since MR agonist is ineffective in the face of mineralocorticoid resistance. Thus, higher doses of oral sodium are often required.

The effectiveness of therapy for either aldosterone deficiency or pseudohypoaldosteronism is monitored by following the growth of the child and measuring plasma electrolytes with a renin level. The goal is to maintain a normal renin level (4–12 ng/mL/h *[10]*). A high renin level indicates the need for increased dietary sodium or an increased dose of fludrocortisone. Children with eunatremia but a high renin level often do not grow well. A consistently suppressed renin level (<1.0) suggests overtreatment and puts the child at risk for hypervolemia and hypertension.

If diagnosed and treated promptly, the prognosis for children with mineralocorticoid deficiency is good. Interestingly, children with either CMO deficiency or autosomal dominant pseudohypoaldosteronism will typically outgrow the obvious salt-wasting stage *(11)*. Thus, by a few years of life, sodium supplementation and/or fludrocortisone may be discontinued, and the child will thereafter maintain eunatremia, usually with a normal renin level. The reasons for this amelioration are still not understood. The decision to wean and stop treatment must be individualized for each patient, however, and monitoring should be continued.

DISORDERS OF EXCESS MINERALOCORTICOID

Introduction

Disorders of mineralocorticoid excess are a rare cause of hypertension in the adult population, since most adults have primary or "essential" hypertension. Whereas in pediatrics, especially in prepubertal children, most hypertension is likely to be secondary to other treatable causes. Thus, although still rare, mineralocorticoid excess should be considered sooner in the evaluation of hypertension in children than it is in adults.

In this chapter, disorders of high renin, high aldosterone hypertension will not be discussed, since these are not primary adrenal disorders and result usually from renal problems.

Primary aldosteronism is the term used for overproduction of aldosterone by the adrenal in the context of suppressed renin and angiotensin levels. It can result from an aldosterone producing adenoma and from idiopathic bilateral hyperplasia of the glomerulosa, seen mostly in adults. A third cause of primary aldosteronism is the genetically inherited condition called glucocorticoid-remediable aldosteronism (GRA), recently renamed familial aldosteronism type I, in which aldosterone production is paradoxically controlled by ACTH. This condition typically presents in childhood.

Other conditions of excess-mineralocorticoid, low-renin hypertension occur when other steroids with mineralocorticoid activity build up to unusually high levels. The principal culprits are DOC and cortisol. Massive overproduction of DOC from the fasciculata is seen in 17α-hydroxylase deficiency, 11β-hydroxylase deficiency, and glucocorticoid resistance. In all three conditions, hyperplasia of the fasciculata results from chronic overstimulation of the adrenal glands by ACTH. This occurs in response to poor cortisol production in the first two disorders, or glucocorticoid receptor defects, in the third. The excess plasma DOC binds and activates MR in target tissues such as the kidney.

The local inactivation of cortisol is mediated by 11β-HSD2, present in mineralocorticoid target tissues, such as the kidney and intestine. Overproduction of cortisol can overwhelm the local metabolism of cortisol to cortisone, thus allowing cortisol to accumulate and bind to MR. Such states of excess cortisol include endogenous Cushing's syndrome, as well as iatrogenic forms due to the ingestion of glucocorticoids with MR-binding activity. However, only a small subset of individuals with Cushing's syndrome have high enough cortisol levels to overwhelm the activity of 11β-HSD2. On the other hand, in glucocorticoid resistance, cortisol levels are frequently two or three orders of magnitude above normal and probably contribute to the effects of high DOC levels in binding to MR and causing hypertension.

In the condition termed "apparent mineralocorticoid excess," cortisol production is normal, or even mildly suppressed, but local levels in mineralocorticoid target tissues are elevated because of deficient activity of 11β-HSD2. This is an autosomal recessive, inherited disorder caused by defects in the gene encoding 11β-HSD2. In its severe form, this is a rare condition, described in only about 50 individuals so far *(12)*. Licorice toxicity can mimic the inherited disorder, as chemicals in this food are specific inhibitors of 11β-HSD2.

In the conditions of high DOC or cortisol levels acting on MR, target tissues respond as they would to aldosterone. Sodium and fluid retention lead to hypervolemia with feedback suppression of renin, angiotensin, and aldosterone production. Thus these conditions cause low-renin, low-aldosterone hypertension, with hypokalemia and metabolic alkalosis.

Only primary aldosteronism and the disorders of 11β-HSD activity will be further addressed in this chapter, as the other conditions are discussed in more detail elsewhere.

Molecular Mechanisms

The molecular basis of aldosterone-producing adenomata is not well defined. These usually occur sporadically and are extremely rare in children *(13,14)*.

GRA is an autosomal dominant, inherited disorder caused by a hybrid of the gene for 11β-hydroxylase (*CYP11B1*) with the gene for aldosterone synthase (*CYP11B2*). These two genes are normally located in tandem on chromosome 8 in humans, with *CYP11B1* upstream of *CYP11B2 (15,16)*. In GRA, crossover between the two genes has occurred because of misalignment of the chromosomes, and a third hybrid gene is found between the two normal genes. The hybrid gene contains the upstream regulatory sequences and various amounts of the 5'-coding region of *CYP11B1* adjacent to 3'-coding sequences of *CYP11B2 (17,18)*. The enzyme produced has all the enzymatic capability of aldosterone synthase but is regulated similarly to 11β-hydroxylase. It is produced in the fasciculata, and its production is stimulated by ACTH, but not by angiotensin or hyperkalemia. Some unusual steroids are produced by the co-localization of aldosterone synthase and 17α-hydroxylase in the same cell in this disorder. Thus, the presence of high blood and urine levels of 18-hydroxycortisol and metabolites of 18-oxocortisol are clues to the diagnosis of GRA.

Apparent mineralocorticoid excess (AME) is caused by mutations in the gene for 11β-HSD2 leading to insufficient activity of the enzyme *(19,20)*. All patients with severe AME detected to date have been homozygotes or compound heterozygotes. A milder homozygous form, with less severe hypertension and less impairment of enzyme activity, was recently diagnosed *(21)*, and further studies pursuing the prevalence of this mutation suggest this form may be more common in certain populations, such as the Mennonites *(12)*. In addition, some heterozygotes may be affected with hypertension *(22)*.

Clinical Presentation

Excess mineralocorticoid activity presents principally with hypertension. The hypertension can range from mild to severe and may be detected in infancy, childhood or adolescence. Both GRA and AME have been detected in infants *(23)*. When presenting in infancy, failure to thrive may be the first sign.

Typically hypokalemia and metabolic alkalosis are also present, but these may not be seen if the patient is on a low-salt diet. Since the typical American diet is not low in sodium, hypokalemia can usually be expected. Interestingly, many patients with GRA have not presented with hypokalemia but seemed unusually sensitive to diuretic therapy, developing severe hypokalemia on this treatment *(23,24)*. With marked hypokalemia, polyuria and polydipsia may occur as a result of resistance of the nephron to the effects of antidiuretic hormone.

Diagnosis

Once a child has been determined to have chronic hypertension, by comparison with age- and sex-adjusted norms, an evaluation for causes of secondary hypertension should commence. The majority of secondary hypertension in pediatrics results from kidney disease. Initial studies would include measurement of electrolytes, blood urea nitrogen, plasma renin, serum and urine creatinine, and urinalysis.

If no evidence of kidney or cardiovascular disease is forthcoming, the evaluation proceeds towards more rare causes of hypertension. A high random renin level rules out primary mineralocorticoid excess, whereas an undetectable random aldosterone level makes primary aldosteronism unlikely. A low potassium level, in the absence of any diuretic therapy, points towards mineralocorticoid excess as a likely etiology. Simultaneously drawn renin, aldosterone, and potassium levels may be revealing and show a high aldosterone level. However, there are many caveats to drawing random renin and aldosterone levels, since these levels may be acutely affected by degree of hydration, amount of salt in the diet, psychologic and physiologic stress, and sudden changes between lying, sitting, and standing. If suspicion is high for mineralocorticoid excess, but the potassium level is normal, electrolytes, renin, and aldosterone levels should be remeasured, drawn fasting in the morning following four days of a high-salt diet of greater than 120 mmol sodium per day. Another useful approach is the measurement of aldosterone and other selected adrenal steroids of interest in a 24-h urine collection, as normative data is available.

If excess aldosterone production is confirmed, imaging of the adrenal should be performed, usually by CT scan, to rule out an adenoma or bilateral hyperplasia. A family history of multiple members diagnosed with hypertension in childhood or adolescence should trigger thoughts of GRA. Tests to confirm GRA include measurement of blood and urine levels of the 18-hydroxycortisol and metabolites of 18-oxocortisol, both of which will be high in GRA. A dexamethasone suppression test is also useful, showing whether aldosterone can be suppressed, which only occurs if GRA is present.

If aldosterone levels are suppressed with a low renin level, congenital adrenal hyperplasia due to 11-β hydroxylase deficiency should be considered, as this is much more common than AME. An ACTH-stimulation test would be useful for diagnosis of the former, while measurement of the of cortisol to cortisone ratio establishes the diagnosis of AME. The ratio will be very high in AME. Before making this diagnosis, care should be taken to evaluate the patient's diet for sources of licorice, or the specific components, glycyrrhizic acid and glycyrrhetinic acid, found in some traditional and herbal formulations.

Another cause of low-renin, low-aldosterone hypertension in children is Liddle's syndrome, caused by activating mutations of the epithelial sodium channel *(25,2)*. Decreased activity in this same channel is seen in autosomal recessive pseudohypoaldosteronism type 1. Liddle's syndrome by contrast shows autosomal dominant inheritance. It is considered when aldosterone, DOC, and cortisol levels are all low, and the cortisol to cortisone is not elevated. In addition, patients will not respond to spironolactone, since the defect lies downstream of the MR.

Treatment

The primary treatment of increased mineralocorticoid activity is clearly to remove the excess mineralocorticoid if possible. The course is most obvious in the case of an aldosterone-producing adenoma, in which surgical excision is advised. Removal of licorice from the diet should cure hypertension owing to ingestion of too much of this food.

Primary aldosteronism caused by GRA is treated with dexamethasone, a glucocorticoid that suppresses ACTH production but has no MR-binding capacity. The dexamethasone suppresses endogenous production of glucocorticoid and ectopic synthesis of aldosterone in the zona fasciculata. Plasma renin levels should eventually rise and allow the zona glomerulosa to take over physiologic production of aldosterone.

Treatment of AME starts with spironolactone to inhibit binding of the excess cortisol to the MR. High doses are usually needed, with gradual escalation, as the patient may become refractory to this medication *(12)*. Other diuretics may be added, and oral potassium supplementation should be considered for hypokalemic patients.

Liddle's syndrome is usually managed by nephrologists and requires a sodium-restricted diet and diuretics such as triamterene.

REFERENCES

1. Pascoe L, Curnow KM, Slutsker L, et al. Mutations in the human CYP11B2 (aldosterone synthase) causing corticosterone methyloxidase II deficiency. Proc Nat Acad Sci USA 1992;89:4996–5000.
2. Mitsuuchi Y, Kawamoto T, Miyahara K, et al. Congenitally defective aldosterone biosynthesis in humans: inactivation of the P-450C18 gene (*CYP11B2*) due to nucleotide deletion in CMO I deficient patients. Biochem Biophys Res Comm 1993;190: 864–869.
3. Geller DS, Rodriguez-Soriano J, Vallo Boado A, et al. Mutations in the mineralocorticoid receptor gene cause autosomal dominant pseudohypoaldosteronism type I. Nat Genet 1998;19:279–281.
4. Chang SS, Grunder S, Hanukoglu A, et al. Mutations in subunits of the epithelial sodium channel cause salt wasting with hyperkalemic acidosis, pseudohypoaldosteronism type I. Nat Genet 1996;12:248–253.
5. Strautnieks SS, Thompson RJ, Gardiner RM, et al. A novel splice-site mutation in the gamma subunit of the epithelial sodium channel gene in three pseudohypoaldosteronism type I families. Nat Genet1996;13:248–250.
6. Hanukoglu A, Bistritzer T, Rakover Y, et al. Pseudoaldosteronism with increased sweat and saliva electrolyte values and frequent lower respiratory tract infections mimicking cystic fibrosis. J Pediatr 1994;125:752–755.
7. Kerem E, Bistritzer T, Hanukoglu A, et al. Pulmonary epithelial sodium-channel dysfunction and excess airway liquid in pseudohypoaldosteronism. N Engl J Med 1999;341:156–162.
8. Kowarski A, Katz H, Migeon, CJ. Plasma aldosterone concentrations in normal subjects from infancy to adulthood. J Clin Endocrinol Metab 1974;38:489–491.

9. Peter M, Sippell WG. Congenital hypoaldosteronism: the Visser-Cost syndrome revisited. Pediatr Res 1996;39(3):554–560.
10. Sassard J, Sann L. Vincent M, et al. Plasma renin activity in normal subjects from infancy to puberty. J Clin Endocrinol Metab 1975;40:524–525.
11. Rappaport R, Dray R, Legrand JC, et al. Hypoaldosteronisme congenital familial par defaut de la 18-OH-dehydrogenase. Pediatr Res 1968;2:456–463.
12. Cerame BI, New MI. Hormonal hypertension in children: 11β-hydroxylase deficiency and apparent mineralocorticoid excess. J Pediatr Endocrinol Metab 2000;13:1537–1547.
13. Li JT, Shu SG, S Chi CA. Aldosterone-secreting adrenal cortical adenoma in an 11-year-old hcild and collective review of the literature. Eur J Pediatr 1994;153:715–717.
14. Abasiyanik, A, Oran B, Kaymakci A, et al. Conn syndrome in a child, caused by adrenal adenoma. J Pediatr Surg 1996;31:430–432.
15. Chua SC, Szabo P, Vitek A, et al. Cloning of cDNA encoding steroid 11β-hydroxylase (*P450c11*). Proc Nat Acad Sci USA 1987;84:7193–7197.
16. Mornet E, Dupont J, Vitek A, et al. Characterization of two genes encoding human steroid 11β-hydroxylase (*P-4501111β*). J Biol Chem 1989;264:20,961–20,967.
17. Pascoe L, Curnow KM, Slutsker L, et al. Glucocorticoid-suppressible hyperaldosteronism results from hybrid genes created by unequal crossovers between *CYP11B1* and *CYP11B2*. Proc Nat Acad Sci USA 1992;89:8327–8331.
18. Lifton RP, Dluhy RG, Powers M, et al. Hereditary hypertension caused by chimaeric gene duplications and ectopic expression of aldosterone synthase. Nat Genet 1992;2:66–74.
19. Wilson RC, Krozowski ZS, Li K, et al. A mutation in the HSD11B2 gene in a family with apparent mineralocorticoid excess. J Clin Endocrinol Metab 1995;80:2263–2266.
20. Mune T, Rogerson FM, Nikkila H, et al. Human hypertension caused by mutations in the kidney isozyme of 11β-hydroxysteroid dehydrogenase. Nat Genet 1995;10:394–399.
21. Wilson RC, Dave-Sharma S, Wei J, et al. A genetic defect resulting in mild low-renin hypertension. Proc Natl Acad Sci USA 1998;95:10200–10205.
22. Li A, Li KXZ, Marui S, et al. Apparent mineralocorticoid excess in a Brazilian kindred: hypertension in the heterozygote state. J Hypertens 1997;15:1397–1402.
23. Rich GM, Ulick S, Cook S, et al. Glucocorticoid-remediable aldosteronism in a large kindred: clinical spectrum and diagnosis using a characteristic biochemical phenotype. Ann Intern Med 1992;116(10):813–820.
24. Grim CE, Weinberger MH. Familial, dexamethasone-suppressible, normokalemic hyperaldosteronism. Pediatrics 1980;65:597–604.
25. Shimkets RA, Warnock DG, Bositis, CM, et al. Liddle's syndrome: heritable human hypertension caused by mutations in the b subunit of the epithelial sodium channel. Cell 1994;79:407–414.
26. Schild L, Canessa CM, Shimkets RA, et al. A mutation in the epithelial sodium channel causing Liddle disease increases channel activity in the Xenopus laevis oocyte expression system. Proc Nat Acad Sci USA 1995;92:5699–5703.

IV THYROID DISORDERS

16 Congenital Hypothyroidism

Cecilia A. Larson, MD

CONTENTS

> INTRODUCTION
> MECHANISM
> CLINICAL PRESENTATION
> DIAGNOSIS
> TREATMENT
> OUTCOME
> SUMMARY
> REFERENCES

INTRODUCTION

Congenital hypothyroidism remains the leading cause of preventable mental impairment worldwide. Despite ongoing efforts to eradicate iodine deficiency, populations remain at risk for iodine deficiency and consequently, high rates of endemic cretinism. In iodine sufficient populations, sporadic congenital hypothyroidism remains among the most common newborn conditions, which if unrecognized and untreated can lead to irreversible mental impairment.

Recognition of iodine deficiency and attempts to eliminate the problem have been ongoing for decades. It is apparent that ongoing surveillance for iodine status is important as dietary deficiency tends to recur in certain populations and regions. While iodine deficiency can cause thyroid disorders in all ages, the fetus and newborn are at special risk for consequences of insufficient iodine owing to the critical thyroxine dependent intervals of neurodevelopment. For this reason, surveillance and treatments aimed at reproductive age women and newborns are of particular importance. Screening for iodine deficiency and its sequelae can be achieved by numerous means (thyroid ultrasonography, urinary iodine measurements, blood thyroid or iodine tests, and newborn screening). Of particular interest is the potential dual role of neonatal thyroid screening to detect both thyroid insufficiency in neonates and to detect populations at risk of iodine deficiency by monitoring the newborn population mean thyroid stimulating hormone (TSH) concentration *(1).*

From: *Contemporary Endocrinology: Pediatric Endocrinology: A Practical Clinical Guide*
Edited by: S. Radovick and M. H. MacGillivray © Humana Press Inc., Totowa, NJ

Even in areas traditionally considered iodine sufficient, such as the US, it is important to have surveillance for iodine status, especially of reproductive-age women and children. In the most recent report on US iodine intake, childbearing-age women demonstrated a significant decline in dietary iodine intake *(2,3)*. It will be important to monitor this trend and track potential consequences in terms of thyroid conditions in these at-risk populations.

Aside from regional iodine deficiency as a cause of hypothyroidism in newborns, certain ethnic groups are at increased risk of developmental thyroid anomalies. Among the groups at increased risk are: Hispanics, Chinese, Vietnamese, Asian Indians, Filipinos, Middle Easterners, and Hawaiians; whereas blacks are at reduced risk (1/3 the risk compared to whites) *(4)*. Thyroid dysgenesis is also twice as common in female newborns as males *(5)*.

While iodine deficiency is the leading world-wide cause for congenital hypothyroidism, in iodine sufficient areas the leading cause of congenital hypothyroidism is thyroid dysgenesis, accounting for about 80% of cases. Any defect in thyroid hormone production, regulation and action can cause hypothyroidism, and Table 1 shows a categorization of types of congenital hypothyroidism. Thyroid hormone synthesis is dependent on sufficient iodine substrate, adequate iodine trapping, oxidation, and organification, as well as sufficient production of thyroglobulin. Release of thyroid hormones from the thyroid gland is accomplished by proteolysis. Thyroid hormone is predominantly protein bound in the circulation, and peripheral conversion to active hormone is accomplished by the deiodinases. The active T_3 binds to its nuclear receptors and transcriptionally activates genes with thyroid hormone-response elements. Regulation of thyroxine production and metabolism is under control of the hypothalamic/pituitary axis (thyrotropin-releasing hormone, and thyroid stimulating hormone). Malfunction of any step of thyroid hormone production or regulation can result in hypothyroidism.

MECHANISM

The thyroid gland forms during the first trimester of development. It has a complex migratory development, arising from the median and lateral anlagen. The median anlage appears during the second week of gestation, expands into a bilobate structure adjacent to the heart and is pulled caudally with the developing heart, completing its migration by the 7th week of gestation. The lateral anlagen derive from the fourth branchial pouches and fuse with the bilobate structure about the time the migration is complete *(6)*. It is notable that many congenital anomalies have been reported in association with congenital hypothyroidism. Some findings (such as the association of congenital hip dislocation) have not been replicated in other studies/populations. The most consistent developmental anomalies associated with congenital hypothyroidism have been cardiac *(7–10)*. The coincidence of timing and location of thyroid and cardiac embryonic development supports the theory of common cause for these anomalies. Since thyroid dysgenesis does not generally recur in families, it has been thought to be a developmental rather than a heritable condition, possibly associated with environmental teratogens. Seasonal variations in incidence of congenital hypothyroidism *(11)* have also been noted, giving further support to critical exposure (such a seasonal viruses) as a contibuting factor to sporadic congenital hypothyroidism. However, as early as 1966, there was a report of dysgenesis in two pairs of monozygotic twins and in a mother and child *(12)*. The discovery of developmental genes that play important roles in embryogenesis and developmental cell

Table 1
Causes of Congenital Hypothyroidism (CH)

Primary hypothyroidism

Thyroid Dysgenesis
    Athyreotic
    Ectopic
    Hypothyreotic (ex hemithyroid)
Thyroid Hormone Dysgenesis- Goitrous Enzyme Defect
    Iodine Deficiency
    Iodine Transporter Defect
    Peroxidase Defect
    Thyroglobulin Synthetic Defect
Peripheral Thyroid Hormone Inactivation
    Tumor Deiodinase Activity
    Iodotyrosine Deiodinase Defect
TSH resistance (normal or hypoplastic gland)
    TSH receptor (TR β)mutations
    Gsα gene mutations
Transient Hypothyroidism
    Maternal Antithyroid Medications
    Maternal Antibodies-maternal thyrotropin receptor blocking antibody (TRB-Ab)
    Iodine
    Idiopathic

Central hypothyroidism

Hypothalamic
Pituitary
Pituitary maldevelopment
Pit-1, TSH β
Medications such as corticosteroids and dopamine

migrations, and the identification of mutations in these types of genes associated with developmental anomalies including thyroid dysgenesis (PAX-8, TTF-2, and connexin, for example) point to a role for genetic predisposition to thyroid dysgenesis *(13–15)*, and may in part explain the observed higher incidence of congenital hypothyroidism among certain ethnic groups. It is likely that both genetic and environmental factors contribute to thyroid developmental anomalies.

Just as thyroid gland development may be caused by genetic and environmental factors, thyroid hormone dysgenesis may be caused by insufficient intake of iodine, or by a number of mostly autosomal recessive defects which affect thyroid hormone synthesis. These include sodium iodide symporter (NIS), responsible for actively transporting iodine into thyroid follicular cells. Numerous NIS mutations have been identified that can cause hypothyroidism, as well as mutations of thyroid peroxidase gene, TSH and its receptor *(17–23)*.

Features of hypothyroidism relate to requirement of sufficient T_3 to bind TR and activate thyroid responsive genes. Thyroid responsive genes are present throughout the body, with specific time intervals of thyroid hormone responsiveness (*see* Fig. 1). Both

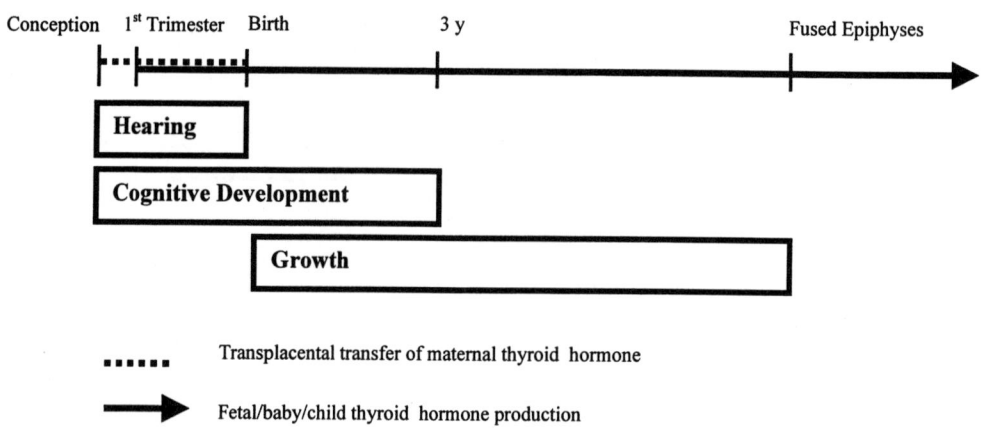

Fig. 1. Critical stages of irreversible thyroid hormone-dependent development.

human and experimental animal data indicate the critical role of thyroid hormone in development. Instances of maternal and fetal hypothyroidism (from iodine deficiency and untreated maternal thyroid-blocking antibodies) point to a critical role of thyroid hormone in neurodevelopment and hearing *(24–27)*. The primary effects in neurodevelopment are on the neural connections and arborization, and myelination, which begins *in utero* and continues until age 3 y *(28–30)*. While bone age delay can begin *in utero*, overall growth is not compromised during gestation with growth retardation appearing postnatally.

CLINICAL PRESENTATION

Congenital hypothyroidism is typically defined as insufficient thyroid hormone production during the newborn period. Most neonates with congenital hypothyroidism appear clinically normal at birth. When signs and symptoms initially present, they are nonspecific, making clinical detection difficult and often delayed. Early signs of possible congenital hypothyroidism include: mottled and dry skin, lethargy, poor feeding, macroglossia, enlarged posterior fontanel (>1 cm), umbilical hernia, jaundice, constipation, hoarse cry, sleepiness, and hypothermia *(31–33)*. Of note, newborns with congenital hypothyroidism are not growth retarded at birth, although bone age may be delayed in severe cases, most commonly with athyreosis. Hypothyroidism of longer duration is associated with decreased linear growth rates and epiphyseal changes. Pseudomuscular hypertrophy, delayed tooth development and developmental delay can also occur.

Acquired hypothyroidism can occur at any age, and frequency increases with age. In the differential of "acquired" hypothyroidism in early childhood is congenital hypothyroidism not detected in the newborn period. This is particularly likely for partial thyroid dysgenesis or dyshormonogesis that is compensated by gland hypertrophy for a variable period of time. Other causes of acquired hypothyroidism are autoimmune thyroiditis and thyroid dysfunction, secondary to thyroid/hypothalamic/pituitary destruction from chemotherapy, radiotherapy, iron or other infiltrative processes. While some signs of hypothyroidism are consistent regardless of age at presentation, such as dry skin, constipation, and lethargy, other signs and sequelae are dependent on the developmental stage during which hypothyroidism occurs. Generally, all aspects of acquired hypothy-

Chapter 16 / Congenital Hypothyroidism

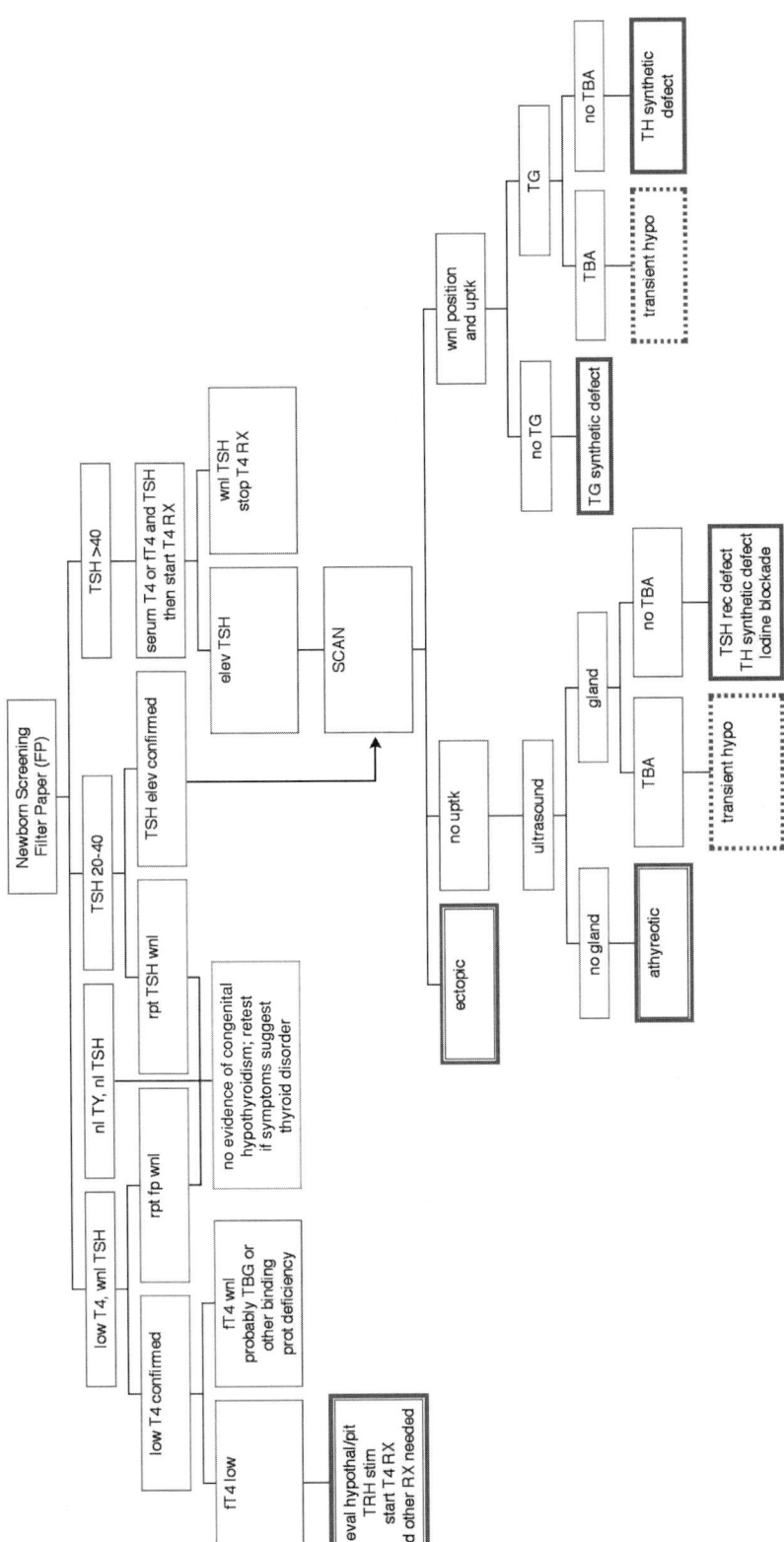

Fig. 2. Work-up of Out-of-Range Thyroid Newborn Screening. Since most cases of congenital hypothyroidism are due to thyroid dysgenesis, early scan and ultrasound will identify the cause in most cases. When family history or physical exam (goiter) suggests dyshormonogenesis, an ultrasound is not generally necessary, and thyroglobulin (TG) testing may be considered sooner in the evaluation. Maternal history of thyroid disease and/or prior affected children may prompt early assessment for thyroid blocking antibodies (TBA).

roidism in adulthood are reversible with thyroxine treatment, and treatment delay does not cause any irreversible effects. In the developing fetus, newborn, and child up to age three, delay in treatment can cause irreversible developmental delays. The most sensitive clinical sign of hypothyroidism in the growing child is growth retardation. Decrease in linear and bone growth are characteristic of hypothyroidism and examination of bone films and the growth curve can be extremely helpful in timing the onset of hypothyroidism.

Manifestations of hypothyroidism do not generally differ by the gender of affected individual (other than menstrual irregularities which can occur in women with hypothyroidism); however, the prevalence of thryoid disease (autoimmune and sporadic dysgenesis) is much greater in females (2:1 ratio for thyroid dysgenesis).

Cardiac malformations have been associated with thryoid dysgenesis, but not with dyshormonogenesis, suggesting a unifying exposure or developmental gene that affects both thyroid gland formation and septation of the embryonic heart *(34)*, rather than *in utero* hypothyroxinemia causing secondary cardiac malformations. TTF-2 has been associated with cleft palate and thyroid dysgenesis *(14)*. Some groups have reported hip dislocation *(9)* though in other series this has not been confirmed . In addition, the following are some of the syndromes associated with congenital hypothyroidism: Pendred Syndrome, pseudohypoparathyroidism and hypoparathyroidism, Beckwith syndrome, Young-Simpson syndrome, and Sotos syndrome. Septo-Optic displasia (SOD) can be associated with varying degrees of hypopituitarism, with growth hormone deficiency occurring with the greatest overall frequency; central hypothyroidism occurs in some cases *(35)*.

Individuals with Trisomy 21 (T21) are at increased risk for congenital hypothyroidism; in some studies, it has been found in 12.5% of Down's newborns *(35,36,38,39–42)*. Congenital hypothyroidism associated with Down's syndrome occurs with equal frequency in affected males and females (unpublished data from New England Newborn Screening Program), and is not associated with dysgenesis, suggesting that T21 does not affect development of the thyroid gland, but rather has an effect on thyroid hormone synthesis and/or gland function. Recent reports suggest zinc deficiency in T21 patients may play a role in minor TSH elevations *(38)*. Individuals with Down's syndrome are also at increased risk of acquired hypothyroidism *(39)*. Since the signs of hypothyroidism can be mistakenly attributed to Down's (macroglossia, developmental delay, growth failure), routine interval TSH screening of all children with Down's is recommended. Although the precise interval for screening has not been established, an approach that would focus on increased screening during the critical developmental phases would be: newborn screening with T_4 and TSH at 2 d, 2 wk, and 2 mo, then serum specimens then q6–12 mo up to 3 yr-of-age, and annually thereafter (sooner if any signs or symptoms of hypothyroidism are noted).

DIAGNOSIS

Newborn Screening

The role of newborn screening is to detect treatable, time-critical, newborn disorders, which if undiagnosed, would lead to significant morbidity and mortality. Newborn screening utilizing dried blood specimens collected on filter paper began in Massachusetts in 1962 with the introduction of the Guthrie Bacterial Inhibition Assay (GBIA) to measure blood phenylalanine levels as a screen for Phenylketonuria (PKU) *(43)*. In the

1970s, the ability to detect thyroxine and thyroid stimulating hormone in dried blood specimens utilizing radioimmunoassay methodology was developed *(44,45)*, and subsequently incorporated into public health newborn screening programs. Currently, there is mandatory universal newborn thyroid screening throughout the US, Canada, much of Europe, Australia, and some form of newborn thyroid screening (but not necessarily universally available) in parts of Asia, the Middle East, and Latin America. Newborn screening for thyroid disease has been one of the great public health success stories. Prior to screening, only one-third of hypothyroid infants were clinically detected before 3 mo-of-age, and the majority of children had severe mental retardation, language, learning and coordination difficulties *(46)*. With the introduction of screening, the age at detection has steadily declined. In the early phases of newborn thyroid screening, the target was to identify and initiate treatment by age 2 mo. Currently with rapid specimen transport of newborn specimens collected on average day of life two and advances in technology allowing rapid T_4/TSH analysis, many screening programs detect and initiate treatment within 1–2 wk-of-age, allowing normal developmental outcome of individuals with congenital hypothyroidism *(47)*. Treatment with thyroxine is curative, making newborn thyroid screening cost effective *(48)*. The incidence of congenital hypothyroidism is approx 1:4000 in North America, though in Massachusetts the incidence has been rising and is currently 1:2000 *(49)*.

TYPES OF THYROID NEWBORN SCREENING STRATEGIES

Primary T_4, secondary TSH: all newborns screened for total thyroxine concentration, with triggered TSH for those with the lowest thyroxine values (below a cut-off value and for a certain percentile of the screened population- for instance all T_4 <13 µg/dL and the lowest decile). This approach allows detection of central and peripheral hypothyroidism *(50–52)*. However, there is a broad range of normal thyroxine concentrations and low thyroxine is common in premature and sick infants and in individuals with thyroxine binding globulin (TBG), or other binding protein, deficiencies. Binding protein deficiency does not require treatment, but is identified as a by-product of this screening strategy.

Primary TSH, with or without secondary T_4: this strategy was initially adopted in European screening programs and provides a mechanism for monitoring for regions of iodine deficiency because it provides information about mean TSH for specific populations *(1)*. Another potential advantage of TSH screening is the theoretical enhanced detection of partially compensated hypothyroidism *(53,55)*; that is, T_4 maintained in the normal range with elevated TSH. In a large study by Dussault in 1983 with simultaneous T_4 and TSH (micromedic T_4 assay and RIA TSH) in 93,000 consecutive filter paper specimens, the T_4 assay had better precision, and there was similar sensitivity in case detections by either primary T_4 or primary TSH screening, with false negatives ($n = 3$) by either approach, including a case of central hypo which was detected only by the T_4 approach *(54)*.

Dual T_4 and TSH: may be the most sensitive approach currently in use allowing detection of central hypothyroidism and euthyroxinemic hypothyroidism, but depending on cut-offs utilized, may result in less specificity and higher recall rates.

Free T_4 (fT_4) is potentially the most sensitive and specific screening strategy. There is report by one program of a fT_4 screening method utilizing filter paper specimens, but it has not been a widely reproducible method to date *(56)*.

As with any laboratory test, the reference range for the normal population and the diseased population has to be established. Determining cut-offs for screening results is complex and should be periodically reassessed *(57)*. This is particularly true of newborn endocrine screening as timing and clinical status can affect the hormone reference range. At parturition and exposure to the cold, extrauterine environment, a neonatal TSH (and consequently T_4) surge occurs within minutes of birth and subsides over the next 24–72 h. This surge also occurs, but in a stunted fashion, in preterm infants *(58–60)*. Newborn screening specimens collected at less than 24h are enriched for mild to moderate TSH elevations that normalize on follow-up (increasing the recall rate); specimens collected at less than 24 h are also at jeopardy of masking hypothyroidism by showing a normal T_4 which subsequently falls (T_4 of maternal origin +/– T_4 surge). The ideal collection time for congenital hypothyroidism screening is probably 3–5 d-of-age to optimize both sensitivity and specificity of screening. In a review of the impact of early discharge on newborn screening, the higher recall rate and cases of missed diagnosis were noted *(61)*. Most screening programs require a follow-up specimen if the initial specimen is collected at <24 h to minimize the chance of a missed diagnosis.

Each laboratory should establish its reference range for its population and testing method.

In the New England Newborn Screening Program, when T_4 measurement was changed from an RIA method to the AutoDELFIA method, a significant increase in mean T_4 for newborns from 13–16 µg/dL was noted, and consequently the absolute T_4 cut-off to trigger TSH testing was raised *(62)*.

WORK-UP OF SCREEN POSITIVE CASES

Whenever notification of out-of-range newborn thyroid screening results are received, it is recommended that the newborn be promptly evaluated with a complete history and physical. History should include note of maternal/family history of thyroid disease, maternal medications (especially anti-thyroid medications or iodine), and baby medications (especially, iodine, steroids, dopamine). Physical examination should include careful inspection for any signs of hypothyroidism, goiter, or sublingual masses (Fig. 2).

Elevated TSH

Because the positive predictive value correlates with the degree of TSH elevation, a general guideline for management of newborn screening results is for TSH < 40 to collect confirmatory serum studies and initiate thyroxine while awaiting confirmatory test results. As a minimum, serum confirmatory studies should include T_4 and TSH.

More modest TSH elevations have a lower positive predictive value. Thus for TSH elevations in the 20–40 range, particularly if the T_4 is in the normal range (>12), a follow-up filter paper or serum specimen is generally sufficient.

Generally accepted case definition for primary hypothyroidism is TSH > 20 (or 25) on more than one specimen, collected after 24 h of age *(64)*.

Low T_4 and Non-elevated TSH

The differential diagnosis of low T_4 and non-elevated TSH includes central hypothyroidism, acute illness, hypothyroxinemia of prematurity, and thyroid binding globulin deficiencies. Central hypothyroidism is rare, occurring 1:50,000-100,000 births *(50,51)*; it has been associated with hypoglycemia (due to adrenal insufficiency) and hypospadias in males, and can be associated with certain syndromes such as SOD and midline craniofacial defects. A general approach to low T_4 is to confirm the finding with another filter paper specimen, and, if confirmed, to proceed to serum fT_4 testing in normal birthweight infants. Since hypothyroxinemia occurs in up to 50% of preterm infants (with 10% having $T_4 < 5$ µg/dL), serial filter paper screening is generally sufficient. Preterm infants are at increased risk for delayed TSH elevations, and this can be detected by performing the serial testing (65).

Role of Additional Confirmatory Testing

Bone age is useful for timing onset of hypothyroidism and for monitoring response to therapy; individuals with significant bone age delay at birth may be at risk for less than optimal outcome, as it may be a marker for *in utero* hypothyroxinemia. In cases of bone age delay, prompt initiation of high thyroxine dose treatment is indicated. With prompt thyroxine, growth will normalize and bone age will also normalize.

Thyroid scan-iodine (I-123) and technetium (Tc99m) scans can be used to determine thyroid location and uptake (62). Iodine scans indicate not only iodine uptake, but also organification of iodine. When the scan indicates athyreosis, or ectopic thyroid (which combined account for about 80% of congenital hypothyroidsim), it indicates need for lifelong thyroxine treatment, and any trials off thyroxine are not indicated. Thyroid scans require the administration of trace amounts of radioactive elements to the child.

Ultrasonography of the thyroid allows examination of the thyroid (without radioactivity) to determine if the thyroid is in the ususal developmental location as a bilobed structure,and if in the usual location, whether it is hypertrophied, suggesting dyshormono-genesis or iodine deficiency. While ultrasound is non-invasive and generally less expensive than other imaging methods, a potential drawback of ultrasonography is that it is often operator dependent.

Thyroglobulin (TG) absence can be associated with athyreosis and thyroglobulin synthetic defects, both of which require lifelong thyroxine replacement.

Thyroid blocking antibodies (TBA), usually of maternal origin, can cause transient hypothyroidism of the newborn (66). The risk for presence of maternal antibodies increases with maternal age, and transient hypothyroidism can recur with subsequent pregnancies. In cases of known maternal thyroid disease, maternal and/or baby antibodies should be considered as an early step in confirmatory testing. Neonatal hypothyroidism due to maternal antibodies is transient, usually lasting only a few months as maternal antibodies decline. Some have advocated routine maternal thyroid screening for all children identified with out of range thyroid newborn screens.

TRH stimulation testing is indicated in cases of suspected central hypothyroidism, associated with low free thyroxine and non-elevated TSH. An exaggerated TSH response to TRH indicates hypothalamic dysfunction and should prompt a further investigation into the status of the hypothalamus and reason for insufficiency, and would generally include MRI of the hypothalamus. Failure to mount a TSH response to TRH indicates pituitary dysfunction, which also warrants further investigation as to its cause and potential association of other pituitary insufficiencies.

While reduced thyroid binding globulin (TBG) levels are indicative of TBG deficiency. In general, the specific measurement of TBG is not necessary, as confirmation of in range free thyroxine level is all that is necessary for follow-up of low T_4, and non-elevated TSH. TBG deficiency in the absence of TSH elevation does not require treatment. Since TBG deficiency in most cases is X-linked, families should be counseled regarding the 1:2 risk of recurrence with subsequent male children.

Special subsets: premature, and low birthweight infants. These infants represent a selected subpopulation at risk for suboptimal longterm outcome *(67,68)*. Whether a portion of this impaired outcome is thyroid hormone dependent is not entirely known. Low T_4 is known to correlate with risk of impaired neurodevelopmental outcome, including increased risk of intraventricular hemorrhage *(69)* and up to 50% of preterm infants are hypothyroxinemic *(70)*. In addition, premature infants are known to have higher iodine requirements, less mature hypothalamic/pituitary axis, and reduced activity of deiodinases (especially in the central nervous system) that convert T_4 to T_3. Thus thyroid hormone, iodine, and TRH treatments have been considered to improve the outcome of preterm babies, but none has demonstrated benefit to date. Additional studies in this area are needed *(71,72)*. Hypothyroxinemia of prematurity generally resolves by 6–10 wk-of-age. However, some preterm infants go on to have delayed TSH elevations. For these reasons, serial screening is recommended for premature infants at 2, 6, and 10 wk-of-age or until they reach 1500 g or are discharged *(65)*.

Acutely ill neonates also tend to have lower total thyroxine values. Because of the crucial role of thyroid hormone in the developing nervous system, some have advocated empiric thyroid hormone treatment in acute illness, and trials of T_3 for cardiac newborns have been performed *(73)*. Treatment has decreased critical care and ionotrope needs, but benefit to neurodevelopmental outcome has not been clearly established. Recovery from acute illness can be associated with transient TSH elevations. Generally, sequential testing can help to distinguish these transient elevations from mild thyroid dysfunction. That is, over time, parallel increases in T_4 and TSH suggest recovery from illness, and TSH should normalize within a week. Transient TSH elevations (without permanent congenital hypothyroidism) are frequently associated with congenital malformations and may represent recovery from acute illness. These elevations tend to be more modest elevations, and are sometimes treated to protect the potentially vulnerable CNS. However, this group warrants a trial off thyroxine after the third birthday to determine whether thyroid dysfunction is persistant.

Blunted TSH response to hypothyroxinemia can occur in babies receiving transfusions, dopamine, and/or high dose steroids. In these cases, serum fT_4 and follow-up thyroid tests post transfusion/treatment may be needed to determine if thyroxine treatment is necessary.

While newborn screening has benefited thousands of newborns in the US (approx 1000 hypothyroid cases/yr), screening has its limitations. As with any screening test, a normal result in the context of signs and symptoms of the disorder should not preclude further diagnostic testing and treatment if indicated. In any newborn or child with signs of potential hypothyroidism, serum T_4 and TSH should be measured *(46,64)*.

TREATMENT

Levothyroxine is the treatment of choice for congenital hypothyroidism Its long half-life allows daily dosing and no consequences of an occasional missed dose. Levothyroxine is converted to the active hormone T_3. In the brain, local T_4 to T_3 conversion is especially important, adding to the rationale for treatment with levothyroxine in pediatric patients. Periodically, combination preparations of T_4 and T_3 have been advocated (74,75), but to date, there is not sufficient evidence to favor this approach, which can be associated with risk of cardiac and other effects of T_3 boluses. Furthermore, all the large-scale outcome studies for treated cases of congenital hypothyroidism have utilized levothyroxine.

Levothyroxine is available as a scored tablet of synthetic hormone in a variety of doses. Adverse consequences of treatment are minimal; in one case, there was report of reversible liver function abnormalities when levothyroxine was used in an individual with antibodies to the medication (76). Prolonged hyperthyroxinemia can cause craniosynostosis (although this has been found in neonatal hyperthyroidism, it is not generally associated with treatment of congenital hypothyroidism) and osteoporosis. These adverse events can be avoided by regular monitoring of thyroid function tests and avoidance of overtreatment.

In treating congenital hypothyroidism, the aim is rapid normalization of total thyroxine (within 1–2 wk of starting treatment); treatment should be initiated at 10–15 µg/kg/d, with the aim to keep the total and free T_4 in the upper half of the normal range. TSH levels generally subside to the normal range within a month of starting treatment, and thereafter should be maintained in the normal range. A rise in TSH while on treatment generally confirms the need for ongoing replacement therapy (provided there has been treatment compliance).

Levothyroxine tablets should be crushed and mixed with some milk and administered by syringe to infants. Soy formulas should be avoided as they interfere with absorption of the medication. Serum T_4 (or fT_4) and TSH should be monitored regularly starting at 2 and 4 wk after medication has been started, every 1–2 mo for the first year, and every 2–3 mo to age 3 yr and every 3 mo until growth is complete. When dose adjustments are made, follow-up testing should be performed in 2–4 wk (64,77).

Resistance (poor absorption, enhanced clearance, pituitary/peripheral resistance) and non-compliance may present with persistant TSH elevation despite thyroxine therapy. In the case of poor absorption and enhanced clearance, the T_4 is usually low. With resistance and non-compliance, the T_4 is usually high or normal. In the noncompliant individual, there can be acute compliance with thyroxine causing the normal or high T_4, but the TSH, which has a longer half life and time to equilibration, will remain elevated, reflecting the prior state of hypothryoxinemia. Random and unannounced sampling of serum can help discover non-compliance. Resistance can be addressed by escalating the dose to determine a sufficient dose to normalize TSH; on occasions, other forms of thyroid hormone are needed for cases of resistance.

In cases of central hypothyroidism, assessment of the adrenal axis should be performed prior to starting levothyroxine to avoid precipitating adrenal crisis.

OUTCOME

There have been numerous studies of cognitive and developmental outcome of children identified with congenital hypothyroidism by newborn screening, and all have demonstrated excellent neurodevelopment and growth when individuals were treated early and with sufficient thyroxine (23,78–89). For the most profoundly hypothyroid cases (athyreosis, maternal antibodies, very low T_4 and high TSH, delayed bone age at diagnosis), there are certain cognitive defects that persist despite adequate treatment, presumably attributable to maternal and fetal hypothyroxinemia. While IQ test scores are generally comparable compared to controls and siblings, there can be subtle defects in memory, attention and visual-spatial processing (82). These defects have not been found in cases of ectopic gland, presumably because there was sufficient thyroid hormone production by the partial gland.

More recent studies of outcome continue to support the notion that early and high thyroxine dosages will yield the maximal outcome, and if possible, treatment should be initiated before 2 wk-of-age.

There are theoretical risks of overtreatment based on the clinical course of neonatal Graves' disease, which can be associated with craniosynostosis, tachycardia, and supraventricular tachyarrythmias, poor weight gain and hyperirritability, and gut hypermotility. However, thyroxine treatment of congenital hypothyroidism does not increase the risk of craniosynostosis or superventricular tachyarrythmias (86), most likely because thyroxine is administered as T_4, which is converted to T_3. Even with high T_4, the T_3 is usually not elevated. Mild effects of excess thyroxine can occur with prolonged high T_4 doses, but in general, these affects are of little clinical consequence.

Thyroid Functional Outcome (Does Treatment Always Need to be Lifelong?)

Since the critical period of thyroid hormone dependent brain development is from fetal development to postnatal age 3 yr, the recommendation is that thyroxine not be withdrawn until after the third birthday. For children confirmed to have ectopic or athyreotic hypothyroidism, no detectable thyroglobulin (prior to starting thyroxine), and for children in whom TSH elevation (>10) has occurred while on thyroxine after 1 yr-of-age, there is no reason to attempt discontinuation of thyroxine. For the remainder of children treated with thyroxine, at the third birthday thyroxine can be discontinued or halved in dose for 30 d with serum thyroxine and TSH determination at that time (90). An elevation of TSH confirms the need for continued thyroxine. If the dose was halved and there was no TSH elevation, the dose should be discontinued for 30 d with repeat thyroid studies. Once discontinuing thyroxine, it is important to advise of the signs and symptoms of hypothyroidism. If they develop, or there are any growth issues, repeat thyroid testing should be performed. Transient hypothyroidism occurs in 5–20% of cases and is more likely in cases of mild newborn screening TSH elevations, children with other malformations, children of mothers with Hashimoto's disease (and presumably transference of maternal antibodies to the baby), and former premature infants.

A more recently recognized area for concern and possible screening is maternal thyroid status early in pregnancy when the developing fetus is dependent on transplacental passage of thyroid hormone (25,26).

SUMMARY

Neurocognitive development, hearing and growth are dependent on sufficient thyroid hormone in fetal, and early child development. Iodine deficiency can affect maternal, fetal and childhood thyroid function and remains the leading cause worldwide for treatable mental retardation. At birth, there may be few signs or symptoms of hypothyroidism, making newborn screening for thyroid function a critical step in detecting congenital hypothyroidism, which is a treatable condition with normal or near normal developmental outcome if sufficient levothyroxine is given early. Individuals at risk for suboptimal outcome are those whose maternal thyroxine supply was insufficient *in utero*, and those whose diagnosis of hypothyroidism was delayed or incompletely treated.

Some children, despite in range newborn screening thyroid tests will develop TSH elevations later, and thus any signs or symptoms compatible with hypothyroidism should be pursued with thyroid testing, regardless of the newborn screening thyroid results.

REFERENCES

1. Delange F. Screening for congenital hypothyroidism used as an indicator of the degree of iodine deficiency and of its control. Thyroid 1998;8(12):1185–1192.
2. Dunn JT. Editorial: What's Happening to Our Iodine? J Clin Endocrinol Metab 1998;83:3398–4000.
3. Hollowell JG, Staehling NW, Hannon H, et al. Iodine Nutrition in the United States. Trends and Public Health Implications: Iodine Excretion Data from National Health and Nutrition Examination Surveys I and III (1971–1974 and 1988–1994. J Clin Endocrinol Metab 1998;83:3401–3408.
4. Waller DK, Anderson JL, Lorey F, Cunningham GC. Risk factors for congenital hypothyroidism: An investigation of infant's birth weight, ethnicity, and gender in California, 1990–1998. Teratology 2000;62(1):36–41.
5. LaFranchi S. Congenital hypothyroidism: etiologies, diagnosis, and management. Thyroid 1999;9(7):735–40.
6. Bongers-Schokking JJ, Koot HM, Wiersma D, Verkerk PH, de Muinck Keizer-Schrama SMPF. Influence of timing and dose of thyroid hormone replacement on development in infants with congenital hypothyroidism. J Pediatr 2000;136:292–297.
7. Stoll C, Dott B, Alembik Y, Koehl C. Congenital anomalies associated with congenital hypothyroidism. Ann Genet 1999;42(1):17–20.
8. Chao T, Wang JR, Hwang B. Congenital hypothyroidism and concomitant anomalies. J Pediatr Endocrinol Metab 1997;10(2):217–221.
9. Oakley GA, Muir T, Ray M, Girdwood RW, Kennedy R, Donaldson MD. Increased incidence of congenital malformations in children with transient thyroid-stimulating hormone elevation on neonatal screening. J Pediatr 1998;132(4):726–730.
10. Roberts HE, Moore CA, Fernhoff PM, Brown AL, Khoury MJ. Population study of congenital hypothyroidism and associated birth defects, Atlanta, 1979–1992. Am J Med Genet 1997;71(1):29–32.
11. Mikai K, Connelly JF, Foley TP Jr, et al. An analysis of the variation of incidences of congenital dysgenetic hypothyroidism in various countries. Endocrinol Jpn 1984;31(1):77–81.
12. Greig WR, Henderson AS, Boyle JA, McGirr EM, Hutchinson JH. Thyroid dysgenesis in two pairs of monozygotic twins and in a mother and child. J Clin Endocrinol Metab 1966;26(12):1309–1316.
13. Macchia PE, Felice MD, Lauro RD. Molecular genetics of congenital hypothyroidism. Curr Opin Genet Dev 1999;9(3):289–294.
14. Macchia PE, Mattei MG, Lapi P, Fenzi G, Di Lauro R. Cloning, chromosomal localization and identification of polymorphisms in the human thyroid transcription factor 2 gene (TITF2). Biochimie 1999;81(5):433–440.
15. Macchia PE. Recent advances in understanding the molecular basis of primary congenital hypothyroidism. Mol Med Today 2000;6(1):36–42.
16. Bakker B, Bikker H, Vulsma T, de Randamie JS, Wiedijk BM, De Vijlder JJ. Two decades of screening for congenital hypothyroidism in The Netherlands: TPO gene mutations in total iodide organification defects (an update). J Clin Endocrinol Metab 2000;85(10):3708–3712.
17. Tatsumi K, Miyai K, Amino N. Genetic basis of congenital hypothyroidism: abnormalities in the TSHbeta gene, the PIT1 gene, and the NIS gene. Clin Chem Lab Med 1998;36(8):659–662
18. Tonacchera M, Agretti P, Pinchera A, et al. Congenital hypothyroidism with impaired thyroid response to thyrotropin (TSH) and absent circulating thyroglobulin: evidence for a new inactivating mutation of the TSH receptor gene. J Clin Endocrinol Metab 2000;85(3):1001–1008.
19. Tiosano D, Pannain S, Vassart G, et al. The hypothyroidism in an inbred kindred with congenital thyroid hormone and glucocorticoid deficiency is due to a mutation producing a truncated thyrotropin receptor. Thyroid 1999;9(9):887–894.
20. Kosugi S, Bhayana S, Dean HJ. A novel mutation in the sodium/iodide symporter gene in the largest family with iodide transport defect. J Clin Endocrinol Metab 1999;84(9):3248–3253.
21. Bieberman H, Liesenkotter KP, Emeis M, Oblanden M, Gruters A. Severe congenital hypothyroidism due to a homozygous mutation of the beta TSH gene. Pediatr Res 1999;46(2):170–173.
22. Gruters A, Kohler B, Wolf A, et al. Screening for mutations of the human thyroid peroxidase gene in patients with congenital hypothyroidism. Exp Clin Cndocrinol Diabetes 1996;104(Suppl 4):121–123.
23. Macchia PE, Lapi P, Krude H, et al. PAX8 mutations associated with congenital hypothyroidism caused by thyroid dysgenesis. Nat Genet 1998;19(1):83–86.

24. Fisher DA. The importance of early management in optimizing IQ in infants with congenital hypothyroidism. J Pediatr 2000;136:273–274.
25. Utiger RD. Maternal Hypothyroidism and Fetal Development. N Engl J Med 1999;341(8):601–602.
26. Haddow JE, Palomaki GE, Allan WC, et al. Thyroid Deficiency During Pregnancy and Subsequent Neuropsychological Development of the Child. N Engl J Med 1999;341(8):549–555.
27. Yasuda T, Ohnishi H, Wataki K, Minagawa M, Minamitani K, Niimi H. Outcome of a baby born from a mother with acquired juvenile hypothyroidism having undetectable thyroid hormone concentrations. J Clin Endocrinol Metab 1999;84(8):2630–2632.
28. Jagannathan NR, Tandon N, Raghunathan P, Kochupillai N. Reversal of abnormalities of myelination by thyroxine therapy in congenital hypothyroidism: localized in vivo proton magnetic resonance spectroscopy (MRS) study. Brain Res Dev Brain Res 1998;109(2):179–186.
29. Masuno M, Imaizumi K, Okada T, et al. Young-Simpson syndrome: further delineation of a distinct syndrome with congenital hypothyroidism, congenital heart defects, facial dysmorphism, and mental retardation. Am J Med Genet 1999;84(1):8–11.
30. Siragusa V, Boffelli S, Weber G, et al. Brain magnetic resonance imaging in congenital hypothyroid infants at diagnosis. Thyroid 1997;7(5):761–764.
31. Price DA, Ehrlich RM, Walfish PG. Congenital hypothyroidism. Clinical and laboratory characteristics in infants detected by neonatal screening. Arch Dis Child 1981;56(11):845–851.
32. Larsson A, Ljunggren JG, Ekman K, Nilsson A, Olin P, Bodegard G. Screening for congenital hypothyroidism. II. Clinical findings in infants with positive screening tests. Acta Paediatr Scand 1981;70(2):147–53.
33. Alm J, Hagenfeldt L, Larsson A, Lundberg K. Incidence of congenital hypothyroidism: retrospective study of neonatal laboratory screening versus clinical symptoms as indicators leading to diagnosis. Br Med J (Clin Res Ed) 1984;289(6453):1171–1175.
34. Devos H, Rodd C, Gagne N, Laframboise R, Van Vliet G. A search for the possible molecular mechanisms of thyroid dysgenesis: sex ratios and associated malformations. J Clin Endocrinol Metab 1999;84(7):2502–2506.
35. Willnow S, Kiess W, Butenandt O, et al. Endocrine disorders in septo-optic dysplasia (De Morsier syndrome)—evaluation and follow up of 18 patients. Eur J Pediatr 1996;155(3):179–184.
36. Aynaci FM, Orhan F, Celep F, Karaguzel A. Frequency of cardiovascular and gastrointestinal malformations, leukemia and hypothyroidism in children with Down syndrome in Trabzon, Turkey. Turk J Pediatr 1998;40(1):103–109.
37. Fort P, Lifshitz F, Bellisario R, et al. Abnormalities of thyroid function in infants with Down syndrome. J Pediatr 1984;104(4):545–549.
38. Bucci I, Napolitano G, Giuliani C, et al. Zinc sulfate supplementation improves thyroid function in hypozincemic Down children. Biol trace Elem Res 1999;67(3):257–268.
39. Selikowitz M. A five-year longitudinal study of thyroid function in children with Down syndrome. Dev Med Child Neurol 1993;35(5):396–401.
40. Cutler AT, Benezra-Obeiter R, Brink SJ. Thyroid function in young children with Down syndrome. Am J Dis Child 1986;140(5):479–483.
41. Rooney S, Walsh E. Prevalence of abnormal thyroid function tests in a Down's syndrome population. Ir J Med Sci 1997;166(2):80–82.
42. Pueschel SM, Jackson IM, Giesswein P, Dean MK, Pezzullo JC. Thyroid function in Down syndrome. Res Dev Disabil 1991;12(3):287–296.
43. Guthrie R, Susi A. 1963. A simple phenylalanine method for detecting phenylketonuria in large populations of newborn infants. Pediatrics 32:338–343.
44. Dussault JH, Laberge C. A new method for detection of hypothyroidism in the newborn. Clin Res 1972;20:918.
45. Klein AH, Agustin AV, Foley TP Jr. Successful screening for congenital hypothyroidism. Lancet 1974;2:77.
46. Hsiao PH, Chiu YN, Tsai WY, Su SC, Lee JS, Soong WT. Intellectual outcomes of patients with congenital hypothyroidism not detected by neonatal screening. J Formos Med Assoc 1999;98(7):512–515.
47. Fisher DA, Dussault JH, Foley TP Jr, et al. Screening for congenital hypothyroidism: results of screening one million North American infants. J Pediatr 1979;94(5):700–705.

48. Barden HS, Kessel R. The costs and benefits of screening for congenital hypothyroidism in Wisconsin. Soc Biol 1984;31(3–4):185–200.
49. Larson C, Hermos RJ, Rojas D, Mitchell ML. Rising Incidence of Congenital Hypothyroidism Detected by Primary T_4 Screening in Massachusetts. Presented June 1999, International Society for Neonatal Screening, Stockholm.
50. Hanna CE, Krainz PL, Skeels MR, et al. Detection of congenital hypopituitary hypothyroidism: Ten year experience in The Northwest Regional Screening Program. J Pediatr 1986;109(6):959–964.
51. Hunter MK, Mandel SH, Sesser DE, Miyahira RS, Rien L, Skeels MR, LaFranchi SH. Follow-up of newborns with low thyroxine and nonelevated thyroid-stimulating hormone-screening concentrations: Results of the 20-year experience in the Northwest Regional Newborn Screening Program. J Pediatr 1998;132(1):70–74.
52. Mandel S, Hanna C, Boston B, Sesser D, LaFranchi S. Thyroxine-binding globulin deficiency detected by newborn screening. J Pediatr 1993;122(2):227–230.
53. Wang ST, Pizzolato S, Demshar HP. Diagnostic effectiveness of TSH screening and of T_4 with secondary TSH screening for newborn congenital hypothyroidism. Clin Chim Acta 1998;22: 274(2):151–158.
54. Dussault JH, Morissette J. Higher sensitivity of primary thyrotropin in screening for congenital hypothyroidism: a myth? J Clin Endocrinol Metab 1983;56(4):849–852.
55. Gruters A, Liesenkotter KP, Zapico M, Jenner A, Dutting C, Pfeiffer E, Lehmkuhl U. Results of the screening program for congenital hypothyroidism in Berlin (1978–1995). Exp Clin Endocrinol Diabetes 1997;105(Suppl 4):28–31.
56. Gruneiro-Papendieck L, Prieto L, Chiesa A, Bengolea S, Bossi G, Bergada C. Usefulness of thyroxine and free thyroxine filter paper measurements in neonatal screening for congenital hypothyroidism of preterm babies. J Med Screen 2000;7(2):78–81.
57. Zurakowski D, DiCanzio J, Majzoub JA. Pediatric Reference Intervals for Serum Thyroxine, Triiodothyronine, Thyrotropin, and Free Thyroxine. Clin Chem 1999;45(7):1087–1091.
58. Dussault JH, Morissette J, Laberge C. Blood thyroxine concentration is lower in low-birth-weight infants. Clin Chem 1979;25(12):2047–2049.
59. Kok JH, Hart G, Endert E, Koppe JG, de Vijlder JJ. Normal ranges of T_4 screening values in low birthweight infants. Arch Dis Child 1983;58(3):190–194.
60. Fisher DA. Thyroid function in very low birthweight infants. Clin Endocrinol 1997;47:1–3.
61. Levy HL. Is early discharge a problem for newborn screening? Early Hospital Discharge: Impact on Newborn Screening, Ed. K Pass, HL Levy, 1995, pp. 23–30. Atlanta: CORN.
62. Hermos R, Rojas D, Delaney A, et al. Rising Mean Thyroxine (T_4) Screening in Massachusetts Newborns. Presented at National Newborn Screening Conference 1999.
63. Sfakianakis GN, Ezuddin SH, Sanchez JE, Eidson M, Cleveland W. Pertechnetate scintigraphy in primary hypothyroidism. J Nucl Med 1999;40(5):799–804.
64. Newborn Screening for Congenital Hypothyroidism: Recommended Guidelines. Pediatrics 1993;91(6):1203–1209.
65. Mandel SJ, Hermos RJ, Lason CA, Prigozhana AB, Rojas DA, Mitchell ML. Late onset hypothyroidism and the very low birthweight infant. Thyroid 2000;10(8):693–695.
66. Brown RS, Bellisario RL, Botero D, et al. Incidence of transient congenital hypothyroidism due to maternal thyrotropin receptor-blocking antibodies in over one million babies. J Clin Endocrinol Metab 1996;81(3):1147–1151.
67. Hack M, Friedman H, Fanaroff AA. Outcomes of Extremely Low Birth Weight Infants. Pediatrics 1996;98(5):931–937.
68. Halsey CL, Collin MF, Anderson CL. Extremely Low-birth-weight Children and Their Peers: A Comparison of School-age Outcomes. Arch Pediatr Adolesc Med 1996;150:790–794.
69. Reuss ML, Leviton A, Paneth N, Susser M. Thyroxine Values from Newborn Screening of 919 Infants Born before 29 Weeks' Gestation. Am J Public Health 1997;87:1693–1697.
70. Paul DA, Leef KH, Stefano JL, Bartoshesky L. Low Serum Thyroxine on Initial Newborn Screening Is Associated With Intraventricular Hemorrhage and Death in Very Low Birth Weight Infants. Pediatrics 1998;101(5):903–907.
71. Van Wassenaer AG, Kok JH, de Vijlder JJ, et al. Effects of thyroxine supplementation on neurologic development in infants born at less than 30 weeks' gestation. N Engl J Med 1997;336(1):21–26.

72. Fisher DA. Hypothyroxinemia in premature infants: is thyroxine treatment necessary? Thyroid 1999;9(7):715–720.
73. Bettendorf M, Schmidt KG, Grulich-Henn J, Ulmer HE, Heinrich UE. Tri-iodothyronine treatment in children after cardiac surgery: a double-blind, randomized, placebo-controlled study. Lancet 2000;356(9229):529–534.
74. Toft AD. Thyroid hormone replacement-one hormone or two? N Engl J Med 1999;340(6):469–470.
75. Bunevicius R, Kazanavicius G, Zalinkevicius R, Prange AJ. Effects of thyroxine as compared with thyroxine plus triodothyronine in patients with hypothyroidism. N Engl J Med 1999;340(6):424–429.
76. Ohmori M, Harada K, Tsuruoka S, Sugimoto K, Kobayashi E, Fujimura A. Levothyroxine-induced liver dysfunction in a primary hypothyroid patient. Endocrinol J 1999;46(4):579–583.
77. Revised guidelines for neonatal screening programmes for primary congenital hypothyroidism. Working Group on Neonatal Screening of the European Society for Paediatric Endocrinology. Horm Res 1999;52(1):49–52
78. Bargagna S, Canepa G, Costagli C, et al. Neuropsychological follow-up in early-treated congenital hypothyroidism: a problem-oriented approach. Thyroid 2000;10(3):243–249.
79. Bargagna S, Dinetti D, Pinchera A, et al. School attainments in children with congenital hypothyroidism detected by neonatal screening and treated early in life. Eur J Endocrinol 1999;140(5):407–413.
80. Barnes ND. Screening for congenital hypothyroidism: the first decade. Arch Dis Child 1985;60(6):587–592.
81. New England Congenital Hypothyroidism Collaborative. Neonatal hypothyroidism screening: status of patients at 6 years of age. J Pediatr 1985;107(6):915–919
82. Rovet JF, Ehrlich R. Psychoeducational outcome in children with early-treated congenital hypothyroidism. Pediatrics 2000;105(3 Pt 1):515–522.
83. Rovet JF. Long-term neuropsychological sequelae of early-treated congenital hypothyroidism: effects in adolescence. Acta Paediatr Suppl 1999;88(432):88–95.
84. Rovet JF. Congenital hypothyroidism: long-term outcome. Thyroid 1999;9(7):741–748.
85. Salerno M, Militerni R, Di Maio S, Bravaccio C, Gasparini N, Tenore A. Eur J Endocrinol 1999;141(2):105–10.
86. Garcia M, Calzada-Leon R, Perez J, et al. Longitudinal assessment of $L-T_4$ therapy for congenital hypothyroidism: differences between athyreosis vs ectopia and delayed vs normal bone age. J Pediatr Endocrinol Metab 2000;13(1):63–69.
87. Report of the New England Regional Screening Program and the New England Congenital Hypothyroidism Collaborative. Pitfalls in screening for neonatal hypothyroidism. Pediatrics 1982;70(1):16–20.
88. New England Congenital Hypothyroidism Collaborative. Effects of neonatal screening for hypothyroidism: prevention of mental retardation by treatment before clinical manifestations. Lancet 1981;2(8255):1095–1098.
89. Mitchell ML, Larsen PR, Levy HL, Bennett AJ, Madoff MA. Screening for congenital hypothyroidism. Results in the newborn population of New England. JAMA 1978;239(22):2348–2351.
90. Davy T, Daneman D, Walfish PG, Ehrlich RM. Congenital hypothyropidism. The effect of stopping treatment at 3 years of age. Am J Dis Child 1985;139(10):1028–1030.

17 Autoimmune Thyroid Disease

*Stephen A. Huang, MD
and P. Reed Larsen, MD*

CONTENTS

INTRODUCTION
CHRONIC AUTOIMMUNE THYROIDITIS
GRAVES' DISEASE
REFERENCES

INTRODUCTION

Autoimmune thyroid disease is the most common autoimmune condition, affecting approximately 2% of the female population and 0.2% of the male population *(1)*. Its overall prevalence peaks in adulthood, but it is also the most common etiology of acquired thyroid dysfunction in pediatrics *(2,3)*. This chapter presents a summary of autoimmune thyroid disease, discussing first chronic autoimmune thyroiditis and then Graves' disease, with an emphasis on their clinical management. Optimal quantities of thyroid hormone are critical to neurodevelopment and growth. By maintaining an appropriate index of suspicion, the clinician can often recognize thyroid dysfunction in its early stages.

CHRONIC AUTOIMMUNE THYROIDITIS

The childhood prevalence of chronic autoimmune thyroiditis peaks in early- to midpuberty and a female preponderance of 2:1 has been reported *(4)*. Presentation is rare under the age of 3 yr, but cases have been described even in infancy *(5,6)*.

Terminology and Definitions

In 1912, Hashimoto described four women with thyromegaly and the apparent transformation of thyroid into lymphoid tissue ("struma lymphomatosa"). These patients comprise the first report of Hashimoto's disease, which we now recognize as a form of chronic autoimmune thyroiditis. Improvements in the measurement of circulating autoantibodies have obviated the need for biopsy in the diagnosis of autoimmune thyroid disease, and the nomenclature itself has been redefined in recent years (Table 1) *(7,8)*. The term thyroiditis is defined as evidence of "intrathyroidal lymphocytic infiltration" with or without follicular damage. Two types of chronic autoimmune thyroiditis (also

From: *Contemporary Endocrinology: Pediatric Endocrinology: A Practical Clinical Guide*
Edited by: S. Radovick and M. H. MacGillivray © Humana Press Inc., Totowa, NJ

Table 1
Classification of Autoimmune Thyroiditis[a]

Type 1 Autoimmune Thyroiditis (Hashimoto's Disease Type 1)
- 1A Goitrous
- 1B Nongoitrous

Status: Euthyroid with normal TSH.

Type 2 Autoimmune Thyroiditis (Hashimoto's Disease Type 2)
- 2A Goitrous (classic Hashimoto's disease)
- 2B Nongoitrous (primary myxoedema, atrophic thyroiditis)

Status: Persistent hypothyroidism with increased TSH.
- 2C Transient aggravation of thyroiditis (example post-partum thyroiditis)

Status: May start as transient, low RAIU thyrotoxicosis, followed by transient hypothyroidism.

Type 3 Autoimmune Thyroiditis (Graves' Disease)
- 3A Hyperthyroid Graves' disease
- 3B Euthyroid Graves' disease

Status: Hyperthyroid or euthyroid with suppressed TSH. Stimulatory autoantibodies to the TSH receptor are present (autoantibodies to thyroglobulin and TPO are also usually present).
- 3C Hypothyroid Graves' disease

Status: Orbitopathy with hypothyroidism. Diagnostic levels of autoantibodies to the TSH receptor (blocking or stimulating) may be detected (autoantibodies to Tg and TPO are also usually present)

[a]Adapted from Williams Textbook of Endocrinology *(8)*.

known as chronic lymphocytic thyroiditis) are causes of persistent hypothyroidism, Hashimoto's disease (goitrous form, Type 2A) and atrophic thyroiditis (nongoitrous form, Type 2B). Both are characterized by circulating thyroid autoantibodies and varying degrees of thyroid dysfunction, differing only by the presence or absence of goiter. The transient disorder of postpartum thyroiditis is believed to be a manifestation of chronic autoimmune thyroiditis (Type 2C) *(9)*. The term chronic autoimmune thyroiditis does not include subacute (deQuervain's) thyroiditis.

Pathophysiology

The activation of CD4 (helper) T-lymphocytes specific for thyroid antigens is believed to be the first step in pathogenesis. Once activated, self-reactive CD4 T cells recruit cytotoxic CD8 T cells as well as autoreactive B cells into the thyroid. The three main targets of thyroid antibodies are thyroglobulin (TG), thyroid peroxidase (TPO), and the thyrotropin receptor (TR). Anti-TPO antibodies have been shown to inhibit the activity of thyroid peroxidase in vitro, but direct killing by CD8 T cells is believed to be the main mechanism of hypothyroidism in vivo *(9)*. Anti-TSH receptor antibodies may contribute to hypothyroidism in a minority of adult patients with the atrophic form of chronic autoimmune thyroiditis, but this has not been proven in children *(10,11)*.

Histologically, goitrous autoimmune thyroiditis is characterized by diffuse lymphocytic infiltration with occasional germinal centers. Thyroid follicles may be reduced in size and contain sparse colloid. Individual thyroid cells are often enlarged with oxyphilic cytoplasm (the Hurthle or Askanazy cell). In contrast, the gland of atrophic autoimmune thyroiditis is small, with lymphocytic infiltration and fibrous replacement of the parenchyma.

Table 2
Symptoms and Signs of Hypothyroidism

Goiter
Growth retardation
Skeletal maturational delay
Pubertal disorders (delay or pseudoprecocity)
Slowed mentation (lethargy and impaired school performance)
Fatigue
Bradycardia (decreased cardiac output)
Constipation
Cold intolerance
Hypothermia
Fluid retention and weight gain (impaired renal free water clearance)
Dry, sallow skin
Delayed deep tendon reflexes

Clinical Presentation

The presentation of chronic autoimmune thyroiditis includes either hypothyroidism, goiter, or both. A goiter or firm thyroid is the first physical sign of chronic autoimmune thyroiditis. Thyromegaly is typically diffuse with a "pebbly" or "seedy" surface that evolves into a firm and nodular consistency *(12)*. As the disease progresses, subclinical and then clinical hypothyroidism appears. Symptoms of hypothyroidism may be subtle, even with marked biochemical derangement (Table 2). The initial history should include inquiries into energy level, sleep pattern, menses, cold intolerance, and school performance. In addition to palpation of the thyroid, assessment of the extraocular movements, fluid status, and deep tendon reflexes are important components of the physical examination. Chronic autoimmune thyroiditis may be the initial presentation of an autoimmune polyglandular syndrome, and the possibility of coexisting autoimmune diseases such as type 1 diabetes, Addison's disease, and pernicious anemia must be addressed by the past medical history and the review of systems.

Growth and pubertal development may be deranged. Similar to other endocrine causes of growth failure, linear progression is compromised to a greater degree than weight gain, and the bone age is delayed (Fig. 1) *(13,14)*. Hypothyroidism typically causes pubertal delay, but may also induce a syndrome of pseudoprecocity manifested as testicular enlargement in boys and breast enlargement and vaginal bleeding in girls *(15–17)*. This differs clinically from true precocity by the absence of accelerated bone maturation and linear growth (Table 2).

Diagnosis

The serum thyrotropin (TSH) concentration is elevated in primary hypothyroidism and its determination is an appropriate screen for thyroid dysfunction. If the differential diagnosis includes central hypothyroidism or if the overall suspicion for hypothyroidism is high, a free T_4 (or fT_4I) should be included on the initial screen. In mild hypothyroidism, serum T_3 can remain in the normal range due to the increased conversion of T_4 to T_3 by type 2 deiodinase and the preferential secretion of T_3 by residual thyroid tissue under the influence of hyperthyrotropinemia *(18,19)*. For these reasons, measurement of

PATIENT 1:

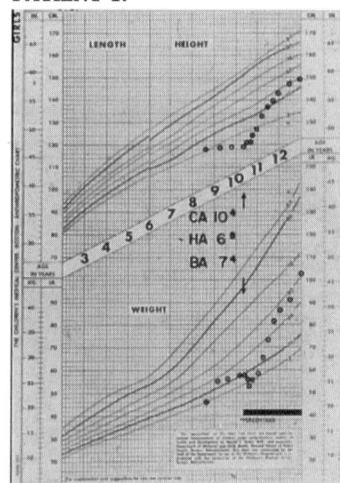
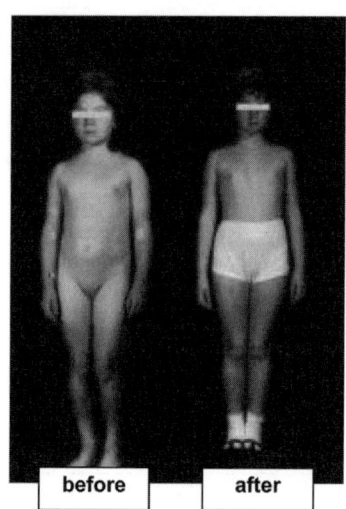

PATIENT 2:

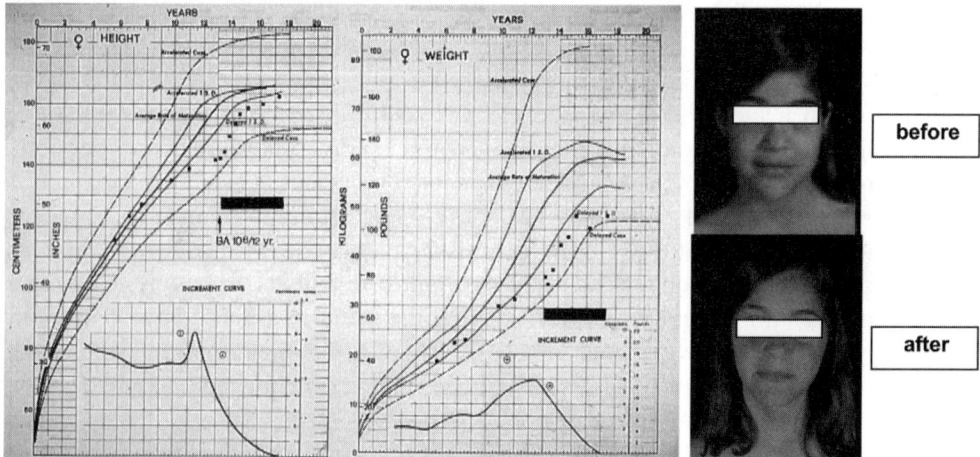

Fig. 1. Two Patients with Chronic Autoimmune Thyroiditis. The growth failure of hypothyroidism characteristically affects height to a greater degree than weight. The initiation of thyroid hormone replacement (solid black bar) is associated with an acute drop in weight due to the mobilization of myxedematous fluid, followed by an acceleration in linear progression or "catch-up growth." Breast development was noted in Patient 1 which regressed after hypothyroidism was corrected. The interval between pre-therapy and post-therapy photographs is one year for patient 1 and six months for patient 2. Charts and photographs are from the files of John F. Crigler, Chief Emeritus of Children's Hospital Endocrinology in Boston.

the serum T_3 concentration is not a useful test in the diagnosis or monitoring of patients with primary hypothyroidism.

The presence of goiter or hyperthyrotropinemia should prompt the measurement of anti-TPO antibodies. Anti-TPO antibodies are the most sensitive screen for chronic autoimmune thyroiditis (20). Little further benefit is gained by the additional measurement of anti-thyroglobulin antibodies, although they may be added if anti-TPO titers are negative *(21)*. The typical patient with hypothyroidism secondary to chronic autoimmune thyroiditis will have an elevated TSH (over 10 μU/mL), a low fT_4I, and positive anti-TPO antibodies. In early stages of the disease, TSH may be normal and anti-TPO antibodies may be positive with goiter (Type 1A). Later, TSH elevation becomes modest (5–10 μU/mL) with a normal fT_4I (biochemical or subclinical hypothyroidism). Up to 90% of patients with hypothyroidism secondary to autoimmune thyroiditis are anti-TPO antibody positive. It should be noted that 10–15% of the general population are positive for anti-TPO antibodies and that low titers (less than 1/100 by agglutination methods or less than 100 IU/L by immunoassays) are less specific for autoimmune thyroid disease *(1)*. If anti-TPO antibodies are absent, less common etiologies of primary hypothyroidism such as transient hypothyroidism (post subacute thyroiditis), external irradiation, and consumptive hypothyroidism should be considered *(22–24)*.

Subclinical hypothyroidism is defined as TSH elevation with normal concentrations of circulating thyroid hormones (T_4 and T_3). The log-linear relationship between serum TSH and free T_4 explains how small reductions in serum free T_4 lead to large deviations in TSH. The majority of these patients are asymptomatic, but studies in the adult population suggest that individuals with the combined risk factors of hyperthyrotropinemia and positive thyroid antibodies (anti-thyroglobulin or anti-TPO) are at high risk for progression to overt hypothyroidism. For this reason, it is our practice to recommend thyroid hormone replacement in all patients with TSH values >10 μU/mL or with TSH values >5 μU/mL in combination with goiter or thyroid autoantibodies *(25)*. Given the critical importance of thyroid hormone in neurodevelopment, persistent hyperthyrotropinemia in infancy should be empirically treated and a trial with reduced therapy considered after the age of 2–3 yr. Similarly, the presence of growth failure may lower the threshold to initiate replacement for persistent hyperthyrotropinemia.

Therapy

Levothyroxine (L-T_4) is the replacement of choice. There are virtually no adverse reactions and its long half-life of 5–7 d allows the convenience of daily administration. Although very rare, case reports have described the development of pseudotumor cerebri around the initiation of levothyroxine in a small number of school-age children *(26)*. Some authors advocate a graded approach to the initiation of levothyroxine *(27)*. Alternatively, a starting dose can be estimated based upon the patient's age and ideal body weight (Table 3) *(4)*. The medication's long half-life insures a gradual equilibration over the course of 5–6 wk. Average daily requirements approximate 100 μg/m^2 per day, but dosing will ultimately be individualized on the basis of biochemical monitoring *(4)*. TSH normalization is the goal of replacement and we aim for a target range of 0.5–3 μU/mL. This will usually be associated with a free T_4 in the upper half of the normal range. Thyroid function tests should be obtained 6 wk after the initiation or adjustment of the levothyroxine dosage. Growth and sexual development should be followed systematically as in any pediatric patient. Once biochemical euthyroidism has been achieved, TSH can be monitored every 4–6 mo in the growing child and yearly once final height has been attained. If noncompliance is suspected as the cause of treatment failure, a free T_4 (or fT_4I) may be measured as a serum TSH greater than twice normal in the context of a normal free T_4 suggests intermittent omission of the medication.

Table 3
Levothyroxine Replacement Doses[a]

Recommended L-T_4 Treatment Doses	
AGE	L-T_4 Dose (µg/kg)
0–3 mo	10–15
3–6 mo	8–10
6–12 mo	6–8
1–3 yr	4–6
3–10 yr	3–4
10–15 yr	2–4
>15 yr	2–3
Adult	1.6

[a] Adapted from LaFranchi, Pediatric Annals 1992 (4).

A variety of conditions or drugs may alter levothyroxine requirements (Table 4). In theory, levothyroxine should be administered at least 30 min before eating or any medication known to impair its absorption. However, from a practical viewpoint, the most important goal is to establish a regular time for levothyroxine administration. Parents of children with chronic autoimmune thyroiditis should be advised that the hypothyroidism will likely be permanent, although exceptions have been reported (28,29). The monitoring of thyroid function is lifelong. A TSH should be checked if pregnancy is diagnosed and the frequency of monitoring should be increased. Levothyroxine requirements increase by an average of 45% during gestation and untreated maternal hypothyroidism may adversely affect the intellectual development of the fetus (25,30).

GRAVES' DISEASE

Robert Graves reported the clinical syndrome of goiter, palpitations, and exophthalmos in 1835. In the adult population, Graves' disease is now recognized as the most prevalent autoimmune disorder in the US, accounting for 60–80% of all patients with hyperthyroidism (31). Hyperthyroidism is relatively rare in children (yearly incidence of 8 per 1,000,000 children less than 15 yr-old and 1 per 1,000,000 children less than 4 yr-old), but Graves' disease is by far the most common etiology (3). Girls are affected four to five times more frequently than boys, although no gender difference is noted under 4 years of age (32,33).

Pathophysiology

Graves' disease shares many features associated with chronic autoimmune thyroiditis, including autoantibodies directed against thyroglobulin, thyroid peroxidase, and the sodium-iodine symporter. Hyperthyroidism is caused by thyroid-stimulating antibodies that bind and activate the thyrotropin receptor, leading to follicular cell hyperplasia and the hypersecretion of thyroid hormone. Lymphocytic infiltration of the thyroid is present,

Table 4
Conditions that Alter Levothyroxine Requirements

Increased levothyroxine requirements

Pregnancy	
Gastrointestinal Disease	Mucosal diseases of the small bowel (e.g., sprue)
	Jejuno-ileal bypass and small bowel resection
	Diabetic diarrhea
Drugs which impair L-T_4 absorption	Cholestyramine
	Sucralfate
	Aluminum hydroxide
	Calcium carbonate
	Ferrous sulfate
Drugs which may enhance CYP3A4 and thereby accelerate levothyroxine clearance	Rifampin
	Carbamazepine
	Phenytoin
	Estrogen (?)
	Sertraline (?)
Drugs which impair T_4 to T_3 conversion	Amiodarone
Conditions which may block Type 1 deiodinase	Selenium deficiency (due to dietary deficiencies as in PKU and cystic fibrosis)
	Cirrhosis

hence its classification as a form of thyroiditis. Occasionally, germinal centers form, which can develop as major sources of intrathyroid autoantibodies. Lymphocytic infiltration and the accumulation of glycosaminoglycans in the orbital connective tissue and skin cause the extrathyroidal manifestations of Graves' ophthalmopathy and dermopathy, respectively.

Clinical Presentation

The presentation of Graves' disease in childhood may be insidious and a careful history will often reveal a several month history of progressive symptoms. Common complaints include nervousness, hyperactivity, heat intolerance, sleep disturbances, and a decline in school performance (Table 5). A goiter is palpable in the majority of cases, characterized by diffuse enlargement which is smooth, firm, and nontender. The pyramidal lobe is often palpable and a bruit may be audible secondary to increased bloodflow through the gland. Extrathyroidal manifestations such as ophthalmopathy and dermopathy are rarer than in adults and tend to be less severe *(32)*. The pediatric literature cites a 25–60% frequency of ocular manifestations, but the majority are mild signs such as lid retraction, "staring", and slight proptosis that can be attributed to the pseudosympathetic hyperactivity of thyrotoxicosis rather than true infiltrative disease of the orbital structures. As expected, these signs improve in most patients after restoration of the euthyroid state *(34)*. Unique to pediatric Graves' disease is the acceleration of linear growth and bone maturation associated with prolonged hyperthyroidism *(35,36)*.

Table 5
Symptoms and Signs of Hyperthyroidism in Children[a]

Goiter
Exophthalmos
Acceleration of linear growth
Nervousness
Increased irritability
Decreased concentration and impaired school performance
Headache
Hyperactivity
Fatigue
Palpitations
Tachycardia
Increased pulse pressure
Hypertension
Heart murmur
Polyphagia
Increased frequency of bowel movements
Weight loss
Heat intolerance
Increased perspiration
Tremor

[a]Adapted from ref. *(50)*.

Diagnosis

The term thyrotoxicosis refers to the manifestations of excessive quantities of circulating thyroid hormone. In contrast, hyperthyroidism refers only to the subset of thyrotoxic diseases which are due to the overproduction of hormone by the thyroid itself. Graves' is the most common etiology of hyperthyroidism and the ability to accurately diagnose it is critical as antithyroid drugs have no role in the treatment of thyrotoxicosis without hyperthyroidism. Thyrotoxicosis is recognized by an elevation of serum free T_4 (or fT_4I) with a decreased serum TSH (typically <0.1 µU/mL). A determination of the fT_3I should be added if TSH is suppressed and the serum free T_4 is normal. In patients with early disease or in iodine-deficient patients, serum free T_4 concentrations may be normal or reduced despite elevated levels of triiodothyronine. These are the only situations in which a serum FT_3I is required to confirm to the diagnosis of thyrotoxicosis. Once biochemical derangement has been documented, it is helpful to address the duration of thyrotoxicosis to facilitate the differentiation of Graves' disease from painless thyroiditis. Onset may be documented by prior laboratory studies or inferred from the history.

The differential diagnosis of thyrotoxicosis includes transient thyroiditis, hyperfunctioning nodule(s), and thyrotoxicosis factitia. In the majority of cases, the presence of a symmetrically enlarged thyroid coupled with the chronicity of symptoms will be adequate to allow a diagnosis, but radionuclide studies using I-123 can provide confirmatory data (Table 6). If thyrotoxicosis has been present for <8 wk, transient thyrotoxicosis secondary to subacute thyroiditis or the thyrotoxic phase of autoimmune/silent thyroiditis should be considered. These forms of thyroiditis are self-limited and refractory to therapy with

Table 6
Differential Diagnosis of Thyrotoxicosis in Children[a]

Causes of Thyrotoxicosis

Thyrotoxicosis associated with sustained hormone overproduction (Hyperthyroidism). High RAIU

Graves' disease
Toxic Multinodular goiter
Toxic adenoma
Increased TSH secretion

Thyrotoxicosis without associated Hyperthyroidism. Low RAIU

Thyrotoxicosis factitia
Subacute thyroiditis
Chronic thyroiditis with transient thyroiditis
   (painless thyroiditis, silent thyroiditis, post-partum thyroiditis)
Ectopic thyroid tissue (struma ovarii, functioning metastatic thyroid cancer)

[a]Adapted ref. *(8)*

---

thionamides. The radioactive iodide uptake (RAIU) will be low, distinguishing them from the more common Graves' disease *(37)*. For thyrotoxicosis present for more than 8 wk, Graves' is by far the most likely etiology. The constellation of thyrotoxicosis, goiter, and orbitopathy is pathognomonic of this condition and no additional laboratory tests or imaging studies are necessary to confirm the diagnosis. If thyromegaly is subtle and eye changes are absent, an I-123 uptake, with or without a scan, should be performed. Autonomous nodules must be large to cause hyperthyroidism (typically 2–3 cm or more in diameter), so radioiodine scanning should be reserved for patients in whom a discrete nodule(s) is palpable. In patients with a toxic nodule, I-123 uptake will localize to the nodule and the signal in the surrounding tissue will be low, secondary to TSH suppression. Thyrotoxicosis factitia can be recognized by a low RAIU and serum thyroglobulin in the presence of thyrotoxicosis and a suppressed TSH.

The sensitivity of serum thyrotropin-receptor antibodies (TRAb) assays is cited to be 75–96% for TBII (a competitive binding assay with TSH) and 85–100% for TSAb measurements (a bioassay of TSH receptor activation) in untreated Graves' disease. A false negative rate of 10–20% has been documented for serum thyrotropin-receptor antibodies in Graves' disease, presumably due to the inadequate sensitivity of the assays or the exclusive intrathyroidal production of autoantibodies *(1,31)*. In practice, the measurement of thyrotropin-receptor antibodies is rarely necessary as the combination of thyrotoxicosis and high RAIU in the absence of a palpable nodule is virtually diagnostic of Graves' disease.

There is a subgroup of patients who have a subnormal but not severely depressed TSH (usually 0.1–0.3 µU/mL) and normal serum concentrations of thyroid hormone. These patients are generally asymptomatic and the term "subclinical hyperthyroidism" has been applied to their condition. The limited screening of TSH determinations in various adult populations indicates a surprisingly high prevalence of 2–16%, although it is unclear how may of these individuals actually have thyroid disease *(38)*. The differential diagnosis is the same as for overt thyrotoxicosis, but the sequelae of untreated subclinical disease in children are poorly defined and no consensus exists as to the indications for therapy *(39)*. In adults over 60 yr-of-age, a low serum TSH concentration has been associated with an increased risk of atrial fibrillation, but no similar risks have been identified in the pediatric population *(40)*. Furthermore, several studies indicate that approximately half of patients with subclinical thyrotoxicosis will experience a spontaneous remission *(41)*. Accordingly, the initial detection of a suppressed TSH concentration without elevated levels of thyroid hormone or associated symptoms should be addressed simply by repeating thyroid function tests in 4–8 wk. Assuming there are no specific risk factors such as a history of cardiac disease, asymptomatic children with subclinical hyperthyroidism can be followed with the expectation that TSH suppression due to transient thyroiditis will resolve spontaneously and that due to Graves' disease or autonomous secretion will declare itself over time.

Antithyroid Medications

The treatment of Graves' hyperthyroidism may be divided into two categories, antithyroid medications and definitive therapy. The thionamide derivatives, Tapazole (MMI) and propylthiouracil (PTU), are the most commonly used antithyroid drugs *(42)*. Both block thyroid hormone biosynthesis and PTU, when used at doses over 450–600 mg per day, has the additional action of inhibiting the extrathyroidal conversion of T_4 to T_3 *(8,43)*. The recommended starting dose is 0.5–1.0 mg/kg per day for MMI and 5–10 mg/kg per day for PTU. For adolescent patients, the following rule of thumb is helpful in the determination of a starting dose:

Starting dose of Tapazole for adolescent patients

Free T_4 index or free T_4	*Tapazole dose*
<1.5 times the upper limit of normal range	10 mg qd
1.5 to 2 times the upper limit of normal range	10 mg bid
>2 times the upper limit of normal range	20 mg bid

Due to its longer half-life, MMI can be administered qd or bid, compared to the tid dosing of PTU. Furthermore, the clinical therapeutic equivalence of 10 mg of Tapazole (one tablet) and 150 mg of PTU (three tablets) facilitates a simpler dosing regimen. Unless the small size of a pediatric patient complicates the titration of MMI dosing, most families appreciate the convenience of once daily administration and it is our first choice for initial therapy. For the specific situations of severe hyperthyroidism or thyroid storm, PTU is the preferred thionamide because of its blockade of T_4 to T_3 conversion through the inhibition of type 1 iodothyronine deiodinase *(8)*. In such patients, a combination of high dose PTU (up to 1200 mg per day divided q 6 h) and inorganic iodine (SSKI three drops po bid for 5–10 d) will speed the fall in circulating thyroid hormones.

Some authors have advocated a "block and replace" strategy of high-dose antithyroid medication (to suppress all endogenous thyroxine secretion) combined with levothyroxine replacement. One report described a lower frequency of recurrence with this approach *(44)*. However, all subsequent studies have failed to duplicate this finding *(45,46)*. This approach offers no therapeutic advantage and is more complicated. For the purpose of simplifying the patient's regimen and minimizing the risk of adverse drug reactions, we prefer monotherapy with a single antithyroid medication. After the fT_4I has fallen to the upper end of normal range, the dose of antithyroid drug should be decreased by one half or one third. Further dose adjustments are guided by serial thyroid function tests, initially relying upon the FT_4I. After pituitary TSH secretion recovers from suppression, the goal of maintenance therapy is TSH normalization.

The first clinical response to medications is 2–4 wk into therapy. Weight loss stops or weight gain occurs. Beta-adrenergic antagonists may be used as an adjunct during this interval but, as the cardiovascular manifestations of hyperthyroidism are generally well-tolerated in the young, we reserve this therapy for symptomatically significant palpitations. Antithyroid drugs are usually well tolerated, but side-effects are seen more commonly in children than in adults. Thirty-six serious complications and 2 deaths in children have been reported to the FDA (47). A recent paper reports an increased incidence of adverse drug reactions in their prepubertal cohort (5 of their 7 patients). One of these children was treated with radioiodine, but the remainder were successfully switched to the alternative antithyroid drug without subsequent side effects (48). Agranulocytosis (defined as a granulocyte count less than 500/µL) is a serious idiosyncratic reaction that can occur with either MMI or PTU. For this reason, a baseline white count should be obtained prior to the initiation of antithyroid drugs, since mild neutropenia may be present in the Graves' patient prior to the initiation of treatment. One study suggests that the occurrence of agranulocytosis with MMI is dose-related, but similar data is unavailable for PTU (49). Families should be counseled that fever, sore throat, or other serious infections may be manifestations of agranulocytosis, and therefore should prompt the immediate cessation of antithyroid drugs, the notification of the physician, and a determination of white blood cell count with differential.

Reports of long term remission rates in children are variable, ranging anywhere from 30–60% (47,50). One year remission rates are considerably less in prepubertal (17%) compared to pubertal (30%) children, but a recent retrospective study of 76 pediatric patients describes a 38% rate of long-term remission achieved with more prolonged courses of antithyroid medication (mean treatment duration of 3.3 yr) (51,52). If the dose of antithyroid medication required to maintain euthyroidism is 5 mg per day of Tapazole (or 50 mg per day of PTU) for 6 mo to 1 yr and the serum TSH concentration is normal, a trial off medication may be offered. Antithyroid drugs can be discontinued and TSH concentrations monitored at monthly intervals. If hyperthyroidism recurs, as indicated by a suppression of TSH, antithyroid medications should be resumed or definitive therapy provided.

Definitive Therapy

The two options for the definitive treatment of Graves' disease are I-131 and thyroidectomy. Both are likely to result in life-long hypothyroidism and there is disagreement in the literature as to their indications. Some centers consider these modalities as options for the initial treatment of pediatric hyperthyroidism (53–55). However, as a remission of Graves' disease occurs in a significant percentage of children, we recommend the long-term use of antithyroid medications until young adulthood. If patient noncompliance prevents the successful treatment of thyrotoxicosis or both antithyroid medications must be discontinued secondary to serious drug reactions, definitive therapy is appropriate.

Thyroid destruction by I-131 is the definitive treatment of choice in adults, but concerns over the potential long-term complications of pediatric radiation exposure have made endocrinologists cautious in applying this approach to children *(8)*. The adult Graves' literature describes an increased relative risk for the development of stomach cancer (1.3 fold) and breast cancer (1.9 fold), but no large, long-term, follow-up studies of patients treated under 16 yr-of-age have appeared *(50)*. It is estimated that more than 1000 children have received I-131 for the treatment Graves' disease. To date, there are no reports of an increase in the incidence of thyroid carcinoma or leukemia in this population *(56–58)*. Despite the reassurances of this literature, experience with X-rays and the Chernobyl nuclear power plant accident indicate that the carcinogenic effects of radiation to the thyroid are highest in young children. This argues for continued surveillance and, for children who fail antithyroid medication, the provision of an I-131 dose adequate to destroy all thyroid follicular cells *(59–61)*. Some institutions administer an empiric dose of 3–15 millicuries, or a dose based upon the estimated weight of the gland (50–200 microcuries per gram of thyroid tissue) *(50,57,58)*. Efficacy is dependent upon both thyroid uptake and mass and it is more logical to prescribe a dose which will provide approximately 200 µCi/g estimated weight in the gland at 24 h. A recent analysis of radioiodine therapy at the Brigham and Women's Hospital included 261 Graves' patients. Successful outcome, defined as hypothyroidism after a single dose of radioiodine, was associated with significantly higher doses of I-131 (178.1 µCi/g compared to 141.3 µCi/g in the treatment failure group, $p<0.01$). Patients who failed single-dose treatment tended to be young with more biochemically severe hyperthyroidism and a history of pretreatment with antithyroid medications *(62)*. Antithyroid drugs should be discontinued for 3 days prior to the administration of I-131. For children who are unable to swallow a capsule, a liquid preparation of I-131 is available.

$$\text{Dose} = \frac{200\ \mu\text{Ci/g} \times \text{g(thy)} \times 100}{\%\ \text{uptake in 24 h}}$$

The frequency of acute side-effects is low although one recent paper describes vomiting in four out of thirty five pediatric patients *(55)*. One prospective study of 443 patients ranging from 15–85 yr-of-age has raised the concern that I-131 may worsen or precipitate the development of Graves' ophthalmopathy in approximately 15% of cases *(63)*. Severe ophthalmopathy is less common in pediatric Graves' disease and, when compounded by the reluctance to use radioiodine in this age group, a study to address the risk of this phenomenon in children is unlikely to be available in the near future. The current pediatric literature suggests that the rate of ophthalmologic exacerbation is similar amongst the various treatment modalities: 3% after I-131; 2% with thionamide derivatives; and 9% after subtotal thyroidectomy *(47)*. A short course of glucocorticoids is appropriate if there is rapid progression of ophthalmopathy or as prophylaxis prior to radioiodine in children with pre-existing moderate to severe ophthalmopathy.

Thyroidectomy is rarely used electively for the definitive therapy of Graves' disease in the US except with massive thyromegaly (over eight times normal size) or for patients in whom coexisting nodules are suspicious for carcinoma by fine needle aspiration. A recent metanalysis of the pediatric literature provided the following analysis of surgical treatment: subtotal thyroidectomy relieved hyperthyroidism in 80% of patients, with

60% becoming hypothyroid. Total thyroidectomy cured hyperthyroidism in over 97% of patients with nearly universal hypothyroidism. The overall complication rate in children included a 2% incidence of permanent hypoparathyroidism, a 2% incidence of vocal cord paralysis, and a 0.08% mortality *(47)*. In the authors' opinion, these average complication rates are unacceptably high given the benign nature of Graves' disease and the other therapeutic options available. One large institution has published a series of 82 children treated surgically over 14 yr with much better results. Bilateral subtotal resection was the most frequently performed operation (86%) and, with a median follow-up of 8.3 yr, they cite a recurrence rate of 6% and *no* cases of permanent recurrent laryngeal nerve palsy, permanent parathyroid disease, or death *(64)*. The difference between the average complication rate and those in a single institution emphasizes the importance of skill and experience in the performance of this procedure *(65)*. While we hesitate to apply average rates of postsurgical complications to every institution, it is clear that referral to a surgeon with a low personal complication rate and extensive experience with subtotal thyroidectomy is required if this is the desired procedure. Postoperative hypothyroidism is expected and should be viewed as a relatively trivial complication, as it is easily treated and all Graves' patients require lifelong monitoring. We suggest that thyroidectomy be considered only for patients who have persistently failed medical management or those whose parents or physicians do not wish to proceed with radioiodine therapy. Based on the results to date, I-131 therapy is an acceptable alternative if the surgical options are undesirable in a given community. I-131 is recommended for all patients who recur following surgery due to the high complication rate of secondary thyroidectomy *(66)*.

Monitoring of Graves' Disease and the Transition to Adult Care

Given the documented risks of surgery and the theoretical risks of radioiodine, prolonged courses of antithyroid medication are appropriate in the treatment of pediatric Graves', especially with the relatively high possibility of remission. We monitor thyroid function tests every 3 mo in the growing child and 3 wk after any medication adjustment with the goal of normalizing the TSH. Physical examination should focus upon heart rate, puberty, linear growth, and vision.

The transition to adulthood should prompt a re-discussion of therapy. For young adults with persistent hyperthyroidism, I-131 is our definitive treatment of choice. We perform an RAIU prior to treatment with the goal of delivering approximately 8 mCi of I-131 into the gland at 24 h. For glands larger than three times normal size, about 11 mCi is required *(62)*. Definitive therapy typically results in permanent hypothyroidism, but allows for a simpler regimen of medication and laboratory monitoring (daily levothyroxine and a yearly TSH measurement). Additionally, prior definitive therapy simplifies the management of female patients during pregnancy.

Neonatal Graves' Disease

Approximately 0.6% of infants born to mothers with a history of Graves' disease will develop neonatal hyperthyroidism due to the transplacental passage of thyroid-stimulating immunoglobulins. Even after definitive treatment by I-131 or thyroidectomy, women with a history of autoimmune thyroid disease are at risk for fetal and neonatal thyroid dysfunction secondary to the persistence of maternal autoantibodies. The care of such women must be coordinated between the high-risk obstetrician and an endocrinologist. Fetal heart rate and growth should be monitored by regular prenatal ultrasounds and the measurement of anti-thyrotropin receptor antibodies during at-risk pregnancies has been recommended as a predictor for the development of fetal/neonatal Graves' *(67)*. Highly experienced ultrasonographers can often visualize the fetal thyroid. The presence of fetal goiter, tachycardia, and intrauterine growth retardation suggests fetal hyperthyroidism. In these rare patients, antithyroid drugs are administered to the mother to control fetal hyperthyroidism. Pediatricians should be aware that the use of maternal antithyroid medications near the time of delivery or the co-transfer of maternal thyrotropin receptor blocking immunoglobulins may delay the appearance of neonatal Graves' *(68)*. For high-risk infants, such as those born to mothers with high levels of thyrotropin stimulating antibodies or those with a history of an affected sibling, it is our practice to obtain thyroid function tests at birth and at 1 and 2 mo-of-age *(69)*. An additional set of labwork at 1 wk-of-age is indicated for infants who have been exposed to maternal antithyroid drugs in the third trimester.

Affected infants are often flushed, diaphoretic, and hyperkinetic. Goiter is common and, when severe, can endanger the infant's airway. Diarrhea, vomiting, poor weight gain, and a transient exophthalmos may be seen. Arrhythmias and/or congestive heart failure can develop and require treatment with digoxin. Serum for confirmatory thyroid function tests (TSH, fT_4I) should be obtained and treatment initiated immediately. Propylthiouracil (5–10 mg/kg per day) or methimazole (0.5–1.0 mg/kg per day) may be administered orally or per nasogastric tube in divided doses every 8 h. Inorganic iodine will speed the fall in circulating thyroid hormone, using saturated solution of potassium iodide (SSKI) (48 mg iodide/drop) at the dose of one drop per day. Iopanoic acid or sodium ipodate have also been used for their iodine content and their capacity to inhibit the activation of T_4 to T_3. As in older patients, adjunctive therapy with beta-blockade (propranolol 2 mg/kg per day) and glucocorticoids (prednisone 2 mg/kg per day) may be helpful in severe cases. The cumulative morbidity of neonatal Graves was estimated to be as high as 25% in the past, although it appears to be considerably lower today *(50)*. Potential long-term morbidity includes growth retardation, craniosynostosis, impaired intellectual function, and central hypothyroidism *(50,70–73)*.

The half-life of maternal immunoglobulin is approximately 14 d, so most cases of neonatal Graves will resolve after 3–12 wk (depending upon the initial levels of thyrotropin-receptor autoantibodies). The differential diagnosis of neonatal thyrotoxicosis includes the McCune-Albright syndrome and activating mutations of the TSH receptor. These nonautoimmune etiologies are exceedingly rare but should be considered if thyrotoxicosis persists beyond 3 mo-of-age.

ACKNOWLEDGMENTS

We are indebted to Dr. John F. Crigler, Chief Emeritus of Children's Hospital Endocrinology in Boston for helpful comments and assistance in the review of this manuscript.

REFERENCES

1. Saravanan P, Dayan CM. Thyroid autoantibodies. Endocrinol Metab Clin North Am 2001;30(2): 315–337, viii.
2. Hunter I, Greene SA, MacDonald TM, et al. Prevalence and aetiology of hypothyroidism in the young. Arch Dis Child 2000;83(3):207–210.
3. Segni M, Leonardi E, Mazzoncini B, et al. Special features of Graves' disease in early childhood. Thyroid 1999;9(9):871–817.

4. Lafranchi S. Thyroiditis and acquired hypothyroidism. Pediatr Ann 1992;21(1):29,32–39.
5. Foley TP Jr, Abbassi V, Copeland KC, et al. Brief report: hypothyroidism caused by chronic autoimmune thyroiditis in very young infants. N Engl J Med 1994;330(7):466–468.
6. Ostergaard GZ, Jacobsen BB. Atrophic, autoimmune thyroiditis in infancy. A case report. Horm Res 1989;31(4):190–192.
7. Davies TF, Amino N. A new classification for human autoimmune thyroid disease. Thyroid 1993;3(4):331–333.
8. Larsen PR, Davies TF, Hay ID. The Thhyroid Gland. In: Williams Textbook of Endocrinology, 9th ed. Wilson JD, Foster DW, Kronenberg HM, Larsen PR, eds. W.B. Saunders Company, Philadelphia, 1998, pp. 389–515.
9. Dayan CM, Daniels GH. Chronic autoimmune thyroiditis. N Engl J Med 1996;335(2):99–107.
10. Matsuura N, Konishi J, Yuri K, et al. Comparison of atrophic and goitrous auto-immune thyroiditis in children: clinical, laboratory and TSH-receptor antibody studies. Eur J Pediatr 1990;149(8):529–533.
11. Takasu N, Yamada T, Takasu M, et al. Disappearance of thyrotropin-blocking antibodies and spontaneous recovery from hypothyroidism in autoimmune thyroiditis. N Engl J Med 1992;326(8):513–518.
12. Foley TP. Disorders of the Thyroid in Childern. In: Pediattric Endocrinology, Sperling MA, ed. W.B. Saunders Company, Philadelphia, 1996, pp. 171–194.
13. Chiesa A, Gruniero de Papendieck L, Keselman A, et al. Final height in long-term primary hypothyroid children. J Pediatr Endocrinol Metab, 1998;11(1):51–58.
14. Boersma B, Otten BJ, Stoelinga GB, et al. Catch-up growth after prolonged hypothyroidism. Eur J Pediatr 1996;155(5): 362–367.
15. Castro-Magana M, Angulo M, Canas A, et al. Hypothalamic-pituitary gonadal axis in boys with primary hypothyroidism and macroorchidism. J Pediatr 1988;112(3):397–402.
16. Jannini EA, Ulisse S, D'Armiento M. Macroorchidism in juvenile hypothyroidism. J Clin Endocrinol Metab 1995;80(8):2543–2544.
17. Anasti, JN, Flack MR, Froehlich J, et al. A potential novel mechanism for precocious puberty in juvenile hypothyroidism. J Clin Endocrinol Metab 1995;80(1):276–279.
18. Lum SM, Nicoloff JT, Spencer CA, et al. Peripheral tissue mechanism for maintenance of serum triiodothyronine values in a thyroxine-deficient state in man. J Clin Invest 1984;73(2):570–575.
19. Bianco AC, Salvatore D, Gereben B, et al. Biochemistry, cellular and molecular biology, and physiological roles of the iodothyronine selenodeiodinases. Endocr Rev 2002;23(1):38–89.
20. Nordyke RA, Gilbert FI, Jr., Miyamoto LA, et al. The superiority of antimicrosomal over antithyroglobulin antibodies for detecting Hashimoto's thyroiditis. Arch Intern Med 1993;153(7):862–865.
21. Foley TP Jr. Mediators of thyroid diseases in children. J Pediatr, 1998;132(4):569–570.
22. Hancock SL, McDougall IR, Constine LS, Thyroid abnormalities after therapeutic external radiation. Int J Radiat Oncol Biol Phys, 1995. 31(5): p. 1165–70.
22a. Huang SA, Fish DA, Dorfman DM, Salvatore D, Kozakewich HP, Mandel SJ, Larsen PR. A 21 year Old Woman with Consumptive Hypothyroidism due to a Vascular Tumor Expressing Type 3 Iodothyronine Deiodinase. Journal of Clinical Endocrinology & Metabolism, 2002;87(10):4457–4461.
23. Huang SA, Tu HM, Harney JW, et al. Severe hypothyroidism caused by type 3 iodothyronine deiodinase in infantile hemangiomas. New England Journal of Medicine 2000;343(3):185–189.
24. Ayling RM, Davenport M, Hadzic N, et al. Hepatic hemangioendothelioma associated with production of humoral thyrotropin-like factor. Journal of Pediatrics 2001;138(6):932–935.
25. Mandel SJ, Brent GA, Larsen PR. Levothyroxine therapy in patients with thyroid disease. Ann Intern Med 1993;119(6):492–502.
26. Van Dop C, Conte FA, Kock TK, et al. Pseudotumor cerebri associated with initiation of levothyroxine therapy for juvenile hypothyroidism. N Engl J Med 1983;308(18):1076–1080.
27. Slyper AH, Swenerton P. Experience with low-dose replacement therapy in the initial management of severe pediatric acquired primary hypothyroidism. J Pediatr Endocrinol Metab 1998;11(4):543–547.
28. Sklar CA, Qazi R, David R. Juvenile autoimmune thyroiditis. Hormonal status at presentation and after long-term follow-up. Am J Dis Child 1986;140(9):877–880.
29. Maenpaa J, Raatikka M, Rasanen J, et al. Natural course of juvenile autoimmune thyroiditis. J Pediatr 1985;107(6):898–904.
30. Haddow JE, Palomaki GE, Allan WC, et al. Maternal thyroid deficiency during pregnancy and subsequent neuropsychological development of the child. N Engl J Med 1999;341(8):549–555.
31. Weetman AP. Graves' disease. N Engl J Med 2000;343(17):1236–1248.
32. Zimmerman D, Lteif AN. Thyrotoxicosis in children. Endocrinol Metab Clin North Am 199827(1): 109–126.

33. Lavard L, Ranlov I, Perrild H, et al. Incidence of juvenile thyrotoxicosis in Denmark, 1982–1988. A nationwide study. Eur J Endocrinol 1994;130(6):565–568.
34. Gruters A. Ocular manifestations in children and adolescents with thyrotoxicosis. Exp Clin Endocrinol Diabetes 1999;107(Suppl 5):S172–S174.
35. Buckler JM, Willgerodt H, Keller E. Growth in thyrotoxicosis. Arch Dis Child 1986;61(5):464–471.
36. Wong GW, Lai J, Cheng PS. Growth in childhood thyrotoxicosis. Eur J Pediatr 1999;158(10):776–779.
37. Deroot LJ, Larsen PR, Henneman G. Acute and Subacute Thyroiditis. In: The Thyroif and Its Diseases, 6th ed. DeGroot LJ, Larsen PR, Henneman G. eds. Churchill Livingstone, New York, pp. 697–709.
38. Marqusee, E., S.T. Haden, and R.D. Utiger, Subclinical thyrotoxicosis. Endocrinol Metab Clin North Am 1998;27(1):37–49.
39. Koutras DA. Subclinical hyperthyroidism. Thyroid 1999;9(3):311–315.
40. Sawin CT, Geller A, Wolf PA, et al. Low serum thyrotropin concentrations as a risk factor for atrial fibrillation in older persons. N Engl J Med 1994;331(19);1249–1252.
41. Utiger RD. Subclinical hyperthyroidism—just a low serum thyrotropin concentration, or something more? N Engl J Med 1994;331(19):1302–1303.
42. Franklyn JA. The management of hyperthyroidism. N Engl J Med 1994. 330(24):1731–1738.
43. Klein I, Becker DV, Levey GS. Treatment of hyperthyroid disease. Ann Intern Med 1994,121(4):281–288.
44. Hashizume K, Ichikawa K, Sakurai A, et al. Administration of thyroxine in treated Graves' disease. Effects on the level of antibodies to thyroid-stimulating hormone receptors and on the risk of recurrence of hyperthyroidism. N Engl J Med 1991;324(14):947–953.
45. McIver B, Rae P, Beckett G, et al. Lack of effect of thyroxine in patients with Graves' hyperthyroidism who are treated with an antithyroid drug. N Engl J Med 1996;334(4):220–224.
46. Lucas A, Salinas I, Rius F, et al. Medical therapy of Graves' disease: does thyroxine prevent recurrence of hyperthyroidism? J Clin Endocrinol Metab 1997;82(8):2410–2413.
47. Rivkees SA, Sklar C, Freemark M. Clinical review 99: The management of Graves' disease in children, with special emphasis on radioiodine treatment. J Clin Endocrinol Metab 1998;83(11):3767–3776.
48. Lazar L, Kalter-Leibovici O, Pertzelan A, et al. Thyrotoxicosis in prepubertal children compared with pubertal and postpubertal patients. J Clin Endocrinol Metab 2000;85(10):3678–3682.
49. Cooper DS, Goldminz D, Levin AA, et al. Agranulocytosis associated with antithyroid drugs. Effects of patient age and drug dose. Ann Intern Med 1983;98(1):26–29.
50. LaFranchi, Hanna CE. Graves Disease in the Neonatal Period and Childhood. In: Werner & Ingbar's The Thyroid. A Fundamental and Clinical Text, Braverman LE, Utiger RD, eds. Lipppincott Williams & Wilkins, Philadelphia, 2000, pp. 989–997.
51. Shulman DI, Muhar I, Jorgensen EV, et al. Autoimmune hyperthyroidism in prepubertal children and adolescents: comparison of clinical and biochemical features at diagnosis and responses to medical therapy. Thyroid 1997;7(5):755–760.
52. Raza J, Hindmarsh PC, Brook CG. Thyrotoxicosis in children: thirty years' experience. Acta Paediatr 1999;88(9):937–941.
53. Ward L, Huot C, Lambert R, et al. Outcome of pediatric Graves' disease after treatment with antithyroid medication and radioiodine. Clin Invest Med 1999;22(4):132–139.
54. Moll GW Jr, Patel BR. Pediatric Graves' disease: therapeutic options and experience with radioiodine at the University of Mississippi Medical Center. South Med J 1997;90(10):1017–1022.
55. Clark JD, Gelfand MJ, Elgazzar AH. Iodine-131 therapy of hyperthyroidism in pediatric patients. J Nucl Med 1995;36(3):442–445.
56. Safa AM, Schumacher OP, Rodriguez-Antunez A. Long-term follow-up results in children and adolescents treated with radioactive iodine (131I) for hyperthyroidism. N Engl J Med 1975;292(4):167–171.
57. Foley TP Jr, Charron M. Radioiodine treatment of juvenile Graves disease. Exp Clin Endocrinol Diabetes 1997;105(Suppl 4):61–65.
58. Cheetham TD, Wraight P, Hughes IA, et al. Radioiodine treatment of Graves' disease in young people. Horm Res 1998;49(6):258–262.
59. Refetoff S, Harrison J, Karanfilski BT, et al. Continuing occurrence of thyroid carcinoma after irradiation to the neck in infancy and childhood. N Engl J Med 1975;292(4):171–175.
60. Baverstock K, Egloff B, Pinchera A, et al. Thyroid cancer after Chernobyl. Nature 1992;359(6390):21–22.
61. Nikiforov Y, Gnepp DR, J.A. Fagin, Thyroid lesions in children and adolescents after the Chernobyl disaster: implications for the study of radiation tumorigenesis. J Clin Endocrinol Metab, 1996. 81(1): p. 9–14.

62. Alexander EK, Larsen PR. High dose of (131)I therapy for the treatment of hyperthyroidism caused by Graves' disease. J Clin Endocrinol Metab 2002;87(3):1073–1077.
63. Bartalena L, Marcocci C, Bogazzi F, et al. Relation between therapy for hyperthyroidism and the course of Graves' ophthalmopathy. N Engl J Med 1998;338(2):73–78.
64. Soreide JA, van Heerden JA, Lo CY, et al. Surgical treatment of Graves' disease in patients younger than 18 years. World J Surg 1996;20(7):794–799; discussion 799–800.
65. Sosa JA, Bowman M, Tielsch JM, et al. The importance of surgeon experience for clinical and economic outcomes from thyroidectomy. Ann Surg 1998;228(3):320–330.
66. Waldhausen JH. Controversies related to the medical and surgical management of hyperthyroidism in children. Semin Pediatr Surg 1997;6(3):121–127.
67. Laurberg P, Nygaard B, Gilnoer D, et al. Guidelines for TSH-receptor antibody measurements in pregnancy: results of an evidence-based symposium organized by the European Thyroid Association. Eur J Endocrinol 1998;139(6):584–586.
68. McKenzie JM, Zakarija M. Fetal and neonatal hyperthyroidism and hypothyroidism due to maternal TSH receptor antibodies. Thyroid 1992;2(2):155–159.
69. Zakarija M, McKenzie JM. Pregnancy-associated changes in the thyroid-stimulating antibody of Graves' disease and the relationship to neonatal hyperthyroidism. J Clin Endocrinol Metab 1983;57(5):1036–1040.
70. Zimmerman D. Fetal and neonatal hyperthyroidism. Thyroid 1999;9(7):727–733.
71. Mandel SH, Hanna CE, LaFranchi SH. Diminished thyroid-stimulating hormone secretion associated with neonatal thyrotoxicosis. J Pediatr 1986;109(4):662–665.
72. Hashimoto H, Maruyama H, Koshida R, et al. Central hypothyroidism resulting from pituitary suppression and peripheral thyrotoxicosis in a premature infant born to a mother with Graves disease. J Pediatr 1995;127(5):809–811.
73. Mandel S, Hanna C, LaFranchi S. Thyroid function of infants born to mothers with Graves disease. J Pediatr 1990;117(1 Pt 1):169–170.

18 Resistance to Thyroid Hormone and TSH Receptor Mutations

Ronald N. Cohen, MD

CONTENTS

RESISTANCE TO THYROID HORMONE (RTH)
TSH RECEPTOR MUTATIONS
CONCLUSION
REFERENCES

RESISTANCE TO THYROID HORMONE (RTH)

Introduction

Resistance to thyroid hormone (RTH) is a syndrome characterized by variable tissue hypo-responsiveness to thyroid hormone. Classically, patients come to attention for a variety of reasons, particularly goiter. Biochemically, the syndrome is characterized by elevated thyroid hormone values in the setting of a non-suppressed thyrotropin (TSH) level. RTH can be further subdivided based on the distribution of tissue resistance: generalized resistance to thyroid hormone (GRTH) and pituitary resistance to thyroid hormone (PRTH). In GRTH, hypo-responsiveness occurs throughout the body, including both the hypothalamic-pituitary-thyroid axis and peripheral tissues. The resistance in the pituitary leads to elevated thyrotropin levels and, in turn, increased thyroid hormone production by the thyroid gland; however, the thyroid hormone produced has reduced activity in the periphery. Therefore, this condition is characterized by a variable degree of compensated thyroid hormone hypo-responsiveness throughout the body. Affected individuals do not exhibit classic signs and symptoms of myxedema even in the setting of reduced thyroid hormone action. Patients with GRTH manifest variable symptoms of delayed growth, hearing defects, and attention-deficit hyperactivity disorder (ADHD) [1]. Patients with PRTH, in contrast, exhibit thyroid hormone hypo-responsiveness mainly in the hypothalamus and pituitary, but less so in peripheral tissues. Therefore, the elevated thyroid hormone levels generated from central resistance lead to a state of systemic hyperthyroidism. PRTH is more accurately called central resistance to thyroid hormone (CRTH) [2], since the defect occurs in both the hypothalamus and the pituitary; the latter term will be used in this review. The majority of patients with

RTH, both GRTH and CRTH, have autosomal dominantly-inherited mutations in the thyroid hormone receptor β gene. A smaller fraction of patients have no recognized mutations to date. Patients have been identified in a wide range of racial and ethnic groups, but the exact geographic distribution of the disorder is not known. It has been estimated that RTH occurs in about 1 case per 50,000 live births *(3)*. Therapeutic strategies for managing RTH are controversial, but in any case treatment must be individualized to the particular patient in question. Unfortunately, most studies of patients with RTH have been done in adults, so approaches for the pediatric population must be deduced in the absence of clear data.

Mechanisms of Resistance to Thyroid Hormone

The thyroid hormone receptor (TR) is a member of the nuclear hormone receptor (NHR) family of transcription factors *(4)*. These transcription factors bind DNA and modulate gene transcription. NHRs each contain a number of distinct domains (*see* Fig. 1): an *N*-terminal activation, or AF-1, domain (A/B domain); a central DNA-binding domain (DBD); and a C-terminal ligand-binding domain (LBD) with a ligand-dependent activation (AF-2) function. In addition to binding ligand, the LBD is involved in homo- and hetero- dimerization and the recruitment of key nuclear cofactors, such as corepressors and coactivators.

The TR and other NHRs bind sequences within the promoters of genes to regulate gene transcription. For the TR, such regions are termed thyroid hormone response elements (TREs) *(5,6)*. TREs can be defined as "positive" or "negative." Gene transcription stimulated by thyroid hormone is characterized by the presence of positive TREs (pTREs); genes that are negatively regulated by thyroid hormone have so-called negative TREs (nTREs). Negative TREs are present in the promoters of the TRH and TSH subunit genes, as well as in certain promoters of genes in the periphery *(7–9)*.

TR action on pTREs has been better characterized than on nTREs. On pTREs, TR binds to DNA response elements in the promoter regions of genes in the presence or absence of the ligand, tri-iodothyronine (T_3) (Fig. 2). In the absence of T_3, the TR binds proteins termed corepressors, such as the nuclear corepressor protein (NCoR) and the silencing mediator of retinoid and thyroid hormone receptors (SMRT) *(10–15)*. These proteins, in turn, bind a protein complex with histone deacetylase function *(16–18)*, leading to basal silencing of gene expression. The binding of T_3 to the TR LBD normally leads to a conformational change in the receptor with resultant loss of corepressor binding, and recruitment of coactivators *(19)*. Coactivators are proteins that stimulate gene expression, in part by increasing the degree of histone acetylation *(20–28)*.

There are two major isoforms of the TR: TRα and TRβ, located on different chromosomes (*see* Fig. 1) *(29,30)*. The gene for TRα is located on chromosome 17; the TRβ gene is located on chromosome 3. Additional isoforms of TRα and TRβ are generated by alternative splicing. For example, TRα2 is an alternatively spliced TRα isoform that has a different LBD than TRα1, such that it does not bind thyroid hormone; its function is unclear. TRβ1 and TRβ2 differ only by their unique amino termini, and contain the same DNA- and ligand-binding domains. A TRβ3 isoform has also recently been described, though its role in TR action has not yet been defined *(31)*.

Although most patients with RTH have mutations in the TRβ gene, a subset of RTH patients without TRβ mutations have been identified. These patients may have mutations

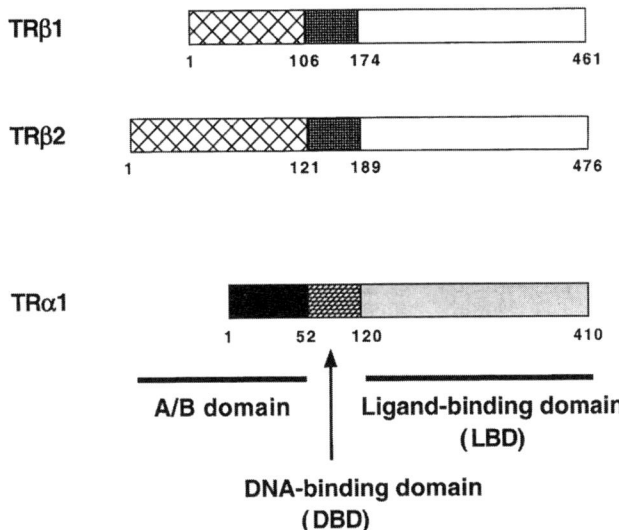

Fig. 1. Thyroid Hormone Receptor Isoforms. The TRα1, TRβ1, and TRβ2 isoforms are shown schematically. Amino acid sequences are indicated. Note that TRβ1 and TRβ2 differ only by their unique N-terminal domains. While the TRα1 domains have significant homology to the TRβ isoforms, they are distinct. The TRα2 isoform is not shown, as it does not bind thyroid hormone; its precise function is unknown.

in TR-associated cofactors *(32)*, though such mutations in these cofactors have not been identified *(33)*. This is an ongoing area of research, and novel mutations will likely be identified in the future. No patients with TRα mutations have yet been identified.

Mutations of TRβ that cause RTH cluster in three "hot spots" of the TRβ gene *(34,35)*. Most of these mutations interfere with the binding of T_3 to the receptor. An example is the Δ337T mutation, which produces a receptor that does not bind T_3. This leads to a situation in which the mutant receptor binds corepressors even in the presence of T_3 (Fig. 2). In a few patients, the defect is not with ligand binding *per se*, but primarily with altered corepressor and/or coactivator recruitment *(36,37)*.

In the vast majority of cases of RTH, the syndrome is inherited in an autosomal dominant fashion *(1)*. Since only one mutant TR is necesssary to generate the disorder, this suggests that the mutant TR interferes with wild-type TR function. This effect has been termed "dominant-negative inhibition." In fact, altering a mutant TR in vitro, such that the receptor no longer dimerizes or binds DNA, impairs dominant-negative inhibition *(38,39)*. Therefore, mutant TRs must maintain certain important TR properties to be able to cause RTH. A mutant TR that cannot bind T_3 but is otherwise functional can maintain the ability to bind NCoR and SMRT. Since T_3 doesn't bind the receptor, the mutant TR cannot alter its conformation to allow for corepressor release (and coactivator recruitment). Therefore, such receptors constitutively bind NCoR and/or SMRT, leading to RTH.

It is not clear why certain TR mutations cause CRTH instead of GRTH. In fact, the notion of CRTH as a distinct clinical entity remains controversial. It has been hypothesized by certain groups that CRTH and GRTH are not distinct, since the same mutation

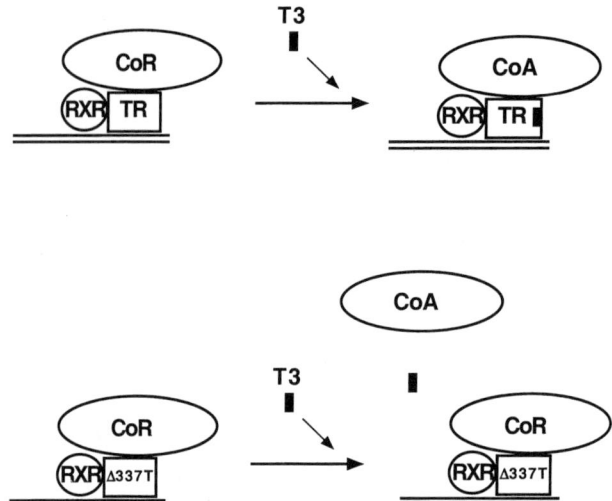

Fig. 2. Role of abnormal TR - corepressor interactions in the pathogenesis of RTH. The thyroid hormone receptor (TR) binds DNA as a TR-TR homodimer or as a heterodimer with the retinoid X receptor (RXR). Normally, the presence of ligand (T_3) results in dissociation of corepressors (CoR) from the TR complex. The Δ337T mutation of TRβ, however, abolishes hormone binding. Even in the presence of T_3, there is no binding of T_3 to the mutant receptor. Thus, the CoR is not dissociated from the TR complex, and coactivators (CoA) are not recruited. This results in loss of T_3-mediated stimulation of gene transcription, as well as constitutive repression.

causes diverse symptoms in different individuals (40). Furthermore, tachycardia is present in many patients, even those with GRTH. The presence of tachycardia in GRTH patients is probably due to the presence of wild-type TRα receptors in the heart even in patients with severe TRβ dysfunction. Therefore, tachycardia cannot be used to reliably distinguish GRTH and CRTH. Certain mutations have also been claimed to cause CRTH in certain individuals and GRTH in others; this has been taken as evidence that CRTH is not a separate disorder. However, patients with presumed CRTH have often not been extensively studied. In fact, a careful evaluation of both clinical and biochemical indices in a patient with RTH suggested that CRTH does exist (41). Also, experiments have revealed that mutant TRs of patients with CRTH behave differently than TRs of patients with GRTH, at least with respect to the TRβ2 isoform (42). The TRβ2 isoform is primarily expressed in the hypothalamus and pituitary, and may therefore play a key role in negative regulation by thyroid hormone. Finally, whether patients are deemed to have a distinct clinical entity (CRTH) or variable resistance across a spectrum of a single disorder (RTH), it seems clear that certain TR mutations cause RTH with a primarily thyrotoxic phenotype.

Transgenic mouse models have clarified the role of the mutant TR in the pathogenesis of RTH. Knock-out of the TRβ receptor produced mice with thyroid function tests consistent with RTH, with elevated TSH and T_4 levels (43). "Knock-in" of mutant TRs found in patients with RTH generate mice with more severe signs and symptoms than that of TR knock-out animals (44,45). These mice also have thyroid tests consistent with more severe RTH. These data point to the fact that RTH is generated not merely from lack of TR action, but from abnormal TR function. In other words, TRs that abnormally bind corepressors are more likely to mediate a significant clinical effect than TRs that are

Table 1
Clinical Characteristics of RTH in Children[a]

A) Physical Exam
  1) Goiter
  2) Tachycardia
  3) Short Stature
B) Associated Symptoms
  1) Neurological
    a) Developmental Delay
    b) Attention Deficit Hyperactivity Disorder (ADHD)
    c) Low IQ
  2) ENT
    a) Deafness
    b) Speech Impediment
    c) Recurrent Ear Infections
  3) Endocrine / Metabolism
    a) Hyperthyroidism (only in patients with CRTH)
    b) Low Body Weight
C) Radiological Findings
  1) Delayed Bone Age
  2) Increased Thyroid ^{123}I Uptake

[a]Clinical findings found in patients with Resistance to Thyroid Hormone, including physical examination abnormalities, associated clinical symptoms, and radiological findings. Derived from data in ref. *1,51*.

merely nonfunctional. In addition, lack of coactivator function can also cause an RTH phenotype in vivo in transgenic mice *(46)*.

Interestingly, knock-out of TRα causes a syndrome of hypothyroidism with low TSH and growth arrest *(47,48)*. No TRα mutations have yet been documented in patients with RTH. The knock-out experiments suggest an explanation: a patient with a dominant negative TRα mutation would not have thyroid function tests (TFTs) consistent with thyroid hormone resistance.

Clinical Presentation

The clinical presentation of RTH is variable (Table 1). The initial family described by Refetoff, et al. *(49)* included an 8 1/2-yr-old girl and a 12 1/2-yr-old boy, both of whom were clinically euthyroid, but had goiter, deaf-mutism, stippled epiphyses (on radiological skeletal survey), and an elevated protein-bound iodine (PBI) level. In contrast to most cases of RTH identified later, this family exhibited an autosomal recessive pattern of inheritance, and affected family members were later found to have a complete deletion of the TRβ allele *(50)*. The heterozygous parents were phenotypically normal, suggesting that a single wild-type TR (in the absence of a mutant TR) is sufficient for thyroid hormone action. As noted above, RTH is usually inherited in an autosomal dominant fashion. This is because the mutant TRs exhibit dominant negative inhibition of wild-type alleles.

Patients with RTH come to medical attention for a variety of reasons. Goiter is the presenting sign in about 38% of cases; less common reasons include learning disabilities, developmental delay, tachycardia, suspected thyrotoxicosis, and elevated thyroxine levels at birth *(3)*. Thyroid function tests are drawn, revealing elevated thyroid hormone levels in the setting of a nonsuppressed TSH (*see* Diagnostic Guidelines).

On physical examination, patients with GRTH tend to have short stature with delayed bone maturation, hearing defects, tachycardia, and goiter *(1)*. In addition, patients often have attention-deficit hyperactivity disorder (ADHD) *(51)*. Infants with RTH may have congenital deafness, congenital nystagmus, neonatal jaundice, and hypotonia *(1)*. In patients with CRTH, however, symptoms of hyperthyroidism predominate. Finally, patients with RTH who have inappropriately underwent thyroidectomy or radioactive iodine treatment may have signs and symptoms of hypothyroidism.

A recent National Institutes of Health study *(52)* prospectively evaluated 42 kindreds with RTH. There was autosomal dominant transmission in 22 kindreds, sporadic transmission in 14, and an unknown transmission in 6. A palpable goiter was identified in 74% of females and 53% of males. Attention-deficit hyperactivity disorder (ADHD) was present in 72% of the males and 43% of females. IQ was about 13 points lower in the patients with RTH compared to controls, and one third of the patients had an IQ <85. Only a few patients had actual mental retardation. Patients with RTH had a higher incidence of speech delay (24%), stuttering (18%), and hearing loss than controls. Although resting pulse was higher in patients with RTH, this correlation did not persist after adjustment for age. Children with RTH had delayed bone maturation. Bone age was delayed in 29% of patients, and 18% had short stature. However, it is not fully clear that RTH is associated with decreased final adult height *(53)*.

Altered CNS function in patients with RTH suggests the importance of thyroid hormone and the TR in CNS development and/or function. As noted above, patients with RTH have a high incidence of ADHD and low IQ levels; however, the ADHD in patients with RTH appears to be distinct from ADHD in patients without RTH *(54)*. Matochik et al. used positron emission tomography (PET) scans to study CNS activity in patients with RTH *(55)*. This study suggested that RTH patients have higher cerebral metabolism in certain key areas of the central nervous system (CNS) during a continuous auditory discrimination task, including the anterior cingulate gyrus and the parietal lobe. These PET scans were also different than would be expected for ADHD patients without RTH. While PET scanning techniques remain solely a research tool for patients with RTH, these results suggest that patients with RTH have discrete areas of altered CNS function, perhaps pointing to an important role of thyroid hormone action in these regions.

A recent prospective study of children with ADHD with and without coexisting RTH examined the role of thyroid hormone therapy (in this case, L-T_3) in ADHD *(56)*. The majority of patients with RTH and ADHD improved when placed on T_3 therapy, whereas patients with ADHD (in the absence of RTH) deteriorated or remained stable. Therefore, T_3 should not generally be given to patients with ADHD in the absence of coexisting RTH. However, such therapy may be beneficial in RTH patients with ADHD. It will be interesting to see if further studies validate this approach.

While a number of unusual coexisting conditions in patients with RTH have been reported, these are most likely not due to thyroid hormone resistance itself, and may occur by chance. These include a bird-like appearance of the face, various vertebral and other skeletal anomalies, short fourth metacarpals, patent ductus arteriosus, and noncommunicating hydrocephalus. These and other coexisting disorders have been extensively reviewed elsewhere *(1)*.

Table 2
Causes of Euthyroid Hyperthyroxinemia[a]

1) Methodological Artifacts
   a) Antibodies to thyrotropin (TSH)
   b) Antibodies to thyroid hormones (T_4, T_3)
2) Binding Protein Abnormalities
   a) Acquired Forms of Increased TBG
      i) Estrogen use / pregnancy
      ii) Liver disease
      iii) Acute intermittent porphyria
      iv) Other drugs (methadone, perphanazine, 5-FU)
   b) Inherited
      i) TBG excess
      ii) Familial dysalbuminemic hyperthyroxinemia (FDH)
      iii) Mutant transthyretin variants
3) T_4 to T_3 Conversion Defects
   a) Acquired
      i) Amiodarone
      ii) Propranolol (high doses)
      iii) Oral cholexystographic contrast agents
   b) Inherited (Deidonase defects)
4) Miscellaneous Causes
   a) Acute psychiatric illness
   b) High altitude
   c) Amphetamine use
   d) Thyroxine therapy
   e) Non-steady state conditions of thyroid hormone testing
5) Resistance to Thyroid Hormone (RTH) (not all cases are euthyroid)

[a] Cause of euthyroid hyperthyroxinemia in the differential diagnosis of Resistance to Thyroid Hormone. Thyrotropin-secreting pituitary edenomas are not included, as they are generally associated with hyperthyroidism.

Diagnostic Considerations

DIAGNOSIS IN CHILDREN AND ADULTS

The initial testing of a patient suspected to have RTH should include routine thyroid function tests. Patients with RTH have elevated thyroid hormone levels in the setting of a non-suppressed TSH level. Because patients with RTH are often (overall) euthyroid, other causes of "euthyroid hyperthyroxinemia" should be excluded (Table 2). First of all, if such thyroid function tests are encountered, they should first be verified. Next, methodological artifacts should be excluded. For example, artifactual elevation of TSH can be seen in the presence of heterophile antibodies *(57)*. Such patients may actually be hyperthyroid, with elevated thyroid hormone levels and (appropriately) suppressed TSH levels (if measured accurately). This problem has been decreased, but not eliminated, with improvements in the TSH assay. Similarly, patients with autoimmune hypothyroidism occasionally have falsely elevated levels of thyroid hormone because of the presence of antibodies that interfere with the measurement of T_4 or T_3. Such artifactual elevations in thyroid function tests can be eliminated in the laboratory by various techniques.

Certain medications, such as amiodarone *(58)* and propranolol (at high doses), inhibit T_4 to T_3 conversion. Decreased T_4 to T_3 conversion may also be seen in patients with deiodinase deficiency. Euthyroid patients with T_4-to-T_3 conversion defects may have elevated T_4 levels and "inappropriately" normal TSH levels; however, these patients have normal TSH and T_3 levels, excluding the diagnosis of RTH.

Patients with defects in thyroid hormone binding proteins, such as TBG, transthyretin, and albumin can also have altered levels of total T_4 and T_3. Euthyroid patients with TBG excess, which can be congenital or acquired (for example, in pregnancy *[59]* and liver disease *[60]*), have elevated total T_4 levels in the setting of a non-suppressed TSH. These patients, though, have normal free T_4 levels, when measured directly or estimated based on thyroid hormone binding ratio (THBR) or T3 resin uptake (T_3RU). They also have normal TSH levels and are euthyroid.

Familial dysalbuminemic hyperthyroxinemia (FDH) is due to the production of albumin variants with Arg-His or Arg-Pro mutations at codon 218 *(61,62)*. These albumin variants have increased affinity for T_4. Therefore, measurement of total serum T_4 is elevated; correction of T_4 based on T_3RU or THBR also yields abnormally high results. Free T_4 levels are falsely elevated when measured by certain analog measurements, but a free T_4 level measured by dialysis will be normal. Serum T_3 levels are normal in FDH, and exclude the diagnosis of RTH.

Therefore, in the patient with elevated thyroid hormone levels and a non-suppressed TSH, methodological artifacts, binding protein defects, and medication effects should be excluded before considering the diagnosis of RTH. A few other conditions, such as acute psychiatric illness *(63)* can also cause abnormal thyroid function tests that can be confused with RTH (Table 2). In the past, RTH was often confused with Graves' hyperthyroidism because of the presence of elevated thyroid hormone levels in the setting of goiter (and often tachycardia). However, with newer guidelines emphasizing the importance of measuring TSH levels in diagnosing primary thyroid disease, this scenario is becoming less common.

Once these various conditions are excluded, the diagnosis is generally one of RTH vs. thyrotroph adenoma *(64)*. Differentiation between these two disorders can be difficult, but the following guidelines can be used to distinguish these disorders:

1) Symptoms of hyperthyroidism

   Thyrotroph adenomas secrete TSH and are associated with hyperthyroidism. In contrast, GRTH patients generally have a variable degree of compensated thyroid hormone hyporesponsiveness. However, patients with CRTH are thyrotoxic, so the presence of thyrotoxicosis does not exclude RTH. In addition, tachycardia is a common finding in patients with RTH (even GRTH), so it cannot be used itself as a screen for symptoms of hyperthyroidism.

2) Alpha subunit measurement

   TSH is composed of a specific beta subunit and a common alpha subunit. The same alpha subunit is also present in the other glycoprotein hormones, luteinizing hormone (LH), follicular-stimulating hormone (FSH), and chorionic gonadotropin (CG). Patients with thyrotroph adenomas generally have higher alpha subunit levels than patients with RTH *(64)*. However, this is not always the case, and a number of patients with thyrotroph adenomas have been identified with values in the normal range.

3) Family history

Thyroid function tests from relatives should be taken because RTH is an inherited condition. In contrast, thyrotroph ademonas are generally sporadic in nature. However, patients with RTH can harbor de novo mutations. Therefore, a lack of family history does not exclude a diagnosis of RTH.

4) Magnetic Resonance Imaging (MRI) abnormalities

Most patients with thyrotroph adenomas have macroadenomas by the time they are diagnosed, so an adenoma is easily visualized on MRI. However, with improved diagnostic accuracy, it may be possible to diagnose thyrotroph adenomas earlier in their clinical course, making radiological visualization more difficult. Furthermore, patients with RTH may have incidental pituitary adenomas, mimicking a thyrotroph adenoma *(65)*. However, the presence of a pituitary macroadenoma makes the diagnosis of thyrotroph adenoma much more likely.

5) Other endocrine abnormalities

Pituitary adenomas often co-secrete multiple hormones. Thus, the presence of hyperprolactinemia or acromegaly points to a likely diagnosis of thyrotroph adenoma.

6) TRH stimulation testing

Patients with thyrotroph adenomas usually have a flat response of TSH in response to exogenous TRH, because TSH secretion is autonomous. In contrast, TSH levels generally rise after a TRH infusion in patients with RTH. TRH testing is often performed in protocols examining T_3 responsiveness in patients with possible RTH.

7) Protocols evaluating clinical and biochemical responses to exogenous T_3

The standard way to confirm a diagnosis of RTH is to give graded doses of T_3, and measure a battery of thyroid hormone-responsive tests. Although patients with thyrotroph adenomas have impaired TSH responses to T_3, they will have intact peripheral responses to T_3. In contrast, patients with RTH have impaired TSH and peripheral responses to exogenous T_3. Unfortunately, the few patients who have CRTH also have intact peripheral responses to T_3, making their diagnosis more difficult. Patients are generally admitted to a clinical research center for the duration of the protocol. The most widely used protocol has been designed by Refetoff et al. In adults, exogenous T_3 is given in an escalating regimen (1):

A) T_3 25 µg po BID × 3 d (50 µg daily dose)
B) T_3 50 µg po BID × 3 d (100 µg daily dose)
C) T_3 100 µg po BID × 3 d (200 µg daily dose).

In pediatric patients, the middle 100 µg daily dose is converted to: 25 µg, for ages 1–3 (8–15 kg BW); 50 µg, for ages 4–9 (16–25 kg BW); and 75 µg, for ages 10–14 (26–45 kg BW, with the other doses altered accordingly.

A variety of clinical parameters are measured: *(1)* body weight, food intake, pulse, basal metabolic rate (BMR), thyroid function tests, prolactin, thyroglobulin, cholesterol, triglycerides, creatinine phosphokinase, ferritin, and sex hormone binding globulin (SHBG). TRH stimulation tests are perfomed at each dose. 24-h urine measurements are performed for creatinine, creatine, urea nitrogen, hydroxyproline, and magnesium. For further discussion of this protocol, the reader is referred to a more detailed description by Refetoff, et al. *(1)*.

Safer, et al. *(41)* used a similar protocol to evaluate patients with CRTH. Adults were given T_3 25 µg BID × 4 d, 50 µg BID × 4 d, and 100 µg BID × 4 d. Biochemical indices, including TSH, ferritin, SHBG, ALT, AST, creatinine phosphokinase, lactic dehydrogenase, total cholesterol, and fasting triglycerides were measured. Similar to Refetoff, et al., TRH stimulation tests, measuring TSH and prolactin responses, were performed. Echocardiograms and sleeping heart rate measurements were obtained for cardiac analysis. Ankle jerk relaxation time was assessed by high speed camera. Neuropsychiatric testing was also performed.

The goals of both protocols are to assess biochemical and physiological thyroid hormone-responsive endpoints. Patients with RTH are expected to exhibit diminished responses to thyroid hormone.

8) Thyroid hormone receptor mutations

Most cases of RTH are associated with mutations in the TRβ gene. Ultimately, the most secure way to make a diagnosis of RTH is to demonstrate: 1) elevated thyroid hormone levels in the setting of a non-suppressed TSH; 2) thyroid hormone hypo-responsiveness; and 3) a TR gene mutation.

NEONATAL CONSIDERATIONS

If a child is born to a parent with RTH and a known TR mutation, the best way to confirm or exclude the diagnosis in the infant is to sequence the TRβ gene in the area of the known mutation. There are two other ways infants with RTH come to medical attention: 1) symptoms consistent with RTH; and 2) abnormal thyroid screening tests. As noted previously, infants with RTH may have congenital deafness, congenital nystagmus, neonatal jaundice, and hypotonia. These symptoms may lead to thyroid function testing, and thus the diagnosis. Alternatively, screening programs that are in place to identify infants with congenital hypothyroidism occasionally identify RTH instead. If T_4 levels are used for screening and are elevated, TSH, total T_3, and free T_4 levels should be measured; neonatal Graves' disease and binding protein abnormalities should be excluded. If TSH levels are used for screening and are elevated, T_4 levels should be measured to distinguish between RTH and congenital hypothyroidism. If the situation is clinically confusing, replacement therapy with levothyroxine 10–15 µg/kg/d is indicated, with evaluation of the response of serum TSH to therapy. However, in certain congenitally hypothyroid patients, serum TSH does not fall as rapidly as expected, due to altered feedback regulation of the hypothalamic-pituitary-thyroid axis. This alteration should not be confused with RTH.

Finally, a fetus with suspected RTH can be tested for TR mutations by chorionic villus sampling and DNA analysis *(66)*; however, the benefits of making the diagnosis at this stage have not been clearly established.

Therapy

No specific therapy is available to correct the underlying defect in RTH. Often, patients with RTH are in a clinical state of compensated thyroid hormone hypo-responsiveness. Thus, in these patients, no specific therapy is indicated. In patients with what appears to be greater peripheral hypo-responsiveness, and thus a degree of clinical hypothyroidism, treatment with thyroid hormone (usually levothyroxine) is reasonable.

The specific dosage must be individualized based on markers of thyroid hormone action (such as SHBG, cholesterol, ferritin, BMR, bone density, and urinary hydroxyproline) *(40)*. In patients that have had their thyroid glands ablated for incorrectly diagnosed hyperthyroidism, treatment with thyroid hormone is often necessary, due to limited thyroid gland reserve. In this case, TSH levels are used to guide therapy. In contrast, in patients with CRTH, the use of beta blockers is indicated to control symptoms. Judicious use of antithyroid medications is indicated if the patient clearly has CRTH, and β-blockers have not controlled symptoms. The use of antithyroid drugs, though, is controversial because of the possibility of thyrotroph hyperplasia.

The use of Triac (3,5,3'-triiodothyroacetic acid), a thyroid hormone analog with relative specificity towards the TRβ1 receptor *(67)*, has been advocated for use in CRTH, but Triac should not be truly considered pituitary-specific. Other agents that have been used to decrease TSH levels include the somatostatin analogs and bromocriptine; however, there has been only limited success with these agents.

A prenatal diagnosis of RTH was recently made *(66)*. In this case, a 29-yr-old pregnant woman with previously diagnosed RTH was noted to have symptoms of anxiety, tachycardia, insomnia, and tremor. Due to concerns about the mother and fetus, prenatal diagnosis was made at 17-wk gestation by PCR and restriction enzyme analysis from DNA obtained from chorionic villi. The fetus and mother were both found to harbor the identical TRβ mutation (T337A). In this case, the pregnant woman was treated with Triac, with beneficial effects on maternal symptoms and fetal goiter size. Cordocentesis was performed to evaluate effects of the medication on fetal thyroid function tests. However, an accompanying editorial to the report *(40)* points out the potential dangers of this approach: cordocentesis led to the need for emergency C-section in this case. The authors propose instead that pregnant woman with RTH and symptoms of hyperthyroidism be treated symptomatically with β-blockers, at least until more information is known.

In children with RTH, special care should be directed towards issues of growth and mental development. In particular, patients with delayed bone age may be candidates for therapy. One approach is to consider treatment in children with the following signs and symptoms: 1) elevated serum TSH levels; 2) unexplained failure to thrive; 3) unexplained seizures; 4) developmental delay; and 5) history of growth or mental retardation in other affected members of the family *(40)*. The latter guideline is based on the probability that the clinical outcome of a pediatric patient with RTH will be similar to other family members affected with the same TR mutation (on similar genetic backgrounds). As noted above, patients with RTH and coexisting ADHD may improve on thyroid hormone therapy *(56)*. In any case, patients who require treatment should be followed closely, with careful evaluation of growth, bone age, and thyroid-responsive biochemical indices.

TSH RECEPTOR MUTATIONS

Introduction

Thyrotropin (TSH) is a member of the glycoprotein family of hormone secreted by the anterior pituitary, along with luteinizing hormone (LH) and follicle-stimulating hormone (FSH) *(68)*. These hormones, along with chorionic gonadotropin consist of noncovalently linked α and β subunits, along with linked carbohydrate chains. While the β subunit of each hormone is unique, they all share a common α subunit. TSH stimulates

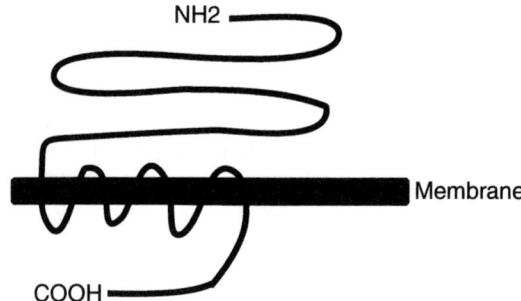

Fig. 3. Schematic diagram of the TSH receptor. The receptor is composed of an *N*-terminal extracellular domain; a trans-membrane region (which spans the plasma membrane seven times); and a cytoplasmic tail.

the growth and function of the thyoid gland, leading to the production of thyroid hormone; therefore, resistance to TSH would be expected to cause hypothyroidism or compensated euthyroid hyperthyrotropinemia. In fact, the first patient reported with resistance to the biological properties of TSH was in 1968 *(69)*, but it was not until 1995 that the first patient with a TSH receptor mutation was documented *(70)*. While activating germline mutations in the TSH receptor have also been identified, leading to syndromes of autosomal dominant hyperthyroidism *(71)*, this chapter will focus on TSH resistance caused by loss-of-function mutations.

Mechanisms of Disease and Clinical Presentation of TSH Resistance

In 1995, Sunthornthepvarakul et al., documented the first case of a TSH receptor mutation leading to TSH resistance *(70)*. The index case was an infant born to unrelated parents, who was found to have an elevated TSH level on routine neonatal screening. Two siblings were also found to have high TSH, but normal thyroid hormone levels. All three were clinically euthyroid. All were found to be compound heterozygotes for mutations in exon 6 of the TSH receptor, corresponding to a portion of the TSH extracellular domain *(70)*. In vitro data suggested that the mutations decreased the biological activity of TSH. Since that time, a number of other patients have been identified with TSH receptor mutations causing TSH resistance. Such patients generally are homozygous for the identified TSH receptor mutations, or, as in the initial family, are compound heterozygotes.

The TSH receptor is a transmembrane G-coupled receptor (Fig. 3). It contains a large extracellular domain with three regions - the middle of these regions (approximately amino acids 58–288) contains the most significant homology to FSH and LH receptors *(72)*. The extracellular domain may inhibit constitutive activity of the receptor *(73)*. Cleavage of the extracellular domain results in two separate subunits (A and B) linked by disulfide bonds, although it is possible that a single-chain form may also exist *(72)*. TSH makes contact with a number of regions within the extracellular domain. The carboxy-terminal portion of the TSH receptor includes the transmembrane domain, which spans the plasma membrane seven times. There is also an 82 amino acid cytoplasmic tail *(72)*. The gene encoding the TSH receptor has been localized to chromosome 14q31 *(74,75)*.

There are two general modes of presentation for patients with loss-of-function germline TSH receptor mutations. The first is similar to the family identified by

Sunthornthepvarakul, et al. *(70)*. In these patients, high TSH levels are necessary to overcome partial TSH resistance. Such patients, however, are euthyroid. Four additional families with these clinical characteristics have been identified by de Roux et al. *(76)*. One patient had a homozygous mutation in codon 162 of the TSH receptor; the other three were compound heterozygotes. Interestingly, one of the mutations (C390W) caused loss of TSH binding; whereas another (D410N) bound TSH normally, but was unable to activate adenylate cyclase. Thus, inactivating mutations of the TSH receptor can interfere with a variety of receptor functions. In addition, mutations affecting signal transduction were found in both the extracellular (D410N) and intracellular (F525L) domains *(76)*. Similar patients with euthyroid hyperthyrotropinemia and TSH receptor mutations have been identified by additional groups *(77,78)*.

In contrast, other TSH receptor mutations cause more extreme hormone resistance. Patients with these mutations present with hypothyroidism, often identified by neonatal screening. For example, Abramowicz, et al., reported two patients, a brother and sister, who were diagnosed with congenital hypothyroidism by neonatal screening *(79)*. Ultrasound evaluation revealed hypoplastic thyroid glands. A homozygous mutation of the TSH receptor in the fourth transmembrane domain (A553T) was found in both patients; the parents and unaffected siblings were found to be heterozygous for the same mutation. In vitro analysis suggested that this receptor bound TSH normally, and was synthesized in normal amounts. However, there were extremely low levels of expression of the mutant receptor at the cell surface, suggesting a mechanism for the extreme TSH resistance *(79)*. At about the same time, a similar patient was reported by another group; this patient was a compound heterozygote of two mutations in exon 10 of the receptor *(80)*. Since that time, other patients with inactivating mutations of the TSH receptor leading to congenital hypothyroidism have also been reported *(81,82)*.

Not all cases of resistance to TSH are caused by mutations in the TSH receptor. When sequenced, the TSH receptor gene (including coding region, intron/ exon junctions, and promoter region) have been found to be normal in some patients with the disorder *(83)*. Interestingly, some of these cases appear to be inherited in an autosomal dominant fashion *(83)*.

Diagnostic Considerations and Therapy

For patients with mild TSH resistance, and thus euthyroid hyperthyrotropinemia, the major differential diagnosis to consider is with subclinical primary hypothyroidism. By definition, subclinical hypothyroidism also presents with elevated TSH levels in the setting of normal thyroid hormone levels. Similarly, patients with more severe TSH resistance, leading to hypothyroidism, will present with thyroid function tests identical to other causes of primary hypothyroidism. Patients with resistance to TSH, however, do not have a goiter, and the disorder is usually inherited in an autosomal recessive pattern.

Patients with severe resistance often present with hypothyroidism detected by neonatal screening programs . Since congenital hypothyroidism is not usually an inherited disorder, a significant family history in the setting of congenital hypothyroidism is suggestive of the possibility of TSH resistance. Furthermore, the thyroid is usually hypoplastic, but not ectopic, in TSH resistance, as can be seen in other causes of congenital hypothyroidism.

Patients with mild TSH resistance and euthyroid hyperthyrotropinemia are in a compensated eumetabolic state. These patients are clinically euthyroid, and do not require treatment, although they should receive genetic counseling. Patients with more severe TSH resistance, leading to hypothyroidism, should be treated with levothyroxine.

CONCLUSION

Hormone resistance leading to thyroid dysfunction occurs at multiple levels of the pituitary-thyroid axis. In milder forms, such resistance presents in a compensated state, and does not require therapy. However, in more severe forms, therapy is required. In particular, therapy in patients with RTH must be individualized, and the metabolic status of the patient must be determined rigorously. In children, special care must be paid to growth, bone development, and mental development in deciding the specific course of therapy. Further studies in children need to be performed so that medical care can be optimized in these patients.

Resistance to thyroid hormone is usually caused by autosomal dominant mutations in the TRβ gene. In contrast, resistance to TSH is usually caused by autosomal recessive mutations in the TSH receptor gene. However, a number of patients with both disorders have been identified without mutations in these genes. Such patients probably harbor mutations elsewhere. Further evaluation of these patients will be important not only to provide optimal medical therapy, but also to gain further insight into the mechanisms of action of thyroid hormone and thyrotropin.

REFERENCES

1. Refetoff S, Weiss RE, Usala SJ. The syndromes of resistance to thyroid hormone. Endocr Rev 1993;14:348–399.
2. Abel ED, Kaulbach HC, Campos-Barros A, et al. Novel insight from transgenic mice into thyroid hormone resistance and the regulation of thyrotropin. J Clin Invest 1999;103:271–279.
3. Refetoff S. Resistance to Thyroid Hormone. In: Braverman LE, Utiger RD, eds. Werner and Ingbar's The Thyroid: A Fundamental and Clinical Text. Lippincott, Williams, and Wilkins, Philadelphia, PA 2000, pp. 1028–1043.
4. Mangelsdorf DJ, Thummel C, Beato M, et al. Overview: the nuclear receptor superfamily: the second decade. Cell 1995;83:835–840.
5. Katz RW, Subauste JS, Koenig RJ. The interplay of half-site sequence and spacing on the activity of direct repeat thyroid hormone response elements. J Biol Chem 1995;270:5238–5242.
6. Umesono K, Murakami KK, Thompson CC, Evans RM. Direct repeats as selective response elements for the thyroid hormone, retinoic acid and vitamin D3 receptors. Cell 1991;65:1255–1266.
7. Hollenberg AN, Monden T, Flynn TR, Boers M-E, Cohen O, Wondisford FE. The human thyrotropin-releasing hormone gene is regulated by thyroid hormone through two distinct classes of negative thyroid hormone response elements. Mol Endocrinol 1995;10:540–550.
8. Tomic-Canic M, Day D, Samuels HH, Freedberg IM, Blumenberg M. Novel regulation of keratin gene expression by thyroid hormone and retinoid receptors. J Biol Chem 1996;271:1416–1423.
9. Bodenner DL, Mrocynski MA, Weintraub BD, Radovick S, Wondisford FE. A detailed functional and structural analysis of a major thyroid inhibitory element in the human thyrotropin b-subunit gene. J Biol Chem 1991;266.
10. Seol W, Choi HS, Moore DD. Isolation of proteins that interact specifically with the retinoid X receptor: two novel orphan nuclear receptors. Mol Endocrinol 1995;9:72–85.
11. Horlein AJ, Naar AM, Heinzel T, et al. Ligand-independent repression by the thyroid hormone receptor mediated by a nuclear receptor co-repressor. Nature 1995;377:397–404.
12. Chen JD, Evans RM. A transcriptional co-repressor that interacts with nuclear hormone receptors. Nature 1995;377:454–457.
13. Sande S, Privalsky ML. Identification of TRACs (T_3 receptor-associating cofactors), a family of cofactors that associate with and modulate the activity of, nuclear hormone receptors. Mol Endocrinol 1996;10:813–825.

14. Ordentlich P, Downes M, Xie W, Genin A, Spinner NB, Evans RM. Unique forms of human and mouse nuclear receptor corepressor SMRT. Proc Natl Acad Sci USA 1999;96:2639–2644.
15. Park EJ, Schroen DJ, Yang M, Li H, Li L, Chen JD. SMRTe, a silencing mediator for retinoid and thyroid hormone receptors- extended isoform that is more related to the nuclear receptor corepressor. Proc Natl Acad Sci USA 1999;96:3519–3524.
16. Alland L, Muhle R, Hou HJ, et al. Role for N-CoR and histone deacetylase in Sin3-mediated transcriptional repression. Nature 1997;387:49–55.
17. Heinzel T, Lavinsky RM, Mullen TM, et al. A complex containing N-CoR, mSin3 and histone deacetylase mediates transcriptional repression. Nature 1997;387:43–48.
18. Nagy L, Kao H-K, Chakravarti D, et al. Nuclear receptor repression mediated by a complex containing SMRT, mSin3A, and histone deacetylase. Cell 1997;89:373–380.
19. Feng W, Ribeiro RCJ, Wagner RL, et al. Hormone-dependent coactivator binding to a hydrophobic cleft on nuclear receptors. Science 1998;280:1747–1749.
20. Onate SA, Tsai SY, Tsai M-J, O'Malley BW. Sequence and characterization of a coactivator for the steroid hormone receptor superfamily. Science 1995;270:1354–1357.
21. Takeshita A, Yen PM, Misiti S, Cardona GR, Liu Y, Chin WW. Molecular cloning and properties of a full-length putative thyroid hormone receptor coactivator. Endocrinology 1996;137:3594–3597.
22. Voegel JJ, Heine MJS, Zechel C, Chambon P, Gronemeyer H. TIF2, a 160 kD transcriptional mediator for the ligand-dependent activation function AF-2 of nuclear receptors. EMBO J 1996;15:3667–3675.
23. Cavailles V, Dauvois S, L'Horset F, et al. Nuclear factor RIP140 modulates transcriptional activation by the estrogen receptor. EMBO J 1995;14:3741–3751.
24. Kamei Y, Xu L, Heinzel T, et al. A CBP integrator complex mediates transcriptional activation and AP-1 inhibition by nuclear receptors. Cell 1996;85:403–414.
25. Torchia J, Rose DW, Inostroza J, et al. The transcriptional co-activator p/CIP binds CBP and mediates nuclear receptor function. Nature 1997;387:677–684.
26. Anzick SL, Kononen J, Walker RL, et al. AIB1, a steroid receptor coactivator amplified in breast and ovarian cancer. Nature 1997;277:965–968.
27. Chen H, Lin RJ, Schlitz RL, et al. Nuclear receptor coactivator ACTR is a novel histone acetyltransferase and forms a multimeric activation complex with P/CAF and CBP/p300. Cell 1997;90:569–580.
28. Monden T, Wondisford FE, Hollenberg AN. Isolation and characterization of a novel ligand-dependent thyroid hormone receptor-coactivating protein. J Biol Chem 1997; 272:29,834–29,841.
29. Sap J, Munoz A, Damm K, et al. The c-erb-A gene protein is a high-affinity receptor for thyroid hormone. Nature 1986;324:635–640.
30. Weinberger C, Thompson CC, Ong ES, Lebo R, Gruol DJ, Evans RM. The c-erb-A gene encodes a thyroid hormone receptor. Nature 1986;324:641–646.
31. Williams GR. Cloning and characterization of two novel thyroid hormone receptor beta isoforms. Mol Cell Biol 2000;20:8329–8342.
32. Weiss RE, Hayashi Y, Nagaya T, et al. Dominant inheritance of Resistance to Thyroid Hormone not linked to defects in the thyroid hormone receptor a or b genes may be due to a defective cofactor. J Clin Endocrinol Metab 1996;81:4196–4203.
33. Reutrakal S, Sadow PM, Pannain S, et al. Search for abnormalities of nuclear corepressors, coactivators, and a coregulator in families with Resistance to Thyroid Hormone without mutations in thyroid hormone receptor b or a genes. J Clin Endocrinol Metab 2000;85:3609–3617.
34. Collingwood TN, Wagner R, Matthews CH, et al. A role for helix 3 of the TRb ligand-binding domain in coactivator recruitment identified by characterization of a third cluster of mutations in resistance to thyroid hormone. EMBO J 1998;17:4760–4770.
35. Safer JD, Cohen RN, Hollenberg AN, Wondisford FE. Defective release of corepressor by hinge mutants of the thyroid hormone receptor found in patients with resistance to thyroid hormone. J Biol Chem 1998; 273:30175–82.
36. Yoh SM, Chatterjee VK, Privalsky ML. Thyroid hormone resistance syndrome manifests as an aberrant interaction between mutant T_3 receptors and transcriptional corepressors. Mol Endocrinol 1997; 11:470–80.
37. Collingwood TN, Rajanayagam O, Adams M, et al. A natural transactivation mutation in the thyroid hormone beta receptor: impaired interaction with putative transcriptional mediators. Proc Natl Acad Sci USA 1997;94:248–253.

38. Nagaya T, Jameson JL. Thyroid hormone receptor dimerization is required for dominant negative inhibition by mutations that cause thyroid hormone resistance. J Biol Chem 1993;268:15,766–15,771.
39. Nagaya T, Madison LD, Jameson JL. Thyroid hormone receptor mutants that cause resistance to thyroid hormone. J Biol Chem 1992;267:13,014–13,019.
40. Weiss RE, Refetoff S. Editorial: Treatment of Reisitance to Thyroid Hormone - Primum Non Nocere. J Clin Endocrinol Metab 1999;84:401–403.
41. Safer JD, O'Connor MG, Colan SD, Srinivasan S, Tollin SR, Wondisford FE. The thyroid hormone receptor-b mutation R383H is associated with isolated central resistance to thyroid hormone. J Clin Endocrinol Metab 1999; 84:3099–3109.
42. Safer JD, Langlois MF, Cohen R, et al. Isoform variable action among thyroid hormone receptor mutants provides insight into pituitary resistance to thyroid hormone. Mol Endocrinol 1997;11:16–26.
43. Forrest D, Hanebuth E, Smeyne RJ, et al. Recessive resistance to thyroid hormone in mice lacking thyroid hormone receptor beta: evidence for tissue-specific modulation of receptor function. EMBO J 1996;15:3006–3015.
44. Kaneshige M, Kaneshige K, Xhu X, et al. Mice with a targeted mutation in the thyroid hormone beta receptor gene exhibit impaired growth and resistance to thyroid hormone. Proc Natl Acad Sci USA 2000;97:13,209–13,214.
45. Hashimoto K, Curty FH, Borges PB, et al. An unliganded thyroid hormone receptor causes severe neurological dysfunction. Proc Natl Acad Sci USA 2001;98:3998–4003.
46. Weiss RE, Xu J, Ning G, Pohlenz J, O'Malley BW, Refetoff S. Mice deficient in the steroid receptor co-activator 1 (SRC-1) are resistant to thyroid hormone. EMBO J 1999; 18:1900–1904.
47. Wikstrom L, Johansson C, Salto C, et al. Abnormal heart rate and body temperature in mice lacking thyroid hormone receptor alpha 1. EMBO J 1998;17:455–461.
48. Fraichard A, Chassande O, Plateroti M, et al. The T_3R alpha gene encoding a thyroid hormone receptor is essential for post-natal development and thyroid hormone production. EMBO J 1997;16:4412–4420.
49. Refetoff S, DeWind LT, DeGroot LJ. Familial syndrome combining deaf-mutism, stippled epiphyses, goiter and abnormally high PBI: Possible target organ refractoriness to thyroid hormone. J Clin Endocrinol 1967;27:279–294.
50. Takeda T, Sakurai A, DeGroot LJ, Refetoff S. Recessive inheritance of thyroid hormone resistance caused by complete deletion of the protein-coding region of the thyroid hormone receptor-β gene. J Clin Endocrinol Metab 1992;74:49–55.
51. Hauser P, Zametkin AJ, Martinez P, et al. Attention deficit-hyperactivity disorder in people with generalized resistance to thyroid hormone. N Eng J Med 1993;328:997–1001.
52. Brucker-Davis F, Skarulis MC, Grace MB, et al. Genetic and clinical features of 42 kindreds with resistance to thyroid hormone: The National Institutes of Health prospective study. Ann Intern Med 1995;123:572–583.
53. Weiss RE, Refetoff SE. Effect of thyroid hormone on growth: lessons from the syndrome of resistance to thyroid hormone. Endocrinol Metab Clin North Am 1996;25:719–730.
54. Stein MA, Weiss RE, Refetoff S. Neurocognitive characteristics of individuals with resistance to thyroid hormone: comparisons with individuals with attention-deficit hyperactivity disorder. J Dev Behav Pediatr 1995;16:406–411.
55. Matochik JA, Zametkin AJ, Cohen RM, Hauser P, Weintraub BD. Abnormalities in sustained attention and anterior cingulate gyrus metabolism in subjects with resistance to thyroid hormone. Brain Res 1996;723:23–28.
56. Weiss RE, Stein MA, Refetoff S. Behavioral effects of Liothyronine ($L-T_3$) in children with Attention Deficit Hyperactivity Disorder in the presence and absence of resistance to thyroid hormone. Thyroid 1997;7:389–393.
57. Kahn BB, Weintraub BD, Csako G, Zweig MH. Facticious elevation of thyrotropin in a new ultrasensitive assay: implications for the use of monoclonal antibodies in "sandwich" immunoassay. J Clin Endocrinol Metab 1988;66:526–533.
58. Martino E, Bartalena L, Bogazzi F, Braverman LE. The effects of amiodarone on the thyroid. Endocr Rev 2001;22:240–254.
59. Burrow GN, A. FD, R. LP. Maternal and fetal thyroid function. N Engl J Med 1994; 331:1072–1078.
60. Huang MJ, Liaw YF. Clinical associations between thyroid and liver diseases. J Gastroenterol Hepatol 1995;10:344–350.
61. Pannain S, Feldman M, Eiholzer U, Weiss RE, Scherberg NH, Refetoff S. Familial dysalbuminemic hyperthyroxinemia in a Swiss family caused by a mutant albumin (R218P) shows an apparent dis-

crepancy between serum concentration and affinity for thyroxine. J Clin Endocrinol Metab 2000;85:2786–2792.
62. Petersen CE, Ha CE, Jameson DM, Bhagavan NV. Mutations in a specific human serum albumin thyroxine binding site define the structural basis of familial dysalbuminemic hyperthyroxinemia. J Biol Chem 1996;271:19,110–19,117.
63. Roca RP, Blackman MR, Ackerley MB, Harman SM, Gregerman RI. Thyroid hormone elevations during acute psychiatric illness: relationship to severity and distinction from hyperthyroidism. Endocr Res 1990;16:415–447.
64. Beck-Peccoz P, Bruckner-Davis F, Persani L, Smallridge RC, Weintraub BD. Thyrotropin-secreting pituitary tumors. Endocr Rev 1996;17:610–638.
65. Safer JD, Colan SD, Fraser LM, Wondisford FE. A pituitary tumor in a patient with thyroid hormone resistance: a diagnostic dilemma. Thyroid 2001;11:281–291.
66. Asteria C, Rajanayagam O, Collingwood TN, et al. Prenatal diagnosis of thyroid hormone resistance. J Clin Endocrinol Metab 1999;84:405–410.
67. Takeda T, Suzuki S, Liu RT, Degroot LJ. Triiodothyroacetic acid has unique potential for therapy of resistance to thyroid hormone. J Clin Endocrinol Metab 1995; 80:2033–2040.
68. Cohen RN, Weintraub BD, Wondisford FE. Chemistry and biosynthesis of thyrotropin. In: Braverman LE, Utiger RD, eds. Werner and Ingbar's The Thyroid. Philadelphia: Lippincott, Williams, and Wilkins, 2000, pp.
69. Stanbury JB, Rocmans P, Buhler UK, Ochi Y. Congenital hypothyroidism with impaired thyroid response to thyrotropin. N Engl J Med 1968; 279:1132–1136.
70. Sunthornthepvarakul T, Gottschalk ME, Hayashi Y, Refetoff S. Brief Report: Resistance to thyrotropin caused by mutations in the thyrotropin-receptor gene. N Engl J Med 1995;332:155–160.
71. Duprez L, Parma J, Van Sande J, et al. Germline mutations in the thyrotropin receptor gene cause non-autoimmune autosomal dominant hyperthyroidism. Nat Genet 1994;7:396–401.
72. Rapoport B, Chazenbalk GD, Jaume JC, McLachlan SM. The thyrotropin (TSH) receptor: interaction with TSH and autoantibdies. Endocr Rev 1998;19:673–716.
73. Zhang M, Tong KPT, Fremont V, et al. The extracellular domain suppresses constitutive activity of the transmembrane domain of the human TSH receptor: implications for hormone-receptor interaction and antagonist design. Endocrinology 2000;141:3514–3517.
74. Rousseau-Merck MF, Misrahi M, Loosfelt H, Atger M, Milgrom E, Berger R. Assignment of the human thyroid stimulating hormone receptor (TSHR) gene to chromosome 14q31. Genomics 1990; 8:233–236.
75. Libert F, Passage E, Lefort A, Vassart G, Mattei MG. Localization of human thyrotropin receptor gene to chromosome region 14q31 by in situ hybridization. Cytogenet Cell Genet 1990;54:82–83.
76. de Roux N, Misrahi M, Brauner R, et al. Four families with loss of function mutations of the thyrotropin receptor. J Clin Endocrinol Metab 1996;81:4229–4235.
77. Russo D, Betterle B, Arturi F, Chiefari E, Girelli ME, Filetti S. A novel mutation in the thyrotropin (TSH) receptor gene causing loss of TSH binding but constitutive receptor activation in a fmily with resistance to TSH. J Clin Endocrinol Metab 2000;85:4238–4242.
78. Clifton-Bligh RJ, Gregory JW, Ludgate M, et al. Two novel mutations inthe thyrotropin (TSH) receptor gene in a child with resistance to TSH. J Clin Endocrinol Metab 1997;82:1094–1100.
79. Abramowicz MJ, Duprez L, Parma J, Vassart G, Heinrichs C. Familial congenital hypothyroidism due to inactivating mutation of the thyrotropin receptor causing profound hypoplasia of the thyroid gland. J Clin Invest 1997;99:3018–3024.
80. Biberman H, Schoneberg T, Krude H, Schultz G, Guderman T, Gruters A. Mutations of the human thyrotropin receptor gene causing thyroid hypoplasia and persistent congenital hypothyroidism. J Clin Endocrinol 1997;82:3471–3480.
81. Tonacchera M, Agretti P, Pinchera A, et al. Congenital hypothyroidism with impaired thyroid response to thyrotropin (TSH) and absent circulating thyroglobulin: Evidence for a new inactivating mutation of the TSH Receptor Gene. J Clin Endocrinol Metab 2000;85:1001–1008.
82. Gagne N, Parma J, Deal C, Vassart G, Van Vliet G. Apparent congenital athyreosis contrasting with normal plasma thyroglobulin levels and associated with inactivating mutations in the thyrotropin receptor gene: Are athyreosis and ectopic thyroid distinct entities? J Clin Endocrinol Metab 1998;83:1771–1775.
83. Xie J, Pannain S, Pohlenz J, et al. Resistance to thyrotropin (TSH) in three families is not associated with mutations in the TSH receptor or TSH. J Clin Endocrinol 1997;82:3933–3940.

19 Thyroid Cancer in Children and Adolescents

Charles A. Sklar, MD
and Michael P. La Quaglia, MD

CONTENTS

INTRODUCTION
PATHOGENESIS OF THYROID CANCER
CLINICAL PRESENTATION
DIAGNOSTIC GUIDELINES
THERAPY
FOLLOW-UP
CONCLUSION
REFERENCES

INTRODUCTION

Thyroid cancer is rare in childhood and adolescence and consists of several histopathologic groups that differ considerably in their clinical behavior. Major pathologic categories include differentiated, medullary, and poorly differentiated thyroid carcinomas. Medullary carcinoma accounts for a small percentage of pediatric thyroid cancers. It is most often diagnosed in children and adolescents affected by MEN IIa, MEN IIb, or Familial Medullary Carcinoma syndromes. These autosomal dominant disorders are known to be caused by mutations in the *RET* proto-oncogene; molecular screening is now available for individuals who, based on family history, are felt to be at risk (*1*). Poorly differentiated thyroid cancers, including anaplastic and insular carcinomas, are fortunately exceedingly uncommon in the pediatric age group but carry a very poor prognosis (*2*). Differentiated thyroid cancers account for the vast majority of thyroid cancers of youth and will be the focus of this review.

Differentiated thyroid cancer is defined by the presence of distinguishable elements of normal thyroid cells. Two subtypes are generally recognized: papillary (including papillary-follicular) and pure follicular. Papillary and papillary-follicular are the most

From: *Contemporary Endocrinology: Pediatric Endocrinology: A Practical Clinical Guide*
Edited by: S. Radovick and M. H. MacGillivray © Humana Press Inc., Totowa, NJ

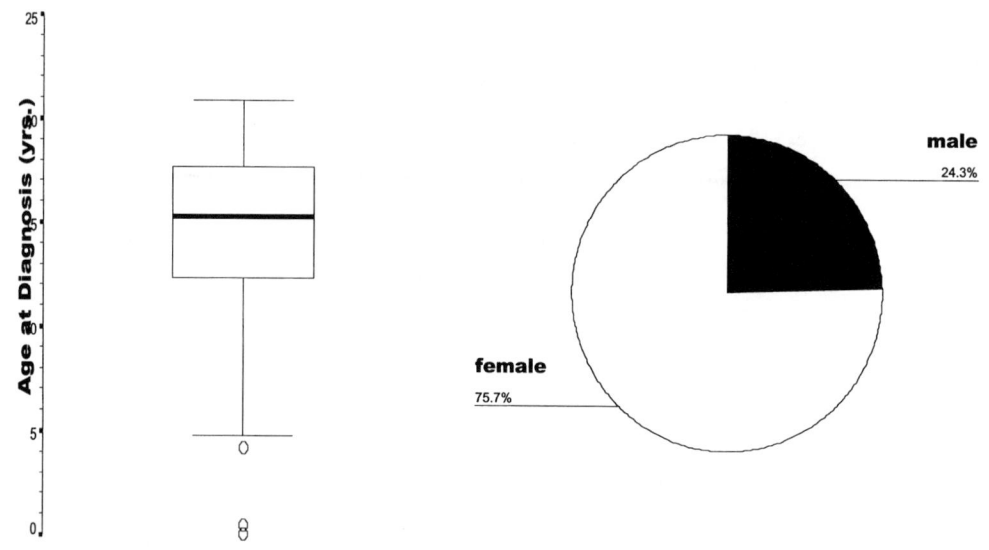

Fig. 1. Distribution by age and sex of 329 cases of differentiated thyroid cancer. Derived from data published in Newman KD, et al. *(6)*.

prevalent subtypes seen in the pediatric population, accounting for 90% of differentiated lesions.

Incidence

Most patients with differentiated thyroid cancer are adults, 40–60 yr-of-age. The age adjusted incidence of thyroid cancer in the pediatric and adult population as a whole is on the order of 30–40 cases per million. The incidence of thyroid cancer in childhood varies by age: it is approx 1.0 case per million in children 5–9 yr-of-age, 3.9 cases per million at ages 10–14, and 14.4 cases per million at ages 15–19 *(3)*. In Connecticut the historic incidence of 1.5/million rose to 3.1 after 1989 at a time when an increased incidence was also observed in Belarus *(4)*.

Patient Characteristics

Differentiated thyroid cancer is a disease seen primarily in adolescents; the median age at diagnosis is around 15 yr (Fig. 1). Proportionally more females are involved compared to males with a female:male ratio varying from 2:1 to 4:1 *(5,6)*.

Predisposing Factors

There is a strong association with the use of ionizing radiation to the head and neck and the subsequent development of differentiated thyroid carcinoma. In 1950, Duffy and Fitzgerald reported that 36% (10/28) of pediatric patients treated for thyroid cancer at the Memorial Sloan-Kettering Cancer Center had been exposed to radiation to the neck region earlier in life *(7)*. Subsequent retrospective reviews showed that irradiation for such benign conditions as thymic enlargement in infancy, infections of the tonsils and adenoids, acne, tinea capitis, or even fluoroscopy increased the risk of development of thyroid carcinoma *(8)*.

Further evidence for an association between thyroid cancer and irradiation comes from epidemiologic studies of populations exposed to atomic fallout and survivors of childhood cancer exposed to therapeutic doses of external beam radiation. Younger patients appear to be more susceptible, particularly individuals exposed prior to age 5 yr. The absolute risk of thyroid cancer in patients receiving cervical radiation in childhood has been estimated from a pooled study of seven series at 4.4 excess cancers per 10,000 person-yr per gray with a relative risk of 7.7 per gray *(9)*. It is important to note that the increased risk of developing thyroid cancer persists even following therapeutic doses to thyroid in excess of 20–30 Gy *(10)*. While the latency period between exposure to radiation and the development of thyroid cancer is usually 10–20 or more years, these cancers can occur as early as 3–5 yr after the radiation.

Although it has been thought that thyroid irradiation secondary to internal isotopes such as ^{131}I is less carcinogenic than external x-rays, recent data from the Chernobyl accident underscore that such exposures, particularly in young children, are capable of inducing thyroid cancers. For those younger than 5 yr at the time of the accident, the incidence of thyroid cancer may be increased 100-fold *(11)*. In contrast, the use of iodine-131 for diagnostic purposes in childhood has not been associated with an increased risk of thyroid cancer *(12)*.

An association between differentiated thyroid cancer and both Gardner's syndrome (lipomas, osteomas, and intestinal polyps) and Cowden's syndrome (multiple hamartomas) have been reported. Ninety-four percent of the Gardner's syndrome patients who develop thyroid cancer are women and 88% of the tumors are papillary with twice the normal incidence of multicentricity *(13)*.

More controversial is the possible association between Hashimoto's thyroiditis and an increased risk of differentiated thyroid cancer in the pediatric age group. While lymphoma of the thyroid does appear to occur more frequently in adults with chronic lymphocytic thyroiditis *(14)*, the evidence supporting an increased risk of differentiated thyroid cancer in these individuals is conflicting and based primarily on anecdotal case reports *(15)*.

PATHOGENESIS OF THYROID CANCER

Several studies have examined the significance of oncogene activation in both benign and malignant thyroid neoplasia. Activation of ras, Gs alpha, trk, and p53 are detected in a small percentage of thyroid nodules *(16)*. None of these appear to be associated with significant clinical outcomes. More recently, a tyrosine kinase oncogene known as RET/PTC has been shown to be present in a high proportion of papillary carcinomas and felt to play a pathogenetic role. Early reports suggested that the various forms of RET/PTC were more prevalent in radiation-induced thyroid cancers compared to sporadic cancers and more common in cancers diagnosed in children compared to those found in adults. Recently both of these findings have, however, come into question *(17)*.

CLINICAL PRESENTATION

Patients with thyroid cancer almost always present with an asymptomatic neck mass or swelling *(5)*. Since 50–90% of pediatric and adolescent patients have involved cervical lymph nodes at diagnosis, in a minority of cases the mass may actually be nodal metastases rather than a palpable thyroid nodule. These nodules may be slow-growing and, initially, may not arouse clinical suspicion. The primary thyroid tumor may be located anywhere in the thyroid gland but isthmic involvement is rare. Although a bilateral cervical mass is not uncommon, the usual presentation is with unilateral disease. A chronic, non-productive cough may be evident in patients with tracheal or recurrent nerve invasion. Hoarseness and dysphagia may also accompany invasive tumors. Obstructive airway symptoms represent an unusual mode of presentation of this disease in childhood. Extrinsic compressive tumors or transtracheal intraluminal tumors, while rare, should always be a consideration in atypical or medically refractory 'asthma' during childhood. Although 10–25% of pediatric subjects with differentiated thyroid cancer will have evidence of distant metastases (primarily pulmonary) at diagnosis (6), it is quite uncommon for these patients to present with symptoms or signs due to metastatic disease.

DIAGNOSTIC GUIDELINES

Once a cervical mass is palpated and clinical suspicion is raised, the workup is relatively straightforward. Initial blood studies should include routine thyroid function studies to determine functional status and thyroid antibodies, which if positive may suggest Hashimoto's thyroiditis. There is no proven value of determining the plasma concentration of thyroglobulin, as it can be elevated in individuals with either malignant or benign lesions of the thyroid. A thyroid ultrasound may be very helpful if there is a question as to the exact nature of the lesion; ultrasound may exclude the possibility of a pure cyst or congenital malformation such as hemiagenesis of the thyroid gland. Additionally, ultrasound can often facilitate the performance of a needle biopsy. While some investigators recommend performing radionuclide scans (such as technetium or ^{123}I) in individuals with a thyroid nodule, most nodules in children will appear cold on scintiscanning, regardless of their ultimate histopathology. We have not found radioisotope scans to be useful in the vast majority of individuals with solitary nodules and no longer employ them as part of our routine, initial work-up. Similarly, the response of a thyroid nodule to TSH suppression with exogenous thyroid hormone has not been shown to be a reliable or sensitive means of differentiating between benign and malignant lesions (18).

Currently, fine needle aspiration biopsy (FNAB) is the cornerstone in the management of solitary thyroid nodules in adults. If performed by experienced personnel, this procedure has a very high sensitivity (80–85%) and specificity (90–95%), with a low (1–5%) false negative rate (19). Limitations include a small but variable number of nondiagnostic specimens and the inability to distinguish between benign and malignant follicular neoplasms. Utilization of the FNAB has dramatically reduced the number of unnecessary open surgical procedures. Historically, some pediatric groups have been reluctant to use FNAB in the initial evaluation of thyroid nodules in children, opting to perform surgery on all such lesions, even though only 15–20% of all solitary thyroid nodules in children and adolescents will prove to be malignant (20). An emerging literature, however, attests to the safety and accuracy of FNAB in children and adolescents (21–23).

Needles of 25–27 gauge are used in children and sampling is done with a 10–20 mL disposable plastic syringe held in one hand. The aspirate should appear orange in color and should be visible as a small drop in the needle hub. The needle tip is moved slightly in and out to loosen cells. Typically up to five or six separate aspirations are performed in a single session to reduce sampling error. The aspirate is smeared on glass microscope slides and immediately treated with cytologic fixative. Analysis by an experienced cytologist is mandatory and an answer is usually available within 24 h or less.

Table 1
Selected Series of Pediatric Thyroid Cancer

Author (ref.)	Year	N	Nodes + (%)	Total or subtotal thyroidectomy (%)	Relapses (%)	Deaths (%)
Exelby (24)	1969	62	87	43	—	6
Liechty (25)	1972	30	77	80	—	6
Richardson (26)	1974	32	50	38	—	6
Buckwalter (27)	1975	58	60	50	7.4	2
Tallroth (28)	1986	37	73	40	14	3
Schlumberger (29)	1987	72	85	40	34	8
La Quaglia (30)	1988	93	71	46	35	0
Zimmerman (31)	1988	58	90	74	31	14
Azizkhan (32)	1991	30	60	60	22	0
Newman (6)	1998	329	74	71	32	0.6
Welch Dinauer (33)	1998	137	39*	82.5*	20*	0.7*
Alessandri (34)	2000	38	60.5	65.8	45	0
Jarzab (35)	2000	109	59	74	15	0
Storm (36)	2001	165	—	—	—	3

*Data from patients with papillary carcinoma only.

In summary, after a careful history and physical examination and routine blood studies, an FNAB (with ultrasound if desired) of suspicious thyroid lesions should be performed. Definitive surgery is required for all lesions with malignant or suspicious cytology and any lesion, regardless of the results of FNAB, that manifests malignant features (e.g., rapid growth, causes compression of local structures). Because FNAB is associated with a small but significant false negative rate, we recommend a repeat FNAB in 6–12 mo for any lesion that either fails to involute or increases in size.

THERAPY

The optimum management of children and adolescents with differentiated thyroid cancer remains an area of some controversy. It is strikingly obvious from Table 1 that mortality in differentiated pediatric thyroid cancer is very low (6,24–36), making it very difficult to prove survival benefit of one therapy versus another. Additionally, as most reports are based on data generated from relatively small patient numbers, the majority of published studies have reduced statistical power and, therefore, limited ability to prove the superiority of a particular management approach. Since mortality is not a feasible endpoint, most authors have used disease recurrence or progression, which occurs in approximately one-third of patients, as an endpoint.

The initial treatment of almost all differentiated thyroid cancers is surgical. There is, however, little agreement concerning the best surgical approach. This is illustrated in Table 1, which lists the larger published series of pediatric thyroid cancer. Even though total/subtotal thyroidectomy, followed by radioiodine treatment has been considered the "gold standard" of therapy for both pediatric and adult thyroid cancers, the risk of major complications (e.g., permanent hypoparathyroidism, hoarseness, facial paralysis, Horner's syndrome, major bleeding, the need for a tracheostomy, or the occurrence of tracheal stenosis) has been shown consistently to increase with more aggressive thyroid

Table 2
Factors Predictive of Outcome (in Univariate or Multivariate Analysis) in Pediatric Thyroid Cancer

Author (ref.)	Year	N	Clinical Variables	Treatment Variables
La Quaglia (30)	1988	93	Age, Histologic subtype	None
Newman (6)	1998	329	Age	Completeness of resection (e.g., presence of residual cervical disease) but not extent of initial surgery
Welch Dinauer (33)	1998	170	Age, size of tumor, focality	None
Welch Dinauer (38)*	1999	37	—	Extent of initial surgery
Alessandri (34)	2000	38	Age	None
Jarzab (35)	2000	109	Age	Extent of initial surgery, Radioactive iodine ($p = 0.07$)

*Data from patients with class 1 papillary thyroid cancer (disease confined to the thyroid gland).

surgery (6,30,37). Risk-based therapy offers an alternative approach to the management of these individuals and attempts to tailor therapy according to the individual's risk of recurrence (6,38). Such an approach, hopefully, will minimize the risks of serious complications, while still providing a high probability of cure.

Predictors of Recurrence or Progression

The clinical and treatment variables that have been found to correlate with outcome in the larger pediatric series are listed in Table 2 (6,30,33–35,39). Because of the extremely low death-rate in childhood and adolescence, the endpoint is usually tumor recurrence in patients with a documented complete response or tumor progression when the initial response cannot be documented. The only variable consistently shown to be of prognostic significance is age at diagnosis, with younger patients demonstrating a higher rate of recurrence (Table 2; Fig. 2). Of note, the presence of distant metastases is not associated with a worse outcome in the pediatric age group (6,40). Extent of initial surgery (i.e., total/subtotal thyroidectomy versus lobectomy) has correlated with outcome in some but not all of the larger series. In a multicenter study that included 329 subjects, progression-free survival was independent of extent of initial surgery (Fig. 3), but did correlate negatively with the presence of residual disease after surgery (6). Treatment with radioactive iodine was associated with a better outcome in only one of the series and this was only of marginal statistical significance (35).

Initial Surgery

The aforementioned data support that lobectomy, with or without modified lymph node dissection, can be used for patients without distant metastases who have small primary tumors (<2 cm) and minimal or absent regional nodal involvement. Patients with primary lesions larger than 3 cm, bilateral thyroid tumors, or those that invade contiguous structures probably should undergo total or subtotal thyroidectomy. Mutilating resections that sacrifice nerves, larynx, or other normal structures should be avoided when invasive tumors are encountered. However, because subsequent ^{131}I treatment will be necessary, a total or subtotal thyroidectomy should be done. Additionally, all patients with documented distant parenchymal metastases should be treated with total or subtotal thyroidectomy in preparation for ^{131}I therapy. Modified lymph node dissection that preserves nervous, vascular, and muscular structures but systematically removes involved nodal echelons should be done in patients with lymph node metastases. Radical neck dissections are contraindicated in the treatment of pediatric differentiated thyroid cancer except under unusual circumstances.

Treatment with ^{131}I

Radioiodine therapy is used to ablate residual normal thyroid tissue after subtotal thyroidectomy or lobectomy and to treat *functioning* metastases from differentiated thyroid carcinoma. Thyroid cancer commonly metastasizes to regional lymph nodes and to the lungs. Bone and central nervous system metastases occur rarely. The thyroid is very efficient at trapping iodide, and this forms the basis for radioiodine therapy. The same is true for functioning metastases. Non-functioning metastases do not take up iodide and are not readily treated with ^{131}I. Because thyroid tumors in children are often locally advanced at diagnosis and bulky cervical nodes may obscure important structures, normal residual thyroid tissue or thyroid tumor might be present even after attempts at total thyroidectomy. As a consequence, functioning metastases may not be detectable by total body imaging using a radioiodine tracer, due to preferential uptake of the iodine by residual thyroid tissue in the neck. Thus, the residual thyroid tissue in the neck needs to be destroyed before a meaningful body scan can be performed.

ABLATION OF RESIDUAL THYROID TISSUE

Residual thyroid tissue can be ablated using radioactive iodine. This will permit better visualization of metastatic disease and will facilitate the treatment of metastases, if present. In general, one can estimate the completeness of surgical removal of the thyroid by measuring thyroid function tests including the plasma thyroxine and TSH value. Ablation can be done without further imaging studies, once an elevated level of TSH (>20 µIU/mL) is documented. In the past, a dose of 75 mCi was given to patients. Thyroid ablation is successful in most cases after a single dose and, rarely, a second or third ablative dose is needed. Alternatively, following dosimetry studies, a dose delivering 30,000 cGy to the residual thyroid bed can be given *(41)*. Outpatient doses of 29 mCi or less result in a high failure rate, necessitating multiple treatments to achieve complete ablation.

TREATMENT OF FUNCTIONING METASTASES

Radioactive iodine is the mainstay of treatment for patients with extensive regional or distant dissemination, despite the lack of definitive data demonstrating long-term benefit. The technique is dosimetry-based and therapeutic administration should be preceded by a diagnostic ^{131}I scan done after definitive surgery or ablation. Approx 6 wk before the ^{131}I scan, patients can be switched to T3 (Cytomel), which has a shorter half-life than T4 and can be stopped a week or two prior to diagnostic scanning. A TSH level greater than 30–40 µIU/mL is necessary to ensure adequate uptake of radioiodine by thyroid tissue. For women of childbearing age, a pregnancy test is done prior to the scan and dosimetry study.

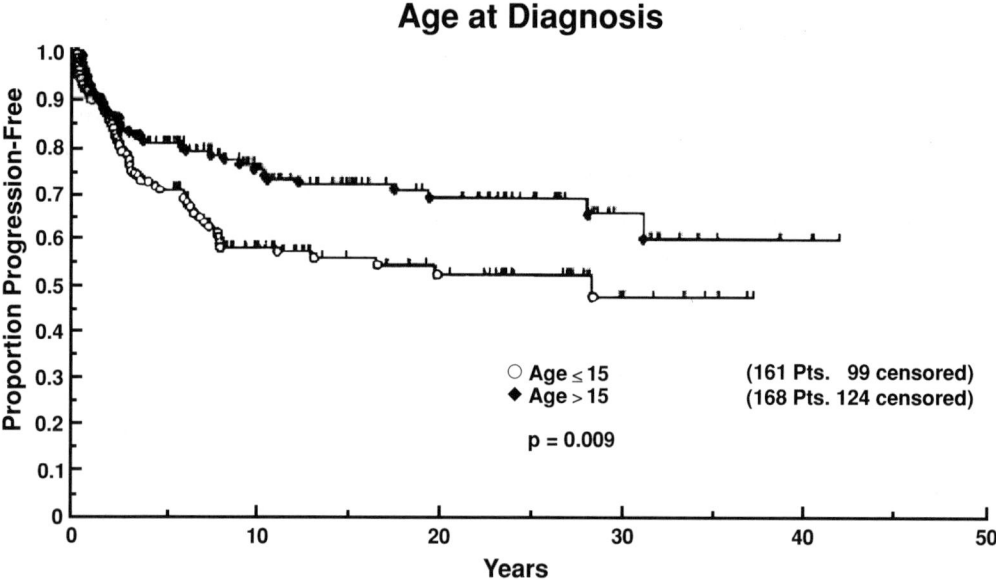

Fig. 2. Association between age at diagnosis and progression-free survival. Reproduced with permission from ref. *(6)*.

In most institutions, a fixed dose of ^{131}I is given to the patients. For patients with regional nodal involvement, demonstrated by the total body scan, 150–175 mCi are given. To treat lung metastases, 175–200 mCi are used, while 200 mCi are used for bone involvement. Alternatively, the dose can be derived from individually performed dosimetry studies *(42)*.

Due to the relatively small number of pediatric thyroid cancer patients treated at a single center, it is difficult to evaluate the impact of radioiodine treatment *(43)*. There are no prospective studies in children that compare therapeutic approaches. Indeed, mortality is so low that the only parameter available for comparison is disease recurrence or progression. It is uncertain whether therapy influences the excellent prognosis. For example, children and young adults with pulmonary metastases do extremely well and 95–100% are alive 10–20 yr after diagnosis *(40)*. Treatment with ^{131}I is associated with disappearance of metastatic disease in 30–50% of subjects, while the remainder, although asymptomatic, will have persistent disease *(44)*. In one study the number of treatments and the cumulative dose of radioactive iodine did not correlate with objective response of the disease *(45)*.

There have been few reported side effects in children treated with radioactive iodine. However, no prospective studies evaluating the efficacy or side effects of radioactive iodine treatments in children have been reported. This is troublesome in that delayed toxicities may take many years to develop. During or shortly after radioiodine therapy mild nausea, emesis, transitory thrombocytopenia, and sialadenitis may occur, particularly when a relatively large therapeutic dose is administered. However, using the doses calculated from our dosimetry studies over many decades at our center, there have been

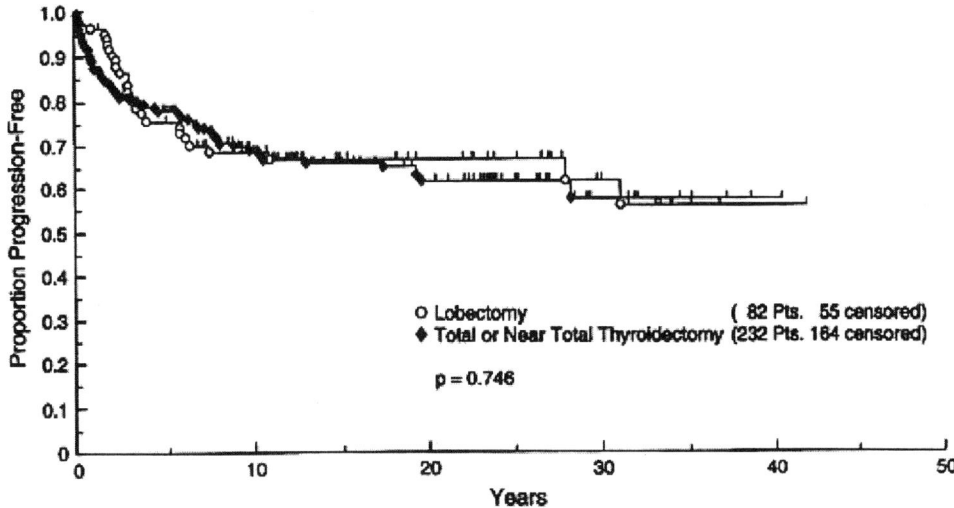

Fig. 3. Comparison of progression-free survival in patients undergoing biopsy or lobectomy to those treated by total or subtotal thyroidectomy. Reproduced with permission from ref. *(6).*

no cases of severe marrow suppression or pulmonary fibrosis as reported in the early studies *(46).*

Red marrow dose in pediatric patients is significantly higher than in adults *(47).* There is no evidence, however, that an increased incidence of bone marrow suppression is observed in pediatric patients. In general, a mild decrease in platelet counts may be encountered about one month after therapy. Complete recovery is expected within a few months. Leukemia and development of solid tumors are major concerns, as ionizing radiation is a well known carcinogen. Most reported cases of radioiodine-associated leukemias are acute *(48),* but chronic myelogenous leukemia has also been reported in patients so treated. The total number of cases of leukemia, including pediatric patients, following ^{131}I therapy worldwide has been quite small. At our center, we have not observed an excess number of leukemias among pediatric patients treated with radioiodine during the past 4 decades.

There is concern that cancer may develop in organs that normally concentrate iodide like the salivary glands, bladder, gastrointestinal tract, and breast. In general, the safety record has been good and development of secondary tumors is rare in thyroid cancer patients treated with radioactive iodine. However, slight increases in the incidence of melanoma and salivary gland cancer have been reported *(49).* In a study by Green et al. *(50)* from Roswell Park, nine female patients who were treated for childhood thyroid cancer from 1960–1988 were reviewed. *In situ* breast cancer developed in two of the four patients treated with radioactive iodine. No cases of *in situ* breast carcinoma were noted in the five patients who did not receive ^{131}I. A recent report found that women with thyroid cancer, particularly premenopausal white women, have a greater than expected risk of developing breast cancer *(51).* This was true independent of treatment with ^{131}I. More studies on the correlation between the incidence of breast cancer and prior radioiodine treatment are necessary.

Aside from nausea, vomiting, xerostomia, or pain in the salivary glands, decreased function of salivary glands may occur. Since the dose delivered to the salivary gland is quite variable and related to the state of hydration, patients under therapy should be encouraged to drink large amounts of fluid and use sour candies or lemons. Frequent bladder emptying is encouraged to lessen radiation exposure to the bladder.

It is known that gonadal damage may be produced by the administration of radioactive iodine *(52)*. A number of studies have addressed the issue of post-treatment fertility *(41)*. In female patients, the fertility rate is not affected, although an increased number of miscarriages following treatments have been reported. In one study, with long follow-up, no adverse effects on female fertility or increased rate of carcinogenesis were observed in children or adolescents treated with radioactive iodine for differentiated cancer of the thyroid *(53)*. A recent study in adult women treated with ^{131}I suggested that they may enter menopause at a slightly younger age than controls *(54)*. To avoid transmitting possible genetic aberrations from the gonadal damage due to ionizing radiation from ^{131}I, patients are advised to avoid conception for 6 mo following treatment using radioactive iodine.

External Beam Radiotherapy

The role of external beam radiation in the management of pediatric thyroid cancer is not well established. Due to potential serious and life-threatening late toxicities *(55)*, external radiation should be avoided in most children and adolescents with differentiated thyroid cancer. Under unusual circumstances (e.g., symptomatic disease that is not amenable to surgery and/or responsive to ^{131}I), radiation therapy may be required.

Thyroid Hormone Suppression

Differentiated thyroid cancers possess TSH receptors and various clinical and laboratory studies suggest that suppression of TSH can reduce growth of the tumors. Most but not all studies demonstrate that TSH suppression is associated with an improved outcome *(56)*. The optimum degree of suppression required remains a source of controversy. Moreover, long-term suppression therapy in adults has been associated with reductions in bone mineral density and impaired cardiac function *(56,57)*. Our current policy is to maintain the TSH level just below the lower limit of normal *(58)*.

FOLLOW-UP

Regular and life-long follow-up is essential, as late recurrences are not uncommon. Additionally, the dose of thyroid hormone will need to be adjusted as the individual grows and develops. We generally recommend visits at least every 6 mo; visits include a complete physical exam and blood studies to assess the degree of TSH suppression and to monitor the plasma concentration of thyroglobulin. Thyroglobulin is produced by differentiated thyroid tissue (normal and neoplastic) and should be very low to undetectable following thyroidectomy and ^{131}I treatments. A rising level of thyroglobulin in an individual with a suppressed TSH level suggests the possibility of either recurrence or progression of thyroid cancer *(59)*. The thyroglobulin level may be difficult to interpret if there are significant circulating titers of anti-thyroglobulin antibodies.

For patients with known or suspected disease, ^{131}I scanning is the most sensitive test available. Preparation for total body scanning has traditionally been accomplished by withdrawing thyroid hormone. Recently, it has been demonstrated that preparation with injections of recombinant human TSH results in scans that are diagnostically equivalent to those obtained after thyroid withdrawal, while avoiding the unpleasant side-effects associated with hypothyroidism *(60)*. Recombinant human TSH is only approved for use in adults at the present time. When radioiodine scanning is not possible or desired, the combination of an ultrasound of the neck and a CT scan of the chest will provide valuable information about the extent of residual disease. It is important *not* to perform the chest CT with contrast, as the iodine load present in the iv contrast will preclude the use ^{131}I for several months.

Following a therapeutic dose of ^{131}I, a follow-up radioiodine scan should be performed in 6–12 mo. Once the scan is negative, it is unclear how often surveillance whole body scans should be done. There is currently no justification for yearly scanning of individuals who lack clinical and biochemical (e.g., low-undetectable thyroglobulin) evidence of active disease.

CONCLUSION

The overall survival for patients with differentiated thyroid cancer presenting in childhood and adolescence is in excess of 90–95%, even for those with distant metastases at diagnosis. Because so few deaths occur in this cohort, the end result is usually measured by the rate of recurrence or progression. Overall the reported recurrence rate for differentiated thyroid carcinoma in childhood and adolescence is 35–40% in large series in which a time-dependent analysis has been performed. Other than younger age at diagnosis, few clinical or treatment variables correlate with risk of disease recurrence. In the absence of randomized, prospective treatment trials, the optimum management of children and adolescents with thyroid cancer will remain unanswered. We recommend a risk-based approach that is tailored to the individual. This necessitates input from a multidisciplinary team, including endocrinology, surgery and nuclear medicine, along with the wishes and preferences of the patient and family.

REFERENCES

1. Vitale G, Caraglia M, Cicarelli A, et al. Current approaches and perspectives in the therapy of medullary thyroid carcinoma. Cancer 2001;91:1797–1808.
2. Hassoun AAK, Hay ID, Goellner JR, Zimmerman D. Insular thyroid carcinoma in adolescents. Cancer 1997;79:1044–1048.
3. Bernstein L, Gurney JG. Carcinomas and other malignant epithelial neoplasms. In: Ries LAG, Smith MA, Gurney JG, Linet M, Tamra T, Young JL, Bunin GR, ed. Cancer Incidence and survival among children and adolescents: United States SEER program 1975–1995. National Cancer Institute, SEER Program NIH Publ. No. 99–4649, Bethesda, MD, 1999, pp. 139–147.
4. Stiller CA. International variations in the incidence of childhood carcinomas. Cancer Epidemiol Biomarkers Prev 1994;3:305–310.
5. Feinmesser R, Lubin E, Segal K, Noyek A. Carcinoma of the thyroid in children-a review. J Pediatr Endocrinol Metab 1997;10:561–568.
6. Newman KD, Black T, Heller G, Azizkhan RG, Holcomb III GW, Sklar C, Vlamis V, Haase GM, La Quaglia MP. Differentiated thyroid cancer: determinants of disease progression in patients <21 years of age at diagnosis. A report from the Surgical Discipline Committee of the Children's Cancer Group. Ann Surgery 1998;227:533–541.
7. Duffy BJ, Fitzgerald P. Thyroid cancer in childhood and adolescence: Report of 28 cases. J. Clin Endocrinol Metab 1950;10:1296–1308.

8. Boice Jr JD. Cancer following irradiation in childhood and adolescence. Med Pediatr Oncol 1996;Suppl1:29–34.
9. Ron E, Lubin JH, Shore RE, et al. Thyroid cancer after exposure to external radiation: a pooled analysis of seven studies. Radiat Res 1995;141:259–277.
10. Sklar C, Whitton J, Mertens A, et al. Abnormalities of the thyroid in survivors of Hodgkin's disease: data from the Childhood Cancer Survivor Study. J Clin Endocrinol Metab 2000;85:3227–3232.
11. Shibata Y, Yamashita S, Masyakin VB, Panasyuk GD, Nagataki S. 15 years after Chernobyl: new evidence for thyroid cancer. Lancet 2001;358:1965–1966.
12. Hahn K, Schnell-Inderst P, Grosche B, Holm LE. Thyroid cancer after diagnostic administration of iodine-131 in childhood. Radiat Res 2001;156:61–70.
13. Bell B, Mazzaferri EL. Familial adenomatous polyposis (Gardner's syndrome) and thyroid carcinoma. a case report and review of the literature. Dig Dis Sci 1996; 38:185-190.
14. Holm LE, Biomgren H, Lowhagen T. Cancer risks in patients with chronic lymphocytic thyroiditis. N Engl J Med 1985;312:601–604.
15. Mauras N, Zimmerman D, Goeliner JR. Hashimoto's thyroiditis associated with thyroid cancer in adolescent patients. J Pediatr 1985;106:895–898.
16. Frauman AG, Moses AC. Oncogenes and growth factors in thyroid carcinogenesis. Endocrine and Metab Clin N Amer 1990;19:479–493.
17. Elesi R, Romei C, Vorontsova T, et al. RET/PTC rearrangements in thyroid nodules; studies in irradiated and not irradiated, malignant and benign thyroid lesions in children and adults. J Clin Endocrinol Metab 2001;86:3211–3216.
18. Gharib H, Mazzaferri EL. Thyroxine suppression therapy in patients with nodular thyroid disease. Ann Intern Med 1998;128:386–394.
19. Gharib H. Current evaluation of thyroid nodules. Trends Endocrinol Metab 1994;5:365–368.
20. Hung W. Well differentiated thyroid carcinomas in children and adolescents: a review. The Endocrinologist 1994;4:117–126.
21. Khurana KK, Labrador E, Izquierdo R, Mesonero CE, Pisharodi LR. The role of fine-needle aspiration biopsy in the management of thyroid nodules in children, adolescents, and young adults; a multi-institutional study. Thyroid 1999;9:383–386.
22. Corrias A, Einaudi S, Chiorboli E, et al. Accuracy of fine needle aspiration biopsy of thyroid nodules in detecting malignancy in childhood: comparison with conventional clinical, laboratory, and imaging approaches. J Clin Endocrinol Metab 2001;86:4644–4648.
23. Arda IS, Yildrim S, Demirhan B, Firat S. Fine needle aspiration biopsy of thyroid nodules. Arch Dis Child 2001;85:313–317.
24. Exelby PR, Frazell EL. Carcinoma of the thyroid in children. Surg Clin N Am 1969;49:249–259.
25. Liechty RD, Safaie-Shirazi S, Soper RT. Carcinoma of the thyroid in children. Surg Gynecol Obstet 1972;134:595–599.
26. Richardson JE, Beaudie JM, Brown CL, Doniach I. Thyroid cancer in young patients in Great Britain. Br J Surg 1974;61:85–89.
27. Buckwalter JA, Thomas CG, Freeman JB. Is childhood cancer a lethal disease? Ann Surg 1975;181:632–638.
28. Tallroth E, Backdahl M, Einhorn J, Lundell G. Lowhagen T, Silfversward C. Thyroid carcinoma in children and adolescents. Cancer 1986;58:2329–2332.
29. Schlumberger M, De Vathaire F, Travagli JP, et al. Differentiated thyroid carcinoma in childhood: long term follow-up of 72 patients. J Clin Endocrinol Metab 1987;65:1088–1094.
30. La Quaglia MP, Corbally MT, Heller G, Exelby PR, Brennan MF. Recurrence and morbidity in differentiated thyroid carcinoma in children. Surgery 1988;104:1149–1156.
31. Zimmerman D, Hay ID, Gough IR, et al. Papillary thyroid carcinoma in children and adults: long-term follow-up of 1039 patients conservatively treated at one institution during three decades. Surgery 1988;104:1157–1166.
32. Azizkhan RG, Askin FB, Reddick RL, Sierk AE, Thomas CG Jr. Papillary and hurthle cell thyroid carcinoma in children: a 40-yr institutional review of prognostic factors, therapy and outcome. Med Pediatr Oncol 1991;19:357–358.
33. Welch Dinauer CA, Tuttle RM, Robie DK, et al. Clinical features associated with metastasis and recurrence of differentiated thyroid cancer in children, adolescents, and young adults. Clin Endocrinol 1998;49:619–628.
34. Alessandri AJ, Goddard KJ, Blair GK, Fryer CJH, Schultz KR. Age is a major determinant of recurrence in pediatric differentiated thyroid carcinoma. Med Pediatr Oncol 2000;35:41–46

35. Jarzab B, Junak DH, Wloch J, et al. Multivariate analysis of prognostic factors for differentiated thyroid carcinoma in children. Eur J Nucl Med 2000;27:833–841.
36. Storm HH, Plesko I. Survival of children with thyroid cancer in Europe 1978–1989. Eur J Cancer 2001;37:775–779.
37. LaQuaglia MP, Telander RL. Differentiated and medullary thyroid cancer in childhood and adolescence. Sem Pediatr Surg 1997;6:42–49.
38. Shaha AR, Shah JP, Loree TR. Low-risk differentiated thyroid cancer: the need for selective treatment. Ann Surg Oncol 1997;4:328–333.
39. Welch Dinauer CA, Tuttle RM, Robie DK, McClellan DR, Francis GL. Extensive surgery improves recurrence-free survival for children and young patients with class I papillary thyroid carcinoma. J Pediatr Surg 1999;34:1799–1804.
40. LaQuaglia MP, Black T, Holcomb GW III, et al. Differentiated thyroid cancer: clinical characteristics, treatment, and outcome in patients under 21 years of age who present with distant metastases. A report from the Surgical Discipline Committee of the Children's Cancer Group. J Pediatr Surg 2000;35: 955–960.
41. Yeh SDJ, LaQuaglia MP. ^{131}I therapy for pediatric thyroid cancer. Sem Pediatr Surg 1997;6:128–133.
42. Maxon HR III, Englaro EE, Thomas SR, et al. Radioiodine-131 therapy for well-differentiated thyroid cancer-a quantitative radiation dosimetric approach: outcome and validation in 85 patients. J Nucl Med 1992;33:1132–1136.
43. Becker DV, Zanzonico PB. Radioiodine therapy in children. In: Robbins J, ed. Treatment of Thyroid Cancer in Childhood, National Institutes of Health, DOE/EH 0406, Bethesda, 1992, pp. 111–125.
44. Brink JS, van Heerden JA, McIver B, et al. Papillary thyroid cancer with pulmonary metastases in children; long-term prognosis. Surgery 2001;128:881–887.
45. Samuel AM, Rajashekharrao, Shah DH. Pulmonary metastases in children and adolescents with well-differentiated thyroid cancer. J Nucl Med 1998;39:1531–1536.
46. Leeper RD. Thyroid cancer. Med Clin North Am 1985;69:1079–76.
47. Reynolds JC. Comparison of ^{131}I absorbed radiation doses in children and adults. A tool for estimating therapeutic ^{131}I doses in children. In: Robbins J, ed. Treatment of Thyroid Cancer in Childhood, National Institutes of Health, DOE/EH 0406, Behtesda, 1992, pp. 127–135.
48. Hall P, Boice JD, Berg G, et al. Leukaemia incidence after iodine-131 exposure. Lancet 1992;340:1–4.
49. Hall P, Holm LE, Lundell G, et al. Cancer risks in thyroid cancer patients. Br J Cancer 1991;64:159–163.
50. Green DM, Edge SB, Penetrante RB, Bakshi S, Shedd D, Zevon MA. In situ breast carcinoma after treatment during adolescence for thyroid cancer with radioiodine. Med Ped Oncol 1995;24:82–86.
51. Chen AY, Levy L, Goepfert Brown BW, Spitz MR, Vassilopoulou-Sellin R. The development of breast carcinoma in women with thyroid cancer. Cancer 2001;92:225–231.
52. Ahmed SH, Shalet SM. Gonadal damage due to radioactive iodine treatment for thyroid carcinoma. Postgrad Med J 1985;61:361–362.
53. Sarkar SD, Beierwaltes H, Gill SP, Cowley BJ. Subsequent fertility and birth history of children and adolescents treated with ^{131}I for thyroid cancer. J Nucl Med 1976;17:460–464.
54. Ceccarelli C, Bencivelli W, Morciano D, Pinchera A, Pacini F. ^{131}I therapy for differentiated thyroid cancer leads to an earlier onset of menopause: results of a retrospective study. J Clin Endocrinol Metab 2001;86:3512–3515.
55. Vassilopoulou-Sellin R, Goepfert H, Raney B, Schultz PN. Differentiated thyroid cancer in children and adolescents: clinical outcome and mortality after long-term follow-up. Head Neck 1998;20:549–555.
56. Dulgeroff AJ, Hershman JM. Medical therapy for differentiated thyroid carcinoma. Endocrine Rev 1994;15:500–515.
57. Biondi B, Fazio S, Cuocolo A, et al. Impaired cardiac reserve and exercise capacity in patients receiving long-term thyrotropin suppressive therapy with levothyroxine. J Clin Endocrinol Metab 1996;81:4224–4228.
58. Burmeister LA, Goumaz MO, Mariash CN, Oppenheimer JH. Levothyroxine dose requirements for thyrotropin suppression in the treatment of differentiated thyroid cancer. J Clin Endocrinol Metab 1992;75:344–350.
59. Ozata M, Suzuki S, Miyamoto T, Liu RT, Fierro-Renoy F, Degroot LJ. Serum thyroglobulin in the follow-up of patients with treated differentiated thyroid cancer. J Clin Endocrinol Metab 1994;79: 98–105.
60. Robbins RJ, Tuttle RM, Sharaf RN, et al. Preparation by recombinant human thyrotropin or thyroid hormone withdrawal are comparable for the detection of residual differentiated thyroid carcinoma. J Clin Endocrinol Metab 2001;86:619–625.

V Calcium and Bone Disorders

20 Abnormalities in Calcium Homeostasis

Ruben Diaz, MD, PhD

CONTENTS

INTRODUCTION
HORMONAL REGULATION OF SERUM Ca^{2+}
HYPOCALCEMIA
HYPERCALCEMIA
REFERENCES

INTRODUCTION

Calcium plays an important role in a number of physiological processes as diverse as bone formation and turnover, neuronal cell excitability, muscle contractility, and blood clotting. Significant shifts in serum calcium concentration have adverse effects on these physiological functions. In children, maintenance of adequate calcium balance is particularly important since bone deposition and growth are closely linked to the availability of calcium. Higher organisms have developed mechanisms to regulate the extracellular concentration of calcium, normally affected by intermittent changes in calcium absorption in the gut, continuous mineral bone turnover, and calcium losses in the urine. Extracellular calcium levels are set within a very narrow range by the concerted action of several regulatory "calciotropic" hormones on calcium handling by the gastrointestinal tract, bone, and kidney. The abnormal function of calciotropic hormones or the failure of any of these organs to handle calcium properly can cause either hypo- or hypercalcemia.

Calcium is among the most abundant mineral ions in the body. Greater than 98% of total calcium is present as mineral salts in bone, but can be mobilized as part of a continuous exchange of calcium between bone and the extracellular compartment during bone remodeling. The remaining fraction of calcium is distributed between the intracellular and extracellular compartments. Calcium in serum exists in three forms: 1) a protein-bound fraction (30–50% of total serum calcium), primarily bound to albumin; 2) complexed with serum anions like phosphate, citrate, and bicarbonate (5–15%); and 3) ionized Ca (Ca^{2+}) (40–60%). Ca^{2+} is the metabolically active form and is the soluble fraction that is tightly regulated. As a result, the concentration of serum Ca^{2+} remains relatively constant with age and dietary intake.

From: *Contemporary Endocrinology: Pediatric Endocrinology: A Practical Clinical Guide*
Edited by: S. Radovick and M. H. MacGillivray © Humana Press Inc., Totowa, NJ

HORMONAL REGULATION OF SERUM Ca^{2+}

Parathyroid Hormone

Changes in serum Ca^{2+} are rapidly sensed by the parathyroid glands *(1)*. There are four paired parathyroid glands, usually positioned in the superior and inferior poles of the thyroid, derived from the 4th and 3rd pharyngeal pouches, respectively. In response to a decrease in serum Ca^{2+}, they secrete parathyroid hormone (PTH), an 84 amino acid polypeptide synthesized and stored in secretory granules. The net effect of PTH on calcium homeostasis is to activate mechanisms that increase serum Ca^{2+} levels *(2)*. PTH promotes calcium mobilization from bone by osteoblast-mediated activation of bone-resorbing osteoclasts. In the kidney's proximal tubule, PTH activates 1-α-hydroxylase to synthesize calcitriol $(1,25(OH)_2D)$, increases the absorption of sodium, calcium, and bicarbonate, while inhibiting phosphate transport and promoting phosphaturia. In the distal tubule, PTH has its most significant effect in the distal convoluted tubule where it activates calcium absorption. In the gut, PTH indirectly promotes, through the action of $1,25(OH)_2D$, the absorption of both calcium and phosphate.

The mechanism that allows parathyroid cells to sense small changes in Ca^{2+} concentration has been recently characterized. Ca^{2+} sensing is mediated by a G protein-coupled, calcium-sensing receptor (CaR) *(3)*. Elevations in serum Ca^{2+} activate the CaR which, in turn, mediates the inhibition of PTH secretion by a yet poorly defined mechanism. Although Ca^{2+} is the major regulator of PTH secretion, other calciotropic factors also affect its secretion. The active form of vitamin D, calcitriol, inhibits PTH synthesis while high serum phosphate has been recently shown to stimulate PTH secretion *(4)*. Profound hypomagnesemia inhibits both PTH secretion and action by affecting intracellular signaling function; hypermagnesemia also inhibits PTH secretion, a process likely mediated by the CaR, since magnesium is also a ligand for this receptor *(1)*. PTH is exquisitely sensitive to degradation both intracellularly in the parathyroid cell and in serum, especially as it traverses the liver and kidney; its serum half-life is less than 8 min. Inactive proteolytic fragments are always present in blood and accumulate to high concentrations in conditions that decrease their clearance (i.e., renal failure). Thus, an accurate measurement of active PTH requires an immunoassay that measures intact PTH, presently achieved by a sandwich immunoradiometric assay (IRMA) or an immunofluorometric assay.

The bioactive site in PTH resides within the first 27 amino acids of the peptide *(2)*. PTH binds to a G protein-coupled receptor (PTH1R) that activates the production of cAMP and, in some cells, the release of intracellular calcium stores via activation of phospholipase C. This receptor is present in osteoblasts and kidney tubular epithelium, cells that play a direct role in calcium homeostasis. Two additional receptors (PTH2R and PTH3R) with some homology to the first characterized receptor have been recently described *(5)*, but their role in calcium homeostasis may not be significant.

At least another peptide has been shown to have PTH-like effects. PTH-related protein (PTHrP) was initially characterized for causing hypercalcemia when secreted by some malignant tumors *(6)*. The amino terminus of this peptide has high homology with the bioactive amino terminus of PTH and binds the PTH receptor. Besides its role as a calciotropic hormone when present in serum in high concentration, PTHrP appears to serve important functions in cartilage formation and the differentiation of several organs, where it is expressed during fetal and postnatal development *(7)*. In the placenta, active transplacental transport of Ca^{2+} appears to be mediated by PTHrP binding to an unidentified receptor *(8)*.

Vitamin D

Vitamin D_3 (cholecalciferol) is produced by photolysis of cholesterol to 7-dehydrocholesterol under UVB irradiation (280–305 nm wavelength) followed by isomerization in the skin *(9)*. It is hydroxylated to 25-hydroxyvitamin D (25OHD) in the liver, a step that is largely substrate dependent, making 25OHD levels a useful index of vitamin D stores. Its serum half-life is 2–3 wk. An additional hydroxylation step by a 1-α-hydroxylase in the renal proximal tubule produces the bioactive form of vitamin D, $1,25(OH)_2D$. PTH, hypocalcemia, and hypophosphatemia are the major inducers of 1-α-hydroxylase activity in the proximal tubule. An increase in $1,25(OH)_2D$ production becomes apparent hours after exposure to a stimulus, and the half-life of $1,25(OH)_2D$ is only several hours. The proximal tubule also has 24-hydroxylase activity; hypercalcemia, hyperphosphatemia and $1,25(OH)_2D$ induce this enzyme, promoting the production of $24,25(OH)_2D$, an inactive metabolite. 1-α-hydroxylation activity is not limited to the proximal tubule. 1-α-hydroxylase is expressed in placenta, a significant source of calcitriol for the fetus, keratinocytes, and activated mononuclear cells. Excess 1-α-hydroxylase activity in mononuclear cells is thought to be responsible for the hypercalcemia and elevation of $1,25(OH)_2D$ levels seen in granulomatous disorders *(10)*.

Vitamin D and its metabolites are transported in serum bound to vitamin D binding protein (DBP), showing greatest affinity for 25OHD. This protein provides a reservoir of vitamin D metabolites and prevents its rapid clearance in the urine. Recently, megalin, a lipoprotein-like receptor that binds DBP, has been shown to mediate the uptake of vitamin D metabolites in the proximal tubule, suggesting a role for this protein in ensuring 25OHD availability for 1-α-hydroxylation in the kidney *(11)*.

Calcitriol promotes the rise of both calcium and phosphate levels in serum *(9)*. $1,25(OH)_2D$ binds to vitamin D receptors (VDR), a member of the retinoid family of nuclear receptors, expressed in intestine, distal renal tubular cells, osteoblasts, parathyroid cells, and other tissues not directly involved in calcium homeostasis. In bone, binding to VDR promotes the activation of osteocalcin and alkaline phosphatase production by osteoblasts, and the differentiation of osteoclasts precursors, having a net effect in mobilizing calcium and phosphate from bone. In the kidney, $1,25(OH)_2D$ facilitates the action of PTH on distal tubule calcium absorption. The major impact of $1,25(OH)_2D$ is in the small intestine where it promotes the absorption of calcium and phosphate in the duodenum and jejunum.

Calcitonin

Calcitonin is a 32 amino acid peptide produced by thyroid parafollicular C cells, and in lesser amounts by other neuroendocrine cells *(12)*. High Ca^{2+} elicits a rise in calcitonin secretion in parafollicular cells, a process mediated by the same calcium-sensing receptor expressed in parathyroid cells *(3)*. In almost all instances, calcitonin antagonizes the effect of PTH on bone and kidney, via its binding to a G protein-coupled receptor of the same family as the PTH receptor. Calcitonin has no measurable effects on intestine handling of mineral ions. Paradoxically, calcitonin levels rise abruptly at birth, despite a drop in serum Ca^{2+} normally seen during the same period, and decrease rapidly after birth *(13)*. In children older than 3 yr, normal serum levels are often below detection unless elicited by hypercalcemia, or in the setting of medullary thyroid carcinoma. The role of calcitonin in normal calcium homeostasis is uncertain, since in the absence of parafollicular cells (i.e., thyroidectomy), no significant alterations in calcium homeostasis have been observed; however, it has a pharmacological role in the acute treatment of hypercalcemia and osteoporosis as a promoter of calcium deposition in bone.

Serum Ca^{2+} "Set Point"

The overall effect of changes in calciotropic hormones on calcium handling by the kidney, gastrointestinal tract and bone is to maintain the extracellular Ca^{2+} concentration around the normal range (usually 1.12–1.23 mmol/L) or set point. As this is primarily achieved by the regulation of PTH secretion in parathyroid cells, the CaR's binding affinity for Ca^{2+} is the major determinant of serum Ca^{2+} set point. Mutations of the CaR have been described that shift its response to serum Ca^{2+}, resulting in a shift of the set point for serum Ca^{2+} *(14)*. Patients harboring inactivation mutations of the CaR, as seen in familial hypocalciuric hypercalcemia (FHH), maintain serum Ca^{2+} concentration above the normal range, since suppression of PTH secretion requires higher concentrations of Ca^{2+}. Conversely, in autosomal dominant hypocalcemia, activating mutations of CaR result in hypocalcemia, as PTH secretion is fully suppressed when serum Ca^{2+} approaches the normal range. Ca^{2+} can also play a direct role in calcium handling by organs involved in calcium homeostasis.

The CaR is highly expressed in the kidney tubule, where Ca^{2+} exerts a direct role in regulating its own absorption in the distal tubule *(3)*; high serum Ca^{2+} inhibits the absorption of luminal calcium. FHH and autosomal dominant hypocalcemia patients have relative hypocalciuria or hypercalciuria, respectively, due to inactivating or activating mutations of the CaR. The CaR is also expressed in the collecting duct and its activation appears to block the expression of water channels on the luminal surface, providing at least one mechanism for the polyuria noted in hypercalcemia. CaRs are also expressed in intestinal epithelia and various bone-derived cells, but its role in calcium homeostasis in these sites has not yet been clearly defined.

Calcium Homeostasis During Fetal and Early Neonatal Period

During fetal development calcium homeostasis is affected by maternal Ca^{2+} levels *(13)*. Serum Ca^{2+} in the fetus is set at a higher concentration (≈0.25 mmol/L higher) than the mother. There is active transport of calcium across the placenta to sustain this gradient, a process that appears to be mediated by PTHrP (likely the midregion fragment of PTHrP), secreted by the fetal parathyroid, among other fetal organs, during pregnancy. Although the parathyroid glands are present as early as the first trimester in gestation, PTH secretion is normally suppressed during fetal development since fetal serum Ca^{2+} levels remain elevated *in utero*. In the fetus, bone mass accretion occurs primarily from 24 wk to full gestation. Maternal serum Ca^{2+} levels and, less significantly, vitamin D status affects the extent of mineralization during this period. The mother is the primary source of vitamin D during this period. Both maternal 25(OH)D and 1,25(OH)$_2$D cross the placenta, while the placenta also produces 1,25(OH)$_2$D.

At birth, there is a fall in serum Ca^{2+} levels, reaching a nadir (1.00–1.17 mmol/L) in the first 24–48 h of life *(15)*. PTH levels are low at birth but rise with the decrease in serum Ca^{2+}. Serum PTHrP levels decrease rapidly in the first day of life. 1,25(OH)$_2$D levels increase concomitantly with the increase in serum PTH. Milk intake provides the primary source of serum Ca^{2+} during the neonatal period. During the initial neonatal period, intestinal calcium absorption is not significantly regulated by $1,25(OH)_2D$; instead, passive absorption mechanisms enhanced by the presence of lactose in milk predominate at this stage *(13)*. The intestine progressively develops increased sensitivity and dependency on vitamin D for adequate calcium absorption. Infant's vitamin D levels correlate best with supplementation and sun exposure and not with breast milk intake, regardless of maternal vitamin D status.

HYPOCALCEMIA

Hypocalcemia develops as a consequence of either reduced influx of calcium from the gastrointestinal tract or bone into the extracellular space, or the excessive loss of calcium from this space into urine, bone, or stool. Causes of hypocalcemia include abnormalities in calciotropic hormone production and action, or improper calcium handling by organs targeted by these hormones (Table 1).

Alterations in Calciotropic Hormones Causing Hypocalcemia

HYPOPARATHYROIDISM

Lack of adequate PTH production is a frequent cause of hypocalcemia in neonates and early childhood. In hypoparathyroidism, decreased PTH levels cause hypocalcemia and hyperphosphatemia. There are sporadic and familial forms of hypoparathyroidism caused by parathyroid agenesis or dysfunction *(16)*. When familial, autosomal dominant, autosomal recessive, and X-linked recessive forms of hypoparathyroidism have been described. In some instances, point mutations of the PTH gene in chromosome 11p15 lead to inappropriate expression of PTH and dyshormonogenesis. A form of autosomal dominant hypoparathyroidism is associated with sensorineural deafness and renal dysplasia. DiGeorge syndrome and its variants are a more generalized embryological abnormality that occurs either sporadically or with variable autosomal dominant penetrance, involving the development of the third and fourth branchial pouches. This complex malformation is associated with dysmorphic facial features and anomalies of the heart and great vessels with variable defects in thymic and parathyroid gland function, often showing dysgenesis of both glands. Deletions and translocations of chromosomes 22q11 and 10p13 have been detected and can be screened in suspected cases *(17)*. Hypoparathyroidism is also common in patients with Barakat syndrome and Kenny-Caffey syndrome, characterized by medullary stenosis of the long bones, short stature, hyperopia, and basal ganglia calcifications. Hypoparathyroidism has also been reported in a number of mitochondrial myopathies (i.e., Kearns-Sayre syndrome) where PTH secretion appears affected by the intracellular metabolic abnormality *(18)*.

Acquired forms of hypoparathyroidism often occur later in infancy and adolescence *(19)*. Infiltrative processes such as excess deposition of iron (thalassemia and hemochromatosis) and copper (Wilson's disease) in the parathyroid can impair the secretion of PTH. Exposure to radiation as part of therapy for hyperthyroidism, or lymphoma has been linked to the onset of hypoparathyroidism as has the surgical removal or compromise of the vascular supply to the parathyroid glands. Autoimmune destruction of the parathyroid gland can be an isolated process or as part of a polyglandular autoimmune disease type 1, an autosomal recessive disorder also associated with hypoadrenocorticism, hypogonadism, thyroid disease, type I diabetes mellitus, pernicious anemia, chronic

Table 1
Differential Diagnosis of Hypocalcemia

Alterations in hormonal response
    Hypoparathyroidism
        Abnormal PTH production
            Parathyroid agenesis/dysfunction
                Familial forms of isolated PTH deficiency
                DiGeorge's Syndrome
                Kenney-Caffey syndrome
                Dyshormonogenesis
            Acquired hypoparathyroidism
                Polyglandular Autoimmune Disease Type I
                Mitcochondrial myopathies
                Disorders of metal ion deposition
                Radiation exposure
                Idiopathic
            Abnormal PTH secretion
                Hypomagnesimia
                Autosomal dominant hypocalcemia
                Critical illness
        Peripheral resistance to PTH
            Pseudohypoparathyroidism types IA, IB, II
            Pseudopseudohypoparathyroidism
    Vitamin D
        Vitamin D deficiency
            Nutritional deficiency
            Liver disease
            Iatrogenic (e.g., phenobarbital use)
        Vitamin D resistance
            Hydroxylase deficiencies
            Vitamin D receptor dysfunction
Alterations of organs involved in calcium homeostasis
    Kidney: Renal failure, Renal tubular acidosis
    Intestine: Malabsorption
    Skeleton: Hungry Bone syndrome

Other causes of hypocalcemia
    High phosphate load
        Tumor lysis syndome
        High phosphate formula
        Rhabdomyolysis
    Ca sequestration or clearance
        Acute pancreatitis
        Drugs: Furosemide, calcitonin
    Decreased ionized calcium
        Exchange blood transfusion
        Alkalosis

active hepatitis, malabsorption, and manifestations of ectodermal dysplasia such as alopecia, vitiligo, mucocutaneous candidiasis, keratopathy, and enamel hypoplasia *(20)*. In this disorder, chronic oral candidiasis is the first manifestation usually in early infancy. The average age of onset for mucocutaneous candidiasis, hypoparathyroidism and adrenal insufficiency is 5, 9, and 14 yr of age, respectively. About half of affected children end up having at least these three manifestations. The presence of intestinal malabsorption complicates the treatment of hypocalcemia, as calcium and vitamin D absorption is often impaired.

Several conditions are characterized by impaired PTH secretion despite the presence of viable parathyroid tissue and PTH synthesis. PTH secretion can be impaired in the presence of severe hypomagnesemia. The etiology of hypomagnesemia can be secondary to intestinal malabsorption or excessive renal wasting as seen in Bartter syndrome and renal tubular acidosis *(21)*. In autosomal dominant hypocalcemia, activating mutations of the CaR shift the curve of inhibition of PTH secretion, changing the set point of serum Ca^{2+} to a concentration that can be sufficiently low to elicit adverse effects. Correction of hypocalcemia causes significant hypercalciuria, as the ability of CaR to decrease tubular absorption of calcium also increases, augmenting the risk of developing urinary stones when compared to other forms of hypoparathyroidism. Finally, PTH secretion has been shown to be impaired in critical illness, perhaps mediated by an interleukin-mediated over-expression of CaR *(22)*.

Tissue insensitivity to PTH has a clinical presentation very similar to hypoparathyroidism. Pseudohypoparathyroidism (PHP) describes various familial disorders, often inherited as autosomal dominant trait, that are characterized by the peripheral resistance to PTH *(23)*. Hypocalcemia occurs despite very elevated PTH levels, but without a concomitant elevation of $1,25(OH)_2D$ levels or increased renal phosphaturia. In patients with type Ia PHP or Albright hereditary osteodystrophy, the characteristic phenotype is short stature, stocky habitus, developmental delay, round face, short distal phalanx of the thumb, brachymetatarsals and brachymetacarpals, dental hypoplasia, and subcutaneous calcifications. Hypocalcemia is often not diagnosed until the middle childhood years. PTH resistance has been characterized by the absence of urinary cAMP after administration of PTH, normally elevated when the kidney is responsive to PTH. Inactivating mutations in the α subunit of the stimulatory protein G_s are responsible for PTH resistance in this condition by presumably preventing the activation of adenylyl cyclase by the PTH receptor. These patients can show additional deficiencies due to the defective action of other peptide hormones that use the same stimulatory G_s to enhance cAMP production. In particular, thyrotropin action is often affected and occasionally hypothyroidism is diagnosed before the hypocalcemia is noted. The action of corticotropin, gonadotropin, glucagon, and GH-releasing hormone, among other hormones, have been shown to be affected. Pseudopseudohypoparathyroidism is used to described patients with the Albright osteodystrophy phenotype without the biochemical abnormalities and may represent the inheritance of the paternal defective gene, suggesting the presence of imprinting in the inheritance of this disorder. Type Ib PHP resembles type Ia except that the $G_{s\alpha}$ subunit is normal, pointing to a defect in another step of the pathway that stimulates cAMP. Type II PHP is another variant where the phenotypic features are absent and infusion of PTH induces the normal elevation of urinary cAMP but without the expected phosphaturia, suggesting a defect distal to cAMP production. To this date, PTH resistance due to mutations of the PTH receptor have not been described.

VITAMIN D DEFICIENCY OR RESISTANCE

If vitamin D stores are depleted, intestinal calcium absorption can decrease sufficiently, causing hypocalcemia. In growing children, the negative calcium balance affects bone deposition, resulting in rickets. The parathyroid response to hypocalcemia is intact, but the elevated levels of PTH cannot compensate for the absence of substrate necessary to produce $1,25(OH)_2D$. Inadequate sun exposure or lack of vitamin D intake can cause a decrease in vitamin D levels. Children with liver disease or taking drugs that enhance the activation of liver hydroxylating enzymes (i.e., phenobarbital) may have impaired 25OHD production or increased turnover to inactive metabolites of 25OHD, respectively. In rare occasions, a deficiency in 1-α-hydroxylase activity in the kidney or the presence of abnormal receptors for $1,25(OH)_2D$, conventionally classified as vitamin D-dependent rickets (VDDR) I and II, respectively, can have the same biochemical consequences and clinical presentation as vitamin D deficiency, including hypocalcemia *(24)*. Patients with VDDR-I do not respond to massive doses of vitamin D or 25OHD. Interestingly, alopecia is often seen in VDDR-II, suggesting a role of vitamin D receptors in hair development and growth.

Other Causes of Hypocalcemia

When calcium handling by the gastrointestinal tract, bone, or kidney is abnormal or not responsive to calciotropic hormones, hypocalcemia can persist despite an appropriate hormonal response (i.e., increased PTH secretion and calcitriol production). The hyperphosphatemia that ensues with renal failure causes hypocalcemia, as excess phosphate complexes with Ca^{2+}, reducing its serum concentration. The lack of calcitriol production in advanced renal failure further aggravates the risk for hypocalcemia by decreasing intestinal calcium absorption. In disorders that have intestinal malabsorption as one of their manifestations or in cases of short gut syndrome, calcium absorption can diminish sufficiently to cause hypocalcemia. In conditions where calcium deposition in bone exceeds nutritional intake (i.e., hungry bone syndrome), as occasionally seen during the treatment phase of severe rickets or following parathyroid surgery for hyperparathyroidism, acute onset of hypocalcemia is not uncommon.

Hypocalcemia can occur in settings where there is a high influx of phosphate or another anion into the extracellular space to complex with Ca^{2+}. The release of high loads of phosphate in tumor lysis syndrome and rhabdomyolysis can cause severe hypocalcemia with deposition of calcium phosphate salts in various tissues. Likewise, an exogenous source of phosphate, as in high phosphate content formula, can have a similar effect in small infants. In acute pancreatitis, calcium is sequestered by free fatty acid complexes, decreasing its effective concentration in serum, while the presence of citrate in exchange blood transfusions or alkalosis can decrease serum Ca^{2+} acutely.

Classification of Neonatal Hypocalcemia

Neonatal hypocalcemia has been traditionally described as "early" when it occurs in the first 72 h of life or "late" when it occurs beyond that period of time *(15)* (Table 2). Infants that are born prematurely or experience asphyxia are particularly prone to experience a period of hypocalcemia in the early neonatal period. Preterm infants may have a deficient increase in PTH secretion to counteract the normal drop in serum Ca^{2+} after birth. In addition, calcium intake is often suboptimal, increasing the risk for hypocalce-

Table 2
Common Causes Neonatal Hypocalcemia

Early

    Asphysia
    Prematurity
    Maternal gestational diabetes
    Hypomagnesemia

Late

    Maternal hyperparathyroidism
    Hyperphosphatemia
    Transient hypoparathyroidism
    Congenital forms of hypoparathyroidism

mia. The role of asphyxia in causing hypocalcemia is poorly defined but may be similar to the hypocalcemia seen in acute illness. Infants of diabetic mothers are also prone to develop hypocalcemia early in the neonatal period. Although both a history of prematurity and asphyxia are usually present in these babies, magnesium deficiency has also been invoked as a likely cause of hypocalcemia, since maternal glycosuria is accompanied by significant magnesium losses predisposing the fetus to total body magnesium deficiency.

Late neonatal hypocalcemia encompasses most of the etiologies described earlier that are commonly seen in childhood. A common cause of hypocalcemia is a transient form of hypoparathyroidism that lasts from a few days to several weeks. These infants appear to have a deficient PTH response to hypocalcemia that improves slowly with time. In some instances, this transient deficiency is due to exposure to maternal hypercalcemia *in utero*. Maternal serum Ca^{2+} should be measured to rule out this possibility. Infants with transient hypoparathyroidism have been shown to have a higher risk to develop hypocalcemia later in life, suggesting that a mild abnormality in parathyroid function may be present.

Diagnosis and Evaluation of Hypocalcemia

Hypocalcemia can be asymptomatic in children and adolescents, especially when it is longstanding, and is often diagnosed in the setting of a routine biochemical screen. Abrupt decreases in serum Ca^{2+} predispose children to more severe symptoms, mostly neurological in nature, that require prompt medical attention. Early neuromuscular symptoms include numbness around the mouth, tingling, paresthesias, muscular cramping (especially after vigorous exercise), and carpopedal spasm. More severe symptoms include seizures, tetany, laryngospasm, and mental status changes. In neonates, symptoms can be more subtle and the only manifestation may be poor feeding and vomiting; however, acute presentations are usually characterized by a history of recurrent seizures, twitching of the extremities, agitation, high-pitched voice, tachypnea, or apnea. In some instances, neonates with acute hypocalcemia may present with cardiac failure.

Infants with acute symptomatic hypocalcemia frequently show hypotonia, tachycardia, and a bulging fontanelle on physical examination. In older asymptomatic children, the physical exam usually reveals no striking abnormality other than hyperreflexia, a positive Chvostek sign (twitching of facial muscles after tapping the facial nerve just in front of the ear), and/or a Trousseau sign (carpopedal spasm with hypoxia after maintaining a blood pressure cuff above the systolic blood pressure for 3–5 min). These findings are not exclusively present in hypocalcemic states; the Chvostek sign can be present in normal adolescents and other ionic abnormalities such as hypokalemia, hyperkalemia, hypomagnesimia, and severe hypo- or hypernatremia can also cause tetany. Hypocalcemia affects cardiac function by impairing myocardial contractility and prolonging the QTc interval, increasing the predisposition to cardiac arrthymias. Ophthalmologic findings can include papilledema, optic neuritis, and subcapsular cataract formation. Calcium deposition in intracranial locations with a preference for basal ganglia is not uncommon in chronic hypocalcemia. Other physical findings in chronic hypocalcemia include coarse hair, dry skin, brittle nails, and defective dentition, all consequences of inadequate serum Ca^{2+}. When hypocalcemia is accompanied by vitamin D deficiency and decreased intestinal calcium absorption, the bone abnormalities commonly seen in rickets are a prominent feature of the physical presentation.

Other findings in the history and physical exam frequently prove useful in the determination of the etiology of hypocalcemia. If the phenotypic features of type I PHP are present, PTH resistance should be suspected, whereas the presence of facial anomalies (i.e., mandibular hypoplasia, hypertelorism, short philtrum, and low set ears), a heart murmur or a history of recurrent infections suggests DiGeorge syndrome. The absence of a thymus shadow on a chest X-ray in a neonate with hypocalcemia should point to this syndrome. A history of mucocutaneous candidiasis, vitiligo, or alopecia may suggest the presence of autoimmune polyendocrinopathy type 1.

Serum calcium concentration should always be obtained and compared to normal values to confirm hypocalcemia. Since calcium is found in both protein bound and ionized forms in serum, conditions that alter protein content and binding affinity affect the Ca^{2+} concentration in serum. In acidic states, calcium is dissociated from albumin and the concentration of serum Ca^{2+} increases, while the reverse occurs in alkaline conditions. In the absence of ionized measurements of calcium, several conversion factors are available to help correct for protein content and pH in blood. Increases or decreases in pH by 0.1 units decreases and increases ionized Ca by 0.03 mmol/L, respectively. Several equations are available to correct total calcium measurements for changes in protein concentration:

Total serum calcium (Ca) (mg/dL) corrected for serum protein (normal range 8.4–10.2)

$$Ca = Ca\ (measured) + 0.8[4 - albumin\ (mg/dL)]$$

$$Ca = Ca\ (measured) / [0.55 + total\ protein\ (g/L)/160]$$

An ionized measurement is the more accurate assessment of serum Ca^{2+} concentration and has currently become more routinely available, especially in the hospital setting. Normal values often range 1.12–1.23 mmol/L in most laboratories. Adequate sampling is imperative to prevent excessive exposure to air or to high amounts of heparin since, in both circumstances, readings are artificially lowered.

As part of a complete evaluation of mineral ion homeostasis, both serum phosphate and magnesium levels should be obtained. Phosphate levels should be compared to normal values adjusted for age. Vitamin D stores can be measured by obtaining 25OHD levels, while $1,25(OH)_2D$ levels provide a good measure of PTH activity. The serum alkaline phosphatase level is a measure of osteoblast activity and bone turnover. It is usually elevated in states of high bone turnover as seen in hyperparathyroidism and rickets. If there is evidence of liver dysfunction, the source of alkaline phosphatase can be distinguished by adequate fractionation of enzyme isoforms. Renal function can be adequately screened by measurement of total protein, electrolytes, bicarbonate, BUN, and creatinine. In addition, urine calcium, phosphate, and creatinine levels provide a measure of mineral ion handling by the kidney, especially when done in conjunction with serum measurements.

Several useful calculations provide a measure of calcium handling before and during therapy:

Ca × Phosphate, if >60 there is a high predisposition to insoluble mineral deposition in joints and tissues.

Urine Ca/Urine Creatinine, if >0.2 the predisposition to calcium deposition in the urinary tract and nephrocalcinosis increases. In healthy neonates and infants, this ratio can be more elevated. Spot measurements are usually adequate, especially if obtained early in the morning and fasting.

TRP (tubular reabsorption of phosphate) = 1 − (Urine phosphate × Serum Creatinine/ Serum phosphate × Urine Creatinine). This measure provides a measure of phosphate retention by the kidney. TmP/GFR = TRP × Serum phosphate (normal range 2.5–4.2 mg/dL), TRP adjusted for glomerular filtration rate.

In most instances, when hypocalcemia has been confirmed, a concomitant measure of serum Ca^{2+} and intact PTH provides an adequate assessment of parathyroid function. In hypocalcemic states, PTH levels should be elevated when parathyroid function is normal. In most laboratories the normal range of serum intact PTH values falls between 10 and 65 pg/mL. If PTH values are below detection level or inappropriately normal for the degree of hypocalcemia, a form of primary hypoparathyroidism is the likely diagnosis. Elevations in serum phosphate would also support this diagnosis. If serum magnesium levels are low, usually below 1.5 mg/dL, hypocalcemia may be due to impaired PTH secretion and action; restoration of normal serum magnesium levels and monitoring of serum Ca^{2+} should be considered before diagnosing an intrinsic abnormality in parathyroid function.

When the PTH level is appropriately elevated in the presence of hypocalcemia, the serum phosphate level provides a measure of PTH action in the kidney. An elevation in serum phosphate, in the setting of normal renal function, would indicate the absence of the expected phosphaturic effect of PTH on the kidney, making a form of PTH resistance or PHP the likely diagnosis. In PHP, PTH levels are frequently very elevated, while calcitriol levels are generally in the normal range or even low despite normal vitamin D stores. To distinguish between different types of PHP, in addition to careful description of the physical phenotype, a PTH infusion with concomitant measurement of urinary cAMP would be required; a test that is seldom performed since PTH is not readily available in most clinical centers. Fortunately, the treatment is currently similar for all forms of PHP and their clinical classification is less critical for adequate management.

If hypocalcemia is accompanied with normal or low serum phosphate levels, a form of vitamin D deficiency should be suspected, a diagnosis that would be supported by physical findings of rickets and an elevated alkaline phosphatase level. Low 25OHD levels would suggest a dietary deficiency, an intestinal malabsorptive process or improper processing by the liver. Normal 25OHD levels would point to a defect in calcitriol production or action. It is not unusual to see very high levels of $1,25(OH)_2D$ in patients with vitamin D receptor defects or VDDR-II disorders.

Management of Hypocalcemia

ACUTE HYPOCALCEMIA

In a symptomatic patient the initial goal is to take the appropriate steps to eliminate symptoms associated with hypocalcemia. In patients whose acid-base status or the infusion of agents that may complex with calcium is responsible for the hypocalcemia, adequate steps to ameliorate these causes should be taken. In acute symptomatic cases or in neonatal hypocalcemia, an intravenous infusion of calcium is the most effective intervention. Calcium gluconate (10% Calcium Gluconate = 9.3 mg Ca/mL), 2 mL/kg can be administered slowly, over a 10 min period to avoid cardiac conduction problems while monitoring the ECG. The dose can be repeated every 6–8 h. To prevent the precipitation of calcium salts, phosphate and bicarbonate infusions should never be given concomitantly A central intravenous access is preferable since inadvertent extravasation of calcium causes severe chemical burns and skin damage.

To maintain normocalcemia, it is occasionally necessary to start a continuous intravenous infusion of calcium (20–80 mg Ca/kg/24 h). This is preferable over frequent boluses as long as there is good intravenous access, since a large fraction of the calcium content in the bolus is lost in the urine during the infusion. The infusion rate should be titrated to achieve a low normal serum Ca^{2+} level. Hypomagnesemia should be corrected when present. $MgSO_4$ (50% solution) 25–50 mg Mg^{2+}/kg in intravenous or intramuscular form every 4–6 h, 10–20 mg Mg^{2+}/kg for the neonate. A maintenance dose of 30–60 mg Mg^{2+}/kg/d as an oral or continuous intravenous infusion could also be given if necessary.

It is preferable to transition patients to oral therapy as soon as possible. In asymptomatic patients, it is likely that the hypocalcemia, even when very severe, has been longstanding and oral therapy should be the first line of therapy. Several forms of calcium supplements (calcium salts of carbonate [40% Ca], citrate [21% Ca], lactate [13% Ca], gluconate [9.4% Ca], glubionate [6.6% Ca]) are available to be used for this purpose. The dose of oral calcium should provide 25–100 mg Ca/kg/d divided every 4–6 h. Milk is also good source of calcium (119 mg Ca/100 mL), but not necessarily appropriate in hyperphosphatemic states since its phosphate content is high (93 mg/100 mL). If calcium losses from bone have been significant, as in untreated cases of nutritional rickets and following parathyroid surgery for hyperparathyroidism, much higher requirements for calcium are often required to sustain the remineralization of bone. In these instances, calcium intake should be increased to meet the additional requirements. Even under optimal conditions where calcium binders are avoided and there is adequate vitamin D supplementation, the intestinal absorption of calcium rarely exceeds 60–70%. Both forms of therapy should be adjusted as needed with monitoring, paying attention to serum Ca^{2+} levels, Ca × Phosphate and Urine Ca/Urine creatinine to avoid the deposition of calcium salts in peripheral tissues and kidney.

CHRONIC HYPOCALCEMIA

The overall goal in management of chronic hypocalcemia is to achieve a serum Ca^{2+} level that does not cause symptoms while avoiding hypercalcemia or excessive hypercalciuria (i.e., Urine Ca/Urine creatinine >0.2), the latter being particularly difficult to achieve in hypoparathyroidism as the absence of PTH limits calcium absorption in the renal distal tubule. In hypoparathyroidism, serum Ca levels <9 mg/dL limits the degree of hypercalciuria. In some patients that normocalcemia has been difficult to achieve without significant hypercalciuria, the addition of a thiazide diuretics has been shown to limit hypercalciuria while increasing serum Ca^{2+} significantly. Correction of hypocalcemia does not need to be so stringent in most forms of PHP since hypercalciuria is rarely seen, even when calcium levels reach high normal values. It is not unusual to require relatively high doses of calcium to overcome longstanding hypocalcemia, especially in PHP; however, calcium requirements are frequently reduced once normocalcemia has been achieved and the degree of hyperphosphatemia has been reduced.

In all forms of hypoparathyroidism, vitamin D administration is an integral part of the therapy once oral supplementation of calcium is initiated. Calcitriol is, in most instances, the adequate choice due to its short half-life and high activity, which limits its toxicity and increases efficacy, respectively. The standard dose of 10–50 ng/kg/d is usually sufficient to promote adequate calcium absorption, but the dose is often increased further if the hypocalcemia remains recalcitrant to oral therapy. Calcitriol is also the adequate choice in the treatment of hypocalcemia secondary to renal failure, liver disease or defects in 1-α-hydroxylase function. In intestinal malabsorption syndromes where there is a deficiency in fat absorption, calcidiol (1–3 μg/kg/d), the more polar vitamin D metabolite can be used. When hypocalcemia is caused by poor vitamin D stores, vitamin D, 1200–1600 U/d, or 50,000 U im should be quite adequate since calcitriol production and action is not defective. Finally, patients with 1-α-hydroxylase deficiency or VDDR-I respond well to calcitriol therapy, while VDDR-II patients with an abnormal vitamin D receptor usually require an exceedingly high dose of calcitriol (up to 1000 μg/d) or chronic parenteral calcium to maintain normal serum Ca^{2+}.

In general, phosphate binders are not required to manage hyperphosphatemia in all forms of hypoparathyroidism; moreover, the use of calcium alone limits intestinal phosphate absorption. The intake of phosphate-rich foods (i.e., dairy products) should not be encouraged. The use of an nonabsorbable antacid when serum phosphate levels remains greater than 6 mg/dL in the older child may be useful to prevent metastatic calcifications.

In chronic forms of hypoparathyroidism, frequent follow up (i.e., every 3–4 mo) to ensure adequate calcium balance may be adequate as is periodical screening of kidney function by urine analysis and ultrasound to rule out the presence of hematuria, kidney stones, and nephrocalcinosis.

NEONATAL HYPOCALCEMIA

The initial treatment of hypocalcemia in neonates with hypothyroidism should be approached as described for all children. As a large proportion of these infants ultimately have a form of transient hypoparathyroidism, initial treatment should be limited to calcium supplementation alone without addition of calcitriol. Since infants depend on maternal or formula milk for their nutrition, a useful approach has been to supplement their milk with calcium. When hyperphosphatemia is significant, the use of a low phosphate content formula (i.e., PM60/40) supplemented with calcium to bring the calcium/phosphate ratio to 4:1 is often sufficient to limit phosphate absorption while supplying sufficient calcium to achieve normocalcemia. The amount of calcium can be slowly tapered as long as the infant remains normocalcemic, and measuring serum Ca^{2+} following each decrease in dose. When a permanent form of hypoparathyroidism has been confirmed (i.e., clear features of DiGeorge syndrome are present or PTH measurements are persistently low) or the hypocalcemia is resistant to oral calcium treatment, calcitriol could be administered to enhance calcium absorption.

HYPERCALCEMIA

Hypercalcemia develops when either there is an increased influx of calcium from the gastrointestinal tract or bone into the extracellular space that exceeds the renal excretory capacity or when there is an enhanced renal tubule absorption of calcium. Causes of hypercalcemia can also be divided into etiologies that involve abnormalities in calciotropic hormones or defects in calcium handling by organs targeted by these hormones (Table 3).

Alterations in Calciotropic Hormones Causing Hypercalcemia
HYPERPARATHYROIDISM

Hyperparathyroidism (HPT) is diagnosed when hypercalcemia is accompanied by elevated PTH levels. HPT is one of the most common causes of hypercalcemia in adults, but it is a relatively uncommon disorder in children and neonates. In one study, only 2 % of 414 cases were less than 19 yr-of-age *(25)*. Furthermore, less than 20% of pediatric cases are diagnosed in children younger than 10 yr. Most cases of HPT (80%) represent a sporadic adenomatous change in one of the parathyroid glands, but a subset of patients show generalized hyperplasia of all glands that can occur sporadically, or as part of the multiple endocrine neoplasia (MEN) type 1 and 2A. Parathyroid carcinoma is an even less common, but more indolent, form of parathyroid cell neoplasia. Parathyroid adenomas show a marked decrease in sensitivity to elevations of serum Ca^{2+}, while hyperplastic glands remain sensitive to Ca^{2+} but secrete more PTH by virtue of the increased cell number.

The underlying cause for sporadic primary HPT is not known, but most tumors are monoclonal in origin; the genetic defect in some of them has been allocated to translocation of cyclin D1 to the proximity of the PTH gene promoter inducing its overexpression *(26)*. Familial forms of HPT, accounting for about 10% of all cases and comprising most cases of hyperplasia, are usually transmitted in autosomal dominant fashion. In type 1 MEN, the affected gene, *menin*, has been mapped to chromosome 11q13 *(27)*. HPT is associated with almost all affected members and is often the first manifestation of the disorder; pancreatic tumors, pituitary adenomas, and neuroendocrine tumors of the gastrointestinal tract are other common manifestations. MEN type 2A is also an autosomal dominant disorder in which HPT occurs in association with medullary carcinoma of the thyroid and pheochromocytoma. The incidence of HPT is only 10–30% and is rarely the first manifestation of the syndrome. The typical presentation is hyperplasia of all glands but adenomatous changes are not uncommon, especially in type 2A. The affected gene is the *RET* proto-oncogene in chromosome 10q11.2 *(28)*.

In conditions where a normal parathyroid is exposed to chronic hypocalcemia (e.g., renal failure, renal tubular acidosis, therapy for hypophosphatemic rickets), the gland can undergo hyperplastic changes with concomitant increases in PTH secretion that cause hypercalcemia and secondary HPT. In severe cases, often in the setting of renal failure, adenomatous changes can also occur (tertiary HPT). A similar but usually less severe and transient form of HPT has been observed in neonates born to mothers with hypoparathyroidism and exposed to low serum Ca^{2+} *in utero*.

Table 3
Differential Diagnosis of Hypercalcemia

Alterations in hormonal response
    Hyperparathyroidism
        Excessive PTH production
            Primary Hyperparathyroidism
                MEN (type I, IIa)
                Sporadic forms
            Secondary/Tertiary Hyperparathyroidism
                Renal failure
                Renal tubular acidosis
                Treatment of hypophosphatemic rickets
            Transient hyperparathyroidism
                Neonatal hyperparathyroidism (secondary to maternal hypoparathyroidism)
        Excessive PTH secretion
            Lithium toxicity
        Calcium-sensing receptor inactivating mutations
            Familial hypocalciuric hypercalcemia (FHH)
            Neonatal severe hyperparathyroidism
        Excessive PTH receptor activity
            Jansen syndrome
    Vitamin D excess
        Nutritional
        Granulomatous disorders
        Neoplasms and lymphomas
Alterations of organs involved in calcium homeostasis
    Skeleton
        Immobilization
        Hyperthyroidism
        Neoplastic bone metastasis
Other causes of hypercalcemia
    Hypercalcemia of malignancy
        PTHrP excess
        Excess cytokine and osteoclast activating factors
    Hypophosphatemia
    High calcium Load (Milk alkali syndrome)
    Vitamin A intoxication
    Drugs (e.g., thiazides)
    William's syndrome
    Hypophosphatasia
    Subcutaneous fat necrosis
    Adrenal insufficiency
    Pheochromocytoma
    Vasoactive intestinal peptide-secreting tumor

Hypercalcemia has been observed in patients treated with lithium *(29)*. PTH levels are elevated, suggesting a form of HPT. Lithium has been shown to decrease the sensitivity of the parathyroid cell to serum Ca^{2+}, by interfering with the signaling mechanisms utilized by the CaR.

In Jansen syndrome, children present with hypercalcemia, a metaphyseal dysplasia and other skeletal findings consistent with HPT. Recently, the genetic defect has been identified as a mutation of the PTH receptor that renders it constitutively active *(30)*. These children have undetectable PTH levels, as their parathyroids respond appropriately to hypercalcemia.

FAMILIAL HYPOCALCIURIC HYPERCALCEMIA

Familial hypocalciuric hypercalcemia is an autosomal dominant disorder characterized by mild, asymptomatic hypercalcemia, increased tubular reabsorption of calcium, and inappropriately normal PTH values, both caused by the presence of an inactivation mutations in one of the alleles coding for the CaR *(14)*. Affected individuals often go undiagnosed until a laboratory screen reveals the hypercalcemia. They do not have the common skeletal and gastrointestinal manifestations seen in primary hyperparathyroidism and are not at risk of developing urinary calcium stones or pancreatitis. The parathyroid glands are normal in appearance and do not show significant hyperplasia in mild forms of the disorder. There is, nevertheless, a broad spectrum of the disorder ranging from mild hypercalcemia to severe, life-threatening hypercalcemia that typically presents in the neonatal period. This severe form, classically described as neonatal severe hyperparathyroidism, is either homozygous for inactivation mutations of the CaR, or heterozygous for a very severe inactivation mutation aggravated by exposure to low Ca^{2+} in fetal development. These infants have very elevated PTH levels and all the manifestations of HPT including hyperplasia of the parathyroid glands. Removal of most parathyroid tissue is often necessary.

VITAMIN D EXCESS

Excessive exposure to vitamin D in the diet or for therapeutic reasons will cause an increase in intestinal calcium absorption and hypercalcemia. In this setting, phosphate absorption also is increased, and PTH levels are appropriately suppressed. Hypercalcemia is similarly present in a number of granulomatous disorders (i.e., sarcoidosis, tuberculosis, leprosy), chronic collagen-vascular inflammatory disorders, and some neoplastic diseases (Hodgkin B cell lymphoma), where there is proliferation and activation of monocytic cells, production of $1,25(OH)_2D$ is increased due to the unregulated expression of 1-α-hydroxylase in these cells *(31)*.

Other Causes of Hypercalcemia

As bone is the repository of greater than 98% of the body's calcium, increased or unregulated bone turnover can easily overcome the renal excretion capacity for calcium. Excess thyroid hormone can promote a disproportional stimulation of osteoclast function causing increased bone resorption and hypercalcemia *(32,33)*. Immobilization, particularly in adolescents and when prolonged for more than 2 wk, results in decreased bone accretion and increased bone resorption initially noted as hypercalciuria. When persistent, frank symptomatic hypercalcemia can occur requiring immediate treatment *(34)*. Increased prostaglandin E secretion by renal tubular cells in Bartter syndrome has been suggested to promote bone resorption *(11)*. Vitamin A excess has been shown to cause hypercalcemia likely mediated by the activation of osteoclast-mediated bone resorption *(35)*.

Malignancy is a rare cause of hypercalcemia in children. When it occurs, it can be the result of metastases to bone with concomitant dissolution of mineral content or the production of lytic factors by the original tumor that promote the mobilization of calcium (i.e., PTHrP, IL-1, IL6, TNF, prostaglandins) *(36)*.

Excessive intake of calcium in milk, calcium containing antacids and alkali can result in absorptive hypercalcemia. Conversely, severe hypophosphatemia associated with parenteral nutrition, and prematurity is associated with a reciprocal increase in serum Ca^{2+} concentration, partly due to increased calcitriol levels and intestinal calcium absorption. Hypercalcemia has also been observed in adrenal insufficiency, pheochromocytoma, and vasoactive polypeptide-secreting tumors by mechanism(s) that have not been well defined.

Hypercalcemia is present transiently during infancy in 15% of children with Williams syndrome, a sporadic disorder linked to the loss of the *elastin* gene in chromosome 7 characterized by a defined facial features (e.g., dolichocephaly, periorbital prominence, bitemporal depression, long philtrum with prominent lips and nasal tip, full cheeks, epicanthal folds, and periorbital prominence) among other physical features. More prominently, up to 30% of affected children have supravalvular aortic stenosis. The etiology of hypercalcemia is unknown; however, mildly elevated calcitriol and calcidiol levels have been reported *(37,38)*. The hypercalcemia often resolves before the first year of life; however, hypercalciuria often persists.

Hypercalcemia, sometimes very severe and life-threatening, has been seen in infants with subcutaneous fat necrosis, a condition seen in neonates, often premature, that have had traumatic births or a history of critical illness with significant poor peripheral perfusion. Subcutaneous fat undergoes necrosis, showing a significant infiltration by mononuclear cells. Although the etiology of hypercalcemia is not known, excessive prostaglandin E production and mononuclear-derived calcitriol, which in some cases have been mildly elevated, have been invoked as causes *(39,40)*.

Diagnosis and Evaluation of Hypercalcemia

Children with mild (total calcium <12 mg/dL) or chronic hypercalcemia frequently go undiagnosed unless a routine biochemical screen reveals the elevation of serum calcium. The predominant manifestation may be failure to thrive with arrest of weight gain and linear growth. In mild hypercalcemia (total calcium 12–13.5 mg/dL), generalized weakness, anorexia, constipation, and polyuria are usually present. In severe hypercalcemia (total calcium >13.5 mg/dL), nausea, vomiting, dehydration, and encephalopathic features including coma and seizures may occur. Neonates with severe hypercalcemia often present in respiratory distress and have hypotonia and apnea. It is not uncommon for relatives and patients to note significant psychological changes ranging from depression to paranoia and obsessive-compulsive behavior.

The physical examination is usually normal in hypercalcemic patients. In patients with MEN 2B, a marfanoid habitus is often present. A parathyroid mass is rarely palpable. When not dehydrated, hypertension may be noted, and a cardiac evaluation may show shortened QTc intervals in ECG tracings. In chronic hypercalcemia, a survey of soft tissues may reveal calcifications in kidney, skin, SQ tissues, cardiac arteries, gastric mucosa. In untreated patients with prolonged HPT, and occasionally reported in untreated children where the diagnosis was never suspected, distinctive skeletal findings showing subperiostal resorption of the distal phalanges, tapering of the distal clavicles, salt and pepper appearance of the skull, bone cysts, and brown tumors (liquefied bone) are the constellation of findings that describe osteitis fibrosa cystica. These findings are readily visible by conventional radiography.

The evaluation of hypercalcemia should include a thorough medical history searching for exposure to drugs, agents, and conditions that can cause hypercalcemia and a family history of hypercalcemia or other associated medical conditions. The approach to the biochemical evaluation is similar to the evaluation described for hypocalcemia and should initially include the measurement of serum intact PTH levels, phosphate, and magnesium together with measurements of urine calcium excretion. Renal function should also be assessed to rule out renal insufficiency, and a urine analysis is useful to look for the presence of hematuria or calcium salt residue.

HPT is diagnosed when hypercalcemia is noted in conjunction with elevated PTH levels. In the absence of secondary causes of HPT, the presence of hypercalciuria is consistent with primary HPT. Hypercalciuria is usually present in HPT since the PTH-mediated increase in tubular calcium resorption does not fully compensate for the increase in calcium concentration in the glomerular filtrate. The degree of hypercalciuria has significant diagnostic value, especially when trying to distinguish mild HPT from FHH, since mild elevations of PTH are often seen in both cases *(14)*. The calculation of 24 h urinary calcium clearance provides a measure of calcium handling by the kidney. Decreased urinary calcium excretion in the presence of mild hypercalcemia should raise the possibility of inactivating mutation of the CaR and FHH. A better measure of hypercalciuria that takes into account changes in glomerular filtration is the calcium clearance ratio ([Urine Ca × Serum creatinine] / [Urine creatinine × Serum Ca]). The clearance ratio in FHH is one third of that in typical primary HPT, and a value less than 0.01 is virtually diagnostic of FHH. Unfortunately, FHH patients do not always show significant hypocalciuria. Mild elevations of magnesium can sometime distinguish FHH from HPT, since serum magnesium is usually in the low normal range in HPT. A family history of asymptomatic hypercalcemia would provide further support for a diagnosis of FHH. Both parents should be evaluated when the diagnosis is suspected in a child. Adequate distinction between HPT and FHH is not trivial since hypercalcemia in FHH has not been associated with any long term adverse outcome and requires no treatment. Furthermore, the surgical removal of parathyroid tissue in FHH, in cases that were thought to represent HPT, does not correct the hypercalcemia.

In cases where the MEN syndrome is suspected, an adequate screen for other hormonal abnormalities in MEN 1 is warranted. Isolated HPT as the first manifestation in MEN 2B is rare, but a genetic screen is currently available to rule mutation in the *RET* gene in suspected cases. In high probability cases, the presence of a pheochromocytoma should be ruled out prior to a parathyroidectomy.

When PTH levels are adequately suppressed in the presence of hypercalcemia, elevated 25OHD levels would suggest vitamin D intoxication. Elevated $1,25(OH)_2D$ without a concomitant elevation of 25OHD points to an ectopic source of 1-α-hydroxylase. In both settings, hyperphosphatemia and marked hypercalciuria are usually present, greatly increasing the predisposition to calcium toxicity. In the absence of elevated PTH and vitamin D metabolites, hypercalcemic patients that have not been exposed to high calcium ingestion or prolonged immobilization should be screened for the secretion of other hypercalcemic factors (i.e., PTHrP, prostaglandin E).

Management of Hypercalcemia

The management of hypercalcemia depends on the severity and cause of the elevation of serum Ca^{2+}. When hypercalcemia is mild and the patient is asymptomatic, no initial treatment may be necessary and medical efforts to reach a diagnosis should be given preference.

When hypercalcemia is severe (total serum calcium >14 mg/dL), or when there are symptoms and signs of cardiac, gastrointestinal, and central nervous system dysfunction, prompt intervention is appropriate. Since patients are usually dehydrated because of the polyuria and anorexia associated with severe hypercalcemia, the initial step is to provide adequate hydration, preferably in the form of isotonic saline at 3000 cc/m^2 for the first 24–48 h. To restore vascular volume, increase glomerular filtration rate and dilute serum Ca^{2+}. After hydration, the loop diuretic furosemide (1 mg/kg every 6 h) can further inhibit the reabsorption of calcium, especially in the presence of sodium, further promoting calciuresis. In comatose patients, hemodialysis should be considered as a means to decrease serum Ca^{2+} more aggressively.

If hypercalcemia does not respond to these initial measures, agents that block bone resorption may be useful as adjuvant therapy. Calcitonin 4 U/kg SQ q 12 h is commonly used for this purpose; however, its efficacy diminishes with continuous administration due to tachyphylaxis. Bisphosphonates, analogs of pyrophosphate that inhibit osteoclast action, have been used, especially when hypercalcemia is primarily driven by the mobilization of calcium from bone as in cases of tumor induced hypercalcemia, severe HPT or immobilization. Both etidronate (7.5 mg/kg/d) and pamidronate (10mg/M^2) could be used, the latter given as a single dose intravenous infusion. It is important to note that the use of bisphosphonates in children has been limited, and their impact on bone growth and development are not well known yet. Agents like plicamycin and gallium nitrate have a similar effects in bone, but their use is associated with significant toxicity and should be avoided if possible.

Additional steps in the management will be partially determined by the etiology of hypercalcemia. When hypercalcemia is due to excess vitamin D ingestion or activity, glucocorticoids (prednisone 1 mg/kg/d) can be very effective since they inhibit both 1-α-hydroxylase activity and intestinal calcium absorption. Ketoconazole (3 mg/kg/d divided in three doses) is also a very effective inhibitor of 1-α- hydroxylase activity, but its use is associated with significant gastrointestinal side effects and can cause adrenal insufficiency.

Pharmacological agents may become available in the near future that can activate the CaR and suppress PTH secretion in affected glands. However, in young patients with well described HPT, preferably confirmed by several measurements of serum calcium and PTH, the surgical removal of the affected gland is ultimately required to control hypercalcemia. A number of imaging techniques (i.e., neck ultrasound, computed tomography, magnetic resonance imaging and radionuclide scanning) have been used to detect a hyperfunctioning gland; however, the reported sensitivities have ranged between 40–90% and may be more informative when used in combination. More recently, ^{99m}Tc-sestamibi scanning has shown some promise, specially in the visualization of adenomas *(41)*. Intraoperative measurements of PTH are now feasible, aiding the surgeon in his search for hyperplastic or adenomatous tissue since successful removal would be reflected by an adequate rapid drop of PTH levels *(42)*. In cases of an isolated adenoma, resection is usually curative. In cases of isolated hyperplasia or secondary HPT, removal of three and one half glands is recommended. Total parathyroidectomy is recommended with autotransplantation of minced parathyroid tissue in the forearm for patients with MEN, where it could easily be removed in cases of recurring hypercalcemia. Post surgical hypocalcemia is common and easily treated with calcium supplements. In cases of severe HPT, hypocalcemia can be more severe and prolonged owing to hungry bone syndrome. These patients have severe phosphate and calcium deficits as mineral bone deposition takes place. The use of both calcium and phosphate supplements together with calcitriol is recommended. In some instances, permanent hypoparathyroidism ensues, requiring life long therapy.

REFERENCES

1. Diaz R, Fuleihan GE, Brown EM. Parathyroid Hormone and Polyhormones: Production and Export. In: Handbook of Physiology, Fray JCS, ed. Oxford University Press, New York, 2000, pp. 607–662.
2. Juppner H, Potts JT. The Roles of Parathyroid Hormone and Parathyroid Hormone-related Peptide in Calcium Metabolism and Bone Biology: Their Biological Actions and Receptors. In: Handbook of Physiology, Fray, JCS Ed. Oxford University Press, New York, 2000, pp. 663–698.
3. Brown EM, MacLeod RJ. Extracellular Calcium Sensing and Extracellular Calcium Signaling. Physiol Rev 2001;81(1):239–297.
4. Slatopolsky E, Dusso A, Brown AJ. The role of phosphorus in the development of secondary hyperparathyroidism and parathyroid cell proliferation in chronic renal failure. Am J Med Sci 1999; 317(6):370–376.
5. Rubin DA, Hellman P, Zon LI, et al. A G protein-coupled receptor from zebrafish is activated by human parathyroid hormone and not by human or teleost parathyroid hormone-related peptide. Implications for the evolutionary conservation of calcium-regulating peptide hormones. J Biol Chem 1999;274(33): 23,035–23,042.
6. Black KS, Mundy GR. Other causes of hypercalcemia:local and ectopic syndromes. InL The Parathyroids, Bilezekian JP, Levine MA, Marcus R, eds. Raven Press, New York, 1994, pp. 341–357.
7. Kronenberg HM, Karaplis AC, Lanske B. Role of parathyroid hormone-related protein in skeletal development. Ann NY Acad Sci 1996;785:119–123.
8. Kovacs CS, Lanske B, Hunzelman JL, et al. Parathyroid hormone-related peptide (PTHrP) regulates fetal-placental calcium transport through a receptor distinct from the PTH/PTHrP receptor. Proc Natl Acad Sci USA 1996;93(26):15,233–15,238.
9. Bouillon R. Vitamin D: From photosynthesis, metabolism, action to clinical applications. In: Endocrinology, DLJ, Jameson JL, Eds. W.B. Saunders, Philadelphia, 2001, pp. 1009–10028.
10. Fuss M, Pepersack I, Gillet C, et al. Calcium and vitamin D metabolism in granulomatous diseases. Clin Rheumatol 1992;11(1):28–36.
11. Friedman PA. Calcium transport in the kidney. Curr Opin Nephrol Hypertens 1999;8(5):589–595.
12. Martin TJ, Moseley JM. Calcitonin. In Endocrinology, DLJ, Jameson JL, eds. W.B. Saunders, Philadelphia, 2001, pp. 999–1008.
13. Kovacs CS, Kronenberg HM. Maternal-fetal calcium and bone metabolism during pregnancy, pueperium and lactation. Endocr Rev 1997;18:832–872.
14. Diaz R, Brown, EM. Familial hypocalciuric hypercalcemia and other disorders due to calcium-sensing receptor muations. In Endocrinology, DLJ, Jameson JL, eds. W.B. Saunders, Philadelphia, 2001, pp. 1121–1132.
15. Carpenter TO. Neonatal hypocalcemia. In: Primer on metabolic bone diseases and disorders of mineral metabolism, Favus MJ, Ed. Lippincott Williams & Wilkins, Philadelphia, 1999, pp. 235–238.
16. Thakker RV. Molecular genetics of hypoparathyroidism. In: The Parathyroids, Bilezekian JP, Levine MA, Marcus R, Eds. 1994, Raven Press, New York. pp. 765–779.
17. Carey AH, Kelly O, Halford S, et al. Molecular genetic study of the frequency of monosomy 22q11 in DiGeorge syndrome. Am J Hum Genet 1992;51(5):964–970.
18. Thakker RV. Molecular genetics of mineral metabolic disorders. J Inherit Metab Dis 1992;15(4): 592–609.
19. Sherwood LM, Santora ACI. Hypoparathyroid states in the differential diagnosis of hypocalcemia. In: The Parathyroids, Bilezekian JP, Levine MA, Marcus R, eds. 1994, Raven Press, New York, pp. 747–752.
20. Whyte MP. Autoimmune aspects of hypoparathyroidism, In: The Parathyroids, Bilezekian JP, Levine MA, Marcus R, Eds. 1994, Raven Press, New York, pp. 753–764.

21. Bettinelli A, Bianchetti MG, Girardin E, et al. Use of calcium excretion values to distinguish two forms of primary renal tubular hypokalemic alkalosis: Bartter and Gitelman syndromes. J Pediatr 1992;120(1):38–43.
22. Cardenas-Rivero N, Chernon B, Stoiko MA, et al. Hypocalcemia in critically ill children. J Pediatr 1989;114(6):946–951.
23. Levine MA. Parathyroid hormone resistance syndromes. In: Primer on metabolic bone diseases and disorders of mineral metabolism, Favus MJ, ed. Lippincott Williams & Wilkins, Philadelphia, 1999, pp. 230–235.
24. Liberman UA, Marx SJ. Vitamin D-dependent rickets. In: Primer on metabolic bone diseases and disorders of mineral metabolism, Favus MJ, Ed. Lippincott Williams & Wilkins, Philadelphia, 1999, pp. 323–328.
25. Langman CB. Hypercalcemic syndromes in infants and children. In: Primer on metabolic bone diseases and disorders of mineral metabolism, Favus MJ, Ed. Lippincott Williams & Wilkins, Philadelphia, 1999, pp. 219–223.
26. Arnold A. Genetic basis of endocrine disease 5. Molecular genetics of parathyroid gland neoplasia. J Clin Endocrinol Metab 1993;77(5):1108–1112.
27. Chandrasekharappa SC, Guru SC, Manickam P, et al. Positional cloning of the gene for multiple endocrine neoplasia-type 1. Science 1997;276(5311):404–407.
28. Mulligan LM, Kwok JB, Healey CS, et al. Germ-line mutations of the RET proto-oncogene in multiple endocrine neoplasia type 2A. Nature 1993;363(6428):458–460.
29. Haden ST, Stoll AL, McCormick S, et al. Alterations in parathyroid dynamics in lithium-treated subjects, J Clin Budoevinal Metab 1997;82(9):2844–2848.
30. Schipani E, Kruse K, Juppner H. A constitutively active mutant PTH-PTHrP receptor in Jansen-type metaphyseal chondrodysplasia. Science 1995;268(5207):98–100.
31. Rigby WF. The immunobiology of vitamin D. Immunol Today 1988;9(2):54–58.
32. Burman KD, Monchik JM, Earll JM, et al. Ionized and total serum calcium and parathyroid hormone in hyperthyroidism. Ann Intern Med 1976;84:668–671.
33. Britto JM, Fenton AJ, Holloway WR, et al. Osteoblasts mediate thyroid hormone stimulation of osteoclastic bone resorption. Endocrinology 1994;134(1):169–176.
34. Bergstrom WH. Hypercalciuria and hypercalcemia complicating immobilization. Am J Dis Child 1978;132(6):553–554.
35. Valentic JP, Elias AN, Weinstein GD. Hypercalcemia associated with oral isotretinoin in the treatment of severe acne. JAMA 1983;250(14):1899–1900.
36. Roberts MM, Stewart AF. Humoral hypercalcemia of malignancy. In: Primer on metabolic bone diseases and disorders of mineral metabolism, Favus MJ, ed. Lippincott Williams & Wilkins, Philadelphia, 1999, pp. 203–207.
37. Garabedian M, Jacqz E, Grillozo H, et al. Elevated plasma 1,25-dihydroxyvitamin D concentrations in infants with hypercalcemia and an elfin facies. N Engl J Med 1985;312(15):948–952.
38. Taylor AB, Stern PH, Bell NH. Abnormal regulation of circulating 25-hydroxyvitamin D in the Williams syndrome. N Engl J Med 1982;306(16):972–975.
39. Sharata H, Postellon DC, Hashimoto K. Subcutaneous fat necrosis, hypercalcemia, and prostaglandin E. Pediatr Dermatol 1995;12(1):43–47.
40. Kruse K, Irle U, Uhlig R. Elevated 1,25-dihydroxyvitamin D serum concentrations in infants with subcutaneous fat necrosis. J Pediatr 1993;122(3):460–463.
41. Chen CC, Holder LE, Scovill WA, et al. Comparison of parathyroid imaging with technetium-99m-pertechnetate/sestamibi subtraction, double-phase technetium-99m- sestamibi and technetium-99m-sestamibi SPECT. J Nucl Med 1997;38(6):834–839.
42. Boggs JE, Irvin JL III, Molinari RS, et al. Intraoperative parathyroid hormone monitoring as an adjunct to parathyroidectomy. Surgery 1996;120(6):954–958.

21 Rickets

The Skeletal Disorders of Impaired Calcium or Phosphate Availability

*Bat-Sheva Levine, MD
and Thomas O. Carpenter, MD*

CONTENTS
>
> INTRODUCTION
> CLINICAL PRESENTATION AND DIAGNOSTIC EVALUATION
> TREATMENT
> REFERENCES

INTRODUCTION

Rickets is a disorder of mineralization of the bone matrix in growing bone; it involves both the growth plate (epiphysis) and newly formed trabecular and cortical bone. In growing children, this disorder, if untreated, may result in severe malalignment of the lower extremities. *Osteomalacia* specifically refers to the lag in mineralization of true bone tissue, independent of changes at the growth plate. Adults subjected to similar pathophysiologic events as children with rickets are said to have osteomalacia, as their growth plates are fused and already mineralized. The terms rickets and osteomalacia should be distinguished from *osteopenia*, which refers to the appearance of overall diminished bone mineral density on radiographs. *Osteopenia* has also been recently used to describe bone mineral density between one and two standard deviations below mean values for peak bone mineral density in adults. *Osteoporosis* is defined as reduced bone tissue per unit volume of whole bone resulting from an imbalance between osteoblastic bone formation and osteoclastic bone resorption. This term has more recently been used to describe bone mineral density two standard deviations or more below the mean. In contrast to a rachitic or osteomalacic lesion, a pure osteoporotic lesion has no excess of unmineralized bone matrix. Of note, some of the underlying causes of rickets in children may also result in osteopenia or osteoporosis.

From: *Contemporary Endocrinology: Pediatric Endocrinology: A Practical Clinical Guide*
Edited by: S. Radovick and M. H. MacGillivray © Humana Press Inc., Totowa, NJ

Table 1
Association of the Causes of Rickets

	Calciopenic	Phosphopenic
Nutritional	Vitamin D deficiency	Phosphate deficiency
	Calcium deficiency	
Inherited	1-alpha-hydroxylase deficiency (Vitamin D-dependent rickets Type I)	Hypophosphatemic rickets (X-linked and autosomal dominant)
	Hereditary resistance to 1,25(OH)$_2$D (Vitamin-D dependent rickets Type II)	Hereditary hypophosphatemic rickets with hypercalciuria
		X-linked hypercalciuiric nephrolithiasis (X-linked recessive hypophosphatemic rickets, Dent's disease)
Other	Malabsorption of Vitamin D	Impaired absorption of phosphate
	Cystic Fibrosis	Severe intestinal disease
	Inflammatory bowel disease	Phospate-binding gels (aluminum-
	Celiac disease	containing antacids)
	Short bowel syndrome	
		Phosphate-wasting renal tubulopathies
	Impairment of hydroxylation of Vitamin D	Heavy metal/toxin exposure
	Severe hepatobiliary disease	Fanconi syndrome
	Severe renal disease	
		Tumor-induced rickets
	Increased catabolism of Vitamin D	
		Associated with various syndromes
	Anticonvulsant therapy	(linear sebaceous nevus syndrome,
		neurofibromatosis, McCune Albright)

The major forms of rickets may be conveniently classified as *calciopenic*—those predominantly resulting from a reduced availability of calcium to the mineralizing skeleton—and *phosphopenic*—those resulting from a reduced availability of phosphate. These major forms of rickets should be distinguished from several *rickets-like* disorders, such as hypophosphatasia and other skeletal dysplasias. Moreover, both the calciopenic and phosphopenic forms of rickets may be subclassified as those resulting from nutritional, inherited, or other causes (Table 1).

In general, most instances of nutritional rickets are calciopenic, whereas heritable causes are usually phosphopenic. Since treatment strategies for the various forms of rickets differ, it is important to identify the precise type of rickets using clues from the patient's medical history, physical examination, and laboratory evaluation. This review describes the various forms of rickets and offers a practical approach to the evaluation and management of this disorder.

CLINICAL PRESENTATION AND DIAGNOSTIC EVALUATION

History/Physical Exam

Despite the notion that nutritional rickets has been eradicated, the incidence of this disorder is more common than most other etiologies encountered. Nutritional deficiency rickets must be excluded as the etiology of any case under evaluation. It is important to consider that calcium deficiency may play a significant role in the development of rickets, and that children with nutritional rickets may have a mixed deficiency of both calcium and vitamin D in their usual diet. This has been particularly evident in view of the association of the disorder with macrobiotic and vegetarian diets, as well as dairy product avoidance. In contrast to calcium deficiency playing a significant role in this process, nutritional phosphorus deprivation is rare. Previous to the 1990s, phosphate deficiency rickets was encountered with some frequency in breast-fed premature infants, however, this group often receives breast milk fortifier products or infant formulas with added mineral content. Abuse of aluminum-containing antacid gels which bind phosphate in the gastrointestinal tract can result in phosphate deficiency, however rarely encountered in children. Exposure to heavy metals or toxic agents may result in phosphate-wasting tubulopathies and should be excluded. Fat malabsorption, and underlying renal or liver disease may be important factors in the development of rickets, and should be considered in obtaining a history. A detailed family history should be obtained with attention to bone diseases and fractures. A history of inborn errors such as those associated with renal Fanconi syndrome should be sought. Finally, in apparent sporadic phosphopenic rickets, an exhaustive search for a tumor should be sought, especially if the patient presents as an older child or an adult.

Rachitic bone deformities are variable, depending on age at onset and the relative growth rate of different bones. The most rapidly growing bones during the first year of life are the skull, the ribs, and the upper limbs; rickets presenting at this age may manifest craniotabes (generalized softening of the calvaria), frontal bossing, widening of the cranial sutures, flaring of the wrists, rachitic rosary (bulging of the costochondral junctions of the ribs), and Harrison grooves (groove extending laterally from the xiphoid process that corresponds to the diaphragmatic attachment). After the first year of life, lower limb deformities become more prominent. Genu varum (bow-leg deformity) often occurs when the age of onset is early childhood and genu valgum (knock-knee deformity) when rickets presents in older children. Bone pain is common in children, and palpable enlargement of the ends of the long bones occurs. In general, the calciopenic forms of rickets manifest both upper and lower extremity involvement, whereas phosphopenic forms involve the lower extremities to a greater extent. Proximal muscle weakness can occur in calciopenic rickets as well, and hypocalcemia can result in carpopedal spasm, laryngeal stridor, seizures, and parasthesias. The severity of growth impairment in childhood rickets generally reflects the extent and duration of lower extremity involvement.

Unique physical findings may accompany rickets in certain specific disorders, such as the alopecia and oligodontia associated with hereditary vitamin D resistance. In X-linked hypophosphatemic rickets (XLH), the skull is often scaphocephalic, and Chiari I malformation, possibly related to severe calvarial osteomalacia and thickening, has been described (for review, see ref. *1*). Adults with XLH may manifest vertebral anomalies such as thickening of the spinous processes, fusion, thickening of facet joints, and spinal canal stenosis. Calcification of tendons and ligaments is also common. Dental abscesses are a frequent occurrence in patients with XLH, due to the undermineralization and expansion of the pulp chamber; this phenomenon results in a diminished barrier to the exterior surface of the teeth and easy access for oral fluids and bacteria to pass through the outer enamel layer and initiate abscess formation. A defect in the regulation of vascular tone also occurs in some patients with XLH, as evidenced by abnormal blood pressure response to exercise and mild ventricular hypertrophy.

Radiographic Abnormalities

The earliest radiographic change of rickets is slight widening of the growth plate. In more severe rickets, fraying, cupping, and widening of the metaphyses occur. In infants, abnormalities are best seen at the costochondral junctions, wrists, and ankles; in older children, the distal femur is likely to exhibit major epiphyseal changes. In adolescence, when the epiphyses begin to fuse, the iliac crest may continue to show rachitic changes, as it is the last epiphysis to fuse. In older children with XLH, asymmetry of the growth plate results due to altered weight-bearing forces through the physis. Osteomalacic changes of the diaphyses include shaft deformities, decreased bone density, coarse spongiosa, thinned compacta, and pseudofractures. As healing of rickets begins, radiodense lines are detectable adjacent to the metaphyses representing rapid calcification of the cartilage.

Biochemical Abnormalities

An initial biochemical investigation should include determination of serum alkaline phosphatase activity as well as serum calcium and phosphate levels. In most cases of rickets increased bone turnover is present, reflected by increased circulating alkaline phosphatase activity. Alkaline phosphatase activity tends to be lower in heritable phosphopenic rickets than the 10 to 15-fold elevations often seen in calciopenic forms. Adults with XLH may have normal alkaline phosphatase levels despite impressive osteomalacia; thus, monitoring levels of this enzyme is not a sensitive indicator of response to therapy. Serum alkaline phosphatase activity is normal in most skeletal dysplasias, however it is abnormally low in hypophosphatasia.

In all forms of calciopenic rickets, serum calcium and phosphate levels tend to be in the low to low-normal range; one can distinguish between the various causes by measurement of vitamin D metabolites. Low serum concentrations of 25-hydroxyvitamin D (25-OHD) are seen in vitamin D deficiency, including nutritional deficiency and malabsorption, however children with nutritional rickets often present with a mixed calcium and vitamin D deficiency and may not have low 25-OHD levels. Partial treatment of vitamin D deficiency may affect the circulating 25-OHD level so that this measure may be normal, and thus not helpful in identifying all cases of nutritional rickets. In the setting of normal levels of 25-OHD, a low $1,25(OH)_2D$ level points to the diagnosis of 1-α-hydroxylase deficiency, and a high $1,25(OH)_2D$ level suggests vitamin D resistance.

A low serum phosphate level and normal serum calcium level suggest the diagnosis of primary hypophosphatemic rickets, and should be followed by an accurate assessment of renal phosphate handling. Obtaining a 2-h urine collection after a 4-h fast for determination of creatinine and phosphate along with concomitant serum creatinine and phosphate levels (best sampled at the midpoint of the timed urine collection) allows one to calculate the tubular reabsorption of phosphate (%TRP). A nomogram *(2)* is used to determine the renal tubular threshold maximum for phosphate, as expressed per glomerular filtration rate (TMP/GFR). A low TMP/GFR in the setting of a low serum phosphate confirms the inappropriate renal phosphate losses characteristic of primary hypophosphatemic rickets.

To distinguish XLH from hypercalciuric variants (HHRH and XLHN) of the disease, urinary calcium excretion should be determined in either a 24-h collection or a briefer timed collection if sufficient volume is obtained. Urinary calcium excretion tends to be low in XLH and in calciopenic forms of rickets. Fanconi syndrome may be associated with glycosuria and aminoaciduria. Proteinuria or microglobulinuria are often present in patients with XLHN. Oncogenic rickets cannot be distinguished biochemically from primary hypophosphatemic rickets, and it must be suspected in all sporadic cases of hypophosphatemic rickets presenting in late childhood or adulthood.

Measurement of PTH levels are useful in the diagnostic evaluation. Moderate to severe hyperparathyroidism is characteristic of calciopenic rickets. On the other hand, in untreated XLH, PTH levels may be normal or modestly elevated; more severe hyperparathyroidism is seen in XLH as a complication of phosphate therapy. Other findings of XLH include normal serum 25-OHD levels, and normal or somewhat low levels of $1,25(OH)_2D$ (inappropriately low in the setting of hypophosphatemia). By contrast, in hypercalciuric variants of hypophosphatemic rickets, the circulating $1,25(OH)_2D$ level appropriately increases in response to hypophosphatemia, resulting in normal to high serum calcium levels and suppressed PTH levels.

Nutritional Rickets

Surprisingly, the incidence of nutritional rickets in the US remains greater than that of inherited forms of rickets. Despite vitamin D supplementation of milk, numerous recent reports have described nutritional rickets occurring with regularity in African-American children with a history of breast-feeding *(3)*. Vitamin D content of human breast milk is relatively low under normal circumstances. There is usually no history of vitamin supplementation in affected children, and such children usually present in the late winter or early spring following a season of limited sunlight exposure. In our experience, many of the children are subsequently weaned to diets with low calcium intake. It is likely the low vitamin D stores are marginal following the breast-feeding in the winter months, and the subsequent shift to a diet low in dairy products compounds the vitamin D deficiency by providing inadequate dietary calcium, which further accelerates the turnover of vitamin D. In contrast to this limited calcium supply, phosphate is nearly ubiquitous in human foodstuffs and nutritional phosphate deficiency is relatively rare. Human milk, although sufficient in phosphate intake for the term infant, does not provide adequate phosphate to preterm infants, who maintain a relatively greater rate of mineral accretion than term babies. Thus, the clinical situation in which pediatricians encounter nutritional phosphate deficiency occurs in the breast-fed premature infant. This problem has been largely alleviated in recent years with breast milk supplements.

Heritable Forms of Calciopenic Rickets

Heritable forms of calciopenic rickets are encountered much less frequently than nutritional rickets. Heritable calciopenic rickets may result from metabolic defects in the vitamin D axis, including inadequate activation of vitamin D and abnormalities of the vitamin D receptor.

1α-Hydroxylase Deficiency

An autosomal recessive form of calciopenic rickets results from abnormal synthesis of the active vitamin D metabolite, $1,25(OH)_2D$. This disorder represents the physiologic loss of function of the renal 25(OH)D 1α-hydroxylase enzyme system that converts 25(OH)D to $1,25(OH)_2D$; mutations in the gene encoding the cytochrome P450 moiety of the enzyme have been identified, rendering a dysfunctional enzyme unable to donate electrons to 25(OH)D *(4)*. This disorder usually has its onset within 4–12 mo of age, when infants with a history of adequate vitamin D intake present with typical features of rickets. The serum 25(OH)D level is typically normal, but the $1,25(OH)_2D$ is low to low-normal, even in patients treated with pharmacologic doses of vitamin D or 25(OH)D.

Hereditary Vitamin D Resistance

Another heritable cause of calciopenic rickets is target tissue resistance to $1,25(OH)_2D$ because of receptor or post-receptor defects. Hereditary vitamin D resistance (also known as vitamin D-dependent rickets type II) is a rare autosomal recessive disorder; a variety of mutations in the gene coding for the vitamin D receptor have been described, including missense mutations in the DNA- or steroid hormone-binding domains of the receptor *(5)*. In addition, mutations resulting in inappropriate truncation of the vitamin D receptor have been identified. In some families with vitamin D resistance, no genetic defect has been clearly identified.

Onset of hereditary vitamin D resistance is typically between 6 mo to 3 yr of age, and the clinical, radiologic, and biochemical features are similar to those observed in 1α-hydroxylase deficiency, except that the circulating levels of $1,25(OH)_2D$ are high. Some kindreds with this disorder have total body alopecia, and other patients may demonstrate oligodontia.

Heritable Forms of Phosphopenic Rickets

X-linked Hypophosphatemic Rickets

Phosphopenic rickets is most frequently due renal tubular phosphate wasting. The prototype disorder, X-linked hypophosphatemic rickets (XLH), is characterized by X-linked dominant inheritance, hypophosphatemia, a low renal tubular threshold for phosphate reabsorption, and impaired generation of $1,25(OH)_2D$ (for review, *see* ref. *1*). The recently-identified mutated gene, *PHEX (6)*, is homologous to known metalloendopeptidases (including neprolysin and endothelin converting enzyme-1); however, the precise role of *PHEX* in the pathophysiology of XLH has not been clearly established. Studies in an animal model, the *Hyp* mouse, indicate that the defect is not intrinsic to the kidney, but rather, that the *PHEX* product is involved in the processing of a circulating humoral factor that influences renal phosphate transport.

XLH usually presents in the second or third year of life with bowing of the legs and short stature. In addition to X-linked transmission, both autosomal recessive and autosomal dominant transmission patterns of hypophosphatemic rickets have been described; the mutation in an autosomal dominant form has recently been mapped to chromosome 12 to a gene on the short arm which encodes a unique growth factor, FGF23 *(7)*.

The XLH phenotype is seen less frequently as an acquired condition, such as in tumor-induced rickets. This disorder is most likely due to a circulating humoral factor secreted by a tumor. Such tumors are often benign and small in size and therefore may escape detection. Candidate factors for mediation of this syndrome include FGF23, FRP4 (friggled related protein 4), and MEPE, a glycosylated matrix protein. Upon resection of these tumors, the clinical and biochemical abnormalities typically resolve. The differential diagnosis of the XLH phenotype also includes rickets observed in the linear sebaceous nevus syndrome, consisting of sebaceous nevi, seizures, and mental retardation. Finally, the phenotype of primary hypophosphatemia may be observed with neurofibromatosis and with the McCune-Albright syndrome.

HEREDITARY HYPOPHOSPHATEMIC RICKETS WITH HYPERCALCIURIA

In contrast to XLH, hereditary hypophosphatemic rickets with hypercalciuria (HHRH) is an autosomal recessive disorder in which there is a primary impairment of renal phosphate handling with an appropriate physiologic response of the 1α-hydroxylase enzyme to the ambient hypophosphatemia. Thus, circulating $1,25(OH)_2D$ levels are elevated, resulting in increased intestinal calcium absorption, suppressed PTH levels, osteopenia, hypercalciuria, and the propensity to develop nephrolithiasis. Mutations in the renal sodium phosphate cotransporter, NaPi2, were not present in several affected families *(8)*. Most cases have been described in North African and Middle Eastern populations, but sporadic cases have been reported elsewhere.

X-LINKED HYPERCALCIURIC NEPHROLITHIASIS

Hypophosphatemic hypercalciuric rickets may occur in the X-linked hypercalciuric nephrolithiasis (XLHN) family of syndromes. Four clinical phenotypes are described, all with X-linked recessive inheritance and proximal renal tubulopathy leading to eventual renal failure. Hypophosphatemic rickets may occur within the spectrum of syndromes of XLHN, particularly in Dent's disease and X-linked recessive hypophosphatemic rickets, in which the rachitic findings can be severe. Various mutations in the voltage-gated chloride channel gene *CLCN5* have been identified in this group of disorders *(9)*, however, the mechanism by which the altered chloride channel results in proximal renal tubular dysfunction and hypercalciuria is not known.

Phosphopenic rickets may occur in association with Fanconi syndrome, a heterogeneous group of disorders characterized by excessive urinary losses of glucose, phosphate, bicarbonate, and amino acids. Some patients with this disorder present with hyperchloremic acidosis in addition to hypophosphatemia and proteinuria. The syndrome may be inherited as a primary tubulopathy, or secondary to such inborn metabolic disorders as cystinosis, tyrosinemia, fructose intolerance, galactosemia, Lowe syndrome, Wilson's disease, or type I glycogen storage disease.

Rickets-like Disorders

Several related conditions manifest rickets-like deformities. These include hypophosphatasia, a rare autosomal recessive disorder characterized by deficiency of tissue and serum alkaline phosphatase (for review, *see* ref. *10*). Four forms of hypophosphatasia have been described, with the severity of the disease being inversely related to the age at presentation: a defective lethal form; an infantile form presenting within the first 6 mo of life with rachitic-like skeletal defects resulting in recurrent respiratory tract infection, poor growth, increased intracranial pressure, and death in 50% of cases; a milder childhood type presenting after 6 mo of age with premature loss of deciduous teeth, rachitic-like lesions, and craniosynostosis; and an adult-onset form with recurrent fractures and pseudofractures. Other skeletal dysplasias include the Schmid type metaphyseal dysplasia, an autosomal dominant disorder due to a mutation in the type X collagen (*COL10A1*) gene *(11)* may resemble metabolic rickets clinically and radiographically. Type X collagen expression is restricted to hypertrophic chondrocytes in areas undergoing endochondral ossification. The deficiency in growth plates can result in a lesion resembling rickets; however, there are no abnormalities in serum calcium, phosphate, and alkaline phosphatase in patients with this skeletal dysplasia.

TREATMENT

Calciopenic Rickets

The immediate goal of medical treatment is to heal the active epiphyseal lesions, thereby preventing progression of bow or knock-knee deformities, which, in untreated disease, may become irreversible and require corrective orthopedic intervention. It should be noted that while this review focuses on tertiary prevention—i.e., management of patients already known to be affected by rachitic disease—efforts need to be expended as well on primary prevention by educating the public and the general pediatric community about the importance of adequate dietary supplementation with vitamin D and calcium. Secondary prevention of nutritional calciopenic rickets has also been proposed in select groups. For example, routine supplementation of the premature infants with 800 IU per day of vitamin D as well as preventive use of breast milk fortifiers to ensure adequate mineral supplementation in the premature infant have been recommended.

Some have also advocated secondary prevention of vitamin D deficiency rickets by targeted screening for vitamin D deficiency rickets in high-risk groups, such as dark-skinned breastfeeding infants, children with low intakes of milk and dairy products, and infants living in areas where colder winter weather precludes outdoor activity. Another group of children recently found to be at risk includes international adoptees from the former Soviet Union; these are children formerly residing in orphanages who are reported to have had limited sunlight exposure and no vitamin supplementation prior to entering the US *(12)*.

The 1998 American Academy of Pediatrics *Pediatric Nutrition Handbook* recommends that all dark-skinned, breast-fed infants and those with inadequate sun exposure be supplemented with 400 IU per day of vitamin D for secondary prevention of rickets *(13)*. Interestingly, an unforeseen consequence of the promotion of breastfeeding may be the "reemergence" of vitamin D deficiency rickets. Currently 1/3 of all American infants are breast-fed at 6 mo of age *(14)*; only 15% of African American infants ever begin breastfeeding *(15)*. The "Healthy People 2010" initiative has set a target of 75%

of American infants breastfeeding in the early postpartum period and 50% by six mo. If this goal is attained, and a major increase in the frequency and duration of breastfeeding were to occur among African Americans, then an epidemic of rickets is inevitable unless widespread vitamin D supplementation is provided to infants of these breastfeeding mothers. Indeed, those with the greatest potential for increased breastfeeding in the U.S. (African Americans) are also those with the highest risk for the development of rickets.

VITAMIN D DEFICIENCY RICKETS

Overt vitamin D deficiency rickets is typically treated with 1000–2000 IU/d of vitamin D. Some prefer the administration of intermediate amounts of oral vitamin D (8,000–16,000 IU/d). After radiographic evidence of healing of rachitic lesions, the dosage can be decreased to 400 IU/d, the generally recognized recommended daily allowance. If there is a concern about compliance, the so-called stoss from of therapy is used, which consists of the administration of a single oral or im dose of 600,000 IU of vitamin D; alternatively, this large oral dose may be divided into two or three doses given several hours apart over a 24-h period. Children with vitamin D deficiency rickets require supplemental calcium, as these children often have a low dietary intake of calcium. In addition, supplemental calcium protects against hypocalcemia, which may arise due to the hungry bone syndrome; the latter occurs during the early stages of vitamin D supplementation, when movement of calcium from the intravascular compartment to the skeletal compartment can exceed the replenishment of circulating calcium. Finally, it has been shown that vitamin D stores may be depleted rapidly in the setting of a concomitantly low dietary intake of calcium *(16)*. Thus, supplemental calcium (usually as calcium glubionate or calcium carbonate) should be included in the therapy of vitamin D deficiency rickets such that the child receives a total daily intake of 30–50 mg/kg/d of elemental calcium.

CALCIUM DEFICIENCY RICKETS

Isolated calcium deficiency, a rare cause of calciopenic rickets in the U.S., responds well to calcium supplementation. In a recent study in Nigerian children, calcium (at a dose of 1000 mg/d), with or without vitamin D supplementation, was more effective than vitamin D alone in achieving biologically important changes in biochemical and radiographic measures of rickets *(17)*. The children with rickets in this study were somewhat older (median age of 46 mo) than would be expected for children presenting with typical vitamin D deficiency, and had adequate sunlight exposure. Most had serum 25-hydroxyvitamin D concentrations within the normal range, thus pointing to calcium deficiency as the primary etiology of the rickets in this population.

1α-HYDROXYLASE DEFICIENCY

Patients with 1 alpha-hydroxylase deficiency are best treated with $1,25(OH)_2D_3$; typical initial dosages range from 0.5–3.0 µg/d, and maintenance dosages range from 0.25–2.0 µg/d. Adequate dietary calcium should be provided. Monitoring for hypercalcemia and hypercalciuria are indicated.

HEREDITARY VITAMIN D RESISTANCE

Patients with hereditary vitamin D resistance have been treated with megadoses of vitamin D or vitamin D metabolites with variable responses to therapy. Parenteral administration of calcium has been shown to completely correct the skeletal abnormalities in severe forms of this disorder. The disorder may be a spectrum of mild disease, responding to dietary calcium supplementation or extremely severe. Treatment should be performed by a pediatrician experienced in the management of metabolic bone disease.

OTHER CAUSES OF CALCIOPENIC RICKETS

For disorders affecting vitamin D absorption in the proximal small intestine and disorders of fat malabsorption, treatment with 5000–10,000 IU of vitamin D daily has been recommended, with monthly follow-up of mineral and vitamin levels so that appropriate adjustments in dosing can be made. Others have suggested the use of the more polar $1,25(OH)_2D_3$, which is, in part, absorbed in water-soluble form and is therefore less dependent on intact fat absorption.

Vitamin D deficiency rickets resulting from impairment of 25-hydroxylation in severe hepatobiliary disease may be treated with high doses of vitamin D (up to 50,000 IU/d) or 25-(OH)D (1–3 mg/kg body weight per day).

Rickets and osteomalacia associated with chronic renal failure is treated with $1,25(OH)_2D_3$ in oral dosages of up to 1.5 mg/d, which can be used to suppress the hyperparathyroidism that often occurs in this disorder. Dietary phosphate intake should be restricted, and hyperphosphatemia is usually treated with calcium carbonate rather than aluminum hydroxide.

Individuals receiving anticonvulsant therapy should receive the recommended dietary allowance of vitamin D (400 IU) from the usual sources for secondary prevention of vitamin D- deficiency rickets, and pharmacologic supplementation may be necessary if overt vitamin D deficiency rickets results.

MONITORING AND COMPLICATIONS OF THERAPY FOR CALCIOPENIC RICKETS

In general, children with nutritional calciopenic rickets should be seen initially every few weeks, with close monitoring of serum calcium, phosphate, alkaline phosphatase, and vitamin D metabolite levels. Radiographic evidence of healing of rachitic lesions may be seen within several weeks to months. Severe complications may occur with the use of vitamin D metabolites in an unmonitored fashion. Most commonly, sequelae from vitamin D intoxication are related to hypercalcemia and hypercalciuria, which have long-term effects on renal function. Therefore, sampling of serum and urinary calcium and creatinine is warranted within 2 wk of the initial dosing and after dose adjustments are made. Patients on stable doses with long-term treatments may have these tests performed every 3–4 mo. If serum calcium becomes greater than 11 mg/dL or the urinary calcium/creatinine ratio is >0.35 mg/dL, adjustments in doses are warranted. Finally, if severe hypercalcemia is present, vitamin D administration should be discontinued, and specific measures for treatment of hypercalcemia should be instituted.

Phosphopenic Rickets

NUTRITIONAL PHOSPHATE DEPRIVATION

Secondary prevention of nutritional phosphopenic rickets by routine use of breast milk fortifier is recommended in premature infants. If rachitic disease related to nutritional phosphate deprivation develops in the premature infant, it can be treated with 20–25 mg of elemental phosphorus/kg body weight per day, given as an oral supplement in 3–4 divided doses. It should be noted that phosphate deprivation may be only one of several components of rickets in the premature infant, and one should ascertain that vitamin D and calcium intakes are adequate as well. If necessary, mineral supplementation may be administered parenterally, and newer amino acid formulations supplemented with the sulfur-containing amino acids taurine and cysteine allow greater quantities of calcium and phosphate to remain in solution in total parenteral nutrition (TPN) formulations. Bone disease in the premature infant may be complex and include a component of osteoporosis as well.

X-LINKED HYPOPHOSPHATEMIC RICKETS (XLH)

Early diagnosis of X-linked hypophosphatemic rickets entails early screening of infants at risk in kindreds known to be affected with this disorder. Serum calcium and phosphate levels, alkaline phosphatase activity, and determination of TRP and TMP/GFR ratio are obtained at 1–2 mo-of-age, and if unrevealing, at 3–4 mo intervals during the first 6–9 mo of life. Early diagnosis is useful in that early therapy is likely to improve long-term outcomes. Mutational analysis is also commerically available.

Treatment of XLH consists of the administration of phosphorus in conjunction with $1,25(OH)_2D_3$, a regimen which has been demonstrated to improve the rachitic lesions at the growth plates and mineralization in trabecular bone *(18)*. Because of the propensity to develop secondary, and in some instances, tertiary hyperparathyroidism with large doses of phosphate, and because of the concern for the complication of vitamin D intoxication, careful attention must be paid to dosing regimens.

In early infancy, 250–375 mg of elemental phosphorus, provided in 2–3 divided doses is usually prescribed; a useful preparation for infants is Phospha-Soda solution containing 127 mg of elemental phosphorus per mL. In older children, it is more convenient to use Neutra-Phos or Neutra-Phos K powder (250 mg elemental phosphorus per packet) dissolved in water. Almost all children will complain of abdominal discomfort or manifest diarrhea soon after the initiation of phosphate therapy, but this usually resolves within days to weeks. Occasionally, administration of phosphate must be suspended and restarted at lower dosages, and very rarely, diarrhea, bloody stools, or persistent dose-related abdominal pain occurs with this therapy, indicating a need for a substantial decrease in the dose. When the child is old enough to chew or swallow a tablet, K-Phos Neutral, or K-Phos #2, each of which contains 250 mg of elemental phosphorus per tablet, is preferred. In the older child an average of 1 g of elemental phosphorus per day is used; it is seldom necessary to prescribe more than 2 g/d. Finally, it should be noted that parents need not wake children in order to administer phosphate throughout the night, as it is clear from nocturnal monitoring studies that serum phosphate levels rise at night, independent of phosphate administration *(19)*.

Administration of $1,25(OH)_2D_3$ is important for a successful outcome of therapy in XLH. This metabolite enhances calcium and phosphate absorption and dampens phosphate-stimulated PTH secretion, however, the mechanism for its skeletal action in XLH is not entirely understood. Starting doses for an infant in the first 2 yr of life are generally 0.25 µg once or twice daily. In early infancy, the oil solvent in a calcitriol capsule can be extracted using a 1 mL syringe and an 18 gauge needle. The liquid can be given to the child in formula or directly into the child's mouth from the syringe after removal of the needle. Others have orally administered the intravenous preparation, Calcijex. This form of $1,25(OH)_2D_3$ is supplied in small glass ampules. Such formulations are awkward for the small child, and parents usually supervise a child swallowing the entire capsule as soon as practical. Recently, calcitriol has become available in a liquid formulation for oral administration; we have not had the opportunity to formally assess the bioavailability of this preparation, but it should be a welcome alternative to capsule extraction. The liquid formulation of dihydrotachysterol is also a reasonable alternative for this very young age group.

Several investigators have examined human growth hormone as a therapeutic agent in XLH, but none have addressed final height in a controlled fashion. Some have shown that growth hormone in combination with standard therapy results in improved circulating phosphate concentrations, and an improvement in height velocity in the short term. Others have shown that children with XLH and very short stature may benefit from adjunctive growth hormone therapy. A recent review of seven trials of growth hormone therapy in XLH involving a total of 77 patients with this disorder *(20)* concluded that the long-term impact of GH treatment on final adult height in patients with XLH remains unknown; thus, at present, GH therapy should be considered an investigational therapy in children with this disease. If this measure is applied it may be important to carefully monitor skeletal age in the patient.

Finally, the effect of $24,25(OH)_2D_3$ in combination with $1,25(OH)_2D_3$ and phosphate has been recently examined. Modest skeletal improvement and parathyroid suppressive effects were observed *(21)*. Use of this metabolite as a specific therapy for secondary hyperparathyroidism in XLH is useful in the short term; other non-hypercalcemic vitamin D analogs and calciomimetic agents should be a promising approach in the near future.

Monitoring and Complications of XLH

Complications of therapy for XLH include hyperparathyroidism, soft-tissue calcification, and hypervitaminosis D. In order to avoid these complications patients should be appropriately monitored. Treatment must provide adequate mineral to improve rachitic lesions, but must not be so excessive that soft-tissue calcification or derangement of parathyroid hormone function will occur. Hyperparathyroidism occurs frequently in XLH *(19)*; thus, PTH levels must be routinely monitored during therapy. The parathyroid glands in XLH have a propensity to readily hypersecrete PTH, and circulating PTH levels may be elevated before the initiation of any therapy in the disease. The further stimulation of PTH secretion by phosphate intake is well-described. Phosphate supplementation should therefore never be given as single therapy in XLH, but always in combination with calcitriol. Prolonged or severe hyperparathyroidism may further compromise renal phosphate retention, provoke hypercalcemia, or enhance calcification of soft tissues. It is possible that chronic exposure to high concentrations of PTH may adversely affect the skeleton. Parathyroidectomy is warranted should complications of this development become significant.

Soft-tissue calcification of the renal medullary pyramids (nephrocalcinosis) is common, and can be detected by renal ultrasonography. This phenomenon is related to the mineral load that the treatment regimen provides. Most compliant patients demonstrate nephrocalcinosis within 3–4 yr of beginning therapy, but in general, no significant clinical sequelae in patients with nephrocalcinosis are usually seen. In one long term survey of several patients with long- standing low-grade nephrocalcinosis a mild, a urinary concentrating defect of limited clinical significance was the only identified abnormality *(22)*. Severe hyperparathyroidism in XLH has been associated with myocardial and aortic valve calcifications. Finally, calcification of the entheses (not thought to be treatment-dependent) and ocular calcifications are described. Hypervitaminosis D is manifest by hypercalcemia and/or hypercalciuria. This complication was formerly encountered with high dose vitamin D therapy, when monitoring of serum and urine biochemistries was infrequently performed. The newer 1α-hydroxylated vitamin D metabolites are more polar, are not stored in fat, and escape from toxic effects more rapidly than with native vitamin D. Unrecognized vitamin D intoxication has resulted in death in XLH, but has not been observed recently.

Children with XLH should be seen every 3–4 mo with concomitant monitoring of serum calcium, phosphate, and alkaline phosphatase. Calcium and creatinine excretion should be determined in a randomly voided urine sample. Circulating PTH should be measured at least twice a year. Accurate height measurements and assessment of the bow defect should be performed at all visits. Radiographs of the epiphyses of the distal femur and proximal tibia are obtained every 2 yr or more frequently if bow deformities fail to correct, or if progressive skeletal disease is grossly evident.

The development of secondary hyperparathyroidism is an indication to alter the calcitriol/phosphate balance by decreasing phosphate or increasing the calcitriol dosage. In the event of a poor clinical response (as assessed by radiographic changes of the epiphyses, or growth rate), an increase in the phosphate dose with a concomitant increase in the calcitriol dose is indicated. Phosphate dosage should NOT be increased on the basis of a decrement in serum phosphate, as the underlying reason for decreases in serum phosphate may be advancing hyperparathyroidism. An inappropriate increase in phosphate dosage generally exacerbates the hyperparathyroidism, and no improvement in serum phosphate is likely. Although some decrement in serum alkaline phosphatase activity usually occurs with initial therapy, the value rarely normalizes until adulthood.

HEREDITARY HYPOPHOSPHATEMIC RICKETS WITH HYPERCALCIURIA

Hereditary hypophosphatemic rickets with hypercalciuria is generally managed by the administration of phosphate salts alone. Bone disease and hypercalciuria require attention. The strategy aims to decrease ambient circulating $1,25(OH)_2D$, thereby decreasing intestinal calcium absorption, while providing phosphate to enhance skeletal mineralization. There is usually no risk of hyperparathyroidism, although experience with monitoring this rare condition is limited. The skeletal disease is complex, involving osteomalacia and osteoporotic defects. It is possible that bisphosphonates may prove to have an important role in adjunctive therapy for this disease. Finally, the importance of generous hydration and avoidance of a high sodium intake is recommended.

Other Causes of Phosphopenic Rickets

Finally, phosphopenic rickets occurring secondary to other renal diseases, such as tubulopathies and Fanconi syndrome, or associated with other systemic diseases, requires specific treatment of the underlying disease. In apparent sporadic phosphopenic rickets, an exhaustive search for a tumor should be sought, especially if the patient presents as an older child or adult, and excision of the tumor will result in resolution of biochemical and skeletal abnormalities.

PSYCHOSOCIAL CONSIDERATIONS

Nutritional rickets is an easily treated disorder and, if diagnosed in a reasonable time frame, is completely reversible before long-standing skeletal damage results. It is important to point out to families that remodeling of the skeleton may require several years, while biochemical changes and acute epiphyseal remodeling occur within weeks to months of the onset of treatment. Many children are initially misdiagnosed with muscular dystrophy, cerebral palsy, or skeletal dysplasia, owing to the common misconception that nutritional rickets no longer occurs in our society.

In contrast to the rapid and complete recovery with treatment of nutritional rickets, inherited forms usually require long-term treatment. 1 α-hydroxylase deficiency usually completely responds to medical therapy, as do many cases of hereditary vitamin D resistance, although life-long therapy is usually required in order to maintain a normal skeleton. In that certain cases of hereditary vitamin D resistance may be unresponsive to high dose $1,25(OH)_2D_3$, and may require intermittent continuous or intravenous calcium therapy, management should always involve a center with considerable experience in the treatment of metabolic bone disease.

XLH is a particularly frustrating disorder to manage over the long term, as current therapy does not correct the underlying defect. A number of long-term complications may occur, including arthritis, spinal canal stenosis, hearing difficulties, impaired fracture healing, and chronic bone pain. Such complications over years have resulted in considerable disability and limited capacity for employment in some individuals. Those in earlier generations where medical therapy has been limited, or in social situations where compliance with treatment has been poor, have been associated with worse outcomes. Psycho-social support is most important in these situations as to avoid depression and other problems such as substance abuse. Individuals with XLH will be better served when improved therapies are available.

REFERENCES

1. Carpenter TO. New perspectives on the biology and treatment of X-linked hypophosphatemic rickets. Pediatr Clin N Amer 1997;44:443–466.
2. Walton RJ, Bijvoet OL. Nomogram for derivation of renal threshold phosphate concentration. Lancet 1975;2:309–310.
3. Kreiter SR, Schwartz RP, Kirkman HN, Charlton PA, Calikoglu AS, Davenport ML. Nutritional rickets in African American breast-fed infants. J Pediatr 2000;137:153–157.
4. Glorieux FH. St-Arnaud R. Molecular cloning of (25-OH D)-1 alpha-hydroxylase: an approach to the understanding of vitamin D pseudo-deficiency. Recent Prog Horm Res 1998;53:341–349.
5. Malloy PJ, Pike JW, Feldman D: Hereditary 1,25-dihydroxyvitamin D resistant rickets. In: Feldman D, Glorieux FH, Pike JW, eds. Vitamin D, Academic, San Diego, 1997, pp. 765–787.
6. The HYP consortium: A gene (PEX) with homologies to endopeptidases is mutated in patients with X-linked hypophosphatemic rickets. Nat Genet 1995;11:130–136.
7. The ADHR Consortium. Autosomal dominant hypophosphatemic rickets is associated with mutations in FGF23. Nature Genetics 2000;26:345–348.
8. Jones AO, Tzenova J, Frappier D, et al. Hereditary hypophosphatemic rickets with hypercalciuria is not caused by mutations in the Na/Pi cotransporter NPT2 gene. J Am Soc Nephrol 2001;12:507–514.
9. Scheinman SJ. X-linked hypercalciuric nephrolithiasis: Clinical syndromes and chloride channel mutations. Kidney Int 1998;53:3–17.
10. Whyte MP. Hypophosphatasia and the role of alkaline phosphatase in skeletal mineralization. Endocr Rev 1994;15:439–461.
11. Warman ML, Abbott M, Apte SS, et al. A type X collagen mutation causes Schmid metaphyseal chondrodysplasia. Nat Genet 1993;5:79–82.
12. Reeves GD, Bachrach S, Carpenter TO, Mackenzie WG. Vitamin D-deficiency rickets in adopted children from the former Soviet Union: An uncommon problem with unusual clinical and biochemical features. Pediatrics 2000;10:1484–1489.
13. Committee on Nutrition. Pediatric nutrition handbook, 4th ed. American Academy of Pediatrics, Elk Grove Village, Illinois, 1998, pp. 275–276.

14. Healthy People 2010: Understanding and Improving Health. US Department of Health and Human Services. November 2000. url:http://www.health.gov/healthypeople/document/html/volume2/16mich.html.
15. Wiemann CM, DuBois JC, Berenson AB. Racial/ethnic differences in the decisions to breastfeed among adolescent mothers. Pediatrics 1998;101.
16. Clements MR, Johnson L, Fraser DR. A new mechanism for induced vitamin D deficiency in calcium deprivation. Nature 1987;62–65.
17. Thacher TD, Fischer PR, Pettifor JM, et al. A comparison of calcium, vitamin D, or both for nutritional rickets in Nigerian children. N Engl J Med 1999;341:563–568.
18. Glorieux FH, Pierre JM, Pettifor JM, Delvin EE. Bone response to phosphate salts, ergocalciferol, and calcitriol in hypophosphatemic vitamin D-resistant rickets. N Engl J Med 1980;303:1023–1031.
19. Carpenter TO, Mitnick MA, Ellison A, et al. Nocturnal hyperparathyroidism: a frequent feature of X-linked hypophosphatemia. J Clin Endocrinol Metab 1994;78:1378–1383.
20. Wilson DM. Growth hormone and hypophosphatemic rickets. J Ped Endocrinol Metab 2000;13:993–998.
21. Carpenter TO, Keller M, Schwartz D, et al. 24,25 Dihydroxyvitamin D supplementation corrects hyperparathyroidism and improves skeletal abnormalities in X-linked hypophosphatemic rickets—a clinical research center study. J Clin Endocrinol Metab 1996;81:2381–2388.
22. Eddy MC, McAlister WH, Leelawattana R, Whyte MP: Diminished renal concentrating ability in children with XLH and ultrasonographic nephrocalcinosis. J Bone Mineral Res 1997;12(Suppl. 1):S393.

VI Reproductive Disorders and Contraception

22 Delayed Puberty

Diane E. J. Stafford, MD

CONTENTS

INTRODUCTION
CLASSIFICATION
REFERENCES

INTRODUCTION

Delayed puberty is defined as the absence of any sign of puberty in a child at a chronological age two standard deviations above the mean age of pubertal development for a given population. By current standards, this is defined as absence of an increase in testicular volume (less than 4 mL) at 14 yr in a boy or absence of any breast development at 13 yr in a girl *(1,2)*. In addition, pathologic abnormalities may be associated with abnormal progression through puberty once initial pubertal changes have begun, and are worthy of further evaluation. In boys, a period of 3.2 +/– 1.8 (mean +/– SD) years is necessary to achieve adult testicular volume after the onset of puberty. In girls, the period from breast budding to menarche is 2.4 +/–1.1 (mean +/– SD) years *(3)*. Therefore, evaluation is warranted if more than 4–5 yr has elapsed from the onset of puberty to adult testicular size in boys or menarche in girls. Further evaluation is necessary to determine the etiology of pubertal delay, and for determination of necessary therapy. Clinical and laboratory assessment is aimed at differentiating a lag in normal pubertal development from abnormalities in need of further investigation and/or therapy.

CLASSIFICATION

Normal puberty is initiated by the onset of pulsatile secretion of gonadotropin-releasing hormone (GnRH) from the hypothalamus. These pulses cause release of luteinizing hormone (LH) and follicular stimulating hormone (FSH) from the pituitary gland. These pituitary gonadotropins then circulate to the gonads and stimulate production of sex steroids. The differential diagnosis of pubertal delay is extensive, but can most easily be divided into three categories: The first group represents temporary delays of puberty that are functional disorders, most commonly, constitutional delay of growth and puberty.

From: *Contemporary Endocrinology: Pediatric Endocrinology: A Practical Clinical Guide*
Edited by: S. Radovick and M. H. MacGillivray © Humana Press Inc., Totowa, NJ

The second is hypogonadotropic hypogonadism, in which hypothalamic or pituitary failure results in deficiency of circulating gonadotropins. Finally, hypergonadotropic hypogonadism results from primary gonadal failure, with subsequent lack of negative feedback of sex steroids at the hypothalamic and pituitary levels resulting in elevated serum gonadotropin levels. Table 1 lists the various etiologies of hypogonadism resulting in delay or failure of pubertal development.

Delays of Pubertal Development

Delays of pubertal development are more common than failure of development, and can most easily be divided into two groups: constitutional delay, and delay caused by underlying chronic disease.

CONSTITUTIONAL DELAY OF PUBERTY

The most common cause of delay is constitutional delay of puberty and growth. These children represent the extreme of the normal physiologic variations in the timing of the onset of puberty. Children with constitutional delay are more likely to be short for age, with a history of relatively normal growth rate, and to have delays in bone maturation. Frequently, there is a family history of late menarche in the mother or sisters or a delayed growth spurt in the father. However, sporadic cases are also seen. The degree of delay in clinical manifestations of puberty is variable, but delay is usually not extreme, falling within the range of 2–4 yr *(3)*. The diagnosis of constitutional delay is made more often in boys than in girls. This may be partly explained by a higher degree of social pressure placed on boys with delayed development, and, subsequently, a higher frequency of referral for evaluation.

CHRONIC SYSTEMIC DISEASE

A variety of chronic diseases are associated with delayed growth and puberty and may be diagnosed in the context of endocrinological evaluation of an otherwise asymptomatic child. Gastrointestinal disorders such as inflammatory bowel disease or celiac disease, as well as chronic renal failure, cardiac disease, and other severe chronic illnesses are causes of pubertal delay (Table 1). These disorders are!ÂDually associated with impaired availability or utilization of fuels, although clinical evidence of malnutrition may be absent. Similarly, patients with nutritional disorders, including anorexia nervosa, may present with delays in growth and/or pubertal development *(4)*. In the case of anorexia nervosa, the cause is most likely both lack of energy intake, as well as a central nervous system effect altering neuroendocrine control of gonadotropins *(5)*. Excessive energy expenditure, such as that seen in young gymnasts and long-distance runners, causes pubertal delay by similar mechanisms *(6,7)*.

ENDOCRINOPATHIES

Other endocrinopathies can also be associated with delays of puberty and growth. Isolated growth hormone deficiency is an important differential diagnosis with constitutional delay of puberty, since both present with decreased growth velocity for chronological age and bone age retardation. Furthermore, growth delay in children with constitutional delay may develop early and, therefore, make the distinction between these two entities more difficult. Acquired hypothyroidism and hyperprolactinemia also may cause delay or arrest in pubertal development. Cushing's syndrome may cause delayed growth and puberty, though it may also result in premature development of sexual hair.

Table 1
Etiologies of Delay or Failure of Pubertal Development

Delays of Puberty
- Constitutional delay of growth and/or puberty
    - Sporadic
    - Familial
- Chronic illness (gastrointestinal disease [inflammatory bowel disease, celiac disease], renal failure, hepatic disease, hematologic abnormalities [sickle cell disease, hemolytic anemia], malignancy, pulmonary disease [asthma, cystic fibrosis])
- Nutritional Disorders
    - Malnutrition
    - Anorexia nervosa
    - Excessive energy expenditure, exercise
- Endocrinopathies
    - Diabetes mellitus
    - Growth hormone deficiency
    - Hypothyroidism
    - Hyperprolactinemia
    - Glucocorticoid excess

Hypogonadotropic Conditions
- Congenital
    - Idiopathic hypogonadotropic hypogonadism
    - Kallman's syndrome
    - GnRH receptor defects
    - LHβ mutations
    - FSHb mutations
    - PROP-1 mutations
    - Adrenal hypoplasia congenita
    - Panhypopituitarism
    - Septo-optic dysplasia
    - Prader-Willi syndrome
    - Laurence-Moon-Biedl syndrome
- Acquired
    - Suprasellar tumors (craniopharyngiomas, etc.)
    - Histiocytosis X
    - Effects of radiotherapy
    - Effects of surgery
    - Cranial trauma
    - Effects of infection

Hypergonadotropic Conditions
- Congenital
    - Males
        - Klinefelter's syndrome (XYY)
        - Noonan's syndrome
        - Gonadal dysgenesis (XO/XY)
        - Defects in testosterone biosynthesis/action
            - Inborn errors of testosterone synthesis
            - 5a-Reductase deficiency
            - Partial androgen insensitivity
        - Anorchia (Vanishing Testis syndrome)
        - Leydig cell agenesis or hypoplasia
    - Females
        - Turner's Syndrome (XO)
        - Gonadal dysgenesis (XO/XY, or XX)
        - Androgen insensitivity
    - Both Sexes
        - Polymalformation syndromes
- Acquired
    - Males
        - Bilateral Orchitis
        - Surgical or traumatic castration
        - Chemotherapy, radiotherapy
    - Females
        - Surgical or traumatic castration
        - Premature idiopathic ovarian failure
        - Autoimmune ovarian failure
        - Chemotherapy, radiotherapy

Hypogonadotropic Hypogonadism

Disorders in this category are characterized by low circulating levels of the pituitary gonadotropins, LH and FSH. This may be the results of genetic defects altering hypothalamic and/or pituitary development, defects in hormonal synthesis or action, or may be acquired due to intracranial disease or trauma.

Idiopathic Hypogonadotropic Hypogonadism

Defects in the production or regulation of gonadotropin-releasing hormone (GnRH) in the hypothalamus, and subsequent lack of LH and FSH production by the pituitary, are the cause of idiopathic hypogonadotropic hypogonadism (IHH). In these individuals, exogenous administration of GnRH usually initiates pubertal development *(8)*. Though the GnRH gene is the most likely candidate for mutations causing GnRH deficiency in IHH patients, no mutations in this gene have been identified in humans to date *(9–13)*.

KALLMAN SYNDROME

Kallman syndrome is a well-recognized form of hypogonadotropic hypogonadism consisting of gonadotropin deficiency accompanied by anosmia. It is frequently transmitted as an X-linked recessive trait, but may also have autosomal dominant inheritance with variable expressivity *(14)*. The X-linked form of Kallman syndrome has been associated with defects in the *KALIG-1* gene, located on the pseudoautosomal region of Xp *(15,16)*. The protein product of the *KALIG* gene has neural cell adhesion molecule properties and provides scaffolding for GnRH neuron and olfactory nerve migration across the cribiform plate to their appropriate synapses *(17)*. In the absence of the KALIG protein, GnRH and olfactory fibers do not synapse properly, producing GnRH deficiency and anosmia. Males with Kallman syndrome may have a variety of other associated anomalies including visual abnormalities, renal agenesis and midline facial defects, congenital deafness, cryptorchidism, and microphallus. Despite the identification of the *KAL* gene, mutations are found in less than 5% of patients with idiopathic hypogonadotropic hypogonadism, suggesting significant heterogeneity in this syndrome *(18)*. Further evidence that other genes cause gonadotropin deficiency with anosmia is supported by the lack of identification of *KAL* gene mutations in female patients with IHH *(17)*.

OTHER INHERITED FORMS OF HYPOGONADOTROPIC HYPOGONADISM (HH)

Several other gene mutations have been shown to produce hypogonadotropic hypogonadism. Mutations in the *AHC* gene are associated with HH and adrenal hypoplasia congenital (AHC), a form of adrenal insufficiency owing to lack of proper adrenal development. The protein product of the *AHC* gene, DAX-1, is predicted to be a transcription factor necessary for proper development of the pituitary gonadotrophs and the adrenal cortex. Adrenal hypoplasia congenita is inherited in an X-linked recessive manner, with the gene located in the region Xp21. Over 50 *AHC* gene mutations have been described in patients with AHC and HH *(19)*. While males are most frequently affected due to the X-linked inheritance pattern, a female patient with HH, but not AHC has been identified in a family of males with AHC and HH and was found to possess an *AHC* gene mutation *(20)*.

An autosomal recessive form of hypogonadotropic hypogonadism has been associated with mutations in the gonadotropin-releasing hormone receptor gene. Patients identified with this defect by Roux et al. *(21)* have incomplete GnRH deficiency, with late progression into puberty followed by decreased libido in the male and amenorrhea in the female. Those identified by Layman et al. *(22)* had complete HH with delayed puberty. This discrepancy most likely relates to functional differences between the mutations involved. Both groups of patients appear to have a level of GnRH resistance with variable responses in gonadotropin levels following stimulation testing.

Defects in the genes coding for the subunits of the pituitary gonadotropins have also been isolated in cases of delayed puberty. Pituitary glycoprotein hormones consist of a common α-subunit encoded by a single gene, and a β-subunit that is specific for LH, FSH, hCG, and TSH. No α-subunit mutations have been described in humans *(17)*. However, β-subunit mutations have been identified in both LHβ- and FSHβ. Weiss et al. *(23)* described a male patient who presented at age 17 with delayed puberty, elevated serum LH levels, but low FSH and testosterone levels. He was found to have an autosomal recessive defect in the *LHβ* gene that produced immunoactive LH, measurable by current assays, but had decreased bioactivity, resulting in delayed puberty. Similarly, mutations have been identified in the *FSHβ* gene, causing delayed puberty and hypogonadism. Matthews et al. *(24)*, and Layman et al. *(25)* each described young women with no evidence of thelarche, undetectable FSH levels and elevated LH. Both young women had no FSH response to GnRH stimulation, but exaggerated rise in LH to menopausal levels. In females, FSH deficiency is expected to produce delayed puberty as a result of lack of follicular development, estradiol production, and maturation of oocytes, as has been described. However, in males, as LH stimulation is responsible for testosterone production, one would predict normal pubertal development, but azoospermia or oligospermia result because of the lack of FSH stimulation *(17)*.

Several patients with combined pituitary hormone deficiency, characterized by deficiencies in growth hormone, TSH, prolactin, and gonadotropins, have been shown to have mutations in the *PROP1* gene *(26,27)*. *PROP1* is a transcription factor felt to be necessary for differentiation of multiple pituitary cell lineages, and its absence results in lack of proper pituitary cellular development.

Leptin deficiency and leptin receptor defects have also been associated with hypogonadism. Patients with defects in leptin production or action typically have extreme obesity, and hyperinsulinemia, in addition to hypogonadism *(17)*.

Associated Syndromes

Hypogonadotropic hypogonadism is also associated with other more complex syndromes. Gross abnormalities of the pituitary gland, such as those seen in panhypopitiutarism and septo-optic dysplasia cause deficiencies in all pituitary hormones including gonadotropins. Hypogonadism is also a frequent feature of other genetic syndromes such as Prader-Willi syndrome and Laurence-Moon-Beidl syndrome, among others. The etiology of gonadotropin deficiency in these syndromes remains unclear, though further investigation of the genetic causes of the underlying syndrome may provide important insights into regulation of this complex system.

Acquired Causes of Hypogonadotropic Hypogonadism

Intracranial disease processes, or therapy designed to treat such diseases are well known causes of hypogonadotropic hypogonadism. Histiocytosis X may be associated with HH, depending on the extent of pituitary involvement. Suprasellar tumors, such as craniopharyngiomas, frequently involve the pituitary and/or hypothalamus. Gonadotropin deficiency may be caused by tumor invasion, or by surgical removal of the tumor with subsequent damage to the pituitary or hypothalamus. Radiation therapy for any intracranial tumor may cause hypogonadism, depending on the field involved and the dose of radiation received by the hypothalamus and pituitary. The exact dose that is required to cause hypothalamic or pituitary dysfunction is unclear. However, hypothalamic GnRH neurons and the pituitary gonadotrophs appear to be less sensitive to radiation effects than somatotrophs, making gonadotropin deficiency unusual in the absence of growth hormone deficiency *(28)*. Cranial trauma causing hypothalamic or pituitary damage, as well as infection involving these areas of the brain are also associated with gonadotropin deficiency.

Hypergonadotropic Hypogonadism

Disorders in this category are characterized by elevated gonadotropin levels. The hypothalamic-pituitary-gonadal axis is activated with the release of GnRH in a pulsatile manner from the hypothalamus, resulting in subsequent increases in LH and FSH, and circulation of these hormones to the gonads. If the gonads cannot properly respond by producing estrogen or testosterone, there is a failure in the normal feedback to the hypothalamus and pituitary, with a compensatory increase in gonadotropin levels above the normal range. Patients present with lack of pubertal development, low serum testosterone or estrogen levels, and inappropriate elevation of LH and FSH.

KLINEFELTER'S SYNDROME

Klinefelter's syndrome is the most frequent form of hypogonadism in males with an incidence of approximately 1:500–1000 males *(29)*. The pubertal delay in this syndrome is caused by seminiferous tubule dysgenesis. These children have a karyotype of 47 XXY or its variants, including mosiacism, 48 XXXY, 49 XXXY, and male 46 XX. They usually enter into puberty at an average age, but do not appropriately progress. Typical phenotypic characteristics include tall stature with long legs and arms, micropenis, small, firm testes, poor muscular development, borderline IQ, and poor social adaptation. Physical examination also typically reveals so-called "eunucoid" proportions with an upper to lower segment ratio of less than one, demonstrating increased long bone growth despite lack of pubertal development.

TURNER'S SYNDROME

Turner's syndrome, characterized by a karyotype of XO or its mosaics, is the most common cause of primary hypogonadism in females. The syndrome is characterized by abnormal karyotype, short stature, webbed neck, low posterior hairline, hypertelorism, and left-sided cardiac defects. Ovarian function varies in girls with Turner's syndrome, giving variable progression through puberty, but patients seldom reach menarche. In girls presenting with short stature and pubertal delay, possible phenotypic features of Turner's syndrome should be evaluated and a karyotype considered.

VANISHING TESTES SYNDROME (CONGENITAL ANORCHIA)

Bilateral anorchia is found in approximately one in 20,000 males. Their external genitalia are normal, implying normal testicular function during the first 14–16 wk of embryonic development. However, at birth, no testicular tissue is present, resulting in the term "vanishing testes." These patients are born with cryptorchidism and either fail to develop secondary sexual characteristics, or have incomplete progression through puberty, depending on the presence of Leydig cell tissue. Unlike males with abdominal crytorchidism, these patients have no increase in testosterone levels following human chorionic gonadotropin administration.

CONGENITAL LEYDIG CELL APLASIA

Male patients with this disorder have poor Leydig cell development, either aplasia or hypoplasia. Several patients with Leydig cell hypoplasia or aplasia have been shown to have mutations in the luteinizing hormone receptor gene *(30–33)*. The degree of masculinization is variable, depending on the particular mutation, ranging from microphallus to genital ambiguity. Testes are small to normal size, FSH levels are normal, with low serum testosterone, but LH levels are elevated, implying resistance. Women identified with LH receptor defects appear to present with amenorrhea *(32)*.

NOONAN'S SYNDROME

Noonan's syndrome shares many phenotypic features with Turner's syndrome including short stature, webbed neck, low posterior hairline, hypertelorism, and hypogonadism. However, patients with Noonan's syndrome have a normal XX or XY karyotype. Females with Noonan's syndrome undergo normal pubertal development and have normal ovarian function. Male patients, in contrast, typically have undescended testes and abnormal Leydig cell function, causing hypergonadotropic hypogonadism. Noonan's syndrome is caused by mutations on the long arm of chromosome 12, and is inherited in an autosomal dominant manner *(34)*.

GONADAL DYSGENESIS

In phenotypic females, pure gonadal dysgenesis is defined by the complete or nearly complete absence of ovarian tissue. Genotype in these girls may be 46 XX, 46 XY, or 45XO/46XY mosaic. In cases of 46 XY, genetic studies have shown microdeletions on either the Y *(35)* or the X chromosome *(36)*. Girls with pure gonadal dysgenesis may have complete lack of pubertal development, or some degree of breast development, but remain amenorrheic. Pelvic ultrasonography reveals a normal, prepubertal uterus, without measurable ovaries. Pure gonadal dysgenesis is also associated with other malformations, as well as trisomy 13 and 18 *(37)*.

Ovarian dysgenesis may also be associated with defects in the FSH receptor gene. These patients are clinically similar to patients with pure ovarian dysgenesis, presenting with variable development of secondary sexual characteristics, primary or early secondary amenorrhea, and high serum FSH and LH levels. However, women with FSH receptor mutations frequently have ovarian follicles present on ultrasound examination, possibly due to residual receptor activity *(38)*.

Gonadal dysgenesis causing male pseudohermaphroditism and hypogonadism is also associated with Denys-Drash syndrome (nephropathy, Wilms tumor and genital abnormalities), and WAGR complex (Wilms tumor, aniridia, genital abnormalities, and mental retardation).

DEFECTS IN TESTOSTERONE BIOSYNTHESIS

Inborn errors of enzymes required in the biosynthetic pathway of testosterone can result in incomplete male sexual differentiation and incomplete progression through puberty. Five enzymes are necessary for testosterone production, three of which are common to the pathway of cortisol production as well. The phenotypic presentation of patients with these defects varies with the location of the enzyme defect in the pathway of steroid production.

Cholesterol side-chain cleavage deficiency (20–22-desmolase) results in total lack of masculinization in males and a severe neonatal salt-losing syndrome. 3β-hydroxysteroid dehydrogenase deficiency presents with adrenal insufficiency with salt-losing and abnormal sexual differentiation. Males have genital ambiguity and females may be normal, or have moderate clitoromegaly. As this enzyme complex is common to synthesis of all active steroid hormones, puberty is incomplete in both sexes *(39)*.

17α-hydroxylase is essential for biosynthesis of androgens, glucocorticoids, and estrogens. Deficiency causes pseudohermaphroditism in genetic males, with elevated LH and FSH and low testosterone levels in puberty. 17,20-desmolase deficiency impairs production of androgens and estrogens with normal cortisol and aldosterone. Genetic males with this deficiency may present with incomplete virilization, or as phenotypic females with absent uterus, and lack of pubertal virilization.

In 17β-hydroxysteroid dehydrogenase deficiency, affected genetic males present with female external genitalia, and moderate labioscrotal fusion. At puberty, breast development is associated with acne, hirsuitism, voice deepening, and amenorrhea. These patients have elevated plasma androstenedione and estrone levels with low or normal testosterone *(39)*.

5α-Reductase Deficiency

5α-reductase enzyme activity is necessary for the conversion of testosterone to dihydrotestosterone (DHT). DHT is necessary for masculinization of the fetal external genitalia. Autosomal-recessive defects in this enzyme result in female external genitalia with male internal genital structures, and a urogenital sinus with a perineal opening. Partial virilization may be seen at puberty because of increases in testosterone production and residual enzymatic activity *(39)*.

Androgen Insensitivity

Androgen insensitivity syndrome (AIS) is a heterogeneous disorder caused by mutations in the androgen receptor gene *(40)*. Phenotype in affected patients varies greatly from normal female to ambiguous forms more closely resembling male (partial androgen insensitivity [PAIS]). This variation is dependent on the location and extent of mutation and the subsequent activity of the androgen receptor *(41)*. Karyotype in these patients is 46 XY, and, under the influence of Mullerian inhibitory substance, they have male internal structures. However, they fail to develop male external genitalia that normally results from androgen effects in embryonic development. Phenotypic females usually enter puberty with breast development as a result of aromatization of testosterone to estrogen, but there is little or no body hair development. However, they frequently present with primary amenorrhea. Phenotypic males will have variable progression through puberty depending on the activity of the androgen receptor.

Acquired Causes of Gonadal Failure

Bilateral testicular torsion, surgical castration and severe trauma to the scrotum and testes are known causes of hypergonadotropic hypogonadism in males. Bilateral orchitis (e.g., mumps) is also an unusual, but known cause of gonadal failure. Exposure to chemotherapeutic agents may cause gonadal failure, but is more likely to affect Sertoli cell development and cause infertility rather than pubertal delay *(42)*. Inclusion of the testis in the direct field of radiation usually causes testicular failure. While exposure to total-body radiation associated with bone marrow transplantation raises concern for possible gonadal failure, at least one recent study showed no clear association with delay in pubertal development *(43)*.

Autoimmune ovarian failure is seen in girls, either as an isolated autoimmune phenomenon, or, more frequently, in association with polyglandular autoimmune disease. Idiopathic premature ovarian failure is also an infrequent cause. As with boys, ovarian failure may also be associated with chemotherapy or radiation therapy, as well as surgical or traumatic injury to the ovary.

Evaluation of Pubertal Delay

HISTORY

A thorough medical history and family history are essential in the evaluation of pubertal delay. In cases of constitutional delay of puberty, a family history of late development may be present in up to 90% of cases. A family history of significant pubertal delay, treatment for such delay or a history of infertility may point to an underlying genetic abnormality. The review of systems must probe for historical details that are consistent with systemic disease or chronic disorders associated with pubertal delay. Review of previous growth data, including weight for height, is essential. Plotting growth data on a longitudinal growth curve (e.g., Bayer and Bayley *(44)*) is useful to demonstrate a pattern of growth consistent with constitutional delay. These patients frequently have slow growth in childhood with normal growth velocity. Growth data may also point to an underlying systemic disorder. Low weight for height may indicate nutritional disorders or underlying gastrointestinal disease. Patients with hypothyroidism, glucocorticoid excess, or Prader-Willi syndrome may have slightly or significantly increased weight for height.

PHYSICAL EXAMINATION

Physical examination should include careful evaluation of pubertal staging, as subtle changes may indicate the spontaneous onset of puberty and alleviate the necessity for further evaluation.

BOYS

Increase in testicular size is usually the first sign of puberty in boys. In general, testicular size greater than 4 mL in volume or a longitudinal measurement greater than 2.5 cm is consistent with the onset of pubertal development. Scrotal skin also changes in texture and reddens in early puberty. Pubic hair development usually correlates with genital development in boys, as both are under androgen control, but pubertal stage is best assessed by evaluating these factors separately *(45)*. Gynecomastia is a common finding in early puberty, but may also be associated with Klinefelter's syndrome or partial androgen insensitivity.

GIRLS

Breast development in girls begins with formation of breast buds. This development is frequently unilateral for several months. Enlargement of the areolar diameter usually accompanies breast budding. Development of axillary and pubic hair may or may not accompany the onset of puberty, as androgens are mainly produced by the adrenal gland, which is under separate control. Under the influence of estrogen, the vaginal mucosa changes from a reddish tint to pink, and a whitish vaginal discharge may be seen.

In addition to height and weight, arm span and lower segment measurements should be performed. The lower segment measurement is the distance from the pubic symphysis to the floor when standing. An upper to lower segment ratio can be determined by subtracting the lower segment measurement from the standing height (upper segment) and evaluating the ratio. During normal pubertal development, this ratio changes from greater than one pre-pubertally (with torso length greater than leg length) to slightly less than or equal to one with increased long bone growth at puberty. In patients with Klinefelter's syndrome, the upper to lower segment ratio is low due to long bone growth, but without significant signs of pubertal development.

A careful neurological evaluation is particularly important in the evaluation of delayed puberty. Neurologic deficits may indicate the presence of central nervous system disease. Physical abnormalities suggestive of genetic syndromes such as Turner's, Noonan's, Prader-Willi, Klinefelter's, and Kallman syndrome as described above should be specifically evaluated, as well as finding which could suggest underlying chronic illness or endocrinopathy.

INITIAL DIAGNOSTIC EVALUATION

In patients with findings suspicious of underlying chronic disease, either by history or physical examination, individual evaluation aimed at the suspected diagnosis should be undertaken. This may include erythrocyte sedimentation rate for evaluation of inflammatory disease, complete blood cell count, electrolytes, renal or liver panel, or gastrointestinal studies.

Bone age evaluation is frequently helpful in the assessment of delayed puberty. Skeletal age more closely correlates with sexual development than does chronological age. A skeletal age of 10 in girls and 12.5 in boys usually correlates with the onset of pubertal development. If bone age is appropriate for chronological age, further evaluation for the etiology of pubertal delay is appropriate. If a patient's bone age is significantly delayed (2 SD), pubertal delay may be caused by underlying chronic disease or endocrinopathy, and further diagnostic evaluation is indicated. In constitutional delay, bone age is usually comparable to height age, and observation may be appropriate.

In patients who are apparently healthy, and have no indications for etiology of delay, most authors recommend initial assessment of serum or urine gonadotropin levels (LH and FSH). If elevated, demonstrating hypergonadotropic hypogonadism, the etiology for gonadal failure should be further investigated based on the differential diagnoses in Table 1. However, low gonadotropin levels may represent constitutional delay, or hypogonadotropic hypogonadism. This distinction may be quite difficult without obvious clinical sign associated with true hypogonadotropic hypogonadism.

LH and FSH pulsatility, as measured by 24 h sampling, has been used in several studies to distinguish between constitutional delay of puberty and hypogonadotropic hypogonadism. Lack of LH pulsatility is associated with hypogonadotropic hypogonadism. While such detailed study is not recommended in the routine evaluation of pubertal delay, these studies may provide useful insight. Odink et al. *(46)* concluded that low FSH levels in children of adolescent age (random FSH of less than or equal to 1.11 in boys, or 2.86 in girls) discriminated patients without LH pulse from those with normal pulses. Thus, random FSH may be a useful tool in distinguishing constitutional delay from hypogonadotropic hypogonadism.

Assessment of estradiol levels is infrequently helpful in early puberty. Elevations are reassuring for onset of early puberty, but levels below the limit of many standard assays may be seen in early puberty. Morning serum testosterone levels may be useful in determination of progression into early puberty. One study determined that an 8 AM serum testosterone level greater than 0.7 nmol/L predicted an increase in testicular size to >4 mL within 1 y in 77% in boys and within 15 mo in 100% of boys. In boys with levels <0.7 nmol/L, only 12.5% of boys progressed to the same point within 1 yr *(47)*.

GnRH stimulation testing is not helpful in distinguishing between constitutional delay of puberty and hypogonadotropic hypogonadism, as both may show pre-pubertal patterns of gonadotropin secretion in response to stimulation. Such testing may be useful in distinguishing gonadotropin gene mutations from other etiologies of hypogonadotropic hypogonadism at a later point in time, but should not be used in routine evaluation.

Karyotype determination, while not routinely indicated, should be carried out if physical examination suggest the presence of a genetic syndrome such as Klinefelter's, Turner's, Noonan's, or Prader-Willi syndrome. It should also be performed in cases of hypergonadotropic hypogonadism to evaluate for karyotypes typically seen in gonadal dysgenesis.

Cranial magnetic resonance imaging should be performed in patient suspected of have intracranial lesions or defects on the basis of initial physical examination. In other patients, such imaging may be considered after further evaluation is completed, but need not be performed as part of the initial evaluation. Similarly, in phenotypic males with cryptorchidism or phenotypic females suspected of having androgen insensitivity, pelvic ultrasound may be part of the initial assessment, though deferred for later evaluation in most cases.

Determination of the etiology of hypogonadotropic hypogonadism, and distinguishing this permanent deficit from constitutional delay may be extremely difficult. As a result, conservative management with observation over 6 mo to 1 yr may be warranted. However, in cases of clearly permanent hypogonadism, therapy should be initiated at a normal pubertal age to avoid the delay of growth and psychological effect of pubertal delay. Cases of probable constitutional delay must be evaluated on an individual basis for psychosocial distress, and subsequent need for intervention.

TREATMENT OF DELAYED PUBERTY

Boys: Testosterone therapy is utilized for induction of puberty in boys with constitutional delay of puberty, hypogonadotropic hypogonadism, and hypergonadotropic hypogonadism. While several preparations of testosterone are available internationally, testosterone esters are the most commonly used. These compounds must be used intramuscularly to avoid hepatic metabolism. Testosterone enanthate and cypionate have longer duration of action than testosterone propionate due to longer side-chain esterification. Following injection, testosterone is hydrolyzed from the ester and becomes metabolically active and identical to endogenous testosterone *(48)*. Two transdermal systems for delivering testosterone are currently available: a scrotal patch and a nongenital patch. When applied daily, both transdermal systems result in similar testosterone concentrations to those seen in normal young men in magnitude and diurnal variation. However, transdermal system are substantially more expensive than testosterone esters and can produce skin reaction at the site of placement *(48)*. Further, while transdermal systems have been used in adults, their effectiveness in induction of puberty remains unclear *(49)*.

Constitutional delay of growth and puberty can cause significant psychosocial stress, particularly in males. As a result, a variety of strategies have been examined for treatment in these cases. Induction of a pubertal growth spurt with oxandrolone has been advocated by some. While the mechanism of action of oxandrolone in unclear, it is a non-aromatizable anabolic steroid that increases growth velocity without promoting excessive skeletal maturation *(49)*. Doses of 1.25 or 2.5 mg/d given orally have been used for up to 1 yr *(49,50)*. In a study by Tse et al., there was no compromise in final adult height as a result of oxandrolone treatment. A randomized placebo-controlled study by Wilson et al. *(51)* similarly found an increase in both height and weight velocity, but found that this increase was not associated with a greater improvement in psychosocial status compared to the control group.

While most physicians advocate a period of "watchful waiting", including periodic evaluation, reassurance, and psychological counseling in boys with probable constitutional delay of growth and puberty, a short course of testosterone therapy may be initiated in order to stimulate pubertal development in some cases. A low dose of testosterone enanthate (50–100 mg given intramuscularly every 4 wk) for 4–6 mo will stimulate linear growth and secondary sexual characteristics without inappropriately accelerating bone age *(48)*. When distinction between constitutional delay and true hypogonadotropic hypogonadism is difficult, a short course of therapy (4–6 mo) followed by discontinuation and monitoring for 4–6 mo for progression of puberty may be of diagnostic use. Enlargement of testicular volume after testosterone treatment becomes extremely obvious in patients with constitutional delay as opposed to those with hypogonadotropic hypogonadism *(49)*. In addition, patients with constitutional delay may continue with pubertal progression following a "jump start" with testosterone therapy *(37)*. However, one 6-mo course may not be sufficient, even in patients with true constitutional delay.

Testosterone esters are also appropriate therapy for permanent hypogonadal states. Testosterone enanthate, administered by intramuscular injection, is the most common method of pubertal induction and maintenance for hypogonadal states. Various schemes have been proposed, but most authors advocate a starting dose of 50 mg every 4 wk. When the pubertal growth spurt is well established, the dose should be gradually increased to a full adult dose of 200 mg every 2 wk. When hypogonadism is diagnosed at a prepubertal age, due to known abnormality, testosterone therapy may be started as early as a bone age of 11–12 yr to decrease the psychological disturbance associated with delays in pubertal development *(52)*.

The side effects of androgen therapy are associated with their physiologic effects. Frequent side effects include acne, oily skin, and some gynecomastia (due to aromatization to estrogen). Beneficial effects include decline in total plasma cholesterol and LDL concentrations, increased lean body mass, and decreased risk of osteoporosis based on improvement in bone mineral density *(48)*.

Girls: Estrogen therapy induces breast development in girls with hypogonadism, with either long-term low doses, or gradual increases in dose providing adequate time for pubertal growth, and gradual breast development. While opinions vary as to the optimum method for achieving normal breast development and longitudinal growth, the scheme proposed here is commonly used by clinicians. In cases where further growth is desired due to short stature, a starting dose of 5 µg ethinyl estradiol given orally on a daily basis is recommended. This low dose may be continued for 12–18 mo, and increase in 5 µg steps every 6 mo to reach a dose of 20–30 µg adult replacement, as desired height is approached *(53,54)*. Alternatively, Premarin (conjugated estrogen) may be used at a dose of 0.3 mg every other day for 6 mo followed by an increase to every day for 6 mo. As breast development and pubertal growth increase, this dose can be increased to 0.625 mg. A progestagen should be added when 15 µg of ethinyl estradiol (or 0.625 mg Premarin) has been reached, or if spotting occurs. This is usually administered as Provera (medroxyprogesterone) at a dose of 5–10 mg for 10–14 d. Dose and duration should be tailored to the individual patient based on occurrence of side effects, such as nausea. The simplest regimen for the adolescent patient in continuous estrogen therapy with medroxyprogesterone added the first 10–14 days of the calendar month. After adult doses of estradiol and medroxyprogesterone are reached, oral contraceptive pill may be substituted for separate preparations of these compounds.

In girls without a uterus, such as in androgen insensitivity or XY gonadal dysgenesis, the same guidelines for estrogen replacement can be used, but there is no need for the addition of progestagen.

Hormonal replacement is associated with some behavioral changes in hypogonadal adolescents. Specifically, boys have an increase in nocturnal emissions and touching behaviors at higher doses *(55)*. However, in at least one study, estrogen or testosterone therapy was found to have minimal effects of behavior problems or mood in adolescents. In this study, low-dose estrogen therapy was associated with an increase in withdrawn behavior *(56)*, but no other association was found when assessed using a variety of behavioral testing tools.

GnRH and Gonadotropin Therapy

In some cases of hypogonadotropic hypogonadism, pulsatile administration of gonadotropin releasing hormone has resulted in induction of puberty *(57)*. However, as a practical matter, such therapy is most frequently used for stimulation of spermatogenesis or induction of ovulation in infertile adult patients. Similarly, gonadotropin therapy has not been commonly used in adolescents, but reserved for therapy for adult infertility.

REFERENCES

1. Marshall WA, Tanner JM. Variations in the pattern of pubertal changes in girls. Am J Dis Child 1969;44:291–301.
2. Marshall WA, Tanner JM. Variations in the pattern of pubertal changes in boys. Am J Dis Child 1970;45:13–21.
3. Argente J. Diagnosis of late puberty. Horm Res 1999;51(Suppl 3):95–100.
4. Warren PW. Effects of undernutrition on reproductive function in the human. Endocr Rev 1983;4:363–377.
5. Warren MP, Van de Wiele RL. Clinical and metabolic features of anorexia nervosa. Am J Ob Gyn 1973;117:435–449.
6. Weimann E, Witzel C, Schwidergall S, Bohles HJ. Perpubertal perturbations in elite gymnasts caused by sport specific training regimes and inadequate nutritional intake. Int J Sports Med 2000;21(3):210–215.
7. Warren MP, Stiehl AL. Exercise and female adolescents: effects on the reproductive and skeletal systems. J Am Med Womens Assoc 1999;54(3):115–120.

8. Crowley W Jr, Filicori M, Spratt D, Santoro N. The physiology of gonadotropin-releasing hormone (GnRH) secretion in men and women. Recent Prog Horm Res 1985;41:473–531.
9. Weiss J, Crowley W Jr, Jameson JL. Normal structure of the gonadotropin-releasing hormone (GnRH) gene is patients with GnRH deficiency and idiopathic hypogonadotropic hypogonadism. J Clin Endocrinol Metab 1989;69:299–303.
10. Layman LC, Wilson JT, Huey LO, Lanclos KD, Plouffe L Jr, McDonough PG. Gonadotropin-releasing hormone, follicule- stimulating hormone beta, and luteinizing hormone beta gene structure in idiopathic hypogonadotropic hypogonadism. Fert Steril 1992;57:42–49.
11. Nakayama Y, Wondisford FE, Lash RW, et al. Analysis of gonadotropin-releasing hormone gene structure in families with familial central precocious puberty and idiopathic hypogonadotropic hypogonadism. J Clin Endocrinol Metab 1990;70:1233–1238.
12. Weiss J, Adams E, Whitcomb RW, Crowley W Jr, Jameson JL. Normal sequence of the gonadotropin-releasing hormone gene in patients with idiopathic hypgonadotropic hypogonadism. Biol Reprod 1991;45:743–747.
13. Layman LC, Lanclos KD, Tho SPT, Sweet CR, McDonough PG. Patients with idiopathic hypogonadoptropic hypogonadism have normal gonadotropin-releasing hormone gene structure. Adolesc Pediatr Gynecol 1993;6:214–219.
14. Santen RJ, Paulsen CA. Hypogonadotropic eunuchoidism. I: clinical study of the mode of inheritance. J Clin Endocrinol Metab 1973;36:47–54.
15. Franco B, Guioli S, Pragliola A, et al. A gene deleted in Kallman's syndrome shares homology with neural cell adhesion and axonal path-finding molecules. Nature 1991;353:529–536.
16. Legouis R, Hardelin J, Levilliers J, et al. The candidate gene for the X-linked Kallmann syndrome encodes a protein related to adhesion molecules. Cell 1991;67:423–235.
17 Layman LC. The molecular basis of human hypogonadotropic hypogonadism. Mol Genet Metab 1999;68:191–199.
18. Georgopoulos NA, Pralong FP, Seidman CE, Seidman JG, Crowley W Jr., Vallejo M. Genetic heterogeneity evidenced by low incidence of KAL-1 gene mutations in sporadic cases of gonadotropin-releasing hormone deficiency. J Clin Endocrinol Metab 1997;82:213–217.
19. Zhang Y-H, Guo W, Wagner RL, et al. DAX1 mutations provide insight into structure-function relationships in steroidogenic tissue development. Am J Hum Genet 199862:855–864.
20. Merke DP, Tajima T, Baron J, Cutler GB. Hypogonadotropic hypogonadism in a female caused by an X-linked recessive mutation in the DAX1 gene. N Engl J Med 340:1248–1252.
21. de Roux N, Young J, Misrahi M, et al. A family with hypogonadotropic hypodonadism and mutations in the gonadotropin-releasing hormone receptor. N Engl J Med 1997;337:1597–1602.
22. Layman LC, Cohen DP, Jin M, et al. Mutations in the gonadotropin-releasing hormone receptor gene cause hypogonadotropic hypogonadism. Nat Genet 1998;18:14–15.
23. Weiss J, Axelrod L, Whitcomb RW, Harris PE, Crowley W Jr, Jameson JL. Hypogonadism caused by a single amino acid substitution in the β subunit of luteinizing hormone. N Engl J Med 1992; 326:179–183.
24. Matthews CH, Borgato S, Beck-Peccoz P, et al. Primary amenorrhea and infertility due to mutation in the β-subunit of follicle-stimulating hormone. Nat Genet 1993;5:83–86.
25. Layman LC, Lee EJ, Peak DB, et al. Delayed puberty and hypogonadism caused by a mutation in the follicle stimulating hormone beta-subunit gene. N Engl J Med 1997;337:607–611.
26. Cogan JD, Wu W, Phillips JAI, et al. The PROP1 2-base pair deletion is a commmon cause of combined pituitary hormone deficiency. J Clin Endocrinol Metab 1998;83:3346–3349.
27. Wu W. Cogan JD, Pfaffle RW, et al. Mutations in PROP1 cause familial combined pituitary hormone deficiency. Nat Genet 1998;18:147–149.
28. Rappaport R, Brauner R. Growth and endocrine disorders secondary to cranial irradiation. Pediatr Res 1989;25(6):561–567.
29. Smyth CM, Bremner WJ. Klinefelter syndrome. Arch Inter Med 1998;158(12):1309–1314.
30. Laue L, Wu SM, Kudo M, et al. A nonsense mutation of the human luteinizing hormone receptor gene in Leydig cell hypoplasia. Hum Mol Genet 1995;4:1429–1433.
31. Kremer H, Kraaij R, Toledo SP, et al. Male pseudohermaphroditism due to a homozygous missense mutation of the luteinizing hormone receptor gene. Nat Genet 1995;9:160–164.
32. Latronico AC, Anasti J, Arnhold IJP, et al. Testicular and ovarian resistance to luteinizing hormone caused by inactivating mutations of the luteinizing hormone-receptor gene. N Engl J Med 1996;334:507–512.

33. Gromoll J, Eiholzer U, Nieschlag E, Simoni M. Male hypogonadism caused by homozygous deletion of exon 10 of the luteinizing hormone (LH) receptor: differential action of human chorionic gonadotropin and LH. J Clin Endocrinol Metab 2000;85(6):2281–2286.
34. Jamieson CR, van der Burgt I, Brady AF, et al. Mapping a gene for Noonan syndrome to the long arm of chromosome 12. Nat Genet 1994;8:357–360.
35. Blagovidow N, Page DC, Huff DE, et al. Ullrich Turner syndrome in a XY female fetus with deletion of the sex-determining portion of the Y chromosome. Am J Med Genet 1989;34:159–162.
36. Scherer G, Chempp W, Baccichetti C, et al. Duplication of an Xp segment that includes the ZFX locus causes sex inversion in man. Hum Genet 1989;81:291–294.
37. Job J-C. Hypogonadism at Adolescence: Lack or Delay of Sexual Development? In: Fima Lifshitz, ed. Pediatric Endocrinology, 3rd Edition, Marcel Dekker, 1996.
38. Aittomaki K, Herva R, Stenman U-H, et al. Clinical features of primary ovarian failure caused by a point mutation in the follicle-stimulating hormone receptor gene. J Clin Endo and Metab 1996;81:3722–3726.
39. Rappaport R, Maguelone GF. Disorders of sexual differentiation. In: Bertrand J, Rappaport R, Sizonenko P, Eds. Pediatric Endocrinology: Physiology, Pathophysiology, and Clinical Aspects, 2nd ed, Williams and Wilkins, 1993.
40. McPhaul MJ. Molecular defects of the androgen receptor. J Steroid Biochem Mol Biol 1999;69(1–6):315–22.
41. Evans BAJ, Hughes IA, Bevan CL, Patterson MN, Gregory JW. Phenotypic diversity in siblings with partial androgen insensitivity syndrome. Arch Dis Child 1997;76:529–531.
42. Bramswig JH, Heimes U, Heiermann E, et al. The effects of different cumulative doses of chemotherapy on testicular function. Cancer 1990;65:1298–1302.
43. Chou RH, Wong GB, Kramer JH, et al. Toxicities of total-body irradiation for pediatric bone marrow transplantation. Int J Radiat Oncol Biol Phys 1996;34(4):843–851.
44. Bayer L, Bayley N. Growth Diagnosis, University of Chicago Press, 1959.
45. Reynolds EL, Wines JV. Physical changes associated with adolescence in boys. Am J Dis Child 1951;82:529–547.
46. Odink RJ, Schoemaker J, Schoute E, Herder E, Delemarre-van de Waal HA. Predictive value of serum follicular-stimulating hormone levels in the differentiation between hypogonadotropic hypogonadism and constitutional delay of puberty. Horm Res 1998;49(6):279–287.
47. Wu FCW, Brown DC, Butler GE, Stirling HF, Kelnar CJH. Early morning plasma testosterone is an accurate predictor of imminent pubertal development in prepubertal boys. J Clin Encrinol Metab 1990;70:26–31.
48. Gambineri A, Pasquali R. Testosterone therapy in men: clinical and pharmacological perspectives. J Endocrin Invest 2000;23:196–214.
49. Brook CGD. Treatment of late puberty. Horm Res 1999;51(Suppl 3):101–103.
50. Tse W, Buyukgebiz A, Hindmarsh PC, Stanhope R, Preece MA, Brook CGD. Long-term outcome of oxandrolone treatment in boys with constitutional delay of growth and puberty. J Pediatr 1990;117(4):588–591.
51. Wilson DM, McCauley E, Brown DR, Dudley R. Oxandrolone therapy in constitutionally delayed growth and puberty. Pediatrics 1995;96(6):1095–1100.
52. Bourguignon J-P. Delayed puberty and hypogonadism. In: Bertrand J, Rappaport R, Sizonenko P, eds. Pediatric Endocrinology: Physiology, Pathophysiology, and Clinical Aspects, 2nd ed, Williams and Wilkins, 1993.
53. Bridges NA, Brook CDG. Disorders of puberty. In: Brook CDG, ed. Clinical Paediatric Endocrinology Blackwell Science, 1995.
54. Rose SR. Induction of puberty in female hypogonadism. The Endocrinologist 1996;6(6):439–442.
55. Finkelstein JW, Susman EJ, Chinchilli VM, et al. Effects of estrogen or testosterone on self-reported sexual responses and behaviors in hypogonadal adolescents. J Clin Endocrinol Metab 1998;83(7):2281–2285.
56. Susman EJ, Finkelstien JW, Chinchilli VM, et al. The effect of sex hormone replacement therapy on behavior problems and moods in adolescents with delayed puberty. J Pediatr 1998;133(4):521–525.
57. Hoffman AR, Crowley WF. Induction of puberty in men by long-term pulsatile administration of low dose gonadotropin-releasing hormone. N Engl J Med 1982;307:1237–1241.

23 Precocious Puberty

Clinical Management

Henry Rodriguez, MD
and Ora H. Pescovitz, MD

Contents

INTRODUCTION AND NORMAL DEVELOPMENT
BENIGN PREMATURE DEVELOPMENT
CENTRAL PRECOCIOUS PUBERTY
PERIPHERAL PRECOCIOUS PUBERTY
CONCLUSION
REFERENCES

INTRODUCTION AND NORMAL DEVELOPMENT

Precocious puberty has been a focus of interest for both the pediatric endocrinologist and the primary pediatrician for many years. Twenty years ago, the development and application of GnRH-agonist (GnRHa) therapy to treat central precocious puberty significantly changed our approach to this disorder. More recently, application of molecular biological techniques has provided us with a better understanding of the intricacies of the regulation of gonadotropin and sex-steroid production characteristic of normal pubertal development and provided us with the tools to elucidate the etiologies of previously uncharacterized disorders of precocious puberty.

The Hypothalamic-Pituitary-Gonadal Axis

The onset of puberty requires the re-activation of the hypothalamic-pituitary-gonadal axis. Maturation of the hypothalamic-pituitary-gonadal axis initially occurs by mid-gestation *(1)*. GnRH or gonadotropin-releasing hormone is a decapeptide secreted by neuroendocrine neurons residing in the supraoptic and ventromedial nuclei of the pre-optic and medial basal hypothalamus. Their nerve termini are found in the lateral portions of the median eminence adjacent to the pituitary stalk. GnRH secretion by these neurons is coordinated in such a way that, when grown in culture, individual cells exhibit pulsatile secretion that becomes synchronous when the cells are placed in physical

From: *Contemporary Endocrinology: Pediatric Endocrinology: A Practical Clinical Guide*
Edited by: S. Radovick and M. H. MacGillivray © Humana Press Inc., Totowa, NJ

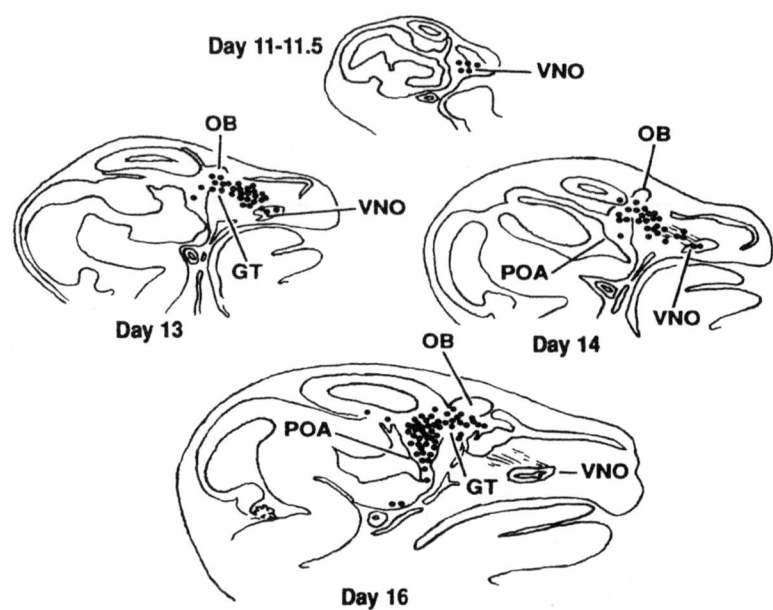

Fig. 1. Ontogeny of the GnRH neurosecretory neurons in the mouse. The migratory route of the GnRH neurons is indicated by the black dots. Their progression is illustrated according to embryonic day of development. At d 11–11.5 the neurons are in the area of the vomeronasal organ (VNO) and the medial wall of the olfactory placode. By d 13 the cell number has increased and their distribution has extended to the olfactory bulb (OB) and the ganglion terminalis (GT). By d 14 the cells approach the preoptic area (POA) and begin to enter the hypothalamus. By d 16 the migration is nearly complete. (Adapted from Schwanzel-Fukuda M, Pfaff DW. Origin of luteinizing hormone-releasing hormone neurons. Nature 1989; 338:161–164; with permission)

proximity to each other. These cells interestingly are one of the few cell-types that originate outside of the central nervous system, in the region of the olfactory placode *(2)*. During fetal development, they migrate with the olfactory neurons to their final location in the hypothalamus (Fig. 1) The initial secretion of GnRH appears unrestrained and occurs between 100–150 days of gestation. The pulsatile secretion is essential to the activation of the pituitary gonadotropes and the pulses must be of sufficient amplitude and frequency to regulate the release of follicle stimulating hormone (FSH) and luteinizing hormone (LH). The frequency of the pulses has been shown to alter the pattern of LH and FSH secretion such that faster frequencies increase gonadotrope release of both LH and FSH, slower frequency pulses increase the secretion of FSH relative to LH, and a constant infusion inhibits the release of both LH and FSH *(3)*. Maturation of negative feedback to the effects of sex steroids occurs after 150 d gestation with a progressive decrease in GnRH secretion resulting in low level GnRH secretion at term *(4,5)*. The GnRH "pulse generator" is highly functional 12 d after birth, presumably secondary to the withdrawal of maternal and placental sex steroid exposure. This leads to prominent FSH and LH release until approximately 6 mo of age in males and 12 mo in females. These gonadotropin levels lead to transient increases in sex steroids in infants that can approximate those seen in mid-puberty *(6)*. Negative feedback control of FSH and LH secretion becomes highly sensitive to sex steroids by 2 yr of age. The role of sex steroid negative feedback in this period has been supported by the observation of high gonadotropin levels in agonadal infants such as those with Turner syndrome (1). Beyond 3–4 yr of age, until puberty, the mechanism by which GnRH secretion is inhibited is less well understood since LH and FSH secretion is suppressed even in the agonadal individual. In part, this finding has led to the hypothesis that there is an "intrinsic CNS inhibitory mechanism" that prevents secondary sexual development until "disinhibition" occurs at the time of puberty. Studies in non-human primates have identified gamma-aminobutyric acid (GABA) as an inhibitory neurotransmitter responsible for restricting GnRH release (7). Reduction in tonic GABA inhibition appears to allow an increase in the response to other neurotransmitters such as glutamate that stimulate GnRH release (8,9).

At the time of the normal onset of puberty, GnRH pulsatile secretion is re-established, presumably following reduction in GABA inhibition of the pulse generator and decreased negative feedback sensitivity to low levels of sex steroids. This leads to increased GnRH pulsatility that is initially sleep-associated. As puberty progresses, there is an increase in LH pulse amplitude during the daytime as well, leading to sex steroid production and progressive development of secondary sexual characteristics. By mid to late puberty, spermatogenesis is established in males and a positive feedback mechanism develops in females resulting in the capacity to exhibit an estrogen-induced LH surge that leads to ovulation.

Normal Pubertal Development

Normal puberty involves activation both the hypothalamic-pituitary-gonadal axis (gonadarche) as well as maturation of the adrenal axis (adrenarche). Adrenarche is associated with an increase of adrenal androgen production that leads to pubarche, or the first appearance of pubic hair. This increase in adrenal androgens begins approximately 2 yr prior to elevations of pituitary gonadotropins and gonadal sex steroids (10,11). Adrenarche and gonadarche are independent events, as evidenced in agonadal children and those with Turner syndrome who exhibit adrenarche, but not gonadarche. The mechanism by which adrenarche is initiated remains unclear despite various theories and investigations over many years. The 17,20-lyase activity of the P450c17 enzyme is dramatically increased, particularly in the zona reticularis of the adrenal cortex leading to increased dehydro-epiandrosterone (DHEA) and androstenedione production. There has been speculation that a pituitary factor is responsible for stimulating the maturation of the zona reticularis, however there are no definitive data to support this claim (12). Preliminary evidence has suggested that post-translational phosphorylation of the P450c17 enzyme may cause the increase in 17,20 lyase activity with a consequent increase in adrenal androgen production (13,14).

The secondary sexual features of puberty in the male are first noted between the ages of 9–14 yr. The first physical sign of puberty is testicular enlargement to greater than 2.5 cm in longest diameter or 3 cc in volume. This is largely due to an increase in Sertoli cell and seminiferous tubular volume with a small contribution by the Leydig cells. Pubic hair appears within a few mo. Tanner stages of genital and pubic hair development are illustrated in Fig. 2. Increasing androgen levels lead to increased oiliness of the hair and skin resulting in acne, adult body odor, deepening of the voice, penile erections, and nocturnal emissions. Normal variations in androgen to estrogen ratios can lead to transient breast budding or gynecomastia in a majority of pubertal boys (15).

Puberty in females is heralded by breast development, or thelarche, between the ages of 8–13 yr. Breast development may be unilateral for 6 mo prior to the development of

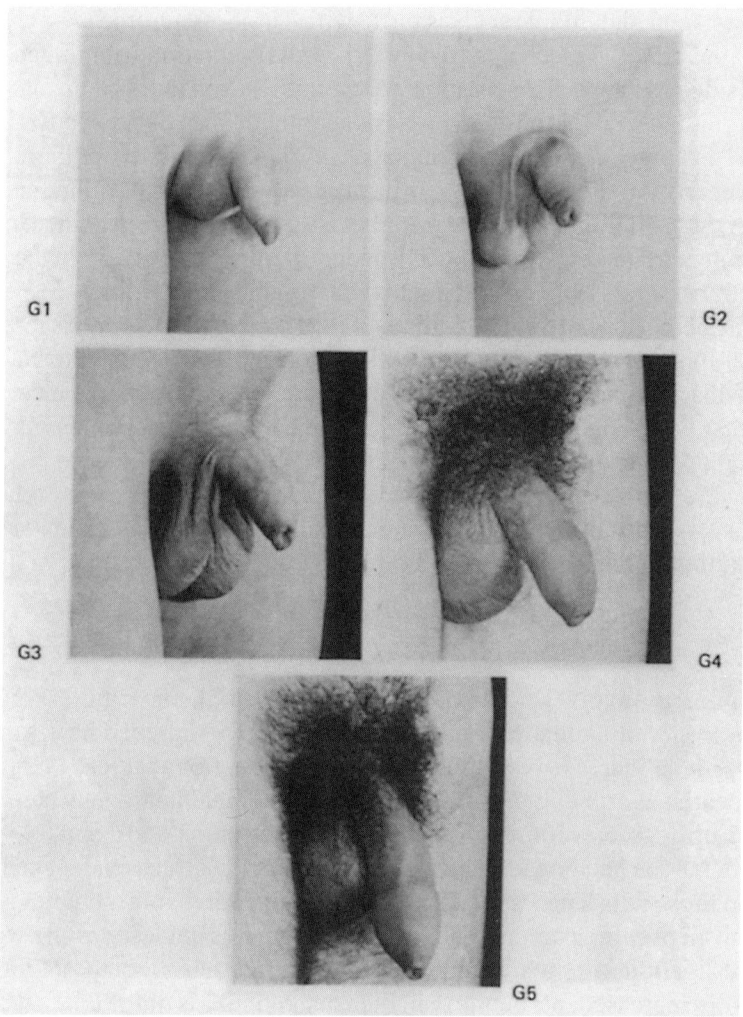

Fig. 2. Tanner stages of male genital and pubic hair development according to Marshall and Tanner and Reynolds and Wines (Photos from Van Wieringen JD, Wafelbakker F, Verbrugge HP, et al. Growth Diagrams 1965 Netherlands: Second National Survey on 0–24 Year Olds. Netherlands Institute for Preventative Medicine TNO. Groningen: Wolters-Noordhoff, 1971; with permission).

the contralateral breast. Pubic hair appears within a few months during Tanner 2 breast development with menarche typically occurring approximately 2 yr after the onset of puberty, during Tanner 4 breast development. This age range was called into question in 1997 by a study coordinated by the American Academy of Pediatrics *(16)*. Analysis of data collected by primary physicians on 17,077 girls of mixed ethnic background suggested that pubarche may occur as early as 5 yr in African-American females and 7 yr of age in Caucasian females. Menarche is not a presenting feature of puberty and its presence should prompt investigation into the possibility of a foreign body or invasive lesion of the vaginal vault, cervix, or uterus. The stages of breast and pubic hair development are summarized in Fig. 3. As indicated in Fig. 4, in contrast to males, the pubertal growth spurt follows shortly after the onset of puberty. This is clearly evident when one

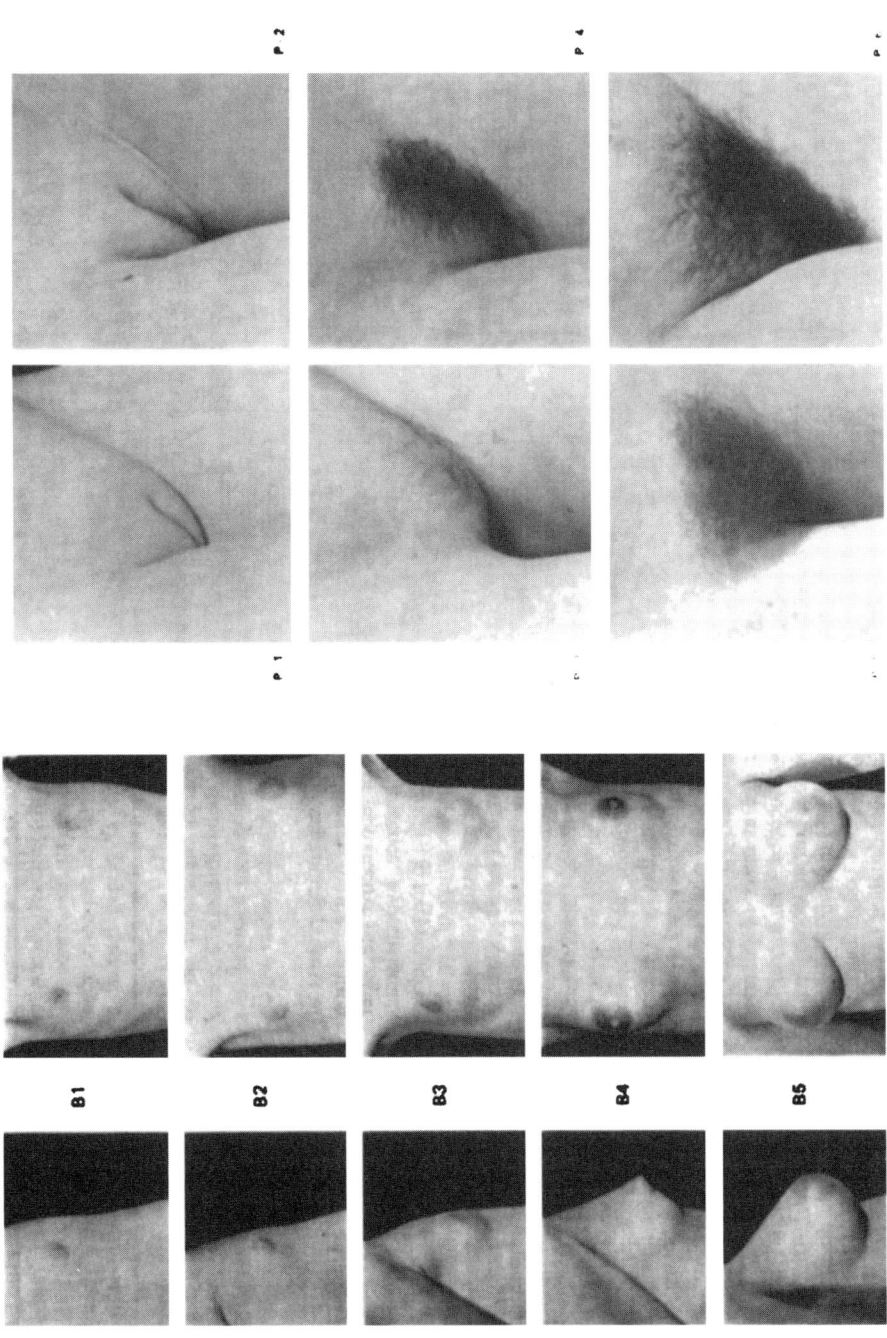

Fig. 3. Tanner Stages of female breast and pubic hair development according to Marshall and Tanner and Reynolds and Wines (Photos from Van Wieringen JD, Wafelbakker F, Verbrugge HP, et al. Growth Diagrams 1965 Netherlands: Second National Survey on 0–24 Year Olds. Netherlands Institute for Preventative Medicine TNO. Groningen: Wolters-Noordhoff, 1971; with permission)

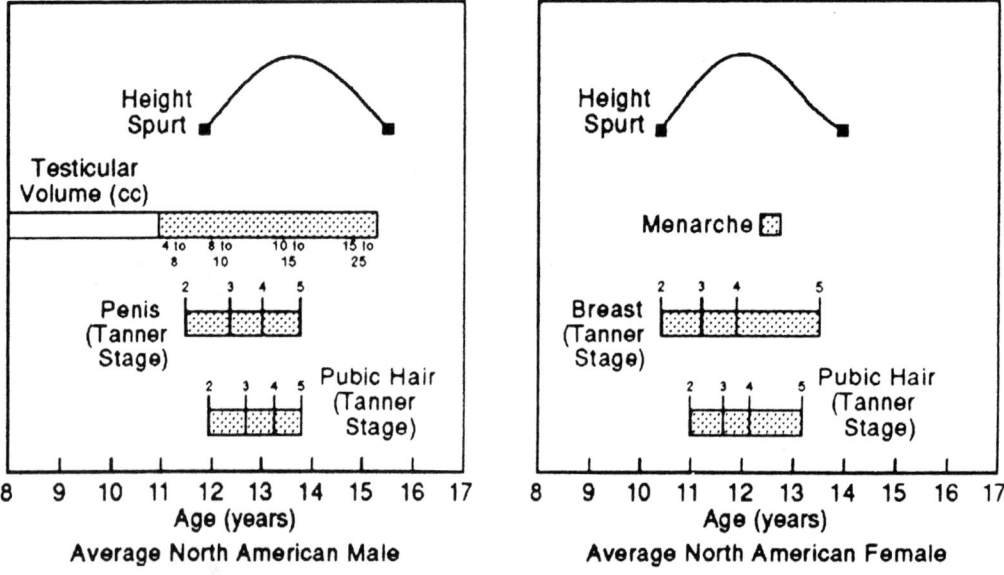

Fig. 4. Sequence of pubertal development in males and females. Relative growth velocity, testicular volume or menarche and Tanner staging are indicated for age. (From Tanner JM. Growth at Adolescence. Oxford, England:Blackwell Scientific Publications;1962:30–36; with permission.)

surveys the relative tall stature of females as compared to males at approx 12 yr of age. Additional features of puberty in the female include growth of the body of the uterus and "estrogenization" of the vaginal mucosa as the epithelium is transformed, the vaginal pH drops (acidifies), and leukorrhea appears. The uterus, as evaluated by pelvic ultrasound, is judged as pubertal in configuration when the body of the uterus is larger than the cervix, with a length >3.5 cm or a volume greater than 18 mL.

Precocious Puberty: Definitions

Recent discussions among pediatricians and pediatric endocrinologists have focused on the determination of the current definition of precocious puberty in females. In 1997, the Pediatric Research in Office settings Network of the American Academy of Pediatrics reported that the onset of puberty in girls in the US is occurring earlier than previous studies have documented *(16)*. The study reported that breast and pubic hair development is occurring 1 yr earlier in Caucasian girls and 2 yr earlier in African-American girls despite no change in the age of menarche. These findings would indicate that girls are entering puberty at an earlier age, but progressing at a slower rate. More recent data by Biro and colleagues on almost 2400 females further demonstrate that adult height in females is associated with age at menarche in both races. The early maturing, more rapidly growing girls are the tallest early on but become the shortest adults *(17)*. This study also highlighted the finding that puberty starts earlier in females with greater body mass index (BMI), specifically with increased adiposity. This is not an insignificant position, as it implies that pubertal development is not precocious in Caucasian females older than 7 yr and African-American girls older than 6 yr. This prompted a review of the literature and the issuance of standards of practice by the Lawson Wilkins Pediatric Endocrine Society *(18)*. The Drugs and Therapeutics and Executive Committees of this body concluded; "recent data demonstrate that in the United States, the onset of puberty in girls is occurring earlier than previous studies have documented, with breast and pubic hair development appearing on average 1 year earlier in white girls and 2 yr earlier in African-American girls." They concluded that aggressive evaluation and treatment are unlikely to be beneficial in African-American females having onset of puberty after 6 yr of age and white females with the onset of puberty after age 7 yr. It must be noted that many in the field of pediatric endocrinology think that the adoption of these new standards is premature and carries the risk of overlooking pathology. In our opinion, until additional studies are performed, premature sexual development in Caucasian girls younger than 8 yr and African-American girls younger than 7 yr deserves a medical evaluation (19).

Precocious puberty is secondary to either central or peripheral mechanisms. Several forms of premature puberty, including both premature thelarche and premature pubarche, are generally considered benign. Premature thelarche is the early appearance of isolated breast development. Premature pubarche is the early appearance of pubic hair, which is most often secondary to premature adrenarche, an "early awakening" of the adrenal gland. Adrenarche occurs in association with increased adrenal androgen production leading to the appearance of pubic hair and other androgen effects such as acne, body odor, and axillary hair development. Central precocious puberty or gonadotropin-dependent precocious puberty results from the premature activation of the hypothalamic-pituitary-gonadal (HPG) axis leading to premature secondary sexual development that proceeds in a fashion similar to normal pubertal progression. Potential triggers of central precocious puberty are listed in Table 1. In contrast gonadotropin-independent precocious puberty occurs in the absence of HPG axis activation and may be secondary to numerous etiologies, including those listed in Table 2. Because of the significant morbidity associated with many of these lesions, determination of the etiology is essential. In addition, any child with premature sexual development is at risk for psychological and social stresses, including sexual abuse. One of the most significant consequences of untreated, rapidly progressive, central precocious puberty is a compromise in final adult height.

BENIGN PREMATURE DEVELOPMENT

Premature thelarche and premature adrenarche may be the consequence of benign, self-limited processes that require no therapeutic intervention. Premature thelarche is limited to modest breast development, but may also include estrogenization of the vaginal mucosa and rarely, vaginal bleeding. Premature adrenarche results in the appearance of pubic and/or axillary hair and occasionally acne and body odor. In general, these conditions are not associated with significant growth acceleration or skeletal maturation. Of note however is increasing attention to studies that question the benign nature of premature adrenarche (20–25).

Premature Thelarche

Premature thelarche is the isolated premature appearance of breast development in girls that occurs during the first 3–4 yr of life (26), with a peak prevalence in the first 2 yr (27, 28). It should be differentiated from neonatal breast hyperplasia which is generally present at birth, is a consequence of gestational hormones, and generally spontaneously resolves within the first few mo of life. Growth acceleration, significant

Table 1
Differential Diagnosis of Gonadotropin-Dependent Precocious Puberty

Idiopathic
    Sporadic
    Familial
    Adoption from developing country
    Following chronic exposure ot sex steroids
Central Nervous System Disorders
    Hypothalamic Hamartoma
    Congenital Anomalies
        Hydrocephalus
        Myelomeningocele
        Midbrain developmental defects
    Cysts
        Arachnoid
        Glial
        Pineal
    Neoplasms
        Astrocytoma
        Craniopharyngioma
        Ependymoma
        Glioma
        Neuroblastoma
        Pinealoma
    Vascular lesion
    Global CNS Injury
    Cranial Irradiation
    Infection
        Abscess
        Encephalitis
        Meningitis
Syndromes
    Neurofibromatosis type 1
    Russel-Silver syndrome
    Williams syndrome
    Klinefelter syndrome
    Cohen syndrome
    Pallister-Hall syndrome
    Solitary maxillary incisor

bone age maturation, or other signs of precocious puberty do not accompany benign premature thelarche *(29)*. The breast development may be unilateral or bilateral with a waxing and waning course. Regression often occurs within 18 mo. However, it has been suggested that complete regression may only be seen if the onset of development is prior to 2 yr of age *(27,28)*. Furthermore, girls with more than Tanner 2 breast development are also less likely to have breast tissue regression *(30)*.

The precise etiology of premature thelarche remains unknown. It has been postulated that in some girls, the glandular breast tissue is particularly sensitive to low levels of circulating estrogen *(31,32)*. It is important to exclude ingestion or exposure to exog-

Table 2
Differential Diagnosis of Gonadotropin-Independent Precocious Puberty

Autonomous Gonadal Function
  McCune-Albright Sundrome
  Peutz-Jeghers Syndrome
  Familial Male Precocious Puberty (Testotoxicosis)
  Ovarian Cysts
Gonadal Tumores
  Ovarian
    Granulosa cell
    Theca cell
    Combination
  Testicular
    Leydig cell
    Sertoli cell
Extogenous Steroid Ingestion/Exposure
hGC Secreting Tumors*
  Hepatoblastoma
  Pinealoma
  Germinoma
    Thymic
    Testicular
  Choriocarcinoma
  Teratoma
Adrenal Disorders
  Congenital adrenal hyperplasia
  Adenoma
  Carcinoma
Severe Primary Hypothyroidism

*hCG is a gonadotropin however, for the purposes of classification of causes of precocious puberty it is generally defined as being a cause of gonadotropin-independent precocious puberty.

enous estrogenic agents such as oral contraceptives or creams in girls with premature thelarche. Environmental pollutants including xenoestrogens, such as plasticizers classified as endocrine disruptors, or phytoestrogens may exhibit estrogenic and antiandrogenic activities and have also been implicated in the etiology of premature breast development (33). Increased levels of sex-hormone-binding globulin (SHBG) levels in conjunction with decreased free testosterone can lead to an alteration of the ratio of androgens to estrogens, and is another postulated etiology for premature thelarche (34). Serial and stimulated gonadotropin measurements in these girls have revealed elevated FSH levels consistent with those seen in early puberty (35–38). It has therefore been suggested that premature thelarche may be a consequence of early and slowly progressive activation of the hypothalamic-pituitary-ovarian axis and thus, may represent part of the continuum of central precocious puberty.

Premature thelarche may be difficult to diagnose in obese females. Adipose tissue over the pectoral area may appear much like breast tissue, and may be difficult to differentiate from glandular tissue. Palpation of the breast may reveal an absence of tissue in the subareolar area, which some clinicians to refer to as "the doughnut sign."

During initial breast development, glandular tissue first appears in the subareolar region and subsequently extends outwards. Ultrasound examination may rarely be useful to make this distinction or to identify a cyst, abscess, or breast tumor *(39)*. Pelvic ultrasound may reveal small ovarian cysts in children with premature thelarche. However, because this finding is usually seen in normal pre-pubertal girls, it is not usually a helpful diagnostic test. On occasion, girls with premature thelarche may have a single, large follicular cyst that produces estradiol. Some of these cysts are self-limited and resorb spontaneously. However, girls prone to ovarian cyst development may have cyst recurrence.

Serial observation and reassurance of the family is all that is necessary for a girl with isolated premature thelarche. A bone age radiograph may be indicated to gauge the extent of estrogen exposure. Evidence of advanced skeletal maturation usually suggests more significant pathology than premature thelarche. It should be kept in mind, however, that the bone age might be slightly advanced in obese children. Although premature thelarche has been viewed as a self-limited variation of normal development, these patients should be followed at three to six month intervals, unless the condition resolves. Long-term studies have indicated that as many as 18% of girls with premature thelarche may progress to central precocious puberty despite their typical presentation *(26, 28,37,40)*.

Premature Pubarche

Premature pubarche is defined as the appearance of pubic and/or axillary hair prior to 8 yr of age. The child with premature pubarche typically presents with the early appearance of pubic and possibly axillary hair. In addition, there may be children that also manifest features of mild hyperandrogenism, including apocrine or adult body odor and comedones. The pubic hair is generally limited to Tanner stage 2 development with few scattered hyperpigmented curly hairs appearing over the labia majora or perineum in females or at the base of the penis in males. The presence of clitoromegaly is highly suggestive of serious pathology and is not seen in benign premature pubarche. Similarly, hirsutism is not a feature of benign premature pubarche. If considerable hirsutism exists, it can be quantified utilizing the Ferriman-Gallwey index (Fig. 5).

Premature pubarche is most commonly a consequence of premature adrenarche, which is more common in females and often observed in children with CNS abnormalities.

As was noted above, work by Herman-Giddens, et al. and the National Heart, Lung, and Blood Institute suggests that puberty and adrenarche may be occurring in younger females, particularly those of African-American descent *(16)*. However, we continue to recommend that caution should be exercised in assigning a diagnosis of "normal variant" pubertal development to females younger than 7–8 yr of age. As many as 20% of girls with premature adrenarche have been reported to progress into central precocious puberty *(41)*. Benign premature adrenarche does not alter normal pubertal progression and is generally thought to be self-limited. However, recent studies suggest that premature pubarche may not be completely benign. These studies indicated higher association with later hyperandrogenism, menstrual irregularities and infertility in females. These studies suggest that premature adrenarche may be the presenting feature of polycystic ovary syndrome (PCOS) *(20)*. Associations between premature adrenarche, elevated adrenal androgens (DHEA-S), and insulin resistance have also been reported in individuals with a history of intrauterine growth retardation (IUGR) *(42–44)*. IUGR, in turn, has been

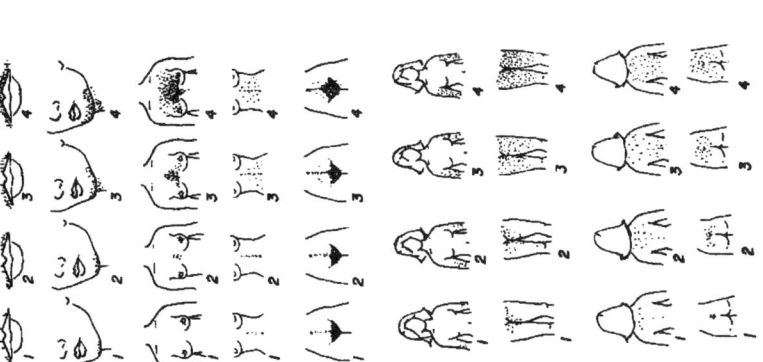

Fig. 5. The Ferriman and Gallwey system for scoring hirsutism. A score of 8 or more indicates hirsutism. (From R Hatch, RL Rosenfield, MH Kim, et al., Hirsutism: Implications, etiology, and management. Am J Obstet Gynecol 1981;140:815, the chart is adapted from D Ferriman and JD Gallwey, Clinical assessment of body hair growth in women. J Clin Endocrinol Metab 1961;21:1440, by permission)

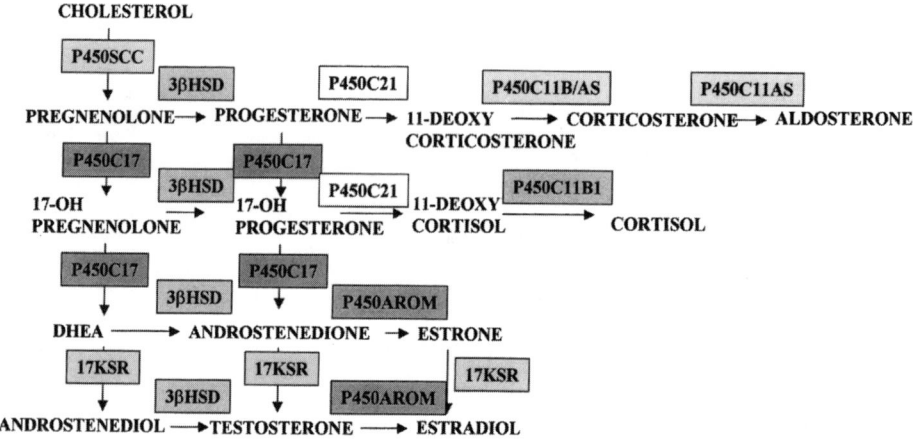

Fig. 6. Biosynthetic pathway of adrenal steroidogenesis.

associated with an increased risk of Syndrome X (insulin resistance, hypertension, and hyperlipidemia) in adult life *(45)*. Since additional prognostic indicators for PCOS and Syndrome X do not exist, long-term follow-up of these individuals may be warranted *(46)*.

Signs of excess virilization such as deepening of the voice, increase in muscle mass, clitoral enlargement in females or testicular/phallic enlargement in males are not features of benign premature adrenarche. When present they should raise the concern of significant pathology. The differential diagnosis includes late-onset or non-classical congenital adrenal hyperplasia (NCAH), rare virilizing adrenal or gonadal tumors, and central precocious puberty in boys. In addition, poorly controlled classical congenital adrenal hyperplasia may cause elevations in androgen levels and excess virilization.

Enzymatic defects in adrenal steroidogenesis may lead to hyperandrogenism. Congenital adrenal hyperplasia is the result of one of several autosomal recessive defects in one of a number of steroidogenic enzymes necessary for cortisol production (Fig. 6). Defects leading to virilization result from the inability to synthesize sufficient quantities of cortisol to adequately suppress hypothalamic corticotropic-releasing-hormone (CRH) and pituitary adrenocorticotropic hormone (ACTH). This leads to elevated ACTH levels that stimulate steroidogenic acute regulatory protein (StAR) and p450SCC leading to an overabundance of intermediary precursors proximal to the enzymatic defect. The excess quantities of these precursors leads to a shunting of hormone production to androgens. Defects in P450c21, P450c11AS, and 3 beta-hydroxysteroid dehydrogenase (3βHSD) lead to increases in adrenal androgen synthesis. Classical defects cause severely compromised or absent enzymatic function causing marked and early hyperandrogenism during fetal development leading to ambiguous genitalia in newborn females. However, partial defects may lead to less severe or absent phenotypic findings in females and may escape detection in male infants. The less severe defects do not lead to substantial mineralocorticoid or glucocorticoid deficiency but instead may cause hyperandrogenism later in life (nonclassical congenital adrenal hyperplasia - NCAH). The incidence of NCAH varies widely depending upon the ethnicity of the population being studied. Rates range from 0.3% in the general population to almost 4% in Ashkenazi Jews *(47)*. Studies of screening for NCAH in females with premature adrenarche report incidences ranging from 6–40% *(46,48,49)*.

Virilizing tumors of the adrenal may rarely present as premature pubarche. Such tumors generally lead to marked virilization, growth acceleration, and skeletal advancement. This occurs in the absence of testicular enlargement in the male.

Evaluation of a child with premature pubarche may not require extensive evaluation. Typically, a bone age x-ray reveals that skeletal maturation is within 2 SD of chronologic age. Androgen levels in premature adrenarche are usually consistent with those seen in Tanner stage 2–3 pubic hair development *(50)*. We recommend obtaining a DHEAS level to help confirm this diagnosis. Clitoromegaly, rapidly progressive or excess virilization and advanced skeletal maturation warrant determination of additional androgen levels including 17-OH progesterone, androstenedione, and testosterone. ACTH stimulation testing with 100 µg of iv/im synthetic ACTH (Cortrosyn) allows one to compare baseline and stimulated levels of adrenal steroid hormone precursors in order to pinpoint possible enzymatic defects. Adrenal computed tomography (CT) scan or ultrasound should be used to identify mass lesions if significant virilization occurs and hormonal evaluation does not reveal an adrenal enzymatic disorder. Tumors may be differentiated from CAH, as they do not typically respond to ACTH stimulation or glucocorticoid suppression.

Therapy, if indicated, is dictated by the etiology of the excess androgens. In the case of NCAH, glucocorticoid replacement therapy is recommended to inhibit excess hypothalamic/pituitary stimulation of adrenal steroidogenesis and consequent hyperandrogenism. Virilizing tumors require surgery, preferably by a pediatric surgeon experienced in such procedures. Although surgical excision is often curative, chemotherapy may be indicated for cases with evidence of tumor extension or for recurrence. The recent association of premature adrenarche and PCOS may support a search for evidence of hyperinsulinism with a consideration of oral contraceptive and/or insulin sensitizers or metformin therapy in postmenarchal females *(51–53)*.

CENTRAL PRECOCIOUS PUBERTY

Central precocious puberty (CPP) is a gonadotropin dependent process. It results from premature activation of the hypothalamic-pituitary-gonadal axis. Secondary sexual development follows the sequence of normal puberty, however beginning at an earlier age. The etiology is most commonly idiopathic in girls, but is identified in the majority of boys *(54,55)*. The reason for this sex difference is unclear. However, it has been proposed that the female axis is more readily activated by various factors. As listed in Table 1, a multitude of CNS abnormalities can lead to CPP, presumably by interrupting the normal prepubertal neuronal pathways that typically inhibit activation of the hypothalamic-pituitary-gonadal axis.

The most common identifiable cause of CPP is a hypothalamic hamartoma. It has been identified in 10–44% of CPP cases *(55)*. These "tumors" are usually benign congenital malformations arising from disorganized central nervous tissue including GnRH neurosecretory neurons. They are best visualized by magnetic resonance imaging (MRI) and typically appear as a pedunculated mass attached to the hypothalamus between the tuber cincreum and the mamillary bodies, just posterior to the optic chiasm *(55,56)*. Rarely, these tumors may be associated with gelastic (laughing) seizures, secondary generalized epilepsy, behavioral difficulties, and variable cognitive deficiencies *(56)*. Most hamartomas rarely enlarge, cause mass effects or increased intracranial pressure and thus, invasive surgery is not indicated. Furthermore, some studies have shown that complete resection of these lesions can fail to halt pubertal progression *(57)*. Like other children with CPP, children with hypothalamic hamartomas respond well to GnRH analog therapy *(56,57)*.

A variety of other CNS lesions can result in central precocious puberty (Table 1). It is believed that they also, cause disruption of tonic inhibitory signals to the hypothalamus, leading to pulsatile GnRH release and activation of the hypothalamic-pituitary-gonadal axis. Such activation has been seen with optic gliomas of the chiasm in neurofibromatosis type 1 *(58)*, CNS developmental defects such as septo-optic dysplasia and myelomeningocele, and in isolated hydrocephalus. High dose cranial irradiation used in the treatment of pediatric malignancies has also been shown to cause precocious puberty in up to 25% of cases *(59)*. CNS irradiation with doses as low as the 18–24 Gy used in CNS prophylaxis therapy for childhood leukemia can also predispose children to central precocious puberty. In these cases, the age of onset of precocious puberty is often correlated with age at the time of radiation therapy.

Central precocious puberty may also arise following exposure of the hypothalamus to elevated sex steroid levels associated with peripheral precocious puberty. We consider this secondary central precocious puberty because the activation of the hypothalamic-pituitary-gonadal axis occurs as a phenomenon secondary to the primary peripheral cause of precocious puberty. Patients with uncontrolled congenital adrenal hyperplasia, virilizing adrenal tumors, McCune-Albright syndrome, familial male precocious puberty, ovarian tumors, and exogenous sex steroid exposure have all been reported to develop central precocious puberty, usually after successful treatment of the primary disorder has lowered the sex steroid levels *(60–63)*. The mechanism responsible for activation of the GnRH neurosecretory neurons in these cases is unknown. It has been hypothesized that "maturation" of the axis leads to disinhibition of the GnRH pulse generator. The degree of bone age advancement appears to be correlated with the onset of CPP. The majority of reported cases have had bone ages in excess of 10 yr at onset of central activation. An exception is the report of a 5 yr old girl who developed CPP at a bone age of only 5.5 yr following removal of an ovarian tumor that had been diagnosed at 7 mo of age.

The evaluation of a child with premature sexual development includes a detailed medical and family history and a history of potential exogenous sex steroid exposure. Prior growth data are invaluable in determining if growth acceleration has occurred. A thorough physical examination to accurately document growth parameters as well to assess for the presence of acne, adult body odor, breast development, axillary and pubic hair, estrogenization of the vaginal mucosa, and physiologic leukorrhea is critical. A bone age determination to evaluate the degree of skeletal maturation is essential for both diagnosis and long-term therapy.

The "gold standard" for detecting activation of the hypothalamic-pituitary-gonadal axis is a GnRH stimulation test. In the most widely utilized version of this test, synthetic GnRH (Factrel®) is administered intravenously and gonadotropin levels are drawn at baseline and at subsequent intervals over one hour. A quiescent axis under tonic inhibition does not respond to a single GnRH stimulus, an activated axis generates a brisk response in gonadotropins and, consequently, sex steroids. Variations on this method have utilized subcutaneous GnRH followed by a single measurement for gonadotropins *(64)* and the use of GnRH agonists, such as leuprolide and nafarelin to induce gonadotropin release *(65–67)*. Although an "LH predominance" is classical in CPP, intermediary responses have been described in early puberty and premature thelarche. Higher sensitivity assays have more recently revealed that circulating LH and FSH levels are pulsatile in prepubertal children, albeit at much lower frequencies and pulse amplitudes *(68–71)*. Peripubertal increases in LH are first seen at night followed by greater increases in daytime levels *(72)*. The recent development of ultra-sensitive LH assays may be sufficient to differentiate prepubertal from pubertal levels of gonadotropins, without the aid of GnRH stimulation of the pituitary gonadotropes, thus replacing the need for a GnRH stimulation test.

If CPP is suspected, a cranial MRI is indicated to determine the anatomy of the hypothalamic-pituitary area and to rule out potential pathology. A bone age radiograph will indicate the degree of sex-steroid exposure and consequent to skeletal maturation with ascertainment of growth potential. Pelvic ultrasonography can reveal adrenal and ovarian lesions and can document ovarian and uterine size. Multiple studies have shown that 53–80% of prepubertal females have small (<9 mm) ovarian cysts. Cyst size does not vary with age, and the finding of multiple cysts within a single ovary is not rare. Pubertal ultrasound findings include a uterine length greater than 3.5 cm and a fundus to cervix ratio of >1 on midline endometrial measurement *(73)*.

Therapy for gonadotropin-dependent precocious puberty must first address the etiology of the disorder. Consultation with experienced pediatric oncologists and/or pediatric neurosurgeons should be sought for potentially invasive CNS lesions. Early exposure of the epiphyses to elevated estrogen in the female and the male (via aromatization of androgens) leads to premature epiphyseal fusion and a compromise in adult height. Thus, a decision to treat a child is primarily based on the risk for adult short stature. Secondarily, treatment is aimed at reducing the rate of progression of secondary sexual development.

Until the early 1980s, therapy for CPP was limited to progestational agents such as medroxyprogesterone acetate (MPA, Provera®). They act by interfering with steroidogenesis and directly inhibiting both GnRH and gonadotrope secretion. Although they were successful in preventing menses and providing at least partial regression of secondary sexual characteristics, they were unsuccessful in slowing skeletal maturation with the resultant effect being a compromise in final height. "Super-agonist" therapy with long-acting GnRH analogs is currently the most widely used and effective therapy for CPP. These agents were initially utilized in the treatment of prostate cancer because they induce a "medical gonadectomy" and limit the further growth of testosterone-responsive tumors. Modification of the GnRH decapeptide in the sixth and tenth positions results in greater receptor affinity with resultant increases in GnRH potency and duration of action. The rapid and sustained binding of these analogs to GnRH receptors typically causes a brief (<4–6 wk) stimulation of gonadotrope release and sex steroid production, followed by a consequent decrease in LH and FSH, which results in a decrease in gonadal sex steroid production and release. The frequent administration required of early generation subcutaneous and intranasal agonists led to difficulties in maintaining compliance and, on occasion, there was actually progression of pubertal development secondary to intermittent agonist administration. Currently, the most widely used agent in the US is Lupron® (depot leuprolide acetate) given as 0.2–0.3 mg/kg im every 28 d. Adequacy of therapy is assessed by clinical, radiographic and biochemical means. Slowing the rate of breast and pubic hair development is common and gonadotropin and sex steroid levels are suppressed *(74)*. The return of ovarian and uterine volumes to age appropriate sizes usually occurs within 6 mo of initiation of therapy. Similarly, testicular volume decreases in boys. Children treated with GnRH analogs achieve significant long-term improvements in adult height when compared with predicted adult height at the start of therapy and with untreated historic controls *(75–77)*. Studies to document final height data are vital because the predicted adult height at the completion of therapy frequently overestimates final height. This may be a consequence of rapid pubertal progression occurring after agonist therapy is discontinued *(78)*.

Following initiation of GnRH agonist therapy, there is a deceleration in growth velocity. On occasion, especially when the bone age is greater than 11 yr, the growth velocity is significantly decreased (<4 cm/yr). This has led to investigation of the role of sex steroids in the GHRH - growth hormone axis *(79,80)*. In a number of studies, addition of growth hormone therapy has been shown to improve growth velocity and predicted adult height *(81)*. The effect on final height remains a topic of debate, but should be clarified within the next few years as ongoing studies are concluded. GnRH agonist therapy may decrease bone mineral density (BMD) somewhat during the course of therapy. However, most reports indicate that BMD remains normal within the range for chronologic age and/or bone age during therapy *(82)* and at the attainment of final height *(83)*. For the individual clinician and patient, it is important to weigh the potential benefit in height against the financial cost of this therapy.

Although there is a single report that suggests an increased risk for the development of PCOS in girls with a history of CPP treated with GnRH agonists, this finding has not been confirmed by other investigators *(84)*.

The decision as to the appropriate time to discontinue GnRHa therapy should be reached by individualized discussions between the physician and the family. The most important factors include the child's predicted adult height and the child's maturity level and ability to adjust to progressive sexual development and, for girls, menstrual cycles. Most girls experience menarche and develop appropriate ovulatory cycles within 1–2 yr of terminating therapy *(85)*.

PERIPHERAL PRECOCIOUS PUBERTY

It is important to differentiate gonadotropin-dependent and gonadotropin-independent forms of puberty because the differential diagnosis and therapeutic approach differ. Peripheral precocious puberty or gonadotropin-independent precocious puberty can arise from a variety of disorders (Table 2). They range from exposure to exogenous sex steroids to carcinomas. The diagnostic and therapeutic approaches to these children are dependent on the sex of the child and whether there are signs of virilization, feminization or both. Prolonged sex-steroid exposure may cause maturation of the hypothalamic-pituitary-gonadal (HPG) axis and lead to CPP secondarily.

Exogenous Sex Steroid Exposure

The evaluation of every child with sexual precocity should include a thorough review of potential exposure to exogenous sex steroids. Ingestion of oral contraceptives, estrogen contaminated foods, and topical exposure to transdermal preparations of estrogens and androgens have all been shown to be capable of causing gonadotropin-independent precocious puberty *(86–88)*. Recent investigations have also suggested that specific environmental pollutants may exhibit estrogenic effects and might be causes of premature sexual development *(33)*.

Ovarian Cysts

Before widespread use of ultrasound imaging, the pre-pubertal ovary was believed to be dormant and the frequency of ovarian cysts among pre-pubertal girls was thought to be low. It is now appreciated that the ovary undergoes continuous change from fetal development to puberty and through adulthood. In utero, follicular cysts develop under maternal, placental, and fetal hormones. Cysts have be been detected as early as 28 wk of gestation. After birth and removal from hormonal stimulus, regression of both follicular and luteinized cysts often occurs. Small follicular cysts (<9 mm) are present throughout childhood *(89)* and 50–80% of prepubertal girls have small cysts detected by ultrasound. Cyst size does not appear to vary with age and multiple cysts within a homogeneous ovary are not uncommon. Cysts are bilateral in up to 23% of cases and usually suggest gonadotropin stimulation rather that intraovarian stimuli. Typically prepubertal cysts do not release appreciable quantities of estrogen however they may become transiently functional, thereby elevating estradiol levels and causing transient breast development.

McCune-Albright Syndrome

McCune-Albright syndrome (MAS) is characterized by the triad of gonadotropin-independent precocious puberty, polyostotic fibrous dysplasia of bone, and irregular café au lait lesions ("Coast of Maine") *(90)*. However, the syndrome is occasionally difficult to diagnose due to its variable phenotypic expression. The clinical findings result from the autonomous hyperactivity of tissues that produce products regulated by intracellular accumulation of cyclic adenosine monophosphate (cAMP). The constitutive over-production of cAMP is caused by an autosomal dominant somatic mutation of the alpha subunit of the stimulatory guanine nucleotide binding protein (G-protein), $G_s\alpha$ *(91,92)*. The guanosine triphosphate (GTP) binding proteins consist of three subunits (α, β, and γ). The activated α-subunit stimulates adenylate cyclase, increasing the production of cAMP. It also acts as a guanosine triphosphatase, catalyzing the hydrolysis of bound guanosine triphosphate to guanosine diphosphate and inactivating the G-protein. Normally, this leads to a decrease of intracellular cAMP and resetting of cellular quiescence. The mutation resulting in MAS leads to unrestrained production of gene products derived from the affected cells. The defect occurs early during embryogenesis and leads to mosaicism. The distribution of the progeny of the affected somatic cell determines the cell types affected and the phenotype of the individual patient.

Mutations of the $G_s\alpha$ gene are found in both endocrine and non-endocrine tissues of patients with MAS *(93)*. The clinical presentation is extremely variable ranging from patients with multiple endocrine and non-endocrine abnormalities to hyperfunction of the ovary alone *(94)*. Affected endocrine organs may include the gonads, thyroid, adrenals, pituitary, and parathyroids *(95–97)*. Non-endocrine disorders may include hepatobiliary dysfunction, hyperplasia of the thymus, spleen, and pancreas, gastrointestinal polyps, and abnormal cardiac muscle cells *(98)*. MAS also can present with only fibrous dysplasia lesions of bone and precocious puberty in the absence of cutaneous lesions *(95)*.

The inheritance of MAS is sporadic and has been reported in all ethnic groups *(99)*. It is most frequently diagnosed in females, although it occurs in both sexes *(100)*. The most common presentation is a girl with precocious puberty secondary to estrogen production of autonomously functioning ovarian tissue *(101)*. Vaginal bleeding may appear as the result of spontaneous cyst regression or unopposed estrogen leading to breakthrough bleeding. Menses have rarely been reported to occur prior to significant breast development *(99)*.

Laboratory evaluation of MAS children with precocious pubertal development reveals periodic elevations of sex steroids with prepubertal gonadotropin levels. GnRH stimulation test results indicate that gonadotropin levels are suppressed, unless sufficient sex steroid exposure has occurred to cause secondary maturation of the HPG axis (central precocious puberty).

The variable presentation of the precocious puberty in children with MAS and the waxing and waning nature of the autonomous gonadal function have made assessment of therapy difficult. In the absence of hypothalamic activation, the precocious puberty of MAS is unresponsive to GnRH analog therapy. However, in cases of "secondary CPP," GnRH agonist therapy has proven beneficial *(62,102)*. Therapeutic interventions have focused on ameliorating the hyperestrogenic state by inhibiting estrogen production or blocking estrogen action. Cyproterone acetate, a steroidal antiandrogen possessing progestin and antiestrogenic effects, has been used in Europe with limited success *(103)*. It has been reported to modestly control breast development and menses; however, growth velocity and skeletal maturation were unaffected. Testolactone, a weak aromatase inhibitor, has been reported to effectively decrease estrogen levels, prevent menses, and also improve predicted height *(104)*. Unfortunately, compliance has been hindered by side effects (headache, diarrhea, and typically transient abdominal cramping), the large number of pills required to achieve adequate dosing, and a rapid increase in serum estradiol levels with cessation of therapy *(105)*. Ongoing studies are investigating the use of potent aromatase inhibitors. Our own experience has suggested that the nonsteroidal estrogen-antiestrogen tamoxifen may have a role in the suppression of estrogen action and precocious puberty in patients with MAS, with results superior to those achieved with aromatase inhibitors (106). Despite these difficulties, female MAS patients can achieve normal menses and fertility and mildly affected patients have achieved normal adult height. The skeletal lesions generally increase in severity and number with increasing age in childhood and then stabilize after puberty. Adult patients may suffer conductive hearing loss secondary to temporal bone sclerosis. In severe cases, Cushing syndrome, growth hormone excess, and the bone disease cause significant morbidity. Anecdotally, there appears to be an increased prevalence of breast cancer in young women who had a prior history of precocious puberty (author's observations).

Familial Male Precocious Puberty

Familial Male Precocious Puberty (FMPP), or testotoxicosis, is a male-limited form of gonadotropin-independent precocious puberty. It is caused by a heterozygous mutation of the LH receptor, leading to constitutive activation in Leydig cells. Mutations have been identified in the first, second, third, fifth, and sixth transmembrane domains, and in the third intracellular loop of the receptor *(107–111)*. The Leydig cell produces testosterone constitutively despite suppressed gonadotropins. Mutations are typically autosomal dominant, however, sporadic mutations have also been identified *(112)*. The finding that females with these mutations do not manifest precocious puberty is not surprising given that both LH and FSH are required for ovarian sex steroid production *(95)*. It is interesting to note that no other signs of LH hypersecretion in females, such as polycystic ovarian syndrome, have been reported.

Boys with FMPP typically present by 4 yr of age with a family history of precocious puberty in males, progressive virilization (acne, pubic and axillary hair, modest testicular enlargement, penile growth, increased musculature, bone age advancement), spermatogenesis, and growth acceleration. The testes are small for the degree of virilization and demonstrate Leydig cell hyperplasia *(113)*. Serum testosterone levels are in the adult male range and baseline and GnRH stimulated gonadotropin levels are suppressed *(114)*. These boys mature rapidly and premature epiphyseal fusion causes short stature. Fertility is generally normal, but oligospermia and testicular dysfunction have been reported in some adult patients *(115–117)*.

Therapy targeting androgen synthesis and action has been fairly effective. Early therapy utilized medroxyprogesterone acetate (MPA) *(118)* to inhibit steroidogenesis. It was modestly effective in decreasing testosterone levels and decreasing growth velocity. However, its effects on glucocorticoid synthesis and testicular morphology limit its application. More effective therapies include ketoconazole *(119)* (an antifungal and inhibitor of the 17,20 lyase activity of P450c17 - Fig. 6), and a combination of spironolactone (an androgen receptor blocker) and testolactone (an aromatase inhibitor) *(120)*. Ketoconazole has been associated with toxicity (rash, nausea, headache, hepatotoxicity, pneumonitis, and renal failure) and requires careful monitoring *(121)*. The addition of an aromatase inhibitor to the anti-androgen treatment is necessary because the elevated androgens may undergo aromatization leading to feminization and an enhanced estrogen effect on skeletal maturation. As in MAS, GnRH agonist therapy is indicated if CPP occurs following long-term sex steroid level elevations *(122)*.

Congenital Adrenal Hyperplasia

Congenital adrenal hyperplasia (CAH) is the result of an autosomal recessive defect in one of a number of steroidogenic enzymes necessary for cortisol production (Fig. 6). As detailed above, non-optimal glucocorticoid therapy of patients with classical CAH, and partial defects in P450c21, P450c11AS, and 3 beta-hydroxysteroid dehydrogenase (3βHSD) insufficient to cause phenotypic changes in the neonate may lead to increased adrenal androgen synthesis later in life and presentation of non-classical CAH (NCAH).

Tumors

Although sex steroid producing tumors are rare in children, their diagnosis is critical. The presentation depends upon the tumor location and the class and quantity of the sex steroids produced.

OVARIAN TUMORS

Primary ovarian tumors are quite rare in children although they comprise approximately 6% of all tumors in adult women. The neoplasms may originate from sex-chord/stromal tissue, epithelium, or the germ-cell line *(123)*. Granulosa-cell tumors account for 5% of all ovarian tumors, but the juvenile variety is the most common before 20 yr of age. The most common presentation of juvenile granulosa cell tumors is precocious puberty, frequently in a precipitous manner of weeks to months. The mean age of presentation is 10 yr, but ovarian tumors have been discovered in infants *(124)*. The majority of ovarian tumors produce estrogen, causing feminization, but they may also produce androgens, causing virilization *(123,125)*. Tumors frequently cause local symptoms including pain, distension, ascites, and mass effects. The frequency of precocious puberty varies but has been reported to be as high as 70% in one series of 17 granulosa/theca cell tumors *(126)*. The diagnosis is usually based upon the identification of a solid ovarian mass and an elevated serum estradiol in conjunction with suppressed gonadotropins. The association between CPP and granulosa cell tumors prompted the recent examination of 4 females with juvenile granulosa cell tumors. No activating mutations were identified in exon 10 and it was suggested that activating mutations at other exons of the FSH receptor or associated G proteins might be responsible for granulosa cell tumors *(127)*. Surgical resection with a unilateral salpingo-oophorectomy is typically the only required therapy and carries a good prognosis, particularly in the case of juvenile granulosa-cell tumors. Pubertal regression should ensue.

TESTICULAR TUMORS

Leydig cell tumors account for only 3% of all testicular neoplasms *(128)*, but they are the most common gonadal stromal tumors associated with precocious puberty in boys. Although 10% of these tumors are malignant, they are typically benign in children. Boys usually present between 5–9 yr of age with virilization, palpable unilateral testicular enlargement, and elevated testosterone levels. The rare Sertoli cell tumor, most commonly seen in Peutz-Jeghers syndrome, may present with gynecomastia in addition to virilization *(129)*. Surgical resection of these tumors will halt pubertal development *(130)*. It should be noted that testicular adrenal rest hyperplasia in the male with poorly controlled CAH may present with testicular enlargement (more commonly bilateral) secondary to the stimulatory effects of elevated ACTH levels. ACTH and GnRH stimulation testing and testicular ultrasound and biopsy may be necessary in order to distinguish adrenal rest tissue from other tumors.

ADRENAL TUMORS

Adrenal tumors typically present with virilization however feminization may occur *(131)*. As noted above in the segment on premature pubarche, adrenal tumors may be differentiated from CAH, as they do not typically respond to ACTH stimulation or glucocorticoid suppression. Adrenal adenomas often produce DHEAS, whereas androstenedione and testosterone are the primary products of carcinomas. Surgical resection is often curative with resolution of the precocious puberty. However, chemotherapy may be required if there is evidence of tumor extension or in the event of recurrence.

hCG-PRODUCING TUMORS

Human chorionic gonadotropin (hCG) and LH possess identical α subunits and similar β subunits. It is therefore not surprising that germ cell tumors secreting hCG may cause precocious puberty. They have been reported to arise in the liver *(132)*, lungs *(133)*, mediastinum *(134)*, pineal gland *(135)*, basal ganglia, thalamus, and hypothalamus *(136)*. In boys, hCG simulates Leydig cell production of testosterone. Precocious puberty in the setting of hCG producing tumors is quite rare in females because both LH and FSH are typically required for ovarian follicular development. The one reported case of a female with a suprasellar germinoma was explained by the demonstration of aromatase activity in the tumor *(137)*. An hCG secreting tumor should be suspected in a boy presenting with marked virilization but without significant testicular enlargement. Hepatoblastomas comprise the majority of these tumors although hCG may arise from pinealomas, intracranial germinomas or choriocarcinomas, and thymic or testicular germ cell tumors *(138)*. Tumor markers that have been quite useful in the diagnosis and follow-up of these tumors include: alpha-fetoprotein, human chorionic gonadotropin

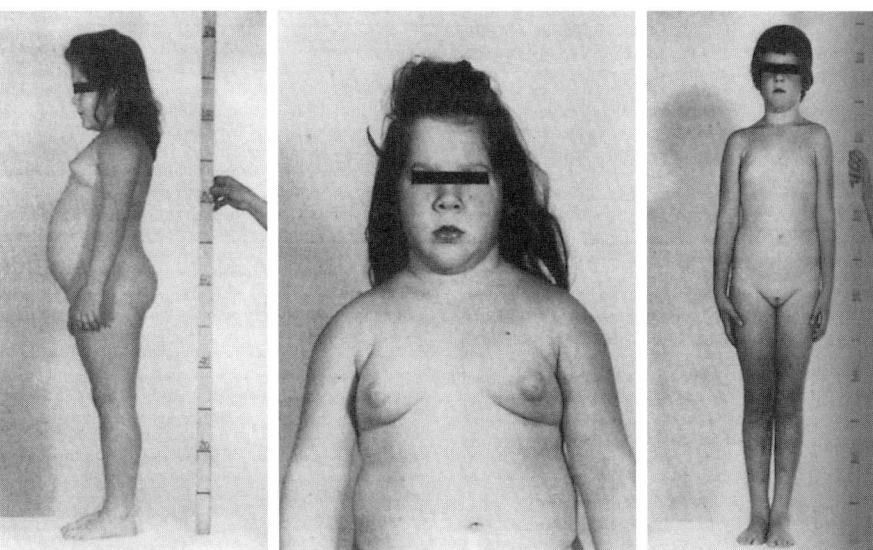

Fig. 7. Left and center, Precocious puberty in a 7 1/2 year old female with severe, chronic hypothyroidism secondary to autoimmune thyroiditis presenting with breast development, vaginal bleeding, and galactorrhea. (height, –1SD; bone age 5 3/12 yr) Right, Identical female after 8 mo of thyroid hormone replacement therapy. Her height increased 7 cm, she had a decrease in breast size, and cessation of galactorrhea. (From Williams Textbook of Endocrinology, 9th Edition. 1998. WB Saunders; with permission.)

(hCG), and pregnancy specific beta 1-glycoprotein *(139)*. The diagnosis of an extra-testicular germ cell tumor should prompt an evaluation for Klinefelter syndrome because such tumors are 50 times more common in these individuals *(140)*. This increased tumor risk has been identified even in those males with low level mosaicism for Klinefelter syndrome *(138)*.

Severe Hypothyroidism

Severe hypothyroidism may rarely present with precocious puberty (Van Wyk-Grumbach Syndrome). The cardinal sign of this disorder is the child presenting with sexual precocity, poor growth and skeletal delay. Girls may present with breast development, galactorrhea, ovarian cysts, and vaginal bleeding *(141,142)* (Fig. 7). Boys may develop testicular enlargement with minimal virilization. Thyroid hormone replacement results in regression of the secondary sexual characteristics with the exception of the macroorchidism *(143)*. The mechanism for the sexual precocity is still somewhat unclear. There is evidence for mechanisms at both the gonadal and pituitary levels; cross-reaction of high levels of TSH and α-subunit can occur at the gonadal FSH receptor *(144)* and stimulation of gonadotrope FSH secretion may occur by elevated TRH levels *(143)*. We have seen several patients with primary hypothyroidism and precocious puberty that had a pubertal gonadotropin profile classical for central precocious puberty.

Gynecomastia

The reported prevalence of pubertal gynecomastia in boys has ranged from 30 to >90% *(145)*. Prepubertal gynecomastia, on the contrary, is quite rare and almost always abnormal. The published data report an age of onset between 2–7 yr with both unilateral

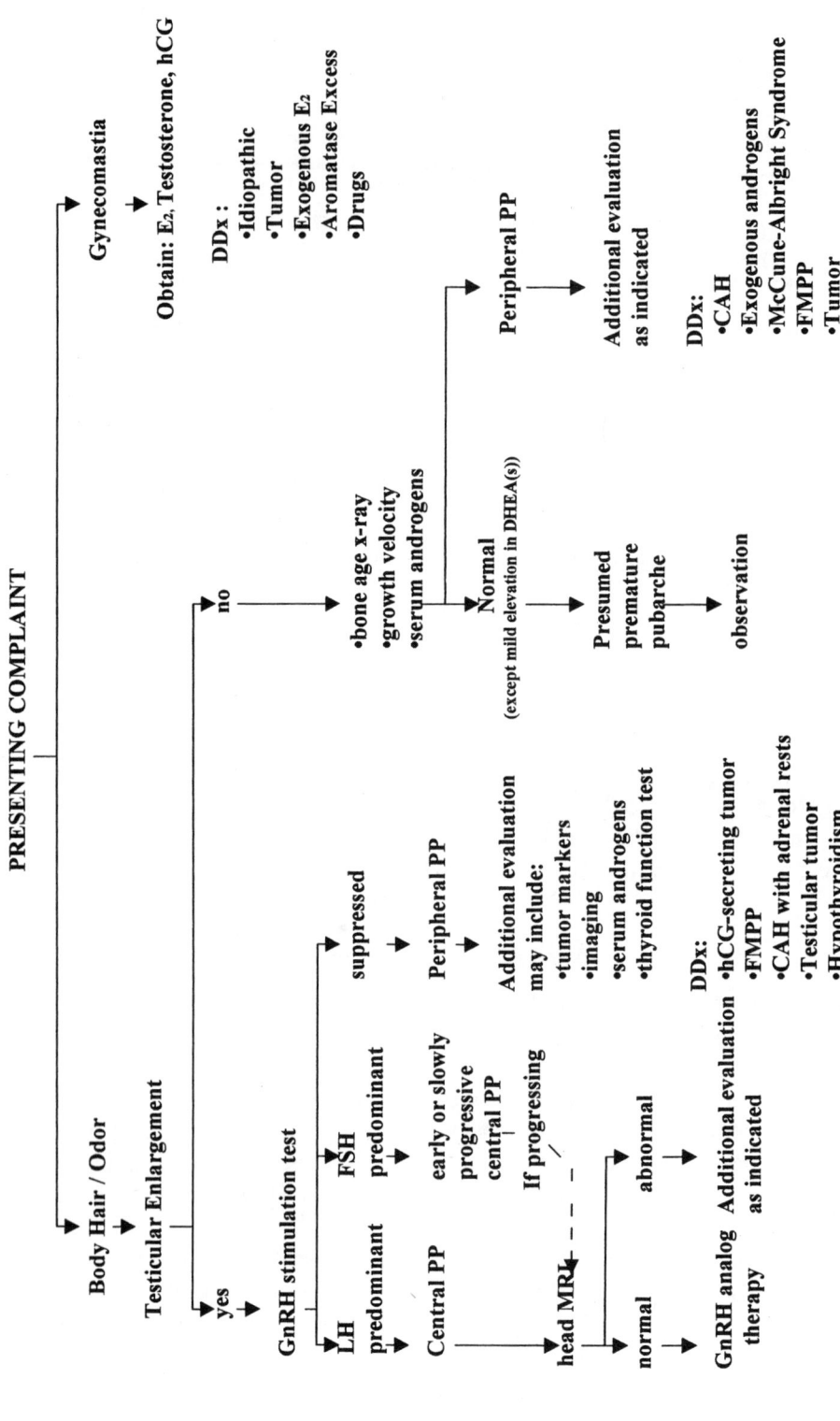

Fig. 8. Diagnostic Approach to Evaluation of Precocious Puberty in Boys. (Adapted from Eugster EA and Pescovitz OH. Precocious Puberty. In: *Endocrinology 4th Edition*, WB Saunders Co., 2000:2011–2021; with permission.)

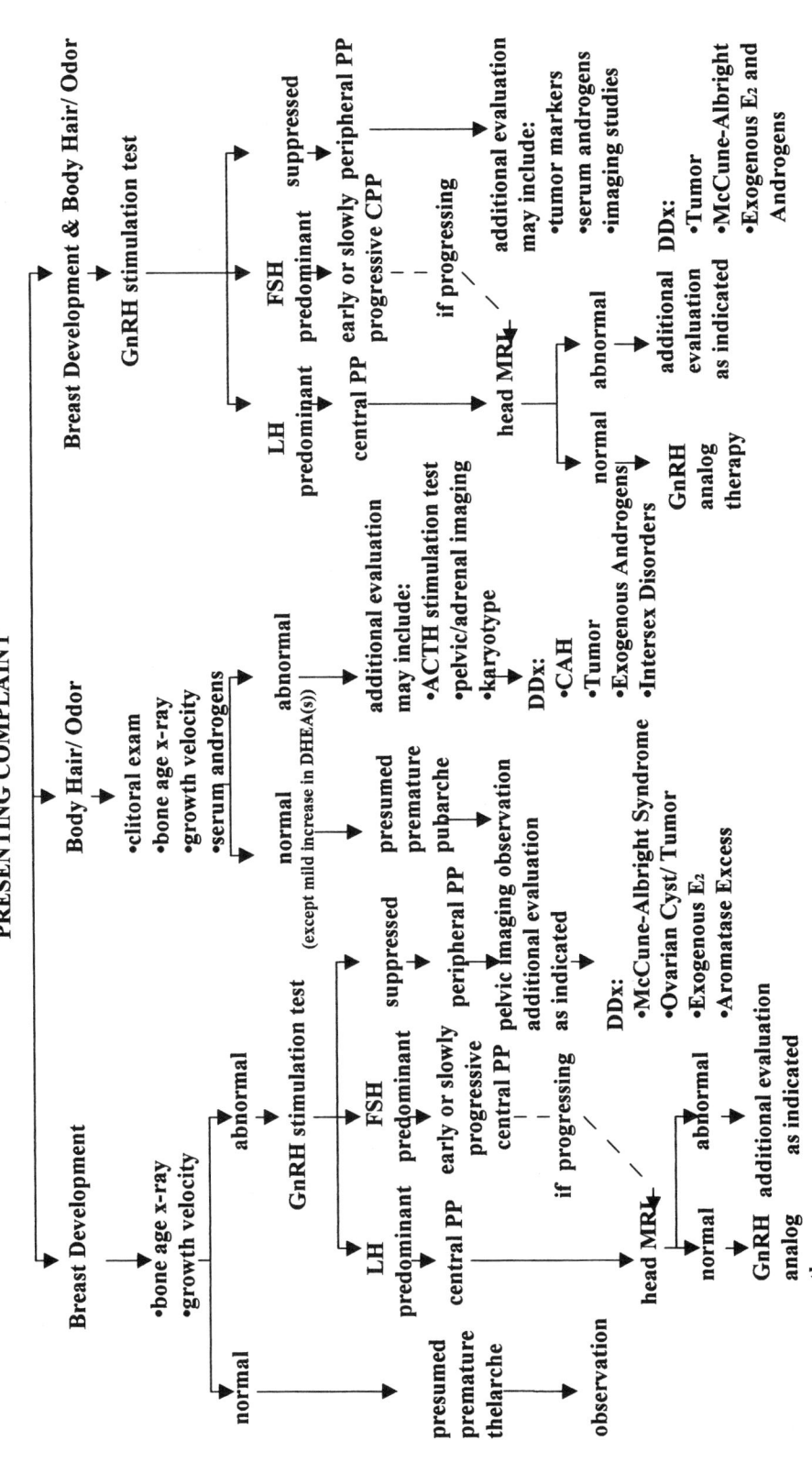

Fig. 9. Diagnostic Approach to Evaluation of Precocious Puberty in Girls. (Adapted from Eugster EA and Pescovitz OH. Precocious Puberty. In: *Endocrinology 4th Edition*, WB Saunders Co., 2000:2011–2021; with permission.)

and bilateral breast development. The etiologies include gonadal, adrenal, and hCG-secreting tumors *(146)*, exogenous estrogen exposure *(88,147,148)*, and "idiopathic" *(149)*. It is likely that some familial cases of gynecomastia are secondary to an aromatase excess syndrome *(150)*. A thorough evaluation for sex steroid origin is required in the male with prepubertal gynecomastia. Tumor excision permits pubertal regression. In the case of idiopathic gynecomastia, surgical excision of glandular tissue is curative. Antiestrogens or aromatase inhibitors are currently being investigated for this indication.

CONCLUSION

Physicians involved in the care of children commonly encounter premature sexual development. The first step in evaluating such a child is the ascertainment of secondary sexual characteristics through a thorough physical examination. Isolated breast development in a female between 12–30 mo of age may be benign premature thelarche. On the other hand, accelerated linear growth and advanced skeletal maturation suggest a more serious or progressive disorder. Isolated virilization in a female indicates excess androgen production. Arriving at a correct diagnosis permits the selection of the appropriate therapy.

Although we have gained much insight into the diagnosis and management of precocious puberty, numerous areas of controversy remain. The age of onset of normal puberty is still being hotly debated. GnRHa therapy has revolutionized treatment for children with central precocious puberty. For some girls with idiopathic central precocious puberty, progression can be quite slow, without an apparent compromise in final height *(151–154)*. Follow-up of these select patients suggests that therapeutic intervention may not be warranted *(41,155,156)*. Advances have been made in the molecular diagnosis of several forms of gonadotropin-independent precocious puberty. However, therapy for these disorders remains suboptimal. While much has been learned, much remains to be discovered.

REFERENCES

1. Grumbach MM, Kaplan SL. Recent advances in the diagnosis and management of sexual precocity. Acta Paediatr Jpn 1988;30(Suppl):155–175.
2. Schwanzel-Fukuda M, et al. Migration of luteinizing hormone-releasing hormone (LHRH) neurons in early human embryos. J Comp Neurol 1996;366:547–557.
3. Plant TM, et al. The arcuate nucleus and the control of gonadotropin and prolactin secretion in the female rhesus monkey (Macaca mulatta). Endocrinology 1978;102(1):52–62.
4. Mueller PL, et al. Hormone ontogeny in the ovine fetus. IX. Luteinizing hormone and follicle-stimulating hormone response to luteinizing hormone-releasing factor in mid- and late gestation and in the neonate. Endocrinology 1981;108(3):881–886.
5. Sklar CA, et al. Hormone ontogeny in the ovine fetus. VII. Circulating luteinizing hormone and follicle-stimulating hormone in mid- and late gestation. Endocrinology 1981;108(3):874–880.
6. Winter JS, et al. Gonadotrophins and steroid hormones in the blood and urine of prepubertal girls and other primates. Clin Endocrinol Metab 1978;7(3):513–530.
7. Zsarmovsky AH, Garcia-Segura TL, Horvath LM, Naftolin BF. Plasticity of the hypothalamic GABA system and their relationship with GnRH neurons during positive gonadotropin feedback in non-human primates in 82nd Annual Meeting of the Endocrine Society. 2000. Toronto, Ontario, Canada.
8. Zhang SJ, MB. GABA-activated chloride channels in secretory nerve endings. Science 1993;259:531–534.
9. Terasawa EF, DL. Neurobiological Mechanisms of the Onset of Puberty in Primates. Endocrine Reviews 2001;22(1):p. 111–151.

10. Dhom G. The prepuberal and puberal growth of the adrenal (adrenarche). Beitr Pathol 1973; 150(4):357–77.
11. Sklar CA, Kaplan SL, Grumbach MM. Evidence for dissociation between adrenarche and gonadarche: studies in patients with idiopathic precocious puberty, gonadal dysgenesis, isolated gonadotropin deficiency, and constitutionally delayed growth and adolescence. J Clin Endocrinol Metab 1980;51(3):548–556.
12. James VHT. The Endocrine function of the human adrenal cortex. Proceedings of the Serono Symposia; v. 18. 1978, London; New York: Academic Press. ix, 628.
13. Zhang LH, et al. Serine phosphorylation of human P450c17 increases 17,20-lyase activity: implications for adrenarche and the polycystic ovary syndrome. Proc Natl Acad Sci USA 1995;92 (23):10,619–10,623.
14. Miller WL, Auchus RJ, Geller DH. The regulation of 17,20 lyase activity. Steroids 1997;62(1): 133–142.
15. Braunstein GD. Gynecomastia. N Engl J Med 1993;328(7):490–495.
16. Herman-Giddens ME, et al. Secondary sexual characteristics and menses in young girls seen in office practice: a study from the Pediatric Research in Office Settings network. Pediatrics 1997;99(4): 505–512.
17. Biro FM, Striegel-Moore RP, Crawford R, Obarzanek PB, Morrison E, JA. Impact of timing of pubertal maturation on growth in black and white female adolescents: the National Heart, Lung, and Blood Institute Growth and Health Study. J Pediatr 2001;138:636–643.
18. Kaplowitz PB, Oberfield SE. Reexamination of the age limit for defining when puberty is precocious in girls in the United States: implications for evaluation and treatment. Drug and Therapeutics and Executive Committees of the Lawson Wilkins Pediatric Endocrine Society. Pediatrics 1999; 104(4 Pt 1):936–941.
19. Rosenfield RL, et al. Current age of onset of puberty [letter]. Pediatrics 2000;106(3):622–623.
20. Ibanez L, et al. Postpubertal outcome in girls diagnosed of premature pubarche during childhood: increased frequency of functional ovarian hyperandrogenism. J Clin Endocrinol Metab 1993; 76(6):1599–1603.
21. Ibanez L, et al. Girls diagnosed with premature pubarche show an exaggerated ovarian androgen synthesis from the early stages of puberty: evidence from gonadotropin-releasing hormone agonist testing. Fertil Steril 1997;67(5):849–855.
22. Ibanez L, de Zegher F, Potau N. Premature pubarche, ovarian hyperandrogenism, hyperinsulinism and the polycystic ovary syndrome: from a complex constellation to a simple sequence of prenatal onset. J Endocrinol Invest 1998;21(9):558–566.
23. Ibanez L, et al. Hyperinsulinaemia, dyslipaemia and cardiovascular risk in girls with a history of premature pubarche. Diabetologia 1998;41(9):1057–1063.
24. Ibanez L, Potau N, De Zegher F. Endocrinology and metabolism after premature pubarche in girls. Acta Paediatr Suppl 1999;88(433):73–77.
25. Ibanez L, Potau N, de Zegher F. Recognition of a new association: reduced fetal growth, precocious pubarche, hyperinsulinism and ovarian dysfunction. Ann Endocrinol (Paris) 2000;61(2):141–142.
26. Volta C, et al. Isolated premature thelarche and thelarche variant: clinical and auxological follow-up of 119 girls. J Endocrinol Invest 1998;21(3):180–183.
27. Ilicki A, et al. Premature thelarche—natural history and sex hormone secretion in 68 girls. Acta Paediatr Scand 1984;73(6):756–762.
28. Pasquino AM, et al. Progression of premature thelarche to central precocious puberty. J Pediatr 1995;126(1):11–14.
29. Mills JL, et al. Premature thelarche. Natural history and etiologic investigation. Am J Dis Child 1981;135(8):743–745.
30. Rosenfield RL. Normal and almost normal precocious variations in pubertal development premature pubarche and premature thelarche revisited. Horm Res 1994;41(Suppl 2):7–13.
31. Jenner MR, et al. Hormonal changes in puberty IV. Plasma estradiol, LH, and FSH in prepubertal children, pubertal females, and in precocious puberty, premature thelarche, hypogonadism, and in a child with a feminizing ovarian tumor. J Clin Endocrinol Metab 1972;34(3):521–530.
32. Escobar ME, Rivarola MA, Bergada C. Plasma concentration of oestradiol-17beta in premature thelarche and in different types of sexual precocity. Acta Endocrinol (Copenh) 1976;81(2):351–361.
33. Colon I, et al. Identification of phthalate esters in the serum of young puerto rican girls with premature breast development [In Process Citation]. Environ Health Perspect 2000;108(9):895–900.

34. Belgorosky A, Chaler E, Rivarola MA. High serum sex hormone-binding globulin (SHBG) in premature thelarche. Clin Endocrinol (Oxf) 1992;37(3):203–206.
35. Pescovitz OH, et al. Premature thelarche and central precocious puberty: the relationship between clinical presentation and the gonadotropin response to luteinizing hormone-releasing hormone. J Clin Endocrinol Metab 1988;67(3):474–479.
36. Wang C, et al. Serum bioactive follicle-stimulating hormone levels in girls with precocious sexual development. J Clin Endocrinol Metab 1990;70(3):615–619.
37. Verrotti A, et al. Premature thelarche: a long-term follow-up. Gynecol Endocrinol 1996;10(4):241–247.
38. Aritaki S, et al. A comparison of patients with premature thelarche and idiopathic true precocious puberty in the initial stage of illness. Acta Paediatr Jpn 1997;39(1):21–27.
39. Orley JN, Goblyos P. Modern imaging methods in paediatric breast examination. Ceska Gynekol 1995;60(3):153–157.
40. Salardi S, et al. Outcome of premature thelarche: relation to puberty and final height. Arch Dis Child 1998;79(2):173–174.
41. Palmert MR, Malin HV, Boepple PA. Unsustained or slowly progressive puberty in young girls: initial presentation and long-term follow-up of 20 untreated patients. J Clin Endocrinol Metab 1999;84(2):415–423.
42. Ibanez L, et al. Precocious pubarche, hyperinsulinism, and ovarian hyperandrogenism in girls: relation to reduced fetal growth. J Clin Endocrinol Metab 1998;83(10):3558–3562.
43. Francois I, de Zegher F. Adrenarche and fetal growth. Pediatr Res 1997;41:440–442.
44. Ibanez L, Potau N, de Zegher F. Precocious pubarche, dyslipidemia, and low IGF binding protein-1 in girls: relation to reduced prenatal growth. Pediatr Res 1999;46(3):320–322.
45. Barker DJ, HC, Fall CH. Type 2 (non-insulin-dependent) diabetes mellitus, hpertension and hyperlipidemia (syndrome X): relation to reduced fetal growth. Diabetologia 1993;36:62–67.
46. Hawkins LC, Blethen FI, SL. The role of adrenocorticotropin testing in evaluating girls with premature adrenarche and hirsutism/oligomenorrhea. J Clin Endocrinol Metab 1992;74:248–253.
47. Speiser PD, Rubenstein R, Piazza P, Kastelan A, New A, MI. High frequency of nonclassical steroid 21-hydroxylase deficiency. Am J Hum Genet 1985;37:650–667.
48. Likitmaskul SC, Donaghue CT, K, Exaggerated adrenarche in children presenting with premature adrenarche. Clin Endocrinol 1995;42:265–272.
49. Temeck JW, et al. Genetic defects of steroidogenesis in premature pubarche. J Clin Endocrinol Metab 1987;64(3):609–617.
50. Sizonenko PC, Paunier L. Hormonal changes in puberty III: Correlation of plasma dehydroepiandrosterone, testosterone, FSH, and LH with stages of puberty and bone age in normal boys and girls and in patients with Addison's disease or hypogonadism or with premature or late adrenarche. J Clin Endocrinol Metab 1975;41(5):894–904.
51. Nestler JJ, DJ. Decreases in ovarian cytochrome P450c17 alpha activity and serum free testosterone after reduction of insulin secretion in polycystic ovary syndrome. N Engl J Med 1996;1996(29): 617–623.
52. Moghetti, P.C., R Negri, C, Metformin effects on clinical features, endocrine and metabolic profiles, and insulin sensitivity in polycystic ovary syndrome: a randomized, double-blind, placebo-controlled 6-month trial, followed by open, long-term clinical evaluation. J Clin Endocrinol Metab 2000;85:139–146.
53. Ibanez LV, Potua C, Marcos N, MV, de Zegher F. Sensitization to insulin in adolescent girls to normalize hirsutism, hyperandrogenism, olgomenorrhia, dyslipidemia, and hperinsulinism after precocious pubarche. J Clin Endocrinol Metab 2000;85:3526–3530.
54. Pescovitz OH, et al. The NIH experience with precocious puberty: diagnostic subgroups and response to short-term luteinizing hormone releasing hormone analogue therapy. J Pediatr 1986;108(1):47–54.
55. Robben SG, et al. Idiopathic isosexual central precocious puberty: magnetic resonance findings in 30 patients. Br J Radiol 1995;68(805):34–38.
56. Mahachoklertwattana P, Kaplan SL, Grumbach MM. The luteinizing hormone-releasing hormone-secreting hypothalamic hamartoma is a congenital malformation: natural history. J Clin Endocrinol Metab 1993;77(1):118–124.
57. Stewart L, Steinbok P, Daaboul J. Role of surgical resection in the treatment of hypothalamic hamartomas causing precocious puberty. Report of six cases. J Neurosurg 1998;88(2):340–345.

58. Habiby R, et al. Precocious puberty in children with neurofibromatosis type 1. J Pediatr 1995;126(3):364–367.
59. Oberfield, S.E., et al., Endocrine late effects of childhood cancers. J Pediatr 1997;131(1 Pt 2):S37–41.
60. Pescovitz OH, et al. True precocious puberty complicating congenital adrenal hyperplasia: treatment with a luteinizing hormone-releasing hormone analog. J Clin Endocrinol Metab 1984;58(5):857–861.
61. Soliman AT, et al. Congenital adrenal hyperplasia complicated by central precocious puberty: linear growth during infancy and treatment with gonadotropin- releasing hormone analog. Metabolism 1997;46(5):513–517.
62. Foster CM, et al. Variable response to a long-acting agonist of luteinizing hormone- releasing hormone in girls with McCune-Albright syndrome. J Clin Endocrinol Metab 1984;59(4):801–805.
63. Holland FJ, SE Kirsch, R Selby, Gonadotropin-independent precocious puberty ("testotoxicosis"): influence of maturational status on response to ketoconazole. J Clin Endocrinol Metab 1987;64(2):328–333.
64. Eckert KL, et al. A single-sample, subcutaneous gonadotropin-releasing hormone test for central precocious puberty. Pediatrics 1996;97(4):517–519.
65. Rosenfield RL, et al. The rapid ovarian secretory response to pituitary stimulation by the gonadotropin-releasing hormone agonist nafarelin in sexual precocity. J Clin Endocrinol Metab 1986;63(6): 1386–1389.
66. Ibanez L, et al. Use of leuprolide acetate response patterns in the early diagnosis of pubertal disorders: comparison with the gonadotropin-releasing hormone test. J Clin Endocrinol Metab 1994;78(1):30–35.
67. Rosenfield RL, et al. Acute hormonal responses to the gonadotropin releasing hormone agonist leuprolide: dose-response studies and comparison to nafarelin—a clinical research center study. J Clin Endocrinol Metab 1996;81(9):3408–3411.
68. Boyar RM, et al. Twenty-four hour patterns of plasma luteinizing hormone and follicle- stimulating hormone in sexual precocity. N Engl J Med 1973;289(6):282–286.
69. Jakacki RK, Sauder RP, Lloyd SE, et al. Pulsatile secretion of luteinizing hormone in children. J Clin Endocrinol Metab 1982;55:453–458.
70. Manasco PU, Muly DM, Godwin SM, et al. Ontogeny of gonadotrophin and inhibin secretion in normal girls through puberty based on overnight serial sampling and comparison with normal boys. Hum Reprod 1997;12:2108–2114.
71. Mitamura RY, Suzuki K, Ito N, Makita Y, Okuno Y, A. Diurnal rhythms of luteinizing hormone, follicle-stimulating hormone, and testosterone secretion before the onset of male puberty. J Clin Endocrinol Metab 1999;84:29–37.
72. Wu FB, Kelnar GE, Stirling CJH, Huhtaniemi HF. Patterns of pulsatile luteinizing and follicle stimulating hormone secretion in prepubertal (midchildhood) boys and girls and patients with idiopathic hypogonadotrophic hypogonadism (Kallman's syndrome): a study using an ultrasensitive time-resolved immunofluorometric assay. J Clin Endocrinol Metab 1991;72:1229–1237.
73. Hall DA, et al. Sonographic monitoring of LHRH analogue therapy in idiopathic precocious puberty in young girls. J Clin Ultrasound 1986;14(5):331–338.
74. Cavallo A, et al. A simplified gonadotrophin-releasing hormone test for precocious puberty. Clin Endocrinol (Oxf) 1995;42(6):641–6.
75. Oerter KE, et al. Effects of luteinizing hormone-releasing hormone agonists on final height in luteinizing hormone-releasing hormone-dependent precocious puberty. Acta Paediatr Suppl 1993;388: 62–68; discussion 69.
76. Oostdijk W, et al. Final height in central precocious puberty after long term treatment with a slow release GnRH agonist. Arch Dis Child 1996;75(4):292–297.
77. Oerter KE, et al. Adult height in precocious puberty after long-term treatment with deslorelin. J Clin Endocrinol Metab 1991;73(6):1235–1240.
78. Bar A, et al. Bayley-Pinneau method of height prediction in girls with central precocious puberty: correlation with adult height. J Pediatr 1995;126(6):955–958.
79. Pasquino AM, et al. Combined treatment with gonadotropin-releasing hormone analog and growth hormone in central precocious puberty. J Clin Endocrinol Metab 1996;81(3):948–951.
80. Saggese G, et al. Effect of combined treatment with gonadotropin releasing hormone analogue and growth hormone in patients with central precocious puberty who had subnormal growth velocity and impaired height prognosis. Acta Paediatr 1995;84(3):299–304.
81. Walvoord EC, Pescovitz OH. Combined use of growth hormone and gonadotropin-releasing hormone analogues in precocious puberty: theoretic and practical considerations. Pediatrics 1999;104(4 Pt 2): 1010–1014.

82. Neely EK, et al. Bone mineral density during treatment of central precocious puberty. J Pediatr 1995;127(5):819–822.
83. Bertelloni S, et al. Effect of central precocious puberty and gonadotropin-releasing hormone analogue treatment on peak bone mass and final height in females. Eur J Pediatr 1998;157(5):363–367.
84. Lazar L, et al. Early polycystic ovary-like syndrome in girls with central precocious puberty and exaggerated adrenal response. Eur J Endocrinol 1995;133(4):403–406.
85. Jay N, et al. Ovulation and menstrual function of adolescent girls with central precocious puberty after therapy with gonadotropin-releasing hormone agonists. J Clin Endocrinol Metab 1992; 75(3):890–894.
86. Saenz CA, et al. Premature thelarche and ovarian cyst probably secondary to estrogen contamination. Bol Asoc Med P R 1982;74(2):16–19.
87. Saenz de Rodriguez CA, Toro-Sola MA. Anabolic steroids in meat and rema premature telarche. Lancet 1982;1(8284):1300.
88. Saenz de Rodriguez CA, Bongiovanni AM, Conde de Borrego L. An epidemic of precocious development in Puerto Rican children. J Pediatr 1985;107(3):393–396.
89. Cohen HE, Eisenberg P, Mandel F, Haller, JO. Ovarian custs are common in premenarchal girls: a sonographic study of 101 children 2–12 yr old. AJM Am J Roentogenol 1992;159(1):89.
90. Albright FB, Hampton AM. syndrome characterized by osteitis fibrosa disseminata, areas of depigmentation and endocrine dysfunction, with precocious puberty in females. N Engl J Med 1937;216:727.
91. Weinstein LS, et al. Activating mutations of the stimulatory G protein in the McCune-Albright syndrome. N Engl J Med 1991;325(24):1688–1695.
92. Shenker A, et al. An activating Gs alpha mutation is present in fibrous dysplasia of bone in the McCune-Albright syndrome. J Clin Endocrinol Metab 1994;79(3):750–755.
93. Shenker A, et al. Severe endocrine and nonendocrine manifestations of the McCune-Albright syndrome associated with activating mutations of stimulatory G protein GS. J Pediatr 1993;123(4):509–518.
94. Pienkowski C, et al. Recurrent ovarian cyst and mutation of the Gs alpha gene in ovarian cyst fluid cells: what is the link with McCune-Albright syndrome? Acta Paediatr 1997;86(9):1019–1021.
95. DiMeglio LA, Pescovitz OH. Disorders of puberty: inactivating and activating molecular mutations. J Pediatr 1997;131(1 Pt 2):S8–12.
96. Mastorakos G, et al. Hyperthyroidism in McCune-Albright syndrome with a review of thyroid abnormalities sixty yr after the first report. Thyroid 1997;7(3):433–439.
97. Cavanah SF, Dons RF. McCune-Albright syndrome: how many endocrinopathies can one patient have? South Med J 1993;86(3):34–37.
98. Lee PA, Van Dop C, Migeon CJ. McCune-Albright syndrome. Long-term follow-up. JAMA 1986;256(21):2980–2984.
99. Holland FJ. Gonadotropin-independent precocious puberty. Endocrinol Metab Clin North Am 1991;20(1):191–210.
100. Benedict PH. Sex precocity and polyostotic fibrous dysplasia. Report of a case in a boy with testicular biopsy. Am J Dis Child 1966;111(4):426–429.
101. Foster CM, et al. Ovarian function in girls with McCune-Albright syndrome. Pediatr Res 1986;20(9):859–863.
102. Schmidt H, Kiess W. Secondary central precocious puberty in a girl with McCune-Albright syndrome responds to treatment with GnRH analogue. J Pediatr Endocrinol Metab 1998;11(1):77–81.
103. Sorgo W, et al. The effects of cyproterone acetate on statural growth in children with precocious puberty. Acta Endocrinol (Copenh), 1987;115(1):44–56.
104. Feuillan PP, et al. Treatment of precocious puberty in the McCune-Albright syndrome with the aromatase inhibitor testolactone. N Engl J Med 1986;315(18):1115–1119.
105. Feuillan PP, Jones J, Cutler GB Jr. Long-term testolactone therapy for precocious puberty in girls with the McCune-Albright syndrome. J Clin Endocrinol Metab 1993;77(3):647–651.
106. Eugster EA, et al. Tamoxifen treatment of progressive precocious puberty in a patient with McCune-Albright syndrome. J Pediatr Endocrinol Metab 1999;12(5):681–686.
107. Shenker A, et al. A constitutively activating mutation of the luteinizing hormone receptor in familial male precocious puberty [see comments]. Nature 1993;365(6447):652–654.
108. Kremer H, et al. Cosegregation of missense mutations of the luteinizing hormone receptor gene with familial male-limited precocious puberty. Hum Mol Genet 1993;2(11):1779–1783.

109. Kraaij R, et al. A missense mutation in the second transmembrane segment of the luteinizing hormone receptor causes familial male-limited precocious puberty. J Clin Endocrinol Metab 1995;80(11): 3168–3172.
110. Gromoll J, et al. A mutation in the first transmembrane domain of the lutropin receptor causes male precocious puberty. J Clin Endocrinol Metab 1998;83(2):476–480.
111. Laue L, et al. Genetic heterogeneity of constitutively activating mutations of the human luteinizing hormone receptor in familial male-limited precocious puberty. Proc Natl Acad Sci USA 1995;92(6): 1906–1910.
112. Latronico AC, et al. A unique constitutively activating mutation in third transmembrane helix of luteinizing hormone receptor causes sporadic male gonadotropin- independent precocious puberty. J Clin Endocrinol Metab, 1998;83(7):2435–2440.
113. Schedewie HK, et al. Testicular leydig cell hyperplasia as a cause of familial sexual precocity. J Clin Endocrinol Metab 1981;52(2):271–278.
114. Clark PA, Clarke WL. Testotoxicosis. An unusual presentation and novel gene mutation. Clin Pediatr (Phila) 1995;34(5):271–274.
115. Reiter EO, et al. Male-limited familial precocious puberty in three generations. Apparent Leydig-cell autonomy and elevated glycoprotein hormone alpha subunit. N Engl J Med 1984;311(8):515–519.
116. Egli CA, et al. Pituitary gonadotropin-independent male-limited autosomal dominant sexual precocity in nine generations: familial testotoxicosis. J Pediatr 1985;106(1):33–40.
117. Kawate N, et al. Identification of constitutively activating mutation of the luteinising hormone receptor in a family with male limited gonadotrophin independent precocious puberty (testotoxicosis). J Med Genet 1995;32(7):553–554.
118. Rosenthal SM, Grumbach MM, Kaplan SL. Gonadotropin-independent familial sexual precocity with premature Leydig and germinal cell maturation (familial testotoxicosis): effects of a potent luteinizing hormone-releasing factor agonist and medroxyprogesterone acetate therapy in four cases. J Clin Endocrinol Metab 1983;57(3):571–579.
119. Holland FJ, et al. Ketoconazole in the management of precocious puberty not responsive to LHRH-analogue therapy. N Engl J Med 1985;312(16):1023–1028.
120. Laue L, et al. Treatment of familial male precocious puberty with spironolactone and testolactone. N Engl J Med 1989;320(8):496–502.
121. Babovic-Vuksanovic D, et al. Hazards of ketoconazole therapy in testotoxicosis. Acta Paediatr 1994;83(9):994–997.
122. Laue L, et al. Treatment of familial male precocious puberty with spironolactone, testolactone, and deslorelin. J Clin Endocrinol Metab 1993;76(1):151–155.
123. Skinner MA, et al. Ovarian neoplasms in children. Arch Surg 1993;128(8):849-53; discussion 853–854.
124. Bouffet E, et al. Juvenile granulosa cell tumor of the ovary in infants: a clinicopathologic study of three cases and review of the literature. J Pediatr Surg 1997;32(5):762–765.
125. Nakashima N, Young RH, Scully RE. Androgenic granulosa cell tumors of the ovary. A clinicopathologic analysis of 17 cases and review of the literature. Arch Pathol Lab Med 1984;108(10):786–791.
126. Cronje HS, et al. Granulosa and theca cell tumors in children: a report of 17 cases and literature review. Obstet Gynecol Surv 1998;53(4):240–247.
127. Bas F, KD, Steinmetz R, Pescovitz OH. Activating Mutations of FSH Receptor in Children with Ovarian Juvenile Granulosa Cell tumors and an Association of These Tumors with Central Precocious Puberty. Pediatr Res 2001;49(6):146A.
128. Masur Y, et al. [Leydig cell tumors of the testis—clinical and morphologic aspects]. Urologe A 1996;35(6):468–471.
129. Diamond FB Jr, et al. Hetero- and isosexual pseudoprecocity associated with testicular sex- cord tumors in an 8 year-old male. J Pediatr Endocrinol Metab 1996;9(3):407–414.
130. Kim I, Young RH, Scully RE. Leydig cell tumors of the testis. A clinicopathological analysis of 40 cases and review of the literature. Am J Surg Pathol 1985;9(3):177–192.
131. Comite F, et al. Isosexual precocious pseudopuberty secondary to a feminizing adrenal tumor. J Clin Endocrinol Metab 1984;58(3):435–440.
132. Heimann A, et al. Hepatoblastoma presenting as isosexual precocity. The clinical importance of histologic and serologic parameters. J Clin Gastroenterol 1987;9(1):105–110.
133. Otsuka T, et al. Primary pulmonary choriocarcinoma in a four month old boy complicated with precocious puberty. Acta Paediatr Jpn 1994;36(4):404–407.

134. Derenoncourt AN, Castro-Magana M, Jones KL. Mediastinal teratoma and precocious puberty in a boy with mosaic Klinefelter syndrome. Am J Med Genet 1995;55(1):38–42.
135. Cohen AR, Wilson JA, Sadeghi-Nejad A. Gonadotropin-secreting pineal teratoma causing precocious puberty. Neurosurgery 1991;28(4):597–602; discussion 602–603.
136. Tamaki N, et al. Germ cell tumors of the thalamus and the basal ganglia. Childs Nerv Syst 1990; 6(1):3–7.
137. Kukuvitis A, Matte C, Polychronakos C. Central precocious puberty following feminizing right ovarian granulosa cell tumor. Horm Res 1995;44(6):268–270.
138. Leschek EW, et al. Localization by venous sampling of occult chorionic gonadotropin- secreting tumor in a boy with mosaic Klinefelter's syndrome and precocious puberty. J Clin Endocrinol Metab 1996;81(11):3825–3828.
139. Englund AT, et al. Pediatric germ cell and human chorionic gonadotropin-producing tumors. Clinical and laboratory features. Am J Dis Child 1991;145(11):1294–1297.
140. Hasle H, et al. Mediastinal germ cell tumour associated with Klinefelter syndrome. A report of case and review of the literature. Eur J Pediatr 1992;151(10):735–739.
141. Van Wyk JG. Syndrome of precocious menstruation and galactorrhea in juvenile hypothyroidism: an example of hormonal overlap in pituitary feedback. J Pediatr 1960;57:416.
142. Lindsay AV, MacGillivray ML. Multicystic ovaries detected by sonography. Am J Dis Child 1980;134:588–592.
143. Bruder JS, Bremner MH, Ridgway WJ, Wierman EC. Hypothyroidism-induced macroorchidism: use of a gonadotropin-releasing agonist to understand its mechanism and augment adult stature. J Clin Endocrinol Metab 1995;80:11–16.
144. Anasti JN, et al. A potential novel mechanism for precocious puberty in juvenile hypothyroidism. J Clin Endocrinol Metab 1995;80(1):276–279.
145. Desforges J. Gynecomastia. N Engl J Med 1993;328(7):490.
146. Coen P. An aromatase-producing sex-cord tumor resulting in prepubertal gynecomastia. N Engl J Med 1991;324(5):317.
147. Halperin DS, Sizonenko PC. Prepubertal gynecomastia following topical inunction of estrogen containing ointment. Helv Paediatr Acta 1983;38(4):361–366.
148. Edidin DL. Prepubertal gynecomastia associated with estrogen-containing hair cream. Am J Dis Child 1982;136(7):587.
149. Latorre HK. Idiopathic gynecomastia in seven preadolescent boys. Am J Dis Child 1973;126:771.
150. Stratakis CA, et al. The aromatase excess syndrome is associated with feminization of both sexes and autosomal dominant transmission of aberrant P450 aromatase gene transcription. J Clin Endocrinol Metab 1998;83(4):1348–1357.
151. Fontoura M, et al. Precocious puberty in girls: early diagnosis of a slowly progressing variant. Arch Dis Child 1989;64(8):1170–1176.
152. Kreiter M, et al. Preserving adult height potential in girls with idiopathic true precocious puberty. J Pediatr 1990;117(3):364–370.
153. Bassi F, et al. Precocious puberty: auxological criteria discriminating different forms. J Endocrinol Invest 1994;17(10):793–797.
154. Leger J, Reynaud R, Czernichow P. Do all girls with apparent idiopathic precocious puberty require gonadotropin-releasing hormone agonist treatment? J Pediatr 2000;137(6):819–825.
155. Brauner R, et al. Adult height in girls with idiopathic true precocious puberty. J Clin Endocrinol Metab 1994;9(2):415–420.
156. Ghirri P, et al. Final height in girls with slowly progressive untreated central precocious puberty. Gynecol Endocrinol 1997;11(5):301–305.

24 Management of Infants Born with Ambiguous Genitalia

Margaret H. MacGillivray, MD
and Tom Mazur, PsyD

CONTENTS

INTRODUCTION
MECHANISMS INVOLVED IN SEXUAL DIFFERENTIATION:
   TISSUES, GENES, AND HORMONES
GLOSSARY OF SEX TERMINOLOGY
CLINICAL APPROACH TO CARE OF INFANTS WITH AMBIGUOUS
   GENITALIA
THE MEDICAL MANAGEMENT OF AMBIGUOUS GENITALIA
REFERENCES

INTRODUCTION

The birth of an infant with ambiguous genitalia is a crisis for parents as well as the primary care physician. In some instances, parents have been forewarned by the results of genetic testing or ultrasound examinations of the uterus during the fetal period. In the absence of prior knowledge, parents must be informed at the first opportunity that the genital ambiguity prevents precise identification of their infant's sex. Because this is an extremely traumatic experience, the physician should emphasize any positive aspects of the infant such as good health including normal cardiac, pulmonary and neurologic function. Also, they are told that chromosome analysis and other diagnostic tests are needed to identify the cause of the problem and to provide a basis for sound sex assignment decisions. They need to be reassured that they will be kept completely informed and that they will help in the decision making process once the tests are completed. Under ideal circumstances, an experienced team of specialists in pediatric endocrinology, pediatric urology, genetics, psychology, and radiology come together promptly to help parents and primary care physicians understand which tests are being ordered and how these studies will help in deciding sex assignment. When the information becomes

From: *Contemporary Endocrinology: Pediatric Endocrinology: A Practical Clinical Guide*
Edited by: S. Radovick and M. H. MacGillivray © Humana Press Inc., Totowa, NJ

available, parents should be given accurate detailed information about the infant's karyotype, genital anatomy, the hormone levels and, when known, the gonadal histology. Parental understanding and involvement are key elements to successful long-term care of the child. Despite every effort to be inclusive, the infant is the sole member of the team with no input during the decision-making process.

From the outset, parents must be given simplified information about the mechanisms controlling sexual differentiation in fetal life in order to understand that males and females share common primordial tissues that eventually are transformed into the sex structures that distinguish a female from a male infant. The roles of specific sex determining genes and gonadal hormones must be discussed. The primary care physician and the team of experts must have current knowledge about this topic if they are to give families an accurate overview of the possible events responsible for the genital findings *(1–9)*.

Traditionally, sex assignment decisions have been influenced by the following factors: 1) potential for sexual functioning, 2) potential for fertility, and 3) requirement for sex hormone replacement during puberty and adulthood. Recent feedback by former patients has emphasized the importance of avoiding surgeries that improve genital appearance but may lead to loss of genital sensation and sexual arousability, or surgeries that may result in genital discomfort that comprises satisfactory sexual functioning. At present, emphasis is being given to preservation of the normal sexual response and to issues of genital comfort, whereas in the past, genital appearance was the main priority.

At present, the medical management of infants born with ambiguous genitalia is undergoing critical reevaluation as to the decision making process of sex of assignment and rearing, timing of surgery, extent and goals of surgery, and the guidelines for optimal physician-parent-patient relationships that span childhood to adulthood *(2–7,10–13)*. The current sparseness of data concerning the long-term outcomes of decisions made in past decades has undermined the confidence previously held by professionals in this field. Until we collect more information, we are obligated to present current options in the context of today's knowledge. The challenge for today's health care provider is how best to maintain open communications with the family as the consequences of medical decisions made during infancy become part of the child's life experience.

It is widely accepted that good outcomes involve having the child feel comfortable in their sex of rearing and with the medical care provided during infancy and early childhood. Certain strategies must be in place: 1) from the outset, physician sensitivity and privacy are of essential importance. These children must not be used as teaching objects, whereby their genital malformations are displayed and discussed in front of medical students, residents, and other uninvolved health professionals; 2) From an early age, these children should be told gradually and age-appropriately about the normal sexual anatomy of boys and girls, since this background eventually provides a context within which they can learn details about their own anatomy. Also, they should be told they will be given sex hormone replacement if they have absent or poorly functioning gonads. Furthermore, they will need advice about adoption if they are unable to reproduce. In some instances, it is reasonable to hold out the hope that someday medical science may make it possible for them to produce a child. A psychologist with expertise in pediatric endocrinology is the best equipped individual to educate and help children and their parents develop the ability to discuss frankly the many issues which arise throughout childhood, adolescence, and adulthood. Family dynamics impact in a major way. Communicative, positive thinking parents are more likely to have a well adjusted child than are couples who cannot accept or support what has happened to their youngster. The latter group will need more intensive counseling from a mental health professional with expertise in this area.

The aims of this chapter are: 1) to provide a concise update on the mechanisms controlling normal and abnormal sexual differentiation since this is essential to the education of the parents; 2) to give a glossary of commonly used sex terminology; 3) to outline practical information about the diagnosis and management of infants born with ambiguous genitalia; and 4) to discuss current differences of opinions about the care of infants born with genital defects. A discussion of infants who are born with disorders of sexual differentiation and normal appearing genitalia will also be included.

MECHANISMS INVOLVED IN SEXUAL DIFFERENTIATION: TISSUES, GENES, AND HORMONES

The Bipotential Gonad

The bipotential gonad is destined to become either a testis or an ovary depending on the sex chromosome constitution of the germ cells (classified as gonadal or primary sex), as well as other critical sex determining determining genes that control the male vs female pathway of sex development. At conception, the genetic sex (XX or XY) of the fetus is determined when a Y or X bearing sperm fertilizes the ovum. Subsequently, the developing germ cells migrate in the early weeks of fetal life from their point of origin near the anal region to their final destination within the primitive gonad.

TESTICULAR DIFFERENTIATION

Testicular differentiation depends primarily on the *SRY* gene located on the short arm of the Y chromosome; its mode of action is not fully understood. Two mechanisms have been proposed: 1) *SRY* activates a cascade of genes needed for male development or 2) SRY inhibits a repressor of male determining genes based on the clinical observations of autosomal recessive inheritance of *SRY* negative XX males. Either mechanism would give the same end result. In the activator model, the male pathway is dominant and the female pathway is the default pathway. In contrast, the repressor model suggests an active female development pathway which must be suppressed by a male gene. The SRY gene product is a 204 amino acid protein (a transcription factor) that binds to and bends the DNA strands, thus allowing access by other transcription factors. In humans, SRY is expressed in the testis and a variety of brain structures; whether this influences sexual behavior is unknown. SRY expression is tightly regulated because it is seen early in development and is very transient. SRY induces Sertoli cell development, followed by differentiation of seminiferous tubules and the formation of Leydig cells. The middle third of the SRY protein has a DNA-binding domain known as the HMG box protein (high mobility group) which belongs to a family of transcription-regulating proteins known as the HMG box proteins. Mutations within the HMG region of the *SRY* gene results in sex reversal due to testicular failure with a female phenotype or genital ambiguity *(1,14,15)*.

SRY is not responsible for all cases of sex reversal in 46 XY females. Nor does it explain the presence of testes in 46 XX males with genital ambiguity. Clearly, other genes must be involved. Only 25% of 46 XY females who present with gonadal dysgenesis (streak gonads) and female phenotype have an SRY mutation. Also, SRY is present in only 10% of 46 XX true hermaphrodites and 10% of 46 XX males with ambiguity. In contrast, among 46 XX males with unambiguous male genitalia and testes, a majority have been found to be SRY positive. It is possible that the role of SRY may be underestimated in some populations of sex reversed individuals if it is present only in the gonad and not in peripheral blood lymphocytes *(1)*.

Recently, some non-Y genes have been discovered to encode proteins, which have similarities to the SRY HMG box region. They have been termed *SOX* genes (an abbreviation for SRY-homeobOX - like genes). One of this family, SOX 9 is essential for Sertoli cell differentiation from cell precursors in interstitium of the primitive gonad. This gene's contribution was discovered when a 46 XY infant with a *SOX 9* mutation presented with skeletal dysplasia (Campomelic Dwarfism), female phenotype (sex reversal), and streak ovarian-like gonads *(15)*. The clinical presentation has been attributed to haploinsufficiency resulting from loss of one copy of *SOX 9*. Since *SOX 9* is located on17q24–25, the female phenotype in 46XY males with this mutation has been classified as autosomal sex reversal. In the testis, SRY is presumed to activate SOX 9 by suppressing DAX 1 that normally inhibits SOX 9; SOX 9 expression in turn mediates Sertoli cell development and testis differentiation. Consequently, *SOX 9* is an autosomal gene which plays a pivotal role in male sexual development (Fig. 1).

OVARIAN DIFFERENTIATION

Ovarian differentiation is poorly understood but recent evidence suggests that the process is actively regulated by a network of genes and transcription factors. It is no longer believed that ovarian development is a passive or default process. Ovarian development appears to depend on suppression of SOX 9 which is a testis-inducing gene, as well as simultaneous activation of ovary inducing genes. The probable candidate genes for suppression of testis differentiation include *DAX 1, SOX 3*, and Wnt 4. Presumably, DAX 1 inactivates SOX 9, thereby blocking testicular development. In the differentiating ovary, Wnt 4 appears to prevent androgen production by precursors of Leydig cells in the interstitium, stabilizes oocytes, and induces Mullerian development. Deletion of Wnt 4 leads to masculinization in both XX mice and XX humans and degeneration of Mullerian duct derivatives *(16)*. Duplication of *SOX 9* is another autosomal cause of 46 XX sex reversal *(17)*. The ovary activating genes have not been completely identified, but are probably located on the X-chromosome and likely have dosage-sensitive functions since Turner syndrome is associated with total or partial absence of an X chromosome and loss of germ cells. The sequence of genetic events in ovarian development is depicted in the following theoretical model: 1) Activation of Dax 1 and SOX 3 antagonizes SF 1 and SOX 9; 2) granulosa cells develop from the supporting cells while Sertoli cell differentiation is blocked; 3) Wnt 4 induces differentiation of Mullerian structures into uterus, fallopian tubes, and upper third of vagina; and d) Wnt 4, produced by ovarian somatic cells, prevents interstitial precursor cells from developing into Leydig cells (1). Hence, no testosterone can be produced by fetal ovary (Fig. 1).

The roles of DAX 1 in the testis and ovary need to be reviewed in more detail. The *DAX 1* gene is located on the X chromosome and males inherit it from their mother's X chromosome. It appears to be an important anti-testis gene in the ovary, but further evidence is needed to substantiate this hypothesis. In the testis, DAX 1 is suppressed by SRY, thereby permitting expression of SOX 9 and male development. However, in 46 XY males who inherit a duplication of DAX 1, SRY cannot suppress fully the double

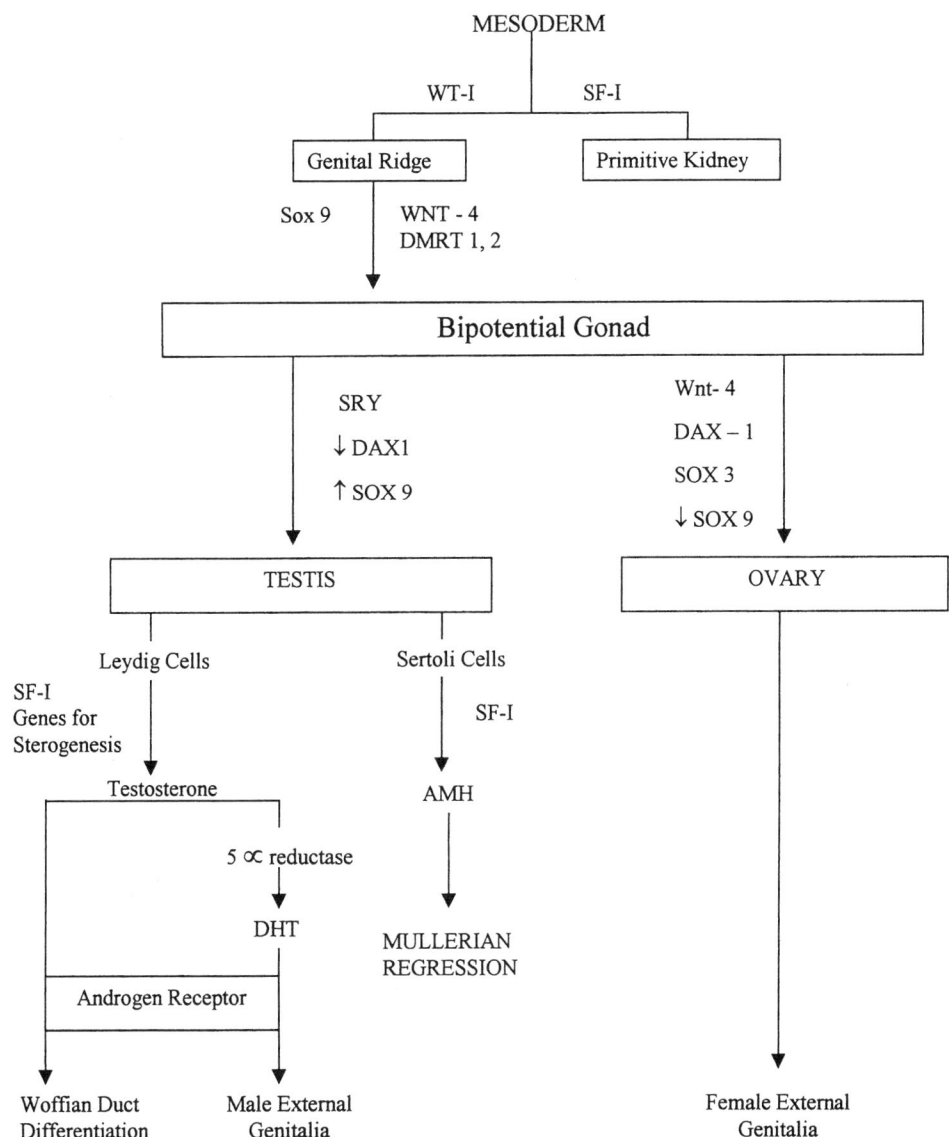

Fig. 1. Pathway of sexual differentiation.

dose of DAX 1, leading to a female phenotype (sex reversal) and gonadal dysgenesis *(18,19)*. The DAX 1 duplication may be located on one X-chromosome or, alternatively, the DAX 1 locus can be normally located on the X chromosome along with a second translocated DAX 1 gene being present on the Y chromosome. The term DAX 1 derives from Dosage- sensitive sex reversal Adrenal hypoplasia congenita critical region of the X chromosome, gene 1.

Other mechanisms have recently been shown to cause 46 XY female phenotype or sex reversal. Wnt 4 appears to act upstream of and in concert with DAX 1. In 46 XY individuals, duplication of Wnt 4 causes upregulation of DAX 1 in the testes, suppression of SOX 9 and female phenotype *(20,21)*. Hence, duplication of either DAX 1 or Wnt 4 causes dosage sensitive 46 XY sex reversal because SRY is unable to suppress DAX 1.

Table 1
Genes Controlling Sexual Differentiation
SEX DETERMINING GENES

Gene/chromosome	Family/function	Clinical phenotype
SRY, Yp11	HMG Protein, Transcription Factor	XY Gonadal Dysgenesis
WT1, 11 p 13	Zinc Finger Protein, Transcription Factor	Denys - Drash S. Frasiers S.
SF1, 9 q 33	Nuclear Receptor Transcription Factor	XY Gonadal Dysgenesis Adrenal Insufficiency
DAX 1, X p 21.3	Nuclear Receptor Transcription Factor	Duplication causes: - XY Sex Reversal Mutation causes: - XY Adrenal Hypoplasia Congenita (AHC) and Gonadotropin Deficiency
SOX 9, 17 q 24	HMG Protein Transcription Factor	Mutation causes: - XY Sex Reversal - Campomelic Dysplasia Duplication causes: - XX Sex Reversal
Wnt- 4, 1p 32.36	Growth Factor	Duplication causes: - 46,XY sex reversal Deletion causes: - Masculinization of 46,XX female

Also, mutations in the SF1 gene and other sex determining genes are known to cause of 46 XY gonadal dysgenesis and female phenotype (Tables 1 and 2).

In 46 XY males, the DAX 1 gene also has a major influence on adrenal development as well as gonadotropin production by the fetal pituitary gland. Hence, 46 XY males lacking DAX 1 present with Congenital Addison Disease (Adrenal Hypoplasia Congenita or AHC) as well as microgenitalia, i.e., micropenis and hypoplastic testes due to hypogonadotropic hypogonadism (22). They do not have ambiguous genitalia. However, their testes are very small and they have a micropenis because of congenital gonadotropin deficiency. In contrast, the genetic female with a DAX 1 gene mutation or a duplication of DAX 1 has normal ovarian development, normal fertility, and normal adrenal gland function. Females are protected because they normally have two DAX 1 genes, and a mutation or a duplication appears to have no consequence on adrenal, pituitary, or gonadal function. However, when an X-chromosome lacking DAX 1 is passed to an 46XY offspring, the male has AHC and hypogonadotropic hypogonadism. Hence 46 XY males need one functional DAX 1 gene in order to have to have normal adrenal function and gonadotropin production. The lack of a functional DAX 1 gene in the testes does not prevent testes differentiation which is controlled by SRY and SOX 9 (15).

In summary, when 46 XY males have two functional DAX 1 genes, the clinical presentation is testicular dysgenesis and sex reversal. The SRY and DAX 1 genes appear to act antagonistically in gonadal differentiation. In normal 46 XY males, SRY inhibits

Table 2
Causes of 46,XY Testicular Dysgenesis

1. XY gonadal dysgenesis
2. Denys-Dash Syndrome WT-1 Mutation
3. Frasier Syndrome WT-1 Mutation, Also Nephropathy, Gonadoblastoma
4. XO/XY Mosaicism - Mixed Gonadal Dysgenesis
5. Campomelic Dysplasia - SOX 9 Mutation
6. DAX - 1 Duplication (DSS Syndrome)
7. Wnt 4 Duplication
8. SF-I Mutation
9. Deletions: 9p–, 10 q–
10. Duplication: x p +

DAX 1 thereby turning off the female pathway and permitting male development to proceed. In normal 46 XX females, SRY is absent; DAX 1 suppresses SOX 9 and activates the female pathway and DAX 1 also inhibits the male pathway. Hence DAX 1 appears to work in two ways in the female fetus: i.e., promoting ovarian development as well as suppressing testis formation. However, more information is needed to identify which of these roles is dominant in the development of the fetal ovary *(1)*.

The Paired Internal Ducts—Wolffian and Mullerian Ducts

Wolffian Duct differentiation into epididymus, vas deferens, seminal vesicles, and ejaculatory ducts in 46 XY males is dependent on the local (paracrine) production of testosterone by the Leydig cells, which is initially regulated by Human Chorionic Gonadotropin (hCG). Genetic males who are agonadal exhibit involution of the Wolffian ducts and also have Mullerian duct development because anti-Mullerian hormone (AMH) is not produced. Normally, AMH is produced by the Sertoli cells in the fetal period and this continues until the age of 8–10 yr in boys. Hence, AMH is a marker of Sertoli cell function in patients with genital abnormalities.

MULLERIAN DUCT

Mullerian Duct differentiation progresses in the absence of AMH, a glycoprotein hormone, and results in the development of the fallopian tubes, uterus, cervix, and upper third of vagina. The Wnt 4 gene appears to play an important role in Mullerian duct differentiation as well as ovarian function during fetal life. Female transgenic mice in whom the Wnt 4 genes are knocked out fail to develop Mullerian structures and lose oocytes. Also, they manifest hypersecretion of ovarian androgens derived from Leydig cell precursors in the interstitium and exhibit masculinization of the Wolffian ducts. Thus, it appears that Wnt 4 acts to suppress androgen production by precursors of Leydig cell in the interstitium of the ovary in addition to being a regulator of mullerian duct development.

The Bipotential External Genitalia

The primordial structures of the male and female external genitalia are identical in the absence of androgens. Thus, the external genitalia of genetic males cannot be distinguished from genetic females at 8 wk of fetal life. Furthermore, female appearing external genitalia will persist if the fetus has no gonads, streak gonads, non-functional testes, androgen insensitivity, or normal ovaries regardless of the sex chromosomes. The outcome and physical appearance is totally androgen dependent. The major embryonic components are:

Genital Tubercle is the precursor of the clitoris or the glans penis.
Urethral Folds develops into the labia minora or the penile shaft and urethra
Labioscrotal or Genital Swellings become the labia majora or the scrotum

Male External Genitalia

Development of male external genitalia depends on the adequacy of testosterone (T) and 5-α-dihydrotestosterone (5α DHT) production as well as functional androgen receptors (AR). The testis is formed by 6–7 wk of fetal life and the leydig cells are initially stimulated by hCG from the placenta in the first trimester and by fetal pituitary LH in the second trimester. Male external genital differentiation is complete by 12 wk; additional penile enlargement in the second trimester is dependent on Leydig cell stimulation by LH from the fetal pituitary gland.

Complete masculinization of external male genitalia requires the conversion of T to 5α DHT; the enzyme responsible for this conversion is 5-α-reductase which is present in the genital tissues. 46 XY infants with 5-α-reductase deficiency have normally functioning testes; the predominantly female phenotype in early childhood is due to defective conversion of T to 5α DHT during early fetal life. In many societies spontaneous sex reassignment to a male gender role usually occurs in puberty because 5α DHT is not an essential androgen for adult male virile muscular development, whereas it is critical for normal external male genital differentiation in fetal life *(23–25)*.

Female External Genitalia

Female external genitalia will be normal except when exposed to androgens in early fetal life. The androgens may be derived from: 1) the mother (ingested or endogenously produced); or from 2) the fetus (Congenital Adrenal Hyperplasia (CAH); or 3) due to homozygous or heterozygous mutations in both aromatase genes which leads to a deficiency of aromatase and failure to convert androgens to estrogens; or 4) to true hermaphroditism; or 5) mixed gonadal dysgenesis *(26–29)*. The degree of virilization is dependent on the quantity, timing, and actions of androgens to which the female fetus is exposed; i.e., clitoromegaly alone vs severe posterior fusion of the labia majora, absence of the labia minora and vaginal orifice, a urogenital sinus and a large phallic appearing clitoris that resembles a hypospadic penis. Rarely, extreme virilization causes complete labioscrotal fusion and a "penile urethra." In the last example, "ambiguity" is not present and the only clue is the absence of palpable gonads often mistakenly thought to represent cryptorchidism. All virilized 46 XX CAH females have a uterus and ovaries and the potential for fertility.

GLOSSARY OF SEX TERMINOLOGY

1. Genetic sex refers to the chromosome make up of the individual, i.e., the sex chromosomes. Normally, the sex chromosomes are XX or XY, but this pattern may differ in true hermaphroditism, mixed gonadal dysgenesis, Klinefelter Syndrome, Turner Syndrome, etc.
2. Gonadal sex refers to the individual's gonad, i.e., ovary, testis, or rarely, ovotestes.

3. Internal sex refers to internal reproductive structures, and to Mullerian or Wollffian derivatives.
4. External sex refers to the external genital structures.
5. Sex of assignment refers to the decision to rear the infant as a boy or a girl.
6. Gender identity is the subjective conviction of an individual as male, female or ambiguous.
7. Gender role refers to public behaviors, manner, and style of dress culturally labeled as masculine or feminine.
8. Sexual orientation refers to the object of one's sexual arousal, i.e., heterosexual, homosexual, or bisexual.
9. Dysgenetic gonad: abnormal development which causes defects in the structure and function of gonads: example, a gonad that is fibrous with poorly differentiated histology as well as decreased or absent function.

CLINICAL APPROACH TO CARE OF INFANTS WITH AMBIGUOUS GENITALIA

If the health professional in charge of the delivery fails to acknowledge the infant's genital birth defect, the primary care physician must assume the responsibility of giving this information to the parents. Parents usually know something is wrong and are at a loss if their health care providers avoid talking with them openly. In most circumstances, the first health professionals to see the infant's genitalia are obstetricians, general practitioners, pediatricians, midwives, and nurses. Physical appearance will not reveal if the infant is: 1) an incompletely virilized genetic male; or 2) a masculinized genetic female; or 3) a true hermaphrodite; or 4) mixed gonadal dysgenesis. If a gonad is palpable, it is highly likely that the infant is either a genetic male, a true hermaphrodite or mixed gonadal dysgenesis. In the past, physicians would try to complete the studies in 3–4 d to shorten the period of anxiety for parents; they would also inform the parents of the sex of assignment decision with little or no input from the family and often with incomplete disclosure as to precise genetic or anatomic information. Sometimes, a Y chromosome was called a shortened X chromosome and the testis was referred to as abnormal ovary when a female sex of rearing was chosen for the baby. The intention was to lessen parental discomfort and facilitate acceptance of their daughter. Not all physicians followed this practice; some were totally frank with families. These practices are being modified in that while urgency is still present, informed parents are willing to accept longer waiting times in order to obtain all the data from the molecular studies and other diagnostic tests because they realize the enormity of their decision on their child's future.

At the outset, the following simple questions will help the physician with the differential diagnosis:

1) Is the infant a genetic female (46 XX) exposed to fetal androgens? (i.e., female pseudohermaphrodite)
2) Is the infant an undervirilized genetic male (46 XY) due to underproduction or underaction of androgens? (i.e., male pseudohermaphrodite)
3) Does the infant have a complex sex chromosome disorder? (such as true hermaphroditism in which 80% of patients have 46 XX chromosomes or possibly mixed gonadal dysgenesis, 45X/46 XY, etc.)
4) Is the genital defect the result of a birth defect in structures that distorts the genitalia? (i.e., epispadius, cloacal exstrophy, or aphallia)

The following is an outline of a protocol we follow at our institution when a baby is born "in house "or is transferred in from a regional hospital. Our team consists of pediatric endocrinologists, pediatric psychologists with extensive endocrine expertise, pediatric urologists, geneticists, radiologists, and the child's primary care physicians.

1) The first physician to receive the consult request alerts the team members that they need to see the infant as soon as possible; i.e., within a few hours. It is important to determine if the baby was announced as a boy or a girl in the delivery room. If a sex assignment already has been made or a name given to the baby, we do not change this information. However, parents are informed that the diagnostic studies may indicate the need to consider reannouncement of the baby's sex. If the infant arrives with no chosen name or sex, the entire staff and parents are asked to refer to the infant as "baby or infant" usually with the family name included, i.e., "baby Jones".

2) The team leader is often the pediatric endocrinologist who organizes the exchange of information with team members and usually examines the infant with the urologist or others. However this changes depending on who is first contacted. In some cases, the team leader has been one of the psychologists. The advice of the urologist is critical because this is the expert who will have to do the penile reconstructive surgery if and when it is necessary. In some centers, a pediatric surgeon rather than a urologist is the surgical expert. Parents are always relieved to learn that their infant will be cared by a team of experts who have cared for many babies with similar problems. They are also told that they will be given details about the studies being carried out, as well as the usual time required to get back the results. Parents are also told they will be given all the test results and they are assured that they will be part of the decision making team when the time arrives to discuss what is best for the baby.

The pediatric endocrinologist or, in some centers, a trained psychologist or geneticist is the usual person to give an overview of the process of sexual differentiation in males and females, stressing the common origins of the sexes and how errors along the pathway change the external genital appearance. Diagrams are helpful. Repetition is essential. Examining the infant with the parents helps them to understand the changes that have led to the ambiguous genital appearance. Sometimes parents want grandparents and close relatives to be involved. A member of the team needs to have daily contact with the primary care physician as this professional will be involved with the child and family for many years. The baby should be protected from curious residents or nurses from other medical services, as this is a stress to the parents. The pediatric psychologist is probably the most important person who will work with parents on a daily basis because they will reveal their most hidden fears to this individual and will tell of other stresses in the family that may complicate the acceptance of their infant. Such frequent contact also allows the parents to grieve over the birth of their infant with serious medical problems. Meetings between the parents and other members of the team at a scheduled time each day goes a long way towards reducing the level of anxiety experienced by families.

3) The endocrinologist and team members promptly schedule diagnostic studies that include hormone assays, genetic studies, ultrasound exams to define pelvic and abdominal structures (uterus, gonads, renal anatomy), and vaginogram, as well as voiding cystourethrogram to define the location of the urethra and the possible presence of the vagina. The endocrinologist must call the genetics and endocrine laboratories to alert them to the urgency of the tests. Also the radiologist must be personally contacted.

4) The team meets to review the results of the diagnostic studies and to arrive at a consensus as to what is best for the infant. Often the cause of the genital defect is identified, but occasionally, a specific etiology is not readily available. Regardless, the team must come

together with a unified decision to present to the parents, fully aware that parents may or may not accept the team's advice as to sex of assignment. We have advised rearing genetic males with hypospadius as boys if they have a reconstructible phallus. Also, we recommend a male sex of rearing if the infant has unambiguous micropenis with or without hypoplastic testes; these infants are given testosterone therapy monthly for 3 mo. The one possible exception to this rule is a micropenis with no corpora present.

5) The final step is to meet with the parents at which time the following occurs:

- Full disclosure of all the test results.
- Discuss pros and cons of sex assignment as male or female: consequences of each choice.
- Give outcome information, re: fertility, need of hormone treatment, psychosexual data if known.
- Answer parents' questions and get their feedback. They may need time to make a decision. We also inform parents that the medical care of their infant will not be compromised should they decide on a sex of rearing that is different than the team's recommendation (i.e., for religious reasons, etc.).
- The sex assignment is made and the name of the baby is announced.

6. Follow-up care is scheduled with team members, re: medical or surgical care. The psychologist sees the family at regular intervals to support and to educate them about when and what to say to their child as time goes by. Eventually the child will meet with the psychologist who, with the parents, will educate him/her about the medical history over time. The goal is total knowledge of the endocrine condition with eventual full participation of the child in their medical care.

THE MEDICAL MANAGEMENT OF AMBIGUOUS GENITALIA

Medical History

The following is needed: maternal health, drug use (body building steroids, testosterone in oral contraceptives, etc.), endocrine status (development of maternal hirsutism or virilization), and family history (infertile non-menstruating hairless adult female relatives suggest androgen resistance which is familial and transmitted by females because the AR gene is on the X chromosome) *(30)*. Also, check for consanguinity in the parents (e.g., homozygous 5-α-reductase deficiency, etc.). Retrieve all data, re: amniocentesis genetic studies for chromosome analysis or ultrasound exams performed prenatally. Discordance between fetal karyotype (46,XY) and ultrasound genital findings (no phallus) may be evidence of androgen resistance or aphalia.

Physical Exam

A gonad located in the inguinal canal by either manual inspection or by ultrasound exam is highly informative. Almost always, an external gonad is a testis. In the absence of an external gonad, the genetic sex of the infant cannot be identified by inspection. It is best to avoid using definitive terms such as penis or scrotum until the diagnostic studies are completed. Instead, the phallic structure (clitoris or penis) is measured and examined for presence of chordee, which is a downward curving phallus due to a shortened ventral surface. The phallic measurement is not easy since it may be hard to measure an erectile mass buried in pubic fat and curved. A tape measure placed from the point of origin on the pubic ramus along the dorsum of the "erectile mass" will give a reasonable estimate of length *(31,32)*. If the stretched length is less than 2.0 cm, the phallus is considered "micro". The width of the erectile tissue and its consistency should also be recorded. The opening or openings should be recorded. The location of a single urethral opening is classified as 1st degree (asymmetric on "glans"), 2nd degree (mid phallic shaft), 3rd degree (junction of phallus with scrotum), or 4th degree (perineal, closer to anus). Not infrequently, the obstetrician has labeled the phallus as a penis with hypospadias. The record should record if a vaginal dimple or entroitus is also present. In 46,XY babies with complete androgen resistance (AR), the urethra and vaginal pouch are in the female positions but there is no uterus. Rarely, 46,XX infants with salt losing CAH (21-OH deficiency) have extreme virilization classified as Prader 5 because they have a penile urethra, a totally fused empty scrotum, and no ambiguity *(33)*. They resemble male infants with cryptorchidism and are at risk for death from salt-losing dehydration and shock.

In most infants with ambiguous genitalia, the labioscrotal folds look like two adjacent sacs separated by an indentation giving the appearance of a "bifid scrotum," either flat or rounded. Gonads may not be palpable. The labioscrotal folds may be smooth or rugated with many linear creases on the surface. The severity of posterior perineal fusion of the labioscrotal folds may be slight or complete; the latter is indistinguishable from a scrotum. Often, the physician is misled as to the actual location of the urethral opening, which may be more posteriorly located but is hidden because the phallus is "enwrapped" in the fused labioscrotal folds.

In addition to the genital appearance, the record should specify the presence or absence of dysmorphic features or skeletal abnormalities. Campomelic dwarfism is a fatal condition in 46,XY infants who have striking skeletal dysplasia and female phenotype (sex reversal).

Diagnostic Tests

The following are tests which are informative:

1. Karyotype (may include SRY, SOX9, DAX 1, Wnt 1, etc.)
2. Serum hormone levels:
   17-OH progesterone
   Testosterone (first weeks of life)
   DHT
   Androstenedione
   17-OH pregnenolone
   LH
   FSH
   DHEAS
   Renin
   Electrolytes after 8–10 d of life
3. Radiologic services:
   ultrasound of pelvis for uterus, gonads
   ultrasound of kidneys for malformations
   ultrasound of inguinal canals for gonads
   urethrogram/vaginogram/voiding cystogram -position of urethra, reflux, presence of vagina.

An algorithm which links the diagnostic tests to clinical diagnosis is provided in Fig. 2.

The most common cause of ambiguous genitalia is 21-OH deficiency in 46 XX genetic females; 75 % are salt losers who will develop a low sodium, high potassium, and marked weight loss during the second week of life. Prior to clinical dehydration, the asymptomatic salt loser can be identified by high renin levels. 46 XY males are at high risk for shock because their genitalia are entirely normal. In the US, screening of newborns for CAH by measuring serum 17 hydroxyprogesterone (OHP) have protected infants from erroneous sex assignment as well as high morbidity and death. Female sex assignment is relatively straight forward in virilized CAH girls because these infants have a uterus and ovaries *(26)*. Vaginal reconstructive or constructive surgery is usually done in late adolescence by an experienced highly trained genital surgeon, although some centers advocate early correction. Infants with a urogenital sinus that connects to the upper vagina usually need early limited surgery to create a vaginal opening and to separate the vagina from the urethra thereby preventing backflow and pooling of urine. Clitoral recession rather than clitoridectomy is the usual practice now and efforts are being made to preserve the glans, the neurovascular bundle and sensory response. However, some young women have complained of discomfort resulting from genital surgery done in past decades. More data is also needed on the outcomes of early vs later vaginal surgery vis a vis vaginal width, depth, and comfort during intercourse. If vaginal surgery is postponed to late adolescence, the female patients have to be mature enough to do all of the postoperative care in order to have a fully functional vagina. The level of maturity and commitment are crucial variables in selecting the timing of surgery. Although many 46 XX CAH individuals with penile urethra have been raised as females following phallectomy and genital reconstructive surgery because they have ovaries and uterus, others have been successfully reared as males and have undergone gonadectomy and hysterectomy *(33)*. There is on going debate as to the best choice for these individuals who actually have unambiguously male external genitalia with female internal sex structures.

The most difficult decisions involve 46,XY infants with micropenis, either isolated or associated with hypospadius. The testes may be normal size, hypoplastic, or dysgenetic. Partial androgen insensitivity is a concern because male genital growth is permanently compromised. At present, many pediatric endocrinologists believe that 46,XY males with isolated unambiguous micropenis and fused scrotum should receive a short course of depot testosterone (25 mg im q month for 3 injections) in infancy and reared in the male role. The outcome of these infants in adult life appears to be reasonably good, even though penis size may not be within the normal range *(34–37)*. Sex reassignment of unambiguous microphallic 46,XY males to a female role is a practice that is being challenged more today within the medical profession. Similar treatment is usually given to 46,XY males with micropenis and hypospadius. This approach has been challenged on the basis that early phallic growth may not be a predictor of subsequent penile growth potential. However, many pediatric endocrinologists and urologists believe that rapid increases in length and width of the phallus are good prognosticators of future penile growth. Also, it facilitates the reconstructive surgery to correct hypospadias. In the most severely affected 46,XY males with negligible phallic tissue, the urologist will likely advise the team and parents that penile reconstruction is not possible. In these circumstances, the parents will make the final decision about accepting a female sex of rearing and the need for gonadectomy and later vaginal construction. However, religious

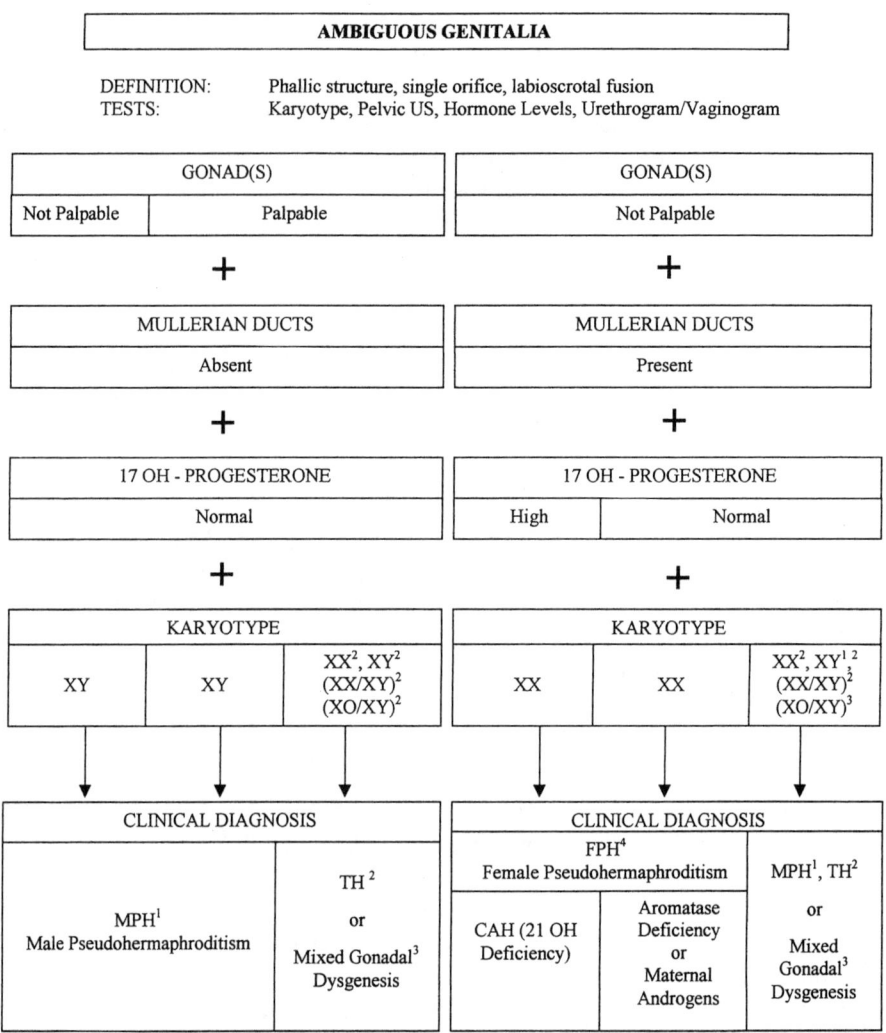

Fig. 2. Differential Diagnosis of Ambiguous Genitalia. The main features included in this diagram are the presence or absence of external gonads, the status of the Mullerian duct derivatives (uterus, etc.), the serum level of 17-hydroxyprogesterone, the karyotype, and possible clinical outcomes using this information. Disorders of sexual differentiation which do not cause ambiguous genitalia are not included in this diagram. Examples are 46,XY androgen resistance, 46,XY 17-α-hydroxylase deficiency, 46,XX males, and 46,XY females. All of these individuals have unambiguous female or male genitalia with discordant sex chromosomes.

MPH[1] = Male Pseudohermaphroditism. These are XY males with testes and incompletely virilized external genitalia due to:

(a) Structurally abnormal dysgenetic malfunctioning testes.
(b) Structurally normal testes that
    (1) Underproduce testosterone due to a defect in the biosynthetic steroidogenic path way; lack of LH receptor, etc.
    (2) Produce normal amounts of testosterone which fails to act on the external genitalia because of a defect in the androgen receptor (androgen resistance)
    or

beliefs may control the decision of parents in that all genetic males must be reared male regardless of penile size or future function. It is essential to give parents all the options as to sex of rearing including the pros and cons of each choice. If language barriers exist, an interpreter must assist communication. In some cultures, a male sex of rearing is considered an advantage regardless of the genital deformities. The medical team needs to be open minded and supportive even though they fear the worst outcome. Parents have to be comfortable with the chosen sex assignment decision since they are responsible for rearing their child. If they oppose the recommendation of the medical team and are forced to accept a decision they disagree with, the emotional well being of the child and family is placed in jeopardy. The level of parental understanding may require prolonged discussions and great patience by the medical team. The trained psychologist is particularly helpful in this situation.

(Continued from Fig. 2 on p. 442)
(3) Because of a deficiency of 5-a-reductase in the fetal genital tissues leading to a lack of 5-a-dihydrotestosterone, the essential androgen needed for male external genital differentiation.

TH[2] = True Hermaphroditism. It is characterized by the simultaneous presence of ovarian and testicular tissue in an individual (germ cell of both gonads). Most TH patients have 46,XX karyotype but 46,XY and 46,XX/46,XY mosaicism are also seen. The appearance of the external genitalia varies from mild to complete virilization depending on the functional capacity of the leydig cells. Also, the presence or absence of the Mullerian duct derivatives (uterus, etc.) is determined by the ability of Sertoli cells to make Anti mullerian hormone (AMH). Very virilized infants with TH are usually reared as male and undergo oophorectomy; they may or may not need later testosterone replacement in puberty and adult life; almost all are infertile because spermatogenesis is lacking in the testes of TH. The function of the fetal testes rather than the karyotype is the main determinant of sex assignment decisions. Female sex assignment is usually chosen if virilization is slight and the infant has a uterus and an ovary.

Mixed Gonadal Dysgenesis[3] is characterized by dysgenetic testes and streak gonads. Many infants have normal male external genitalia and others present with mild to severely virilized ambiguous genitalia. Subsequent short stature is common and the phenotypic features of Turner Syndrome are variably present.

FPH[4] = Female Pseudohermaphroditism. These are females with 46,XX chromosomes, ovaries, and uterus and virilized external genitalia. The most common cause is androgen production from the fetal adrenal gland due to 21 hydroxylase deficiency (CAH, 75% are salt losers) which interferes with the synthesis of cortisol and aldosterone but leaves the androgen steroidegenic pathway intact. The degree of virilization is classified using the Prader criteria. A penile urethra in a 46,XX CAH female is classified as Prader 5. This means the external appearance is entirely male whereas internally a uterus and ovaries are present. Other causes of FPH are:

(a) Androgens ingested by mother during gestation or produced by a maternal androgen-secreting tumor.
(b) Aromatase deficiency (p450 aromatase) is an autosomal recessive disorder which results from homologous or heteralogous mutation in the p450 aromatase genes. Consanguinity in parents may exist. Aromatase is a critical enzyme for estrogen production from precursor androgens. Aromatase deficiency in the fetus and placenta blocks the conversion of fetal androgens to estrogen leading to virilization of the female fetus as well as the mother during gestation. The 46,XY male fetus is not affected. During childhood, the 46,XX female does not exhibit androgen excess until onset of puberty when progressive virilization occurs. Estrogen replacement suppresses the elevated levels of gonadotropins and androgens and improves bone mineral density.

Disorders of sexual differentiation may be present in infants with normal or nearly normal external genitalia *(2,30)*. For example, 46,XY males who have complete androgen resistance (AR) or 17-α-hydroxylase (P450C17 or CYP17) deficiency are born with normal appearing female genitalia. 46,XY females with complete AR present either in childhood with a hernia containing a testis or in late adolescence or adulthood because of primary amenorrhea and absence of sexual hair. 46,XY females with 17-α-hydroxylase deficiency present with primary amenorrhea and hypertension due to ACTH mediated excess of mineralocorticoids from the adrenal glands. This condition is an autosomal recessive condition and consanguinity may be present in the parents. These patients fail to make all sex steroids because this enzyme plays a pivotal steroidogenic role in both the testis and adrenal glands. They are hairless and sometimes are misdiagnosed as androgen resistant (AR) females. The sertoli cells of the testes function normally, explaining why they lack of a uterus. A 46,XX female with the same genetic defect will also lack sex hormones and be hypertensive but she will menstruate when given estrogen replacement because she has a uterus. Androgen replacement in patients with 17-α-hydroxylase deficiency will result sexual hair growth that distinguishes them clinically from androgen resistant individuals.

Current Issues

The overall care of infants with ambiguous genitalia is currently undergoing re-examination by both the medical profession and by the lay public. In the past, 46,XY infant males with micropenis, with or without hypospadius, were often reassigned to a female sex of rearing *(38,39)*. This recommendation was based on the belief that it was easier to make a functional vagina than a functional penis. Thus, a female sex of rearing was predicted to result in a more favorable psychosexual outcome. The proponents of this recommendation appreciated the influences of intrinsic genetic forces (i.e., nature) as well as the impact of environmental factors (i.e., nurture) but reasoned that the environmental influences within the family were more dominant than the genetic forces if the sex reassignment was done within the first year of life *(40)*. With this strategy, the genital reconstructive surgery in infancy was done without a prior trial of testosterone therapy to enlarge the micropenis because it was believed that the penile response to treatment would not accurately predict the size of the penis in adulthood. Also, it was held that a micropenis at birth was synonymous with a micropenis at death. The validity of this premise had been undermined by follow- up studies of male infants with micropenis reared male who have reported satisfactory sexual function as adult men, even though they expressed concerns about their penis size *(34–37)*. Furthermore, some formerly male infants with micropenis who were sex reassigned and reared female have criticized the medical profession for performing surgical procedures to make female appearing external genitalia. These women now complain of genital discomfort and a lack of sexual arousability in adult life *(41)*. If this outcome is reported by larger numbers of patients, the rationale for female sex assignment decisions will be one which is not supported by scientific evidence. At present, the most vocal feedback has come from dissatisfied adults born with intersex who founded The Intersex Society of North America (ISNA) in 1994 *(42)*. They recommend avoidance of genital surgery in intersex infants without the patient's consent unless it is necessary for the child's health and comfort, and they advocate full disclosure of medical information given in a supportive emotional environment. Legally, parents have the authority to approve surgery for their infant with intersex because the infant is incapable of giving assent. However, it is evident that the challenge of creating a comfortable, adequately sized, sexually responsive vagina was significantly underestimated in past.

What have we learned in the past 4 decades about 46,XY infant males who were reassigned to a female sex of rearing? We know now that female sexual arousability and functioning is far more complicated than was assumed previously; it requires the preservation of erectile tissue and neural and vascular anatomy. Hence, a constructed vagina that lacks intravaginal sensory responses or the ability to lubricate will not likely result in satisfactory adult female sexual function. We also know that the clitoris is an important sexual organ; total clitoridectomy in virilized 46,XX female infants with CAH leads to a significant reduction of sexual sensation in adulthood. In addition, one recent follow-up study of 58 adult male pseudohermaphrodites from Johns Hopkins University has reported that a majority of those assigned either male or female were satisfied with the gender to which they had been assigned and with their sexual functioning *(43)*. A previous study of 46,XY adult pseudohermaphrodites by Money and collaborators also showed that most intersex individuals remained with their assigned gender, but the chances of adult patient initiated gender re-reassignment were higher in 46,XY patients reared female changing back to male gender identity than in those reared male changing to a female gender *(44,45)*. These outcomes are at variance with the experience reported by the ISNA group.

Has the poor prognosis previously given for 46,XY infant males with micropenis been proven by scientific evidence or outcomes research? Adult penis size is still seriously considered when decisions are made as to sex of rearing because a functional penis is essential for penis-vaginal intercourse. The current practice of administering testosterone, 25 mg im monthly for 3 injections, to male infants with micropenis before advising parents as to the need to consider reassignment to a female sex of rearing means that parents must accept longer periods of uncertainty before a final decision about the sex of rearing is made. Most families have the courage to tolerate this stressful experience because of the finality of the decision. We still need more information about the growth potential, erectile qualities, and minimal size requirement for a functional penis. Nevertheless, recent data indicate that males born with a small penis that never fully catches up in size are able to have satisfactory heterosexual adult experiences *(34–37)*. This means that we no longer should assume that a normal adult penis size is prerequisite for a man to be well adjusted and sexually active. Parents need to know that while penis size may not be fully restored to a normal adult range, the growth potential of an infant's penis is greater than was previously believed. Also, parents need information about the positive and negative aspects of choosing a female sex of rearing, since that decision will mandate vaginal construction in late adolescence and lack of guarantees, re: sexual arousability.

At present, there is general agreement as to the urgent need of feedback from former patients reared male or female to obtain additional information as to their level of satisfaction or dissatisfaction and their overall psychosocial/psychosexual adjustment. Many changes in the approach to the care of these children are taking place *(46,47)*. First, clitoral recession is the usual procedure rather than clitoridectomy or clitoral amputation in virilized 46,XX infants with CAH or other causes of androgen exposure. Second, improved surgical techniques are being developed to minimize genital discomfort and enhance sexual arousability in adulthood. Third, vaginal construction is usually postponed until adolescence, in order to have the patient fully involved in accepting the surgery as well as the responsibility for the post-operative care. Fourth, greater efforts are now being made to include the child in the decision making process if surgery is contemplated during the childhood and adolescent years. When all is said and done, the health professionals and parents chose the sex of assignment for an infant with ambiguous genitalia, but this does not guarantee that the child's gender identity will be in agreement with the chosen gender role.

Many important questions are still unanswered because we lack adequate follow-up information about adult patients. To what extent does androgen imprinting influence gender identity? The famous Joan-John patient was not an intersex infant, but rather a healthy male infant born with normal male external genitalia who had a circumcision accident at 7 mo that led to the loss of his penis; he also had a healthy twin brother. John was reared male until 17 mo when it was decided to reassign him to a female gender and he was renamed Joan; genital feminizing surgery was not done until he was 21 mo. In adulthood, Joan self re-reassigned herself to a male identity and took the name of John. The lateness of the sex reassignment at 17 mo and the prolonged period of a male sex of rearing coupled with normal male hormone levels in early childhood combine to make this a unique case that cannot be extrapolated to the care of 46,XY newborns with intersex *(48–52)*. We need more information about the gender identity of 46,XY males born with agenesis of the penis and normal testes and or male infants with perinatal traumatic loss of the penis in order to evaluate the significance of androgen imprinting on the development male gender identity *(53,54)*. The available outcome data on male infants with penile ablatio or cloacal exstrophy of the bladder who were reared female is conflicting, in that some, but not all individuals returned to a male gender. Androgen exposure has a major influence on gender-role behavior, but does not appear to be the primary determinant of gender identity *(55,56)*. For example, severe genital virilization of the 46,XX fetus with CAH because of high levels of androgens in utero is associated with tomboyish behavior and a higher prevalence of homosexuality, but the subsequent gender identity of these patients is female. Rarely do these virilized girls undergo a gender change from female to male *(57)*. Also, it is known that transexuals (male to female or vice versa) have a gender identity conflict, yet they were born endocrinologically normal with normal genitalia. Hence, the development of gender identity is a complex and incompletely understood phenomenon.

Concept of Sexual Dimorphism

Is the theory of sexual dimorphism a valid concept, i.e., is society comprised only of males or females? This simple idea has prevailed in Western culture since antiquity. Fausto-Sterling has challenged this belief by substituting five categories of gender (male, female, true hermaphrodite, female pseudohermaphrodite, and male pseudohermaphrodite). This theory lacks practical relevance. Very little has changed in the way gender identity is practiced. Most individuals consider themselves male, female, or bisexual. Gender identity is not synonymous with genital anatomy. The best example of this is the transsexual individual. At present we do not fully understand the forces controlling an individual's gender identity, even though we accept the interplay between genetic/hormonal /unknown factors and environmental influences *(11,58–65)*.

The following comments address recent attempts to conceptualize sex as a function of the genetic constitution of an organism and new efforts to re-interpret the meaning of genital malformations. The argument has been made that there are multiple genotypic sexes in humans and other mammalian species; hence the dimorphic concept of sex is scientifically inadequate to incorporate the variability in the genotypic makeup of individuals with disorders of sexual differentiation and the resulting clinical phenotypic diversity. This concept is the basis for the argument that genital malformations because of hermaphroditism, pseudohermaphroditism, and virilizing congenital adrenal hyperplasia should not be considered intersex conditions, but rather as expected variance of genotypic sex *(66)*. The end result of this line of reasoning is to abandon the dimorphic concept of sex (i.e., male and female) and substitute the concept of multiple sexes. It is argued that the dimorphic concept of sex has been one of the reasons for the current controversies in clinical management of intersex conditions.

The above interpretation of multiple genotypic sexes is not validated by evidence derived from molecular research, which details the precise contribution of many autosomal and sex chromosomal genes during each step in the process of fetal sexual differentiation. While it may be politically acceptable to deny the presence of a genetic defect, it is neither accurate nor scientifically sound to claim that genital malformations are the result of expected variance of genotypic sex. Patients are entitled to accurate explanations about the cause of their genital condition. When all goes well, there are only two outcomes of normal sexual differentiation in humans; i.e., male or female *(67)*. At present, we are able to identify most of the gene mutations that cause phenotypic variability in infants with disorders of sexual differentiation. The scientific proof for the existence multiple genotypic sexes and biologic phenotypic variability requires that normal molecular processes result in a diversity of phenotypic outcomes. Such is not the case; the phenotypic variability is always the result of abnormal gene function. It is our opinion that the concept of multiple genotypic sexes and expected biologic variability of phenotype will not simplify the care of infants born with genital defects. More importantly, this hypothesis is not validated by molecular genetic evidence. Until this debate is resolved, it is essential that health professionals adhere to scientific principles and maintain mutual respect for differing points of view. The ultimate goal is to educate and support our patients so that they will participate in all of life's experiences, fully understanding the past events in their medical care.

REFERENCES

1. Vilain E. Genetics of sexual development. Ann Rev Sex Res 2000;1:1–25.
2. Grumbach MM, Conte FA. Disorders of sex differentiation. In: Williams Textbook of Endocrinology (Wilson JD, ed.) Sanders, 1998.
3. Witchel SS, Lee PA. Ambiguous genitalia. In: Pediatric Endocrinology (Sperling MA, ed.) WB Sanders, Philadelphia, 1996, pp. 31–50.
4. Lee PA. Should We Change our Approach to Ambiguous Genitalia. The Endocrinologist 2001;11: 118–123.
5. Quigley CA. Chapter 140 In: Genetic Bases of Sex Determination and Differentiation, 4th ed. (De Groot LJ, ed.) Saunders, Philadelphia, 2001, pp. 1926–1946.
6. Migeon CJ, Berkovitz G, Brown T. Sexual differentiation and ambiguity. In: The Diagnosis and Treatment of Endocrine Disorders in Childhood and Adolescence (Kappy MS, Bilzzard RM, Migeon CJ, eds.) Charles C. Thomas, Springfield, 1994; pp. 659–662.
7. Root A. Genetic errors of sexual differentiation. Adv Pediatr 1999;46–67.
8. McElreavey K, Barbaux S, Ion A, Fellous M. The genetic basis of murine and human sex determination: A review. Heredity 1995;75:599–611.
9. McElreavey K, Fellous M. Sex determination and the Y chromosome. Am J Med Genet 1999;89:176.
10. Zucker KJ. Intersexuality and gender identity differentiation. Ann Rev Sex Res 1999;10:1–69.

11. Meyer-Bahlburg HFL. Gender assignment and reassignment in 46 XY pseudohermaphrodites and related conditions. J Clin Endocrinol Metab 1999;4:3455–3458.
12. Meyer-Bahlburg HFL. Gender assignment in intersexuality. J Psychol Hum Sex 1998;10:1–21.
13. Udry JR. Biological Limits of Gender Construction. Am Sociol Rev 2000;65:443–457.
14. Koopman P, Gubbay J, Vivian N, Goodfellow PN, Lovell-Bodge R. Male development of chromosomally female mice transgenic for Sry. Nature 1991;117–121.
15. Koopman P. Sry and Sox 9: Mammalian testes-determining genes. Cell Mol Life Sc 1999;55:839–856.
16. Vainio S, Keikkila M, Chin N, McMahon AP. Female development in mammals is regulated by Wnt-4 signalling. Nature 1999;397:405–409.
17. Huang B, Wang S, Ning Y, Lamb AN, Bartley J. Autosomal XX sex reversal caused by duplication of SOX 9. Am J Med Gen 1999;87:349–359.
18. Bardoni B, Zanaria E, Guioli S, et al. A dosage-sensitive locus at chromosome Xp21 is involved in male to female sex reversal. Nat Genet 1994;7:497–501.
19. Arn P, Chen H, Tuck-Miller CM, Mankinen C, Wachtel G, Li S et al. SRXX; A sex reversing locus in Xp21.2–p22.11. Hum Genet 1994;93:389–393.
20. Wieacker P, Missbach D. Sex reversal in a child with karyotype 46 XY, dup (1) (pp22.3 p32.3). Clin Genet 1996; 49:271–273.
21. Jordan BK, Mohammed M, Ching ST, Dilot E, Chen XN, Dewing P. Upregulation of Wnt-4 signaling and dosage-sensitive sex reversal in humans. Am J Hum Genet 2001;68:1102–1109.
22. Zanaria E, Muscatelli F, Bardoni B, et al. An usual member of the nuclear hormone receptor super family responsibility for x-linked adrenal hypoplasia congenita. Nature 1994;372:635–641.
23. Imperato-McGinley J, Guerrero L, Gautier T, et al. Steroid 5-α reductase deficiency in man: An inherited form of male pseudohermaphroditism. Science 1974;186:1213.
24. Peterson RE, Imperato-McGinley J, Gautier T, Sturla E. Male pseudohermaphroditism due to steroid 5 alpha reductase deficiency. American Journal of Medicine 1977;62:170–191.
25. Imperato-McGinley J, Peterson RE, Gautier T, et al. Androgens and the evaluation of male-gender identity among male pseydohermaphrodites with 5 α reductase deficiency. N Engl J Med 1979;300(1233).
26. White PC, Speiser PW. Congenital adrenal hyperplasia due to 21-hydroxylase deficiency. Endocr Rev 2000;21:245.
27. Morishima A, Grumbach MM, Simpson ER, Fisher C, Qin K. Aromatase deficiency in male and female siblings caused by novel mutation and the physiological role of estrogens. J Clin Endocrinol Metab 1995;80:3689–3697.
28. Müller J, et al. Management of males with 45X/46XY gonadal dysgenesis. Horm Res 1999;52:11.
29. Sarafoglou K, Ostrer H. Familial sex reversal: A review. J Clin Endocrinol Metab 2000;85:483–493.
30. Quigley CA, DeBellis A, Marschke KB, el-Awady MK, Wilson EM, French FS. Androgen receptor defects: Historical, clinical, and molecular perspectives. Endocr Rev 1995;16:271–321.
31. Committee on Genetics Endocrinology and Urology, American Academy of Pediatrics. Evaluation of the newborn with developmental anomalies of the external genitalia. Pediatrics 2000;106:138.
32. Feldman KW, Smith DW. Fetal phallic growth and penile standards for newborn male infants. J Pediatr 1975;86:395.
33. Lee PA, Witchel SF. Adult 46XX males with adrenal hyperplasia: Outcome data. Pediatr Res 2000;47:134A.
34. Bin-Abbas B, Conte FA, Grumbach MM, Kaplan SL. Congenital hypogonadotropic hypogonadism and micropenis: effect of testosterone treatment on adult penile size- why sex reversal is not indicated. J Pediatr 1999;134:579–583.
35. Reilly JM, Woodhouse CR. Small penis and the male sexual role. J Urol 1989;142:569–571.
36. Van Wyk JJ, Calikoglu AS. Should boys with micropenis be reared as girls? J Pediatr 1999;134: 537–538.
37. Mazur T, Sandberg DE, Perrin MA, et al. Patients with micro or small penis reared male: Adult quality of life and psychosocial outcomes The Endocrine Society Annual Meeting Toronto, ON 2000.
38. Money J, Lehne GK, Pierre-Jerome F. Micropenis: gender, erotosexual coping strategy, and behavioral health in nine pediatric cases followed to adulthood. Compr Psychiatry 1985;26:29–42.
39. Money J, Mazur T, Abrams C, Norman BF. Micropenis, family mental health, and neonatal mangment: a report on 14 patients reared as girls. J Prev Psychiatry 1981;1(17):27.
40. Money J, Ehrhardt AA. Man and Woman, Boy and Girl. Differentiation and Dimorphism of Gender Identity from Conception to Maturity. Baltimore: 1972, pp.117–146.
41. Chase C. Surgical progress is not the answer to intersexuality. J Clin Ethics 1998;9:385–392.

42. Intersex Society of North America. Recommendations for Treatment: Intersex Infants and Children. 1985. San Francisco, ISNA. Ref Type: Pamphlet
43. Meyer-Bahlburg HFL, Migeon CJ, Berkovitz GD, Gearhart JP, and Wisniewski AB Satisfaction with gender and genital status and attitude to management policies in adult 46 XY pseudohermaphrodites International Academy Sex Research 25th Annual Meeting Stony Brook, NY, 1999.
44. Money J, Devore H, Norman BF. Transition: Longitudinal outcome study of 33 male hermaphrodites assigned girls. J Sex Marit Ther 1986;12:165–181.
45. Money J, Norman BF. Gender identity and gender transposition: Longitudinal outcome of 24 male hermaphrodites assigned as boys. J Sex Marit Ther 1987;13:75–92.
46. Schober JM. A surgeon's response to the intersex controversy. J Clin Ethics 1998;9:393–397.
47. Creighton S. Surgery for intersex. J R Soc Med 2001;94:218–220.
48. Colapinto J. As Nature Made Him: The Boy Who Was Raised as a Girl. New York: HarperCollins, 2000.
49. Diamond M, Sigmundson HK. Sex reassignment at birth. Long-term review and clinical implications. Arch Pediatr Adolesc Med 1997;151:298.
50. Diamond M. Sexual identity and sexual orientation in children with traumatized or ambiguous genitalia. J Sex Res 1997;34:199–211.
51. Diamond M. Critical evaluation of the ontogeny of human sexual behavior. Q Rev Biol 1965;40: 147–175.
52. Diamond M, Sigmundson HK. Management of intersexuality: guidelines for dealing with persons with ambiguous genitalia. Arch Pediatr Adolesc Med 1997;151:1046–1050.
53. Money J. Ablatio penis: nature/nurture redux. In: Sin, Science, and the Sex Police: Essays on Sexology and Sexosophy (Money J, ed.) Prometheus Books, Amherst, NY, 1999: pp. 297–326.
54. Bradley SJ, Oliver GD, Chermick AB, Zucker KJ. Experiment of nurture: Ablatio penis at 2 months, sex-reassignment at 7 months, and a psychosexual follow-up in young adulthood. Pediatrics 1998;102.
55. Ehrhardt AA, Evers K, Money J. Influence of androgen and some aspects of sexually dimorphic behavior in women with the late-treated adrengenital syndrome. Johns Hopkins Med J 1968;123:115–122.
56. Ehrhardt AA, Epstein R, Money J. Fetal androgens and female gender identity in the early treated adrenogenital syndrome. Johns Hopkins Med J 1968;122:160–167.
57. Meyer-Bahlburg HFL, Gruen RS, New MI, et al. Gender change from female to male in classical Congenital Adrenal Hyperplasia. Horm Behav 1996;30:319–322.
58. Meyer-Bahlburg HFL. Variants of gender differentiation. In: Outcomes in Developmental Psychopathology (Steinhausen HC, Verhulst FE, eds). Oxford University Press, New York, 1999, pp. 298–313.
59. Kessler SJ. Lessons for the Intersex. Rutgers University Press, Piscatway, 1998.
60. Fausto-Sterling A. Sexing the Body: Gender Politics and the Construction of Sexuality. Basic Books, New York, 2000.
61. Herdt G (ed). Third Sex, Third Gender: Beyond Sexual Dimorphism in Culture and History. Zone Books, New York, 1996.
62. Reiner WG. Sex assignment in the neonate with intersex or inadequate genitalia. Pediatr Adolesc Med 1997;151:1044.
63. Dreger AD. Hermaphrodites and the Medical Intervention of Sex. Harvard University Press, Cambridge, MA, 1998.
64. Howe EG. Special issue Intersexuality J Clin Ethics 1998;9:4.
65. Wisniewski AB, Migeon CJ, Meyer-Bahlburg HFL, et al. Complete androgen insensitivity syndrome: Long-term medical, surgical, and pyschosexual outcome. J Clin Endocrinol Metab 2000;85: 2664–2669.
66. McCullogh LB A framework for the ethically justified clinical management of intersex conditions Pediatric Gender Reassignment: A Critical Reapprasial Dallas, TX 1999.
67. Sax L. How common is intersex? A response to Anne Fausto, Sterling, J Sex Research 2002;39:174–178.

25 Menstrual Disorders and Hyperandrogenism in Adolescence

Robert L. Rosenfield, MD

CONTENTS
INTRODUCTION
ETIOLOGY
DIFFERENTIAL DIAGNOSIS
MANAGEMENT
REFERENCES

INTRODUCTION

The menstrual disorders that concern endocrinologists are primary amenorrhea (failure of menses to begin at a normal age), *secondary amenorrhea* (cessation of menstrual periods for 4 mo or more after initially menstruating), *oligomenorrhea* (less than 9 menstrual periods a year), and *dysfunctional uterine bleeding* (anovulatory bleeding which is abnormally frequent or excessive) *(1)*. Menses which occur excessively frequently (at more often than 22 d intervals) are also suggestive of anovulatory cycles.

Adolescents require special consideration for three reasons. The first is because of the normal variation in the age of onset of puberty. The National Child Health Survey (NCHS) in the 1960s found menarche to occur at 12.7 ± 1.0 yr of age in the US *(2)*. A more recent prospective study in Cincinnatti, Ohio found that menarche occurred at 12.6 yr in Caucasians and 12.0 yr in Negros *(3)*. Breast development has been estimated from NCHS data to begin at 10.75 ± 1.0 (SD) yr of age in North America *(4)*. The second is that menarche will be delayed if puberty is delayed in onset, although there is a tendency for puberty to be of shorter duration when it begins relatively late *(5,6)*. The third is that physiologic anovulation must also be taken into consideration. Adolescents often have long periods of anovulation before they establish a menstrual pattern that is normal by adult standards. About half of menstrual cycles are anovulatory in the 2 yr after menarche *(7)*. If irregular cycles persist for 2 yr after menarche, an approximate 67% probability of ongoing menstrual irregularity exists. The normal menstrual cycle length varies with age, the interval between menstrual cycles decreasing in the first several years after menarche (Fig. 1) *(8)*.

From: *Contemporary Endocrinology: Pediatric Endocrinology: A Practical Clinical Guide*
Edited by: S. Radovick and M. H. MacGillivray © Humana Press Inc., Totowa, NJ

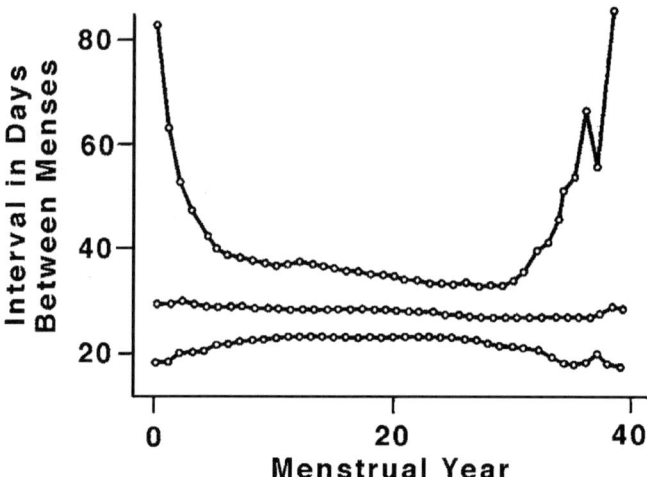

Fig. 1. Menstrual cycle lengths throughout reproductive life from menarche to menopause. Tenth, fiftieth, and ninetieth percentiles are shown. Reproduced with permission from ref. *(8).*

ETIOLOGY

Two general types of disorders cause these menstrual abnormalities: those that are associated with genital tract disorders and, more often, those that result from anovulation. The etiology of menstrual disorders is given in Table 1 *(9).*

Genital Tract Disorders

Failure of the onset of menses can result from structural abnormalities of the genital tract that do not have an endocrinologic basis. If the uterus is intact, hydrometrocolpos will occur, however. The vagina may have an imperforate hymen. The vagina or uterus may be congenitally aplastic. Varying degrees of vaginal and uterine aplasia are associated in the Rokitansky-Kustner-Hauser syndrome *(10).* This syndrome seems to occur as a single gene defect or as an acquired teratogenic event that sometimes affects differentiation of the urinary tract.

Uterine aplasia may also result from those intersex syndromes in which anti-Müllerian hormone secretion by testicular tissue has occurred. For this reason, primary amenorrhea may be the presenting symptom of phenotypic girls with complete androgen resistance (testicular feminization syndrome) or congenital deficiency in one of the enzymes necessary for testicular testosterone secretion. It is also a complaint in patients with ambiguous genitalia due to partial versions of these disorders or due to 5α-reductase deficiency.

Intrauterine adhesions (Asherman's syndrome) may result from trauma, such as postcurettage or as a complication of radiation therapy of pelvic disease or chronic inflammatory disease *(11).*

Abnormal bleeding, on the other hand, can result from genital tract trauma or infection. The most common examples of these are sexual abuse and foreign body. Bleeding may also result from genital tract tumors.

Anovulatory Disorders

Anovulatory disorders are otherwise the most common cause of menstrual disorders, and the most common cause of these is pregnancy. Anovulatory disorders can be catego-

Table 1
Causes of Adolescent Menstrual Disorders[a]

ABNORMAL GENITAL STRUCTURE
    Aplasia[b]
        Hymenal
        Vaginal
        Müllerian
        Intersex
    Endometrial adhesions
    Ambiguous Genitalia
        Intersex
        Pseudointersex
ANOVULATORY DISORDERS
    Hypoestrogenism: FSH Elevated
        Primary ovarian failure
            Congenital
                Chromosomal disorders
                Genetic disorders
                Resistant ovaries
                Bioinactive gonadotropin
                Steroidogenic block
            Acquired
                Oophorectomy
                Radiotherapy or chemotherapy
                Oophoritis
                Idiopathic
    Hypoestrogenism: FSH Not Elevated
        Gonadotropin deficiency
            Congenital
            Acquired
                Organic
                Functional (non-organic)
    Delayed puberty
        Constitutional delay[b]
        Growth-retarding disease
    Primary ovarian failure
        Complete, if BA <11 yr[b]
        Incomplete, if BA >11 yr
    Virilization
    Estrogenized: FSH Not Elevated
        Pregnancy
        Functional hypothalamic anovulation
            Athletic amenorrhea
            Psychogenic amenorrhea
            Idiopathic functional hypothalamic amenorrhea
            Post-pill amenorrhea
        Secondary hypothalamic anovulation
            Chronic disease
            Undernutrition or obesity
            Cushing's syndrome
            Hypothyroidism
            Hyperprolactinemia
        Hyperandrogenism

[a] Adapted with permission from ref. (9).
[b] Cause only primary amenorrhea

rized according to whether or not the patient is hypoestrogenic and whether or not gonadotropins, particularly serum follicle stimulating hormone (FSH) levels, are elevated (Table 1). Anovulation often results from various degrees of hypogonadism. If hypogonadism is complete and is present prior to the onset of neuroendocrine puberty, it causes sexual infantilism. If hypogonadism is slightly less severe or becomes manifest in the early teenage years, it may permit some feminization, but too little to permit the onset of menses. In either case, primary amenorrhea results. Milder, partial, or incomplete forms of hypogonadism may cause either secondary amenorrhea or oligomenorrhea. At its mildest, hypogonadism may present with the anovulatory symptoms of dysfunctional uterine bleeding or with excessively frequent periods due to short luteal phase.

Hypoestrogenism with elevated FSH indicates primary ovarian failure (hypergonadotropic hypogonadism). The causes include both hereditary and acquired disorders. Chromosomal disorders are well-known causes of ovarian failure. Gonadal dysgenesis due to sex chromosome abnormalities, particulary deficiency of genes on the X-chromosome causing Turner syndrome, is the most common cause of primary ovarian failure, with an incidence of about 1 in 2500 live born girls. About 5% of Turner syndrome patients present with secondary amenorrhea, even though they have congenitally dysgenetic ovaries *(12)*. Autosomal aneuploidy *(13)* or gene mutations *(14,15)* can also cause gonadal dysgenesis. Fragile X-chromosome premutation is associated with some cases of X-linked premature ovarian failure *(16)*. Premature ovarian failure may result from hereditary gonadotropin resistance: LH receptor and FSH receptor mutations have recently been found to cause autosomal recessive gonadotropin resistance *(17)*. These have been associated with a spectrum of defects ranging from primary amenorrhea to oligomenorrhea. Partial gonadotropin resistance is common in the Albright osteodystrophy form of pseudohypo-parathyroidism because of the generalized defect in G-protein signal transduction *(18)*. On rare occasions, bioinactive gonadotropins may simulate primary gonadal failure *(19,20)*. Steroidogenic blocks in estradiol biosynthesis can also cause secondary amenorrhea *(21)*. Acquired ovarian failure commonly results from irradiation, chemotherapy, trauma to the ovary, or autoimmune disease. Unexplained acquired ovarian failure has an autoimmune basis in approx one-third of cases *(22)*.

Hypoestrogenism without elevated FSH levels usually indicates secondary ovarian failure (gonadotropin deficiency, hypogonadotropic hypogonadism) because a normal gonadotropin level is inappropriate in the setting of hypoestrogenism. Gonadotropin deficiency can be congenital or acquired. Congenital gonadotropin deficiency can occur in association with cerebral, hypothalamic, or pituitary dysfunction, or as an isolated defect *(20)*. Congenital hypopituitarism may be due to a chromosomal disorder (such as in Prader-Willi syndrome), be due to single gene mutations (as in Prop-1 deficiency), or be associated with congenital brain defects of unknown origin. Congenital isolated gonadotropin deficiency may result from autosomal recessive disorders, of which gonadotropin releasing hormone (GnRH) receptor deficiency is more common in women than the anosmia-associated Kallmann's syndrome *(23)*.

Acquired gonadotropin deficiency may be organic or functional (non-organic). Organic acquired gonadotropin deficiency can be a consequence of tumors, trauma, autoimmune hypophysitis *(24)*, degenerative disorders involving the hypothalamus and pituitary *(25)*, irradiation *(26)*, or chronic illness of virtually any organ system *(27)*. Functional hypogonadotropinism is commonly caused by eating disorders *(28)*. Anorexia nervosa is the prototypic form, but bulimia nervosa, the binge-eating/purging variant, is easily overlooked because the weight is often normal and vomiting surreptitious. In these disorders, low body fat blunts the secretion of leptin, which is important for the function of the GnRH pulse generator *(29)*. Stress-related neurotransmitter dysfunction causes proopiomelano-cortin overproduction and a mild state of cortisol excess *(30)*. Hyperprolactinemia can also cause functional gonadotropin deficiency, as discussed below.

Delayed puberty seems to be a persistance of the prepubertal state of physiologic isolated gonadotropin deficiency. It may be secondary to chronic disease of virtually any organ system or, most commonly, it may occur as a familial extreme variation of normal which is termed "constitutional delay in growth and pubertal development".

Gonadotropin deficiency can also be mimiced by primary ovarian failure in two circumstances. The most common is in children who are too young to have undergone neuroendocrine puberty, as indicated by a bone age <11 yr. Gonadotropin levels may also not be elevated in premature ovarian failure because gonadotropin levels may be normal as the ovary begins to fail during the menopausal transition *(31,32)*. Suppression of gonadotropins and estrogens occurs in frankly virilizing disorders.

Menstrual disturbance in the presence of adequate estrogenization is probably the single most common problem that is encountered. Pregnancy, hypothalamic anovulation, with its diverse causes including hyperprolactinemia, and hyperandrogenism are the considerations.

Hypothalamic anovulation occurs in patients who secrete sufficient gonadotropin tonically to estrogenize normally, but have disorders that interfere with the ability to produce a midcycle surge of luteinizing hormone. In this group of disorders, there are disturbances of cyclic or pulsatile GnRH release that interfere with the positive feedback mechanism. Functional hypothalamic amenorrhea is often seen in the setting of weight loss, athletic stress, or psychogenic stress. Even when these factors are not obvious, idiopathic functional hypothalamic amenorrhea bears resemblance to anorexia nervosa *(33)*. Post-pill amenorrhea may be suspected after the long-term use of hormonal contraceptives. However, this entity usually results from an undetected antecedent anovulatory disturbance or an intercurrent illness, so a work-up is required.

Chronic disease of virtually any organ system can mimic gonadotropin deficiency or hypothalamic anovulation. Obesity is thought to cause amenorrhea via the overproduction of estrogen from plasma precursors in adipose tissue *(34)*. Glucocorticoid excess causes amenorrhea by multiple mechanisms, prime among which is interference with gonadotropin responsiveness to GnRH *(30,35)*. Thyroid disorders are well-known causes of menstrual irregularity *(36)*.

Hyperprolactinemia requires special consideration since it varies greatly in its presentation. This is because it engenders variable degrees of gonadotropin deficiency. Prime among the multiple mechanisms is disruption of GnRH pulsatility *(37,38)*. Galactorrhea is present in about half of the patients, particularly those with residual estrogen production. The causes of hyperprolactinoma are diverse, and include hypothalamic or pituitary disorders, drugs, hypothyroidism, renal or liver failure, peripheral neuropathy, stress, and idiopathic. It is not only in the differential diagnosis of hypogonadotropic hypogonadism and hypothalamic amenorrhea, it may cause short or inadequate luteal phase (characterized by menstrual cycles less than 22 d), dysfunctional uterine bleeding, or a hyperandrogenic picture.

Hyperandrogenism is the most frequent cause of anovulation, after pregnancy, so it is considered in more detail next.

Table 2
Causes of Hyperandrogenism[a]

Functional Gonadal Hyperandrogenism
    Primary (dysregulational) functional ovarian hyperandrogenism[b]
    Secondary polycystic ovary syndrome
- Poorly controlled classic congenital adrenal hyperplasia
- Syndromes of severe insulin resistance
- Ovarian steroidogenic blocks

    Adrenal rests
    Hermaphroditism
    Chorionic gonadotropin-related
Functional Adrenal Hyperandrogenism
    Primary (dysregulational) functional adrenal hyperandrogenism[c]
    Congenital adrenal hyperplasia
    Prolactin or growth hormone excess
    Dexamethasone-resistant functional adrenal hyperandrogenism
- Cushing's syndrome
- Cortisol resistance
- Apparent cortisone reductase deficiency

Peripheral Androgen Overproduction
    Obesity
    Idiopathic hyperandrogenism
Tumoral Hyperandrogenism
Androgenic Drugs

[a]Adapted with permission from ref. *(39)*.
[b]Common form of PCOS.
[c]Uncommon form of PCOS.

Hyperandrogenism

Androgen excess arises from abnormal ovarian or adrenal sources in the vast majority of cases. It occasionally appears to be caused by abnormalities in the peripheral formation of androgen, rarely by tumors or by self-administration. The causes of hyperandrogenism are listed in Table 2 *(39)*.

POLYCYSTIC OVARY SYNDROME (PCOS)

PCOS is the most common cause of androgen excess presenting at or after the onset of puberty. The classic Stein-Leventhal form accounts for nearly half the cases of chronic hyperandrogenism. This is characterized clinically by various combinations of amenorrhea, hirsutism, and obesity, and endocrinologically by hyperandrogenemia, as well as polycystic ovaries or elevation of serum LH *(39–41)*. About two-thirds of patients with classic PCOS, so defined, have hirsutism (or the hirsutism equivalents, acne vulgaris or pattern alopecia), two-thirds have anovulatory symptoms (which vary from amenorrhea to dysfunctional uterine bleeding to unexplained infertility), and half are obese. Thus, only about a third of otherwise classic cases have the full-blown clinical picture (Fig. 2). Approximately eighty percent have the characteristic PCOS-type of primary functional ovarian hyperandrogenism (FOH), and half have the characteristic PCOS-type of primary functional adrenal hyperandrogenism (FAH). Acanthosis nigricans, a sign of insulin resistance, may be prominent.

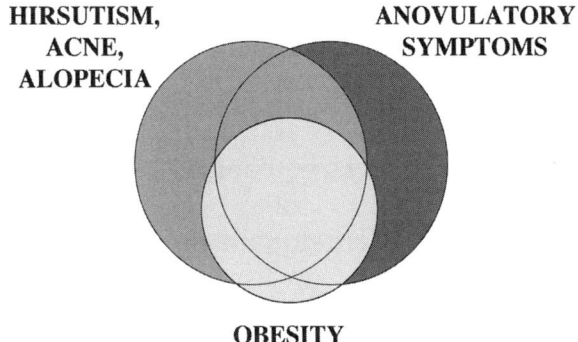

Fig. 2. Manifestations of polycystic ovary syndrome in approximate proportion to their relative incidence and coincidence. Cutaneous symptoms include hirsutism, acne or acanthosis nigricans. Anovulatory symptoms include amenorrhea, oligomenorrhea, dysfunctional uterine bleeding, and infertility. Reproduced with permission from ref. (39).

Atypical cases (nonclassic PCOS) that do not meet the classic laboratory criteria but possess the characteristic PCOS-type of FOH, or occasionally FAH, account for most remaining cases of chronic hyperandrogenism. FOH occurs alone in approximately one-third of cases, FOH and FAH coexist in approximately one-third, and FAH occurs alone in approximately one-quarter. The more obese the patient, the less likely serum LH is to be elevated, probably because insulin excess exerts a co-gonadotropic effect. As a group, PCOS is accompanied by insulin-resistant hyperinsulinemia, but this is not uniformly present.

PCOS in adolescents has clinical and endocrine features similar to those of adults (42). In addition, there may be a history of premature onset of pubic hair, breast development, obesity, and/or pseudoacromegaly. Although the typical ovarian dysfunction is often found in the perimenarcheal phase of development (42), it may not be demonstrable until 3 yr after menarche (43).

Pathophysiology. The central abnormality in primary FOH seems to be intraovarian androgen excess. The intraovarian androgen concentrations arising in FOH are higher than in most adrenal causes of androgen excess and seem responsible for the ovarian abnormalities: intraovarian androgen excess appears to stimulate excessive growth of small follicles while hindering the follicular maturation involved in the emergence of a dominant follicle, as well as causing thecal and stromal hyperplasia.

The PCOS-type of FOH was demonstrated to be characterized by 17-hydroxyprogesterone (17-OHP) hyperresponsiveness to GnRH agonist stimulation without evidence of a steroidogenic block and by subnormal dexamethasone suppression of plasma free testosterone and 17-OHP in the presence of normal adrenocortical suppression. Dexamethasone suppression and GnRH agonist test results are 65–85% concordant. The PCOS-type of FAH consists of moderately excessive 17-ketosteroid responses to ACTH without evidence of a steroidogenic block. This FAH had earlier often been mistaken for nonclassical 3β-hydroxysteroid dehydrogenase deficiency, now known to be a rare disorder. Although FAH has also been suspected of being "exaggerated adrenarche," this explanation now seems unlikely for several reasons, one of which is that the adrenarche marker dehydroepiandrosterone sulfate (DHEAS) is elevated in only about 20% of cases.

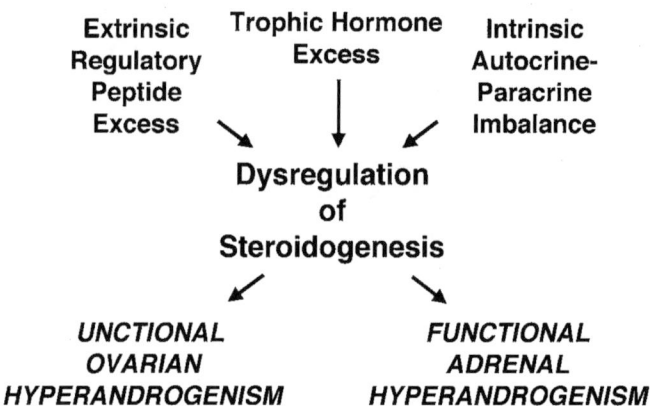

Fig. 3. Model of factors causing the common types of functional ovarian and adrenal hyperandrogenism. A mild degree of androgen excess can arise from excess trophic hormone (LH or ACTH) stimulation. Disturbances either extrinsic or intrinsic to these endocrine glands can amplify the effect of normal levels of trophic hormones. Extrinsic regulatory peptide excess is exemplified by hyperinsulinemia. Intrinsic peptides capable of inappropriately up-regulating steroidogenesis include IGFs. Reproduced with permission from ref. *(41)*.

These studies have led to the hypothesis that primary FOH and primary FAH are due to abnormal regulation (dysregulation) of steroidogenesis. Dysregulation is postulated to result from imbalance among various intrinsic and extrinsic factors involved in the modulation of trophic hormone action (Fig. 3). Within the ovary, there appear to be flaws in the processes which normally coordinate androgen and estrogen secretion. This causes the ovaries to hyperrespond to LH, rather than undergoing down-regulation in response to LH stimulation. Recent evidence suggests that the majority of cases have an intrinsic theca cell defect that causes widespread, but not global, overexpression of steroidogenic enzymes *(44)*. This raises the possibility that the fundamental defect in PCOS may be one of transcriptional co-regulation of a panoply of processes.

Insulin excess appears to be an important extrinsic factor in dysregulation, and treatments which lower insulin levels reduce the androgen excess. The insulin/insulin-like growth factor (IGF) system seems to act in synergism with trophic hormones to cause ovarian or adrenal androgen excess. The ovaries and adrenal glands function as if responding to the hyperinsulinemic state in spite of the resistance to the effects of insulin on skeletal glucose metabolism. This paradox remains to be resolved.

Excessive LH secretion was once thought to be central to the pathogenesis of PCOS due to a complex cycle of events in which peripheral conversion of adrenal androstenedione to estrone sensitized gonadotropes to GnRH ("estrone hypothesis"). However, LH excess does not appear to be causative since it is not a consistent feature of the syndrome, although the syndrome is gonadotropin-dependent.

Pathogenesis. The cause of PCOS is unknown, but there is considerable interest in the possibility that PCOS may arise as a complex genetic disorder in which an intrinsic ovarian genetic trait interacts with other congenital or environmental factors to cause dysregulation of steroidogenesis *(39,45–47)*. Proposed ovarian predisposing traits include polycystic ovaries, steroidogenic enzyme polymorphisms *(45,47)*, or a serine phosphorylase enhancer. In this model, a "second hit" is required to precipitate the syndrome. For example, polycystic ovaries in seemingly normal women produce excessive androgens, but to a subclinical extent *(48–50)*. Asymptomatic mothers with polycystic ovaries (or the postulated male equivalent, premature male pattern baldness) transmit this trait to offspring in autosomal dominant fashion, and affected daughters manifest the *syndrome* only if it is precipitated by another factor. An important precipitant seems to be insulin-resistant hyperinsulinemia: this may arise on an environmental basis (e.g., dietary obesity or puberty) or a genetic one (e.g., type 2 diabetes mellitus). PCOS clearly has a relationship to adult-type diabetes mellitus. Approximately one-third of patients have a parent with diabetes mellitus, and PCOS patients have a high incidence of diabetes-like defects in insulin secretion, insulin sensitivity, and glucose tolerance *(51,52)*. Other proposed precipitating factors include premature adrenarche, heterozygosity for congenital adrenal hyperplasia *(53)*, a predisposition to LH excess ("hyperpuberty"), and intrauterine growth retardation *(54)*. Prenatal androgenization may program the female fetus to develop LH excess, ovarian hyperandrogenism, amenorrhea, and insulin resistance *(55–57)*.

OTHER CAUSES OF FUNCTIONAL OVARIAN HYPERANDROGENISM

FOH can be secondary to several disorders (Table 2). Extraovarian androgen excess (as in poorly controlled congenital adrenal hyperplasia) and ovarian steroidogenic blocks (such as 3β-hydroxysteroid dehydrogenase, 17β-hydroxysteroid dehydrogenase, or aromatase deficiency) are causes. Excessive stimulation of the LH receptor may well mediate the hyperandrogenism reported with chorionic gonadotropin-related ovarian dysfunction during pregnancy and with partially resistant ovarian follicles *(58)*. All known forms of extreme insulin resistance, including the hereditary cases which are due to insulin receptor mutations, as well as acromegaly *(59)*, are accompanied by PCOS, apparently by excessively stimulating the IGF-I signal transduction pathway to escape from desensitization to LH. Functional ovarian hyperandrogenism may also result from adrenal rests of the ovaries in congenital adrenal hyperplasia or from true hermaphroditism. PCOS has also been reported as a complication of the impaired steroid metabolism that occurs as a complication of portasystemic shunting *(60)*.

OTHER CAUSES OF FUNCTIONAL ADRENAL HYPERANDROGENISM

Less than 10% of adrenal hyperandrogenism can be attributed to the well-understood disorders listed in Table 2. Congenital adrenal hyperplasia arises from an autosomal recessive deficiency in the activity of any one of the adrenocortical enzyme steps necessary for the biosynthesis of corticosteroid hormones *(61)*. Mild enzyme deficiency causes nonclassical ("late-onset") presentations, which lack the genital ambiguity of classic congenital adrenal hyperplasia and cause adolescent or adult-onset of anovulatory symptoms and/or hirsutism. Women with the nonclassical disorder may have polycystic ovaries and high serum luteinizing hormone levels, but FOH seems to be unusual except in the presence of adrenal rests of the ovaries *(55)*. Nonclassical 21-hydroxylase deficiency is the most common form of congenital adrenal hyperplasia and accounts for about 5% of hyperandrogenic adolescents in the general population. Deficiency of 3β-hydroxysteroid dehydrogenase (3β-HSD) or 11β-hydroxylase are forms of congenital adrenal hyperplasia which have on rare occasions presented in adolescence.

Dexamethasone-resistant forms of hyperandrogenism, such as Cushing's syndrome, cortisol resistance, or apparent cortisone reductase deficiency *(62)*, are even more unusual than nonclassic congenital adrenal hyperplasia. Prolactin excess causes adrenal hyperandrogenism *(63).* Cushing's and hyperprolactinemia sometimes occur in association with polycystic ovaries *(64,65).*

OTHER CAUSES OF HYPERANDROGENISM

In approx 8% of hyperandrogenic patients, a cause cannot be ascertained after thorough testing. This is idiopathic hyperandrogenemia. Few of these patients have menstrual abnormalities. Obesity seems to explain some of these cases, because adipose tissue has the capacity to form testosterone from androstenedione. Obesity may simulate PCOS by causing amenorrhea, acanthosis nigricans, and hyperandrogenemia *(41)* Other idioipathic cases may be due to hereditary quirks in peripheral metabolism of steroids. Tumor and exogenous ingestion of anabolic steroids are more rare causes of virilization.

DIFFERENTIAL DIAGNOSIS

Primary amenorrhea is defined as absence of a spontaneous menstrual period by 15.0 yr of age. Work-up should be undertaken earlier if breast budding has not occurred by 13 yr of age. A diagnostic approach to primary amenorrhea is shown in Fig. 4 *(66).* The history should include a search for clues to chronic disease or eating disorder, The key features on physical examination are whether puberty is delayed, or indeed whether it has even begun, whether the child is underweight *(67,68),* and the normalcy of the external genitalia. The key initial laboratory tests in the sexually *immature* patient are bone age radiograph and screening tests for chronic disease. The key initial laboratory tests in the sexually *mature* patient are pregnancy test, plasma testosterone, and pelvic ultrasound examination.

In patients with secondary amenorrhea or oligomenorrhea, secondary sex characteristics will have matured because the occurrence of menarche indicates a substantial degree of development of the reproductive system. Clues to the diagnosis may be obtained from the history and examination. In their absence, a pregnancy test and serum gonadotropin levels, particularly FSH, are the key tests with which to initiate the work-up, as shown in Fig. 5 *(69).*

If a sexually mature girl with secondary amenorrhea or oligomenorrhea has a negative work-up to this point (Fig. 5), or if she has other menstrual irregularities, further investigation for an anovulatory disorder should be undertaken (Fig. 6) *(70).* Dysfunctional uterine bleeding is an alternate presentation of anovulatory cycles; it occurs in anovulatory women whose ambient estradiol levels are over approximately 40 pg/mL *(71).* If bleeding is not controlled by trials of progestin or OCP, sexual abuse, bleeding disorder, and genital tract tumor should be considered *(72).* The history of a woman with anovulatory symptoms should be carefully reviewed for evidence of the nutritional disorders and the physical or emotional stress that are common causes of these complaints. The examination should particularly focus on the possibility of intracranial disorders, galactorrhea, and evidence of hirsutism or its equivalents. A chronic disease panel is indicated in all anovulatory patients. The work-up can be directed differently according to whether the patient is hypoestrogenic or hyperprolactinemic. GnRH testing is indicated in hypoestrogenic cases. GnRH agonist testing yields similar results and in addition allows assessment of gonadotropin reserve in gonadotropin deficiency and also permits assessment of ovarian responsiveness to gonadotropins *(32,73,74).* Imaging of either the ovaries or the brain is usually indicated.

Hyperandrogenism may be present without hirsutism. Hirsutism is defined as excessive male-pattern hair growth in woman. In approximately one-third of cases, there are not even the common hirsutism equivalents of acne vulgaris or pattern alopecia; this seems to be due to considerable individual variability in pilosebaceous unit sensitivity to androgens. Conversely, a small percentage of hirsute women have idiopathic hirsutism, that is, hirsutism without androgen excess. Therefore, it is important to document hyperandrogenism in the settings of either anovulatory symptomatology or hirsutism. We recommend screening for hyperandrogenism with measurement of plasma total and free testosterone as well as plasma DHEA sulfate. A very high plasma testosterone level (>200 ng/dL) or DHEA sulfate level (>700 µg/dL) is suspicious for tumor. Subtle androgen excess is more often detected by a plasma free than a total testosterone determination; unfortunately, the free testosterone assay methodology is variable and there is no international standard. Another key study with which to initiate the investigation of androgen excess is a pelvic ultrasound examination. The main purpose of the ultrasonographic examination is to exclude tumor, because the presence of polycystic ovaries is not specific for PCOS (55,64,65), nor are polycystic ovaries necessary for the diagnosis of PCOS.

The tack taken to screen for adrenal causes of hyperandrogenism differs widely among clinics (75,76). Clearly, it is both costly and impractical to measure multiple steroids on multiple occasions. It is our opinion that if key historical or physical features and the initial round of laboratory tests have not pointed to a specific cause of androgen excess, diagnostic screening is accomplished in a way that will be definitive for PCOS in the majority of cases by performing an outpatient dexamethasone androgen-suppression test, according to the algorithm presented in Fig. 7 (77). A single blood sample after a few days of dexamethasone yields results diagnostic of PCOS in a majority of cases, whereas without dexamethasone pretreatment, an 8:00 AM level of 17-hydroxyprogesterone may not be definitive in ruling out congenital adrenal hyperplasia and a cortisol at that time may not be sufficiently low (below 10 µg/dL) to rule out Cushing's syndrome. We reserve ACTH testing, which is expensive if comprehensive, for the subset of patients with dexamethasone-suppressible androgen excess. There has been considerable confusion about the interpretation of moderately abnormal responses of DHEA and 17-OHP to this test. The experience to date indicates that mutations indicative of nonclassic congenital adrenal hyperplasia cannot be documented unless one of the steroid intermediates rises over 7 SD above average in response to ACTH testing (78,79). If the source of androgen excess cannot be localized by these tests, one may occasionally find an ovarian source by a GnRH agonist challenge test (42,80). If no source for the androgen excess can be found, one is dealing with idiopathic hyperandrogenism.

MANAGEMENT

Appropriate therapy depends on first reaching an accurate diagnosis. All too often, oral contraceptive pills (OCPs) are used indiscriminantly to treat menstrual disorders because, with the notable exception of uterine/endometrial disorders, they will induce regular menstrual periods with a high degree of reliability. However, the role of OCPs in long-term management is limited: for one thing they do not permit conception, for another, the patient may be lulled into thinking that this treatment is curative and thus defer a more defininitive diagnostic work-up.

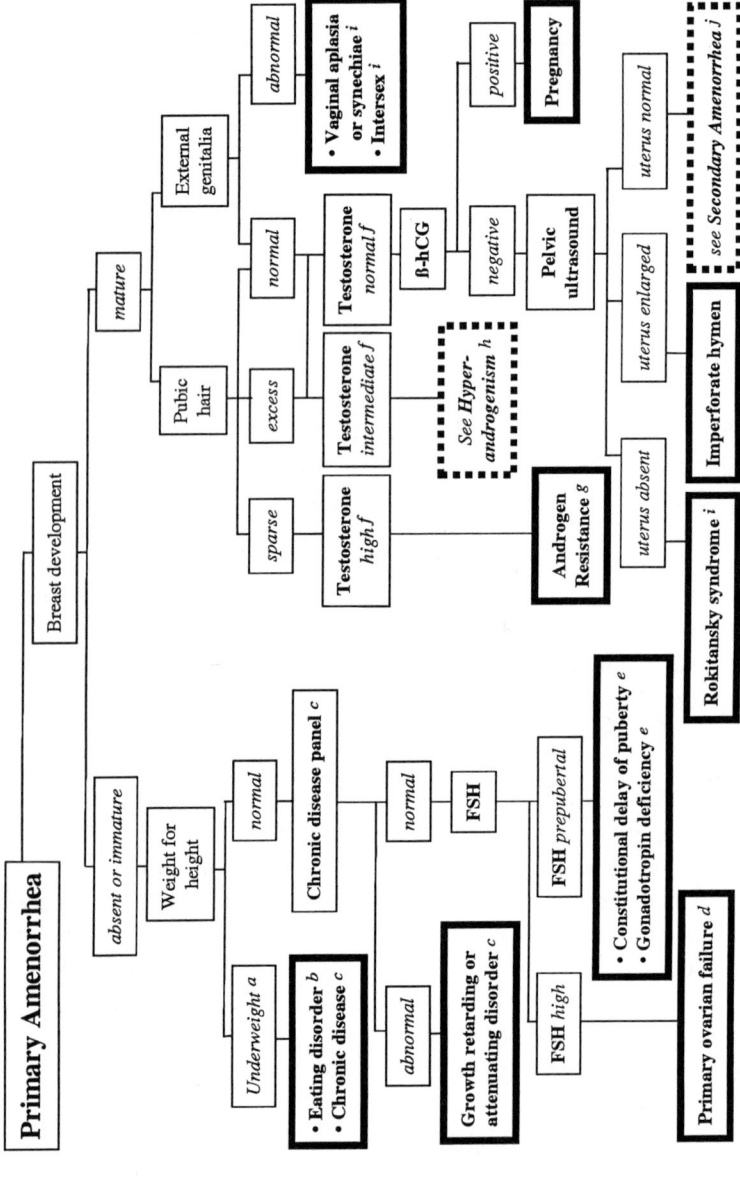

Fig. 4. Differential diagnosis of primary amenorrhea. Adapted with permission from ref. (66).

[a]Underweight is defined in prepubertal children by weight below 10th percentile of body fatness for height or BMI <10th percentile, in pubertal girls by weight below 10th percentile of body fatness for height age. Body fat less than 10–15% of body mass is the critical parameter, and this may not be reflected accurately by weight-for-height parameters in athletes who have a disproportionately great muscle mass.
[b]Anorexia nervosa is a symptom complex consisting of amenorrhea, voluntary starvation, and a self-delusional disturbance in the perception of body fatness. Body fat determination by dual photon x-ray absorptiometry or bioimpedence monitoring may be necessary to document low body fat in bulimia nervosa.

[c]In the absence of specific symptoms or signs to direct the work-up, laboratory screening tests for chronic disease should include: bone age radiograph, complete blood count, differential, sedimentation rate, comprehensive metabolic panel, celiac panel, thyroid panel, cortisol and insulin-like growth factor-I levels, and urinalysis.

[d]The differential diagnosis of primary ovarian failure is shown in the next figure (secondary amenorrhea and oligomenorrhea).

[e]Congenital gonadotropin deficiency is closely mimiced by the more common extreme variation of normal, constitutional delay of puberty. History and examination may yield clues to the congenital nature of congenital hypogonadotropic hypogonadism, such as anosmia (Kallmann's syndrome), midline facial defect (congenital hypopituitarism), or extreme short stature (congenital hypopituitarism). The work-up of gonadotropin deficiency is discussed further in relation to the later figure for the differential diagnosis of anovulatory disorders.

[f]Plasma total testosterone of normal sexually mature females is 20–70 ng/dL (0.7–2.4 nM), that of normal adult males is >320 ng/dL (>11 nM). Plasma free testosterone is a more accurate measure of the bioavailable testosterone (see Hirsutism).

[g]Androgen resistance is characterized by a male plasma testosterone level (when sexual maturation has concluded), male karyotype (46, XY), and absent uterus. External genitalia may be ambiguous (partial form) or normal female phenotype (complete form).

[h]The differential diagnosis of hyperandrogenism is shown in the last figure in this series.

[i]Vaginal aplasia in a girl with normal ovaries may be associated with uterine aplasia (Rokitansky-Kustner-Hauser syndrome). The distal vagina may be normal, with aplasia of the upper vault, or there may be complete vaginal aplasia. When the vagina is blind and the uterus aplastic, this disorder must be distinguished from androgen resistance and, if the external genitalia are ambiguous, other causes of intersex.

[j]Secondary amenorrhea differential diagnosis is given in the next figure.

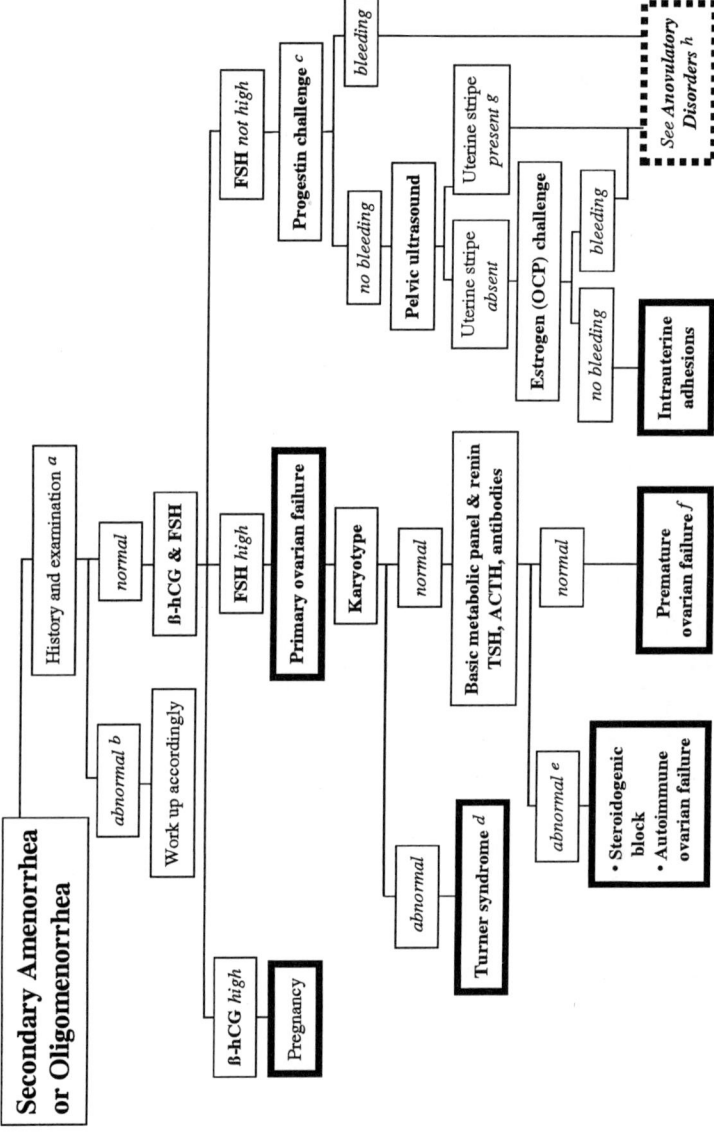

Fig. 5. Differential diagnosis of secondary amenorrhea or oligomenorrhea. Adapted with permission from ref. (69).

[a]Secondary sex characteristics are mature because the occurrence of menarche indicates a substantial degree of development of the reproductive system. Once breast development has matured, the breast contour does not substantially regress, even in the absence of ovarian function.

[b]Clues to disorders causing anovulation abound. The history may reveal excessive exercise, symptoms of depression, radiotherapy to the brain or pelvis, or rapid virilization. Physical findings may include hypertension (forms of congenital adrenal hyperplasia, chronic renal failure), short stature (hypopituitarism, Turner syndrome, pseudohypopara-thyroidism), abnormal weight for height (anorexia nervosa, obesity), decreased sense of smell (Kallmann's syndrome), optic disc or visual field abnormality (pituitary tumors), cutaneous abnormalities (neurofibromatosis, lupus), goiter, galactorrhea, hirsutism, or abdominal mass.

[c]Withdrawal bleeding in response to a 5–10 d course of medroxyprogesterone acetate 10 mg hs suggests the cumulative effect of an integrated estradiol level over 40 pg/mL. However, this is not entirely reliable, so in the interests of making a timely diagnosis it is often worthwhile to go directly on to the further studies.

[d]Patients missing only a small portion of an X-chromosome may not have the Turner syndrome phenotype. Indeed, among 45,X patients the classic Turner syndrome phenotype is found in less than one-third (with the exception of short stature in 99%). Ovarian function is sufficient for 10% to undergo some spontaneous pubertal development and for 5% to experience menarche.

[e]Ovarian insufficiency is associated with mineralocorticoid excess in 17-hydroxylase deficiency and with mineralocorticoid deficiency in lipoid adrenal hyperplasia. Autoimmune ovarian failure may be associated with tissue-specific antibody-associated hypothyroidism, adrenal insufficiency, hypoparathyroidism, and/or diabetes mellitus. Non-endocrine autoimmune disorders may occur, such as mucocutaneous candidiasis, celiac disease, and chronic hepatitis.

[f]The history may provide a diagnosis: cancer chemotherapy or radiotherapy, for example. Specific tests to distinguish among the causes of premature ovarian unexplained by the above tests are generally available only on a research basis. Diverse antiovarian antibodies have been identified; some antibodies are destructive, others are blocking. Other known causes of premature menopause include heritable disorders, such as X-chromosome fragile site and point mutations, as well as gonadotropin-resistance syndromes such as LH receptor mutation and pseudohypoparathyroidism. A pelvic ultrasound which shows preservation of ovarian follicles carries some hope for fertility.

[g]A thin uterine stripe suggests hypoestrogenism; a thick one suggests endometrial hyperplasia, as may occur in polycystic ovary syndrome.

[h]The further differential diagnosis of anovulatory disorders continues in the next figure.

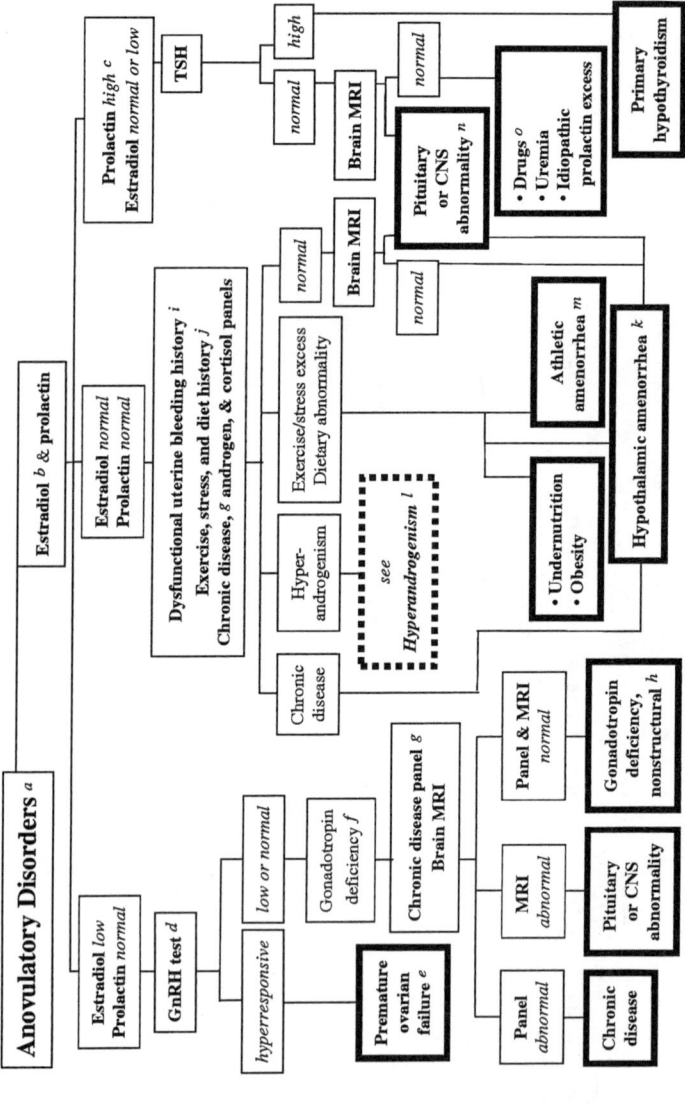

Fig. 6. Differential diagnosis of anovulatory disorders. Adapted with permission from ref. (70).

[a]Anovulatory disorders should be considered in any girl with unexplained amenorrhea or oligomenorrhea, irregular menstrual bleeding, short cycles, or excessive menstrual bleeding. The work-up (including history and examination, a pregnancy test, and determination of gonadotropin levels) should be initiated as indicated in the previous figure.

[b]Hypoestrogenism is suggested if plasma estradiol is persistently <40 pg/mL, vaginal cytology lacks superficial cells, or vaginal bleeding does not occur in response to progestin withdrawal.

[c]Galactorrhea is found in half of hyperprolactinemic females. Hyperprolactinemia is heterogeneous in its presentation. Some have normoestrogenic anovulation; this may be manifest as hypothalamic anovulation, dysfunctional uterine bleeding, or short luteal phase. On the other hand, some are hypoestrogenic due to gonadotropin deficiency, some are hyperandrogenic.

^{d}Baseline gonadotropin levels may not be low in gonadotropin deficient patients, particularly according to polyclonal antibody-based assays. Gonadotropin releasing hormone (GnRH) testing is usually performed by assaying LH and FSH before and 0.5–1.0 h after the administration of 1 µg/kg GnRH intravenously. GnRH agonist testing may alternatively be performed by administering 10 µg/kg leuprolide acetate subcutaneously, assaying LH and FSH at 0, 0.5–1; sampling may additionally be performed at 4 h to assess gonadotropin reserve, and at 0 and 24 h to assess the ovarian steroid response.

^{e}Baseline gonadotropin levels may be normal as the ovary begins to fail, as in menopause, but an exaggerated FSH response to GnRH and subnormal E2 response to acute GnRH agonist challenge are characteristic. A pelvic ultrasound is indicated to determine whether preservation of ovarian follicles offers hope for fertility.

^{f}Responses to GnRH may vary from nil to normal in gonadotropin deficiency. Normal LH and FSH responses indicate inadequate spontaneous hypothalamic GnRH compensation for the hypoestrogenic state.

^{g}Chronic disease screening tests should include complete blood count with differential, sedimentation rate, comprehensive metabolic panel, celiac panel, thyroid panel, insulin-like growth factor-I level, and urinalysis.

^{h}Gonadotropin deficiency may be congenital or acquired, organic or functional. Congenital causes include midline brain malformations or specific genetic disorders such as Prader-Willi syndrome, Laurence-Moon-Biedl syndrome, or Kallmann syndrome. Kallmann's, the association of anosmia with gonadotropin deficiency, is less frequent in females than males (1:5 sex ratio), reflecting the predominance of the X-linked disorder. Special MRI views often demonstrate absence of the olfactory tracts. Acquired gonadotropin deficiency may be secondary to a variety of organic CNS disorders, varying from hypothalamic-pituitary tumor to radiation damage to empty sella syndrome. Autoimmune hypophysitis is a rare disorder, sometimes accompanying a polyendocrine deficiency syndrome. The prototypic form of functional gonadotropin deficiency is anorexia nervosa. Idiopathic hypogonadotropic deficiency may sometimes occur in families with anosmia, suggesting a relationship to Kallmann's syndrome.

^{i}Dysfunctional uterine bleeding or menorrhagia not controlled by progestin or OCP therapy additionally requires a pelvic ultrasound examination, coagulation work-up (including platelet count, prothrombin time, thromboplastin generation test, and bleeding time), and consideration of the possibility of sexual abuse.

^{j}The equivalent of 4 miles/d or more is generally required before amenorrhea occurs.

^{k}Hypothalamic amenorrhea is a diagnosis of exclusion. Functional hypothalamic amenorrhea may be stress- or undernutrition-related, psychogenuc, or idiopathic. It may be secondary to chronic illness or result from obesity or diverse types of endocrine dysfunction. Research studies show subnormal LH pulsatility or estrogen-induceability of the LH surge.

^{l}Hyperandrogenism differential diagnosis is outlined in the next figure.

^{m}The low body fat content of athletic amenorrhea may not be reflected by weight for height because of high muscularity. Dual photon absorptiometry scan may be useful in documenting body fat below 10–15%.

^{n}Hyperprolactinemia may be caused by prolactinomas which secrete excess prolactin or may be secondary to interruption of the pituitary stalk by large hypothalamic-pituitary tumors or other types of injury. The latter cause variable pituitary dysfunction, which may include secondary hypothyroidism.

^{o}Drugs, particularly those of the phenothiazone or tricyclic type, may induce hyperprolactinemia. A rare "big" form of prolactin has been reported which is of no functional significance. Uremia also causes hyperprolactinemia.

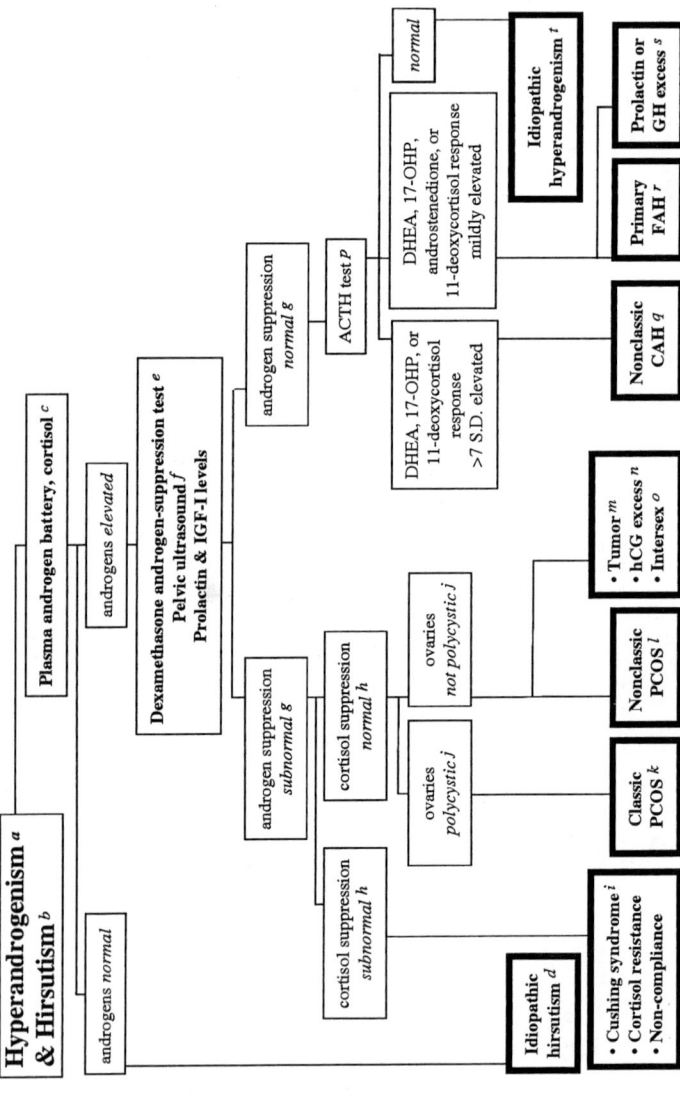

Fig. 7. Differential diagnosis of hyperandrogenism and hirsutism. Adapted with permission from ref. (77).

[a]Androgen excess is not necessarily expressed as hirsutism. Acne vulgaris, seborrhea, pattern alopecia, hyperhidrosis, or hidradenitis suppurativa are "hirsutism equivalents" and may be alternative signs of hyperandrogenism. Acanthosis nigricans and obesity are manifestations of the insulin resistance that is often associated with androgen excess. In some hyperandrogenic cases, there is no cutaneous symptomatology ("cryptic hyperandrogenism") and androgen excess is suspected only because of obesity or anovulatory symptoms.

[b]Hirsutism is excessive sexual hair growth on the spectrum found in men. A small amount of sexual hair growth in a male pattern is normal (Ferriman-Gallwey score below 8). Hirsutism must be distinguished from hypertrichosis. Hypertrichosis is excessive hair growth in a non-sexual pattern. Hair is more prominent on the forehead or shoulders than elsewhere, though it may be generalized. Hypertrichosis is not due to androgen excess. It may be due to certain drugs (e.g., phenytoins, diazoxide, minoxodil, cyclosporine) or chronic illness (e.g., malnutrition). Alternatively, it may be constitutional.

[a]Plasma free testosterone is the single most sensitive test for the detection of androgen excess. It is abnormal more often than plasma total testosterone because a low level sex hormone binding globulin (SHBG), the major determinant of the bioavailable fraction of plasma testosterone, is common in hirsute females. Free testosterone is calculated from measurement of total testosterone and SHBG. Low SHBG is a marker of hyperandrogenism and hyperinsulinemia. Normal ranges for both methods are method-dependent. Dehydroepiandrosterone sulfate (DHEAS) is the main marker of adrenal hyperandrogenism. A 17-hydroxyprogesterone (17-OHP) level is usually not warranted at the initial visit, being uninterpretable unless drawn in the early morning, before 8:00 AM and during the early follicular phase of the cycle or while anovulatory. However, under these conditions, a value over 50 ng/dL (1.5 nM) is suggestive of hyperandrogenism, and congenital adrenal hyperplasia is suggested by a value over 400 ng/dL and virtually assured by a level over 1200 ng/dL. Some authorities also measure androstenedione as a marker of hyperandrogenism. A random cortisol value below 10 μg/dL (276 nM) is good evidence against endogenous Cushing's syndrome. Serum LH excess is a nonspecific finding of little clinical value in hyperandrogenism, so it is not listed here. The physician should be aware that most laboratories establish the normal range for androgens in the early morning, at which time plasma levels are normally higher than the rest of the day, and in the follicular phase of the cycle, at which time they are lower than in the preovulatory phase of the cycle.

[d]Idiopathic hirsutism literally signifies lack of a hyperandrogenic basis for the problem, hence, a constitutional hypersensitivity of the pilosebaceous unit to normal amounts of androgen. The term is often misused as equivalent to idiopathic hyperandrogenemia.

[e]Dexamethasone is given in a dose of 1 mg/m² in four divided doses (0.5 mg qid in adult) for 4 d and plasma cortisol, free testosterone, 17-OHP, and DHEAS are measured on the morning of the 5th day after the final dexamethasone dose. For individuals weighing 100 kg or more, dexamethasone should be given for 7 d.

[f]Ultrasonographic visualization of the ovaries by the vaginal route yields better definition than by the abdominal route, but this is not a generally acceptable technique in the virginal child.

[g]Dexamethasone suppression of ACTH-dependent adrenal function normally causes plasma total testosterone to fall below 35 ng/dL, DHEAS to fall by 75% to below 80 μg/dL, and 17-OHP to fall to less than 50 ng/dL. Total testosterone is not as discriminating a criterion as free testosterone below 8 pg/mL (unfortunately, a method-dependent criterion) or 17-OHP below 50 ng/dL (when amenorrheic or in follicular or amenorrheic phase of menstrual cycle). Subnormal androgen suppression with normal adrenocortical suppression indicates a source of androgen other than an ACTH-dependent adrenal one. To convert mass units to SI units, multiply testosterone by 0.0347 (nM), DHEAS by 0.271 (μM), and 17-PROG by 0.0303 (nM).

[h]Normally cortisol falls below 1.0 μg/dL (27.6 nM).

[i]Subnormal cortisol suppression is most often due to noncompliance with taking the dexamethasone tablets. Cushing's syndrome is an infrequent cause of hyperandrogenism and requires a more definitive work-up. Hyperandrogenism has been reported in the rare conditions of cortisol resistance and cortisone reductase deficiency.

[j]An excessive number (10 or more in the maximal ovarian plane) of "microcysts" (typically 3–8 mm diameter) together with an increase in ovarian stroma is a conservative ultrasonographic criterion for a polycystic ovary. An alternative criterion is an increase in ovarian size (volume over 11 cc or >550 mm² area contained within the circumference of the maximal plane of an ovary) in the absence of an excessive number of cysts.

[k]Classic polycystic ovary syndrome (PCOS) is a symptom complex with various combinations of hirsutism or its equivalents, anovulation, and obesity. It has classically been diagnosed by the presence of one or more polycystic ovaries or a high serum LH level. Approximately 80% of cases have subnormal 17-androgen suppressibility according to a dexamethasone androgen-suppression test and a characteristic type of ovarian dysfunction, which consists of 17-OHP hyperresponsiveness to a GnRH agonist or hCG challenge. Dexamethasone test criteria are more highly concordant with GnRH agonist challenge test

(*continued on page 470*)

criteria (65–85%) than with ultrasound or LH criteria (50%).

^{l}Nonclassic PCOS is defined here as atypical chronic hyperandrogenism which lacks the characteristic ultrasonographic or gonadotropic findings of classic PCOS. Most have the typical PCOS-type of functional ovarian hyperandrogenism on dexamethasone suppression or GnRH agonist testing.

^{m}The baseline pattern of plasma androgens may yield a clue to the type of tumor. A DHEAS level over 700 µg/dL which is poorly suppressible by dexamethasone is suspicious of an adrenal tumor. Disproportionate elevations of the ratio of plasma androstenedione to testosterone is typical of virilizing tumors. MRI or CT scan of the abdomen may be indicated in such cases.

^{n}Human chorionic gonadotropin excess during pregnancy is a rare cause of virilization. It results from luteoma of pregnancy or hyperreactio luteinalis of pregnancy.

^{o}True hermaphroditism may mimic PCOS. These patients may only have a clearly elevated plasma testosterone level in response to a midcycle LH surge, hCG, or GnRH agonist test.

^{p}The standard ACTH test is performed by infusing 250 µg ACTH$_{1-24}$ intravenously over a period of one minute and obtaining a blood sample before injection and 1 h later.

^{q}Congenital adrenal hyperplasia (CAH) cannot be confirmed upon mutation analysis unless the steroid intermediates immediately prior to the enzyme block rise over 7 SD above average in response to ACTH. For 17-OHP, this is over 1200 ng/dL, for DHEA this is over 3000 ng/dL.

^{r}Primary functional adrenal hyperandrogenism (FAH) is a term for idiopathic, ACTH-dependent (dexamethasone-suppresible), adrenal hyperandrogenism in which modest rises in DHEA, 17-OHP, and the like do not meet the criteria for the diagnosis of congenital adrenal hyperplasia. Primary FAH often coexists with functional ovarian hyperandrogenism in PCOS. This is the only demonstrable source of androgen excess in a minority of patients with nonclassic PCOS.

^{s}Hyperprolactinemia should be worked-up as outlined in the previous figure.

^{t}Idiopathic hyperandrogenemia is distinguished from idiopathic hirsutism. About 8% of chronic hyperandrogenemia remains unexplained after intensive investigation which includes GnRH agonist testing to detect the occasional case of ovarian hyperandrogenism that is not detected by the dexamethasone test.

Hypoestrogenism is the proximate cause of many cases of amenorrhea and oligomenorrhea. If the patient is sexually immature, there are a few important considerations before initiating estrogen replacement therapy: is there an underlying disorder that requires *medical* therapy, is there an underlying disorder that requires *surgical* therapy, and is *short stature* present?

Chronic diseases such as cystic fibrosis, heart failure, cirrhosis, chronic renal failure, regional enteritis, or systemic lupus erythematosis will not respond well to hormone replacement therapy unless the underlying disorder can be controlled. The hypoestrogenism of anorexia nervosa, other eating disorders, and athletic amenorrhea, as well as some cases of hypothalamic amenorrhea, will correct with behavior modification. In severe anorexia nervosa, rehydration and metabolic stabilization are the first priorities, and management of the psychiatric problem is the next *(81)*. Estrogen treatment of patients with eating disorder will mask the psychopathology that underlies the menstrual disturbance, and estrogen treatment of patients with short stature may compromise height potential. Panhypopituitary patients require replacement of growth hormone and cortisol deficits to obtain a normal degree of breast development.

Surgical considerations arise in several settings, particularly those involving genital tract disorders and gonadotropin deficiency. Surgery is required if vaginal synechieae do not lyse spontaneously with estrogenization, and is required for vaginal aplasia or imperforate hymen. Some cases of intrauterine adhesions respond to hysteroscopic lysis of intrauterine adhesions *(11)*. Gonadotropin deficiency may be caused by an intracranial disorder such as hypothalamic-pituitary tumor. In such cases, if growth was not an issue preoperatively, it may become an issue if hypopituitarism develops post-operatively.

Stature is an important consideration in sexually immature teenagers with both hypogonadotropic and hypergonadotropic hypogonadism, and nowhere is it more important than in Turner syndrome. The dose of estrogen in standard OCPs will inhibit growth and lead to premature fusion of the epiphyses in sexually immature patients. Estrogen replacement must be undertaken in such a way as to preserve height potential. Therefore, unless the patient has already achieved a stature they find acceptable, a bone age radiograph should be obtained to predict adult height. Maximizing height potential requires growth hormone therapy in some, and this should be initiated before the induction of puberty if this is feasable from a psychosocial perspective; further discussion of growth hormone therapy is beyond the scope of this chapter. Oxandrolone (2-oxo-17α-methyldihydro-testosterone [Anavar®]) 0.0625 mg/kg/d is an adjunctive growth-stimulatory therapy, particularly in synergism with growth hormone, without causing clitoromegaly *(82)*; its usage is limited by its modest efficacy and the small risk of hepatotoxicity.

Optimal estrogen replacement therapy in the sexually immature girl requires the induction of puberty in a physiologic manner with an extremely low dose of estrogen to maximize growth. If this is done properly, the girl will not experience menarche for 1–2 yr. A physiologic form of treatment is to begin with intramuscular depot estradiol 0.2 mg/mo and increase the dose by 0.2 mg every 6 mo. Optimal dosimetry is achieved by diluting the stock solution (5.0 mg/mL) in cottonseed oil under sterile conditions. Midpubertal sex hormone production is approximated by delivering 1.0–1.5 mg of estradiol per month, which typically induces menarche within 1 yr *(83)*. A reasonable alternative regimen begins with 5 µg ethinyl estradiol (one-fourth of the smallest available tablet) by mouth daily for 3 wk out of 4 *(84)*. Conjugated estrogen doses as low as

0.325 mg daily inhibit the growth response to growth hormone *(85)*. Adult estrogen replacement typically requires administration of depot estradiol 2.5 mg im monthly, transdermal estradiol 37.5 µg daily, ethinyl estradiol 20 µg or conjugated estrogen 0.625 mg po daily for 3 wk out of 4. Physiologic considerations suggest that progestin is unnecessary early in the induction of puberty: normally progesterone is not secreted by the ovary in substantial amounts until ovulation results in formation of a corpus luteum, and normally half of cycles are anovulatory for the first 2 yr after menarche. Therefore, progestin replacement does not seem physiologic until menstrual bleeding becomes irregular or until 1 yr after menarche.

In sexually mature adolescents with menstrual irregularities, it is often convenient and effective to begin with a course of medroxyprogesterone acetate (Provera®) 10 mg orally hs for approx 1 wk out of the month. In the beginning, this may be of some diagnostic help, because a positive response, withdrawal bleeding beginning a few days after completion of the course of therapy, only occurs if there has been substantial estrogenization. In the perimenarcheal girl who responds well to this, progestin therapy may be repeated in 2–3 mo cycles in order to detect the emergence of spontaneous menses that signals the resolution of the physiologic anovulation of adolescence. This treatment seldom causes side effects and has never been incriminated as a cause of post-pill amenorrhea; thus, it has the appeal of potentially disturbing the developing neuroendocrine system less than OCPs. However, patients must be made aware that this is not a contraceptive treatment.

Hypoestrogenism in sexually mature girls may be managed by its replacement or by administration of an oral contraceptive. OCPs are the most convenient option, since the currently available ones carry very little risk of venous thromboembolic disease *(86)*, and the progestational component protects against endometrial hyperplasia *(87)*. Those containing the lowest dose of estrogen that will result in normal menstrual flow are preferable, all else being equal. The lowest estrogen dosage currently available in combination OCPs in the US is 20 µg ethinyl estradiol (e.g., with 1.0 mg norethindrone acetate in Loestrin 20 1/21® and with 0.15 mg desogestrel in Mircette®). Obese patients tend to require higher doses of estrogen. However, patients sensitive to estrogen because of such conditions as hypertension, migraine, or lymphedema, are best advised to use a more physiologic type of therapy, estradiol itself in a form delivered systemically, bypassing the liver: for this purpose one may use depot estradiol given intramuscularly, depot estradiol with medroxyprogesterone acetate (Lunelle®), or estradiol patches. When using estrogen alone, a progestin is administered for the last 1–2 wk of each course of estrogen (e.g., medroxyprogesterone acetate 5–10 mg daily); the more progestin administered, the less the risk of endometrial hyperplasia, but the greater the risk of premenstrual symptoms. As in the sexually immature, when hypoestroestrogenism results from stress or eating disorders, behavioral modification and psychological counseling are indicated rather than estrogen replacement therapy, and concomitant hormonal deficiencies must be corrected.

Dysfunctional uterine bleeding can usually be treated with cyclic progestin. However, estrogen is required to stop an acute episode. It can be given in high dosage with progestin as OCPs, one tablet 3–4 times daily for 7 d. Treatment is then stopped for 5 d, and the patient warned that heavy withdrawal bleeding with cramps may occur. Therapy with 1 tablet daily for a few cycles should then be started to prevent recurrence of dysfunctional bleeding.

Excessive menstrual bleeding to the point of anemia is termed menorrhagia. OCP therapy will decrease menstrual blood loss by about 50% in anemic subjects. Antiprostaglandins, such as naproxin 500 mg twice a day, decrease blood loss nearly as well. A patient who is hypovolemic because of rapid, heavy dysfunctional bleeding should be hospitalized and treated with intravenous fluids and blood products as necessary. Premarin in a dose of 25 mg intravenously every 3–4 h for 3–4 doses is customary. When medical management fails, a bleeding diathesis or uterine structural abnormality should be considered. If heavy bleeding persists, curettage should be performed by a gynecologist.

Hyperprolactinemia may be due to hypothyroidism or drugs, in which case specific therapy is indicated. Otherwise, whether idiopathic or tumoral, it usually responds to dopaminergic agonists *(88–90)*. Hyperprolactinemia will be maximally suppressed within 1 mo and the menstrual cycle normalized within 3 mo by an effective regimen. Pergolide in a dosage of 50–100 µg once or twice daily or cabergoline 0.5–1.0 mg once or twice weekly will usually control galactorrhea and shrink prolacinomas. To minimize nausea it is best to start with a low dose at bedtime. Transphenoidal resection of prolactinomas is required if the patient's conditon or eyesight is critical and for the rare treatment failures.

Hyperandrogenic states that are amenable to specific therapy are congenital adrenal hyperplasia, Cushing syndrome, virilizing tumors, hermaphroditism, acromegaly and hyperprolactinemia. Glucocorticoids are indicated for the treatment of congenital adrenal hyperplasia. The sequelae of glucocorticoid therapy can typically be minimized by using a modest bedtime dose (about 5–7.5 mg prednisone); this will reduce adrenal androgen secretion selectively without causing adrenal atrophy. We generally aim to suppress DHEA sulfate to below the adult range, but not completely. Significant glucocorticoid deficiency can be excluded by finding a cortisol level of 18 µg/dL or more 30 min after administering a very low dose (1.0 µg/1.73 m^2) of ACTH (cosyntropin) *(91)*. Control of androgens in congenital adrenal hyperplasia may not suffice unless nocturnal progesterone excess is also controlled *(92)*. This treatment will typically normalize the menstrual pattern in nonclassic congenital adrenal hyperplasia, but the effect in classic congenital adrenal hyperplasia is more problematic, since nonclassic PCOS complicates many of these cases, apparently as the result of congenital or perinatal masculinization *(55)*. Glucocorticoids are occasionally beneficial in PCOS in which there is a large component of adrenal dysfunction (primary FAH), but should not be used for more than 3 mo if menses remain abnormal *(93)*.

The most common cause of hyperandrogenism is PCOS, and, in the absence of understanding its fundamental etiology, its management depends upon the symptomatology. The anovulation of PCOS may be managed with progestin alone, as discussed above, in adolescents who are not concerned about hirsutism or hirsutism equivalents. Ordinarily, however, the skin manifestations are an issue or menstrual irregularity is not well-controlled, so OCP therapy is usually used in PCOS. A nonandrogenic OCP should be used for the treatment of hyperandrogenic anovulation. A new generation of oral contraceptives is now available containing nonandrogenic progestins such as norgestimate and desogestrel *(94)*; norgestimate combined with 35 µg ethinyl estradiol in Ortho-Tri-Cyclen®, has received Food and Drug Administration approval for the treatment of acne. The progestin in Demulen 1/50®, ethynodiol diacetate, also has a low androgenic potential, and is useful for very obese patients who require a larger dose of estrogen. Fertility may become important for patients with anovulatory disorders. Such patients are generally referred to a reproductive endocrinologist.

Endocrinologic treatment of hirsutism, acne, or pattern alopecia is indicated if standard cosmetic or dermatologic measures short of isotretinoin or minoxidil fail. It consists of interrupting one or more of the steps in the pathway of androgen action. OCPs are effective in typical PCOS patients in whom FOH is the predominant source of androgen excess. They lower plasma free testosterone levels by reducing serum gonadotropin levels, increasing SHBG levels, and modestly lowering DHEAS levels. They will improve acne within 3 mo and arrest progression of hirsutism in most PCOS patients. Similar results can probably be obtained with chronic GnRH agonist therapy to suppress gonadotropin secretion, but this would only seem indicated in patients who cannot tolerate OCPs, and then it would require low-dose, physiologic estradiol add-back to maintain vaginal lubrication and to prevent osteoporosis.

Antiandrogens are required for substantial reversal of hirsutism. The maximal effect of these agents on hirsutism takes 9–12 mo because of the long growth cycles of sexual hair follicles. Spironolactone has been shown to be effective to the extent of lowering hirsutism score by about one-third, with considerable individual variation, and is probably the most potent and safe antiandrogen available in the US. We recommend starting with 100 mg bid, then reducing the dosage for maintenance therapy after the maximal effect has been achieved. This dosage is usually well tolerated; fatigue and hyperkalemia at higher doses may limit its usefulness, however. It is potentially teratogenic to fetal male genital development and may cause menstrual disturbance; therefore it should be prescribed with an oral contraceptive. Cyproterone acetate is the major antiandrogen in use; it is only available outside the US. It is also a potent progestin and it has been combined with ethinyl estradiol as an antiandrogenic contraceptive (Diane®). Flutamide is a more specific antiandrogen of similar efficacy; however, its usage has been limited by its expense and the possible side effect of hepatocellular toxicity. Although it may permit ovulation, the dangers of causing genital ambiguity in male offspring limit its utility for this purpose. It is not clear that the type 1 5α-reductase inhibitor finasteride has any advantages over the antiandrogens.

Treatments which reduce insulin resistance improve hyperandrogenemia and ovulation in PCOS. Antiandrogens have only a modest effect on metabolic abnormalities *(95)*. Weight reduction is indicated in obese hyperandrogenemic patients. The new insulin-lowering agents are a promising means of normalizing menstrual status *(96)*, but if the elevation in androgens is great, they will not become normal. These agents include metformin, thiazolidinediones, and D-chiro-inositol. All of these modalities have been reported to improve androgen levels and ovulatory status. Metformin appears to have the most utility of these agents in the management of adolescents because it tends to bring about some weight loss, albeit to a modest degree. Metformin is effective only to the extent that weight is lost *(51)*.

PCOS is a risk factor for the early development of non-insulin dependent (type 2) diabetes mellitus and dyslipidemia in these patients, and nearly half of them have a primary relative with this disorder *(52)*. Therefore, glucose tolerance should be monitored regularly.

Psychological support is an important aspect of the management of teenagers with menstrual disorders. Girls with delayed puberty, whether it has an organic or functional basis, can almost always be assured that they will feminize and, if a uterus is present, that they will experience menses. Girls can be reassured that menstrual abnormalities will be regulated. In addition, patients with Turner syndrome or similar primary hypogonadism disorders can hold hope for the the ability to carry a pregnancy, and patients with hypogonadotropic hypogonadism and chronic anovulatory disorders can hold hope for the ability to conceive, though in both situations this will require special care by a reproductive endocrinologist.

REFERENCES

1. Warren M. Evaluation of secondary amenorrhea. J Clin Endocrinol Metab 1996;81(2):437–442.
2. MacMahon B. Age at Menarche. United States Vital Health Statistics, 1973. vol 11.
3. Lucky A, Biro F, Simbartl L, Morrison J, Sorg N. Predictors of severity of acne vulgaris in young adolescent girls: Results of a five-year longitudinal study. J Pediatr 1997;130(1):30–39.
4. Tanner JM, Davies PS. Clinical longitudinal standards for height and height velocity for North American children. J Pediatr 1985;107(3):317–329.
5. Marshall W, Tanner J. Variations in pattern of pubertal changes in girls. Arch Dis Child 1969;44:291.
6. Marti-Henneberg C, Vizmanos B. The duration of puberty in girls is related to the timing of its onset. J Pediatr 1997;131(4):618–621.
7. Apter D, Bützow T, Laughlin G. Hyperandrogenism during puberty and adolescence, and its relationship to reproductive function in the adult female. In: Frajese G, Steinberger E, Rodriguez-Rigau L, eds. Reproductive Medicine. Raven Press, New York, 1993:265–275.
8. Treloar A, Boynton R, Benn B, Brown B. Variation of human menstrual cycle through reproductive life. Int J Fertil 1967;12:77–84.
9. Rosenfield RL. Chap 14, The ovary and female maturation. In: Sperling M, ed. Pediatric Endocrinology. 1st ed. Saunders, Philadelphia, PA, 1996;329–385.
10. Golan A, Langer R, Bukovsky I, Caspi E. Congenital anomalies of the müllerian system. Fertil Steril 1989;51:747–754.
11. March C. Acquired intrauterine adhesions. In: Adashi E, Rock J, Rosenwaks Z, eds. Reproductive Endocrinology, Surgery and Technology. Philadelphia: Lippincott-Raven, 1996:chap 75; pp 1475–1488.
12. Saenger P. Turner's syndrome. N Engl J Med 1996;335(23):1749–1754.
13. Cunniff C, Jones K, Benirschke K. Ovarian dysgenesis in individuals with chromosomal abnormalities. Hum Genet 1990;86:552–556.
14. Pelletier J, Bruening W, Kashtan C, et al. Germline mutations in the Wilms' tumor suppressor gene are associated with abnormal urogenital development in Denys-Drash syndrome. Cell 1991;67:437–447.
15. Peters H, Byskov A, Grinsted J. Follicular growth in fetal and prepubertal ovaries of humans and other primates. Clin Endocrinol Metab 1978;7:469.
16. Vianna-Morgante A, Costa S, Pares A, Verreschi I. FRAXA premutation associated with premature ovarian failure. Am J Med Genet 1996;64:373–375.
17. Layman LC, McDonough PG. Mutations of follicle stimulating hormone-beta and its receptor in human and mouse: genotype/phenotype. Mol Cell Endocrinol 2000;161(1-2):9–17.
18. Namnoum AB, Merriam GR, Moses AM, Levine MA. Reproductive dysfunction in women with Albright's hereditary osteodystrophy. J Clin Endocrinol Metab 1998;83(3):824–829.
19. de Zegher F, Jaeken J. Endocrinology of the carbohydrate-deficient glycoprotein syndrome type 1 from birth through adolescence. Pediatr Res 1995;37:395.
20. Layman LC. Genetics of human hypogonadotropic hypogonadism. Am J Med Genet 1999;89(4):240–248.
21. Bose HS, Pescovitz OH, Miller WL. Spontaneous feminization in a 46,XX female patient with congenital lipoid adrenal hyperplasia due to a homozygous frameshift mutation in the steroidogenic acute regulatory protein. J Clin Endocrinol Metab 1997;82(5):1511–1515.
22. Lieman H, Santoro N. Premature ovarian failure: a modern approach to diagnosis and treatment. The Endocrinologist 1997;7:314–321.
23. Beranova M, Oliveira LMB, Hall JE, et al. GnRH receptor mutations in idiopathic hypogonadotropic hypogonadism (IHH): Impact of clinical subphenotyping and mode of inheritance. Clinical Science: Endocrine Genetics. Toronto, Canada: The Endocrine Society, 2000.
24. Komatsu M, Kondo T, Yamauchi K, et al. Antipituitary antibodies in patients with the primary empty sella syndrome. J Clin Endocrinol Metab 1988;67:633.
25. Hendricks SA, Lippe BM, Kaplan SA, Bentson JR. Hypothalamic atrophy with progressive hypopituitarism in an adolescent girl. J Clin Endocrinol Metab 1981;52:562.

26. Rappaport R, Brauner R, Czernichow P, et al. Effect of hypothalamic and pituitary irradiation on pubertal development in children with cranial tumors. J Clin Endocrinol Metab 1982;54:1164.
27. Van den Berghe G, de Zegher F, Bouillon R. Clinical review 95: Acute and prolonged critical illness as different neuroendocrine paradigms. J Clin Endocrinol Metab 1998;83(6):1827–1834.
28. Becker AE, Grinspoon SK, Klibanski A, Herzog DB. Eating disorders. N Engl J Med 1999; 340(14):1092–1098.
29. Magoffin DA, Huang CTF. Leptin and reproduction. The Endocrinologist 1998;8:79–86.
30. Chrousos G, Gold P. The concepts of stress and stress system disorders. Overview of physical and behavioral homeostasis. JAMA 1992;267:1244–1252.
31. Razdan A, Rosenfield R, Kim M. Endocrinologic characteristics of partial ovarian failure. J Clin Endocrinol Metab 1976;43:449.
32. Winslow KL, Toner JP, Brzyski RG, Oehninger SC, Acosta AA, Muasher SJ. The gonadotropin-releasing hormone agonist stimulation test—a sensitive predictor of performance in the flare-up in vitro fertilization cycle. Fertil Steril 1991;56:711–717.
33. Laughlin GA, Dominguez CE, Yen SS. Nutritional and endocrine-metabolic aberrations in women with functional hypothalamic amenorrhea. J Clin Endocrinol Metab 1998;83(1):25–32.
34. Edman CD, MacDonald PC. Effect of obesity on conversion of plasma androstenedione to estrone in ovulatory and anovulatory young women. Am J Obstet Gynecol 1978;130:456–461.
35. Lado-Abeal J, Rodriguez-Arnao J, Newell-Price JDC, et al. Menstrual abnormalities in women with Cushing's disease are correlated with hypercortisolemia rather than raised circulating androgen levels. J Clin Endocrinol Metab 1998;83:3083–3088.
36. Winters SJ, Berga SL. Gonadal dysfunction in patients with thyroid disorders. The Endocrinologist 1997;7:167–173.
37. Sauder S, Frager M, Case C, Kelch R, Marshall J. Abnormal patterns of pulsatile luteinizing hormone secretion in women with hyperprolactinemia and amenorrhea: Responses to bromocriptine. J Clin Endocrinol Metab 1984;59:941.
38. Colao A, Lombardi G. Growth-hormone and prolactin excess. Lancet 1998;352(9138):1455–1461.
39. Rosenfield RL. Current concepts of polycystic ovary syndrome. Baillière's Clin Obstet Gynaecol 1997;11:307–333.
40. Ehrmann DA, Barnes RB, Rosenfield RL. Polycystic ovary syndrome as a form of functional ovarian hyperandrogenism due to dysregulation of androgen secretion. Endocr Rev 1995;16:322–353.
41. Rosenfield RL. Ovarian and adrenal function in polycystic ovary syndrome. Endocrinol Metab Clin N Am 1999;28(2):265–293.
42. Rosenfield RL, Ghai K, Ehrmann DA, Barnes RB. Diagnosis of polycystic ovary syndrome in adolescence. Comparison of adolescent and adult hyperandrogenism. Fertil Steril 2000;13(Suppl 5): 1285–1289.
43. Ibañez L, Potau N, Zampolli M, Street ME, A C. Girls diagnosed with premature pubarche show an exaggerated ovarian androgen synthesis from the early stages of puberty: evidence from gonadotropin-releasing hormone agonist testing. Fertil Steril 1997;67:849–855.
44. Wickenheisser JK, Quinn PG, Nelson VL, Legro RS, Strauss III JF, McAllister JM. Differential activity of the cytochrome P450 17α-hydroxylase and steroidogenic acute regulatory protein gene promoters in normal and polycystic ovary syndrome theca cells. J Clin Endocrinol Metab 2000;85:2304–2311.
45. Franks S, Gharani N, Waterworth D, et al. Genetics of polycystic ovary syndrome. Mol Cell Endocrinol 1998;145(1-2):123–128.
46. Legro RS, Driscoll D, Strauss 3rd JF, Fox J, Dunaif A. Evidence for a genetic basis for hyperandrogenemia in polycystic ovary syndrome. Proc Natl Acad Sci USA 1998;95(25):14,956–14,960.
47. Nayak S, Lee PA, Witchel SF. Variants of the type II 3beta-hydroxysteroid dehydrogenase gene in children with premature pubic hair and hyperandrogenic adolescents. Mol Genet Metab 1998; 64(3):184–192.
48. Gilling-Smith C, Willis DS, Beard RW, Franks S. Hypersecretion of androstenedione by isolated theca cells from polycystic ovaries. J Clin Endocrinol Metab 1994;79:1158–1165.
49. Gilling-Smith C, Story H, Rogers V, Franks S. Evidence for a primary abnormality of thecal cell steroidogenesis in the polycystic ovary syndrome. Clin Endocrinol 1997;47:93–99.
50. Chang PL, Lindheim SR, Lowre C, et al. Normal ovulatory women with polycystic ovaries have hyperandrogenic pituitary-ovarian responses to gonadotropin-releasing hormone-agonist testing. J Clin Endocrinol Metab 2000;85(3):995–1000.

51. Ehrmann DA. Relation of functional ovarian hyperandrogenism to non-insulin dependent diabetes mellitus. Baillière's Clin Obstet Gynaecol 1997;11:335–347.
52. Ehrmann DA, Barnes RB, Rosenfield RL, Cavaghan MK, Imperial J. Prevalence of impaired glucose tolerance and diabetes in women with polycystic ovary syndrome. Diabetes Care 1999;22:141–146.
53. Witchel SF, Lee PA, Suda-Hartman M, Hoffman EP. Hyperandrogenism and manifesting heterozygotes for 21-hydroxylase deficiency. Biochem Mol Med 1997;62(2):151–158.
54. Ibañez L, Potau N, Francois I, deZegher F. Precocious pubarche, hyperinsulinism, and ovarian hyperandrogenism: relation to reduced fetal growth. J Clin Endocrinol Metab 1998;83(10):3558–3562.
55. Barnes RB, Rosenfield RL, Ehrmann DA, et al. Ovarian hyperandrogenism as a result of congenital adrenal virilizing disorders: Evidence for perinatal masculinization of neuroendocrine function in women. J Clin Endocrinol Metab 1994;79:1328–1333.
56. Speiser PW, Serrat J, New MI, Gertner JM. Insulin insensitivity in adrenal hyperplasia due to nonclassical steroid 21-hydroxylase deficiency. J Clin Endocrinol Metab 1992;75(6):1421–1424.
57. Abbott DA, Dumesic DA, Eisner JR, Colman RJ, Kemnitz JW. Insights into the development of polycystic ovary syndrome (PCOS) from studies of prenatally androgenized female Rhesus monkeys. Trends in Endocrinology and Metabolism 1998;9:62–67.
58. Meldrum D, Frumar A, Shamonki I, et al. Ovarian and adrenal steroidogenesis in a virilized patient with gonadotropin-resistant ovaries and hilus cell hyperplasia. Obstet Gynecol 1980;56:216.
59. Kaltsas GA, Mukherjee JJ, Jenkins PJ, et al. Menstrual irregularity in women with acromegaly. J Clin Endocrinol Metab 1999;84(8):2731–2735.
60. Speiser PW, Susin M, Sasano H, Bohrer S, Markowitz J. Ovarian hyperthecosis in the setting of portal hypertension. J Clin Endocrinol Metab 2000;85(2):873–877.
61. Ritzén E. Adrenogenital syndrome. Curr Opin Pediatr 1992;4:661–667.
62. Jamieson A, Wallace AM, Andrew R, et al. Apparent cortisone reductase deficiency: a functional defect in 11beta-hydroxysteroid dehydrogenase type 1. J Clin Endocrinol Metab 1999;84(10):3570–3574.
63. Glickman SP, Rosenfield RL, Bergenstal RM, Helke J. Multiple androgenic abnormalities, including elevated free testosterone, in hyperprolactinemic women. J Clin Endocrinol Metab 1982;55:251.
64. Kaltsas GA, Korbonits M, Isidori AM, et al. How common are polycystic ovaries and the polycystic ovarian syndrome in women with Cushing's syndrome? [In Process Citation]. Clin Endocrinol (Oxf) 2000;53(4):493–500.
65. Futterweit W, Krieger DT. Pituitary tumors associated with hyperprolactinemia and polycystic ovary disease. Fertil Steril 1979;31:608–613.
66. Rosenfield RL, Bourguignon JP. Primary amenorrhea and abnormal genital anatomy. In: Hochberg Z, ed. Practical Algorithms in Pediatric Endocrinology. Basel: S Karger, AG, 1999:26–27.
67. Frisch RE, McArthur JW. Menstrual cycles: fatness as a determinant of minimum weight for height necessary for their maintenance or onset. Science 1974;185(4155):949–951.
68. Rolland-Cachera MF, Sempe M, Guilloud-Bataille M, Patois E, Pequignot-Guggenbuhl F, Fautrad V. Adiposity indices in children. Am J Clin Nutr 1982;36(1):178–184.
69. Rosenfield RL, Bourguignon JP. Secondary amenorrhea. In: Hochberg Z, ed. Practical Algorithms in Pediatric Endocrinology. Basel: S Karger, AG, 1999:28–29.
70. Rosenfield RL, Bourguignon JP. Anovulatory disorders. In: Hochberg Z, ed. Practical Algorithms in Pediatric Endocrinology. Basel: S Karger, AG, 1999:30–31.
71. Rebar R, Connolly H. Clinical features of young women with hypergonadotropic amenorrhea. Fertil Steril 1990;53:804–810.
72. Wathen PI, Henderson MC, Witz CA. Abnormal uterine bleeding. Med Clin North Am 1995;79(2):329–344.
73. Goodpasture J, Ghai K, Cara J, Rosenfield R. Potential of gonadotropin-releasing hormone agonists in the diagnosis of pubertal disorders in girls. Clin Obstet Gynecol 1993;36:773–785.
74. Ibañez L, Potau N, Zampolli M, et al. Use of leuprolide acetate response patterns in the early diagnosis of pubertal disorders: comparison with the gonadotropin-releasing hormone test. J Clin Endocrinol Metab 1994;78:30–35.
75. American College Obstetricians and Gynecologists. Hyperandrogenic chronic anovulation. ACOG Technical Bulletin 1995;202(2):1–10.
76. American College Obstetricians and Gynecologists. Evaluation and treatment of hirsute women. ACOG Technical Bulletin 1995;203(3):1–8.
77. Rosenfield RL, Sippell WG. Hirsutism. In: Hochberg Z, ed. Practical Algorithms in Pediatric Endocrinology. Basel: S Karger, AG, 1999:32–33.

78. New M. Steroid 21-hydroxylase deficiency (congenital adrenal hyperplasia). Am J Med 1995;98 (Suppl A):2S–8S.
79. Pang S. Congenital adrenal hyperplasia. Bailliére's Clin Obstet Gynaecol 1997;11:281–306.
80. Ibañez L, Potau N, Zampolli M, et al. Source localization of androgen excess in adolescent girls. J Clin Endocrinol Metab 1994;79(6):1778–1784.
81. Beaumont P, Russell J, Touyz S. Treatment of anorexia nervosa. Lancet 1993;341:1635.
82. Rosenfeld RG, Frane J, Attie KM, et al. Six-year results of a randomized prospective trial of human growth hormone and oxandrolone in Turner syndrome. J Pediatr 1992;121:49–55.
83. Rosenfeld RL, Fang VS. The effects of prolonged physiologic estradiol therapy on the maturation of hypogonadal teenagers. J Pediatr 1974;85:830–837.
84. Ross JL, Long LM, Skerda M, et al. The effect of low dose ethinyl estradiol on six monthly growth rates and predicted height in patients with Turner syndrome. J Pediatr 1986;109:950.
85. Chernausek SD, Attie KM, Cara JF, Rosenfeld RG, Frane J. Growth hormone therapy of Turner syndrome: the impact of age of estrogen replacement on final height. Genentech, Inc., Collaborative Study Group. J Clin Endocrinol Metab 2000;85(7):2439–2445.
86. Farmer RD, Lawrenson RA, Todd JC, et al. A comparison of the risks of venous thromboembolic disease in association with different combined oral contraceptives. Br J Clin Pharmacol 2000; 49(6):580–590.
87. Woodruff J, Pickar J. Incidence of endometrial hyperplasia in postmenopausal women taking conjugated estrogens (Premarin) with medroxyprogesterone acetate or conjugated estrogens alone. Am J Obstet Gynecol 1994;170:1213–1223.
88. Molitch ME, Thorner MO, Wilson C. Management of prolactinomas. J Clin Endocrinol Metab 1997;82(4):996–1000.
89. Freda PU, Andreadis CI, Khandji AG, et al. Long-term treatment of prolactin-secreting macroadenomas with pergolide. J Clin Endocrinol Metab 2000;85(1):8–13.
90. Verhelst J, Abs R, Maiter D, et al. Cabergoline in the treatment of hyperprolactinemia: a study in 455 patients. J Clin Endocrinol Metab 1999;84(7):2518–2522.
91. Kannisto S, Korppi M, Remes K, Voutilainen R. Adrenal suppression, evaluated by a low dose adrenocorticotropin test, and growth in asthmatic children treated with inhaled steroids. J Clin Endocrinol Metab 2000;85(2):652–657.
92. Rosenfeld RL, Bickel S, Razdan AK. Amenorrhea related to progestin excess in congenital adrenal hyperplasia. Obstet Gynecol 1980;56:208.
93. Azziz R, Black VY, Knochenhauer ES, Hines GA, Boots LR. Ovulation after glucocorticoid suppression of adrenal androgens in the polycystic ovary syndrome is not predicted by the basal dehydroepiandrosterone sulfate level. J Clin Endocrinol Metab 1999;84(3):946–950.
94. DeCherney A, Speroff L. Next generation of contraception: oral contraceptives in the 1990s. Am J Obstet Gynecol 1992;167 (suppl): (4), part 2(4, part 2).
95. Ibañez L, Potau N, Marcos MV, de Zegher F. Treatment of hirsutism, hyperandrogenism, oligomenorrhea, dyslipidemia, and hyperinsulinism in nonobese, adolescent girls: effect of flutamide. J Clin Endocrinol Metab 2000;85(9):3251–3255.
96. Hasegawa I, Murakawa H, Suzuki M, Yamamoto Y, Kurabayashi T, Tanaka K. Effect of troglitazone on endocrine and ovulatory performance in women with insulin resistance-related polycystic ovary syndrome. Fertil Steril 1999;71(2):323–327.

26 Contraception

Helen H. Kim, MD

CONTENTS

    INTRODUCTION
    NON-HORMONAL METHODS OF CONTRACEPTION
    HORMONAL METHODS OF CONTRACEPTION
    HORMONAL CONTRACEPTION: NON-CONTRACEPTIVE BENEFITS
        OF HORMONAL CONTRACEPTION
    CONCLUSION
    NEW DELIVERY METHODS
    REFERENCES

INTRODUCTION

Contraception refers to reversible methods for the prevention of pregnancy. Although contraception may not seem like a pediatric issue, approximately one million teenagers become pregnant each year in the US, and the majority of these are unplanned. The US has the highest teenage pregnancy rate of all developed countries despite the fact that teenage pregnancy rates have declined during the 1990s. The overall pregnancy rate for women, aged 15–19, was 98.7 per 1000 in 1996 *(1)*. Given the magnitude of the problem, contraception needs to be addressed with all adolescents to prevent unplanned pregnancies.

Unplanned pregnancies may be particularly deleterious in women with endocrine disease. Pregnancy increases thyroxine requirements in many women with primary hypothyroidism *(2)* so careful monitoring during pregnancy is necessary to ensure adequate treatment. Hypothyroidism during pregnancy has been associated with both maternal and fetal morbidity *(3)*. Adequate thyroid replacement is thought to be critical for child neuropsychological development, since undiagnosed or inadequately treated hypothyroidism during pregnancy was found to be associated with lower IQ in the children *(4)*. There is also evidence that good metabolic control of diabetes at the time of conception may reduce the risk of spontaneous abortions *(5)* and possibly reduce the risk of fetal malformations *(6)*.

Realistic choice of contraceptive method appears to be particularly important in the adolescent population. Although many forms of hormonal and non-hormonal contraception are available (Table 1), each contraceptive method has its own set of limitations

From: *Contemporary Endocrinology: Pediatric Endocrinology: A Practical Clinical Guide*
Edited by: S. Radovick and M. H. MacGillivray © Humana Press Inc., Totowa, NJ

Table 1
Available Contraceptive Methods

Non-Hormonal Contraception

Behavioral	Withdrawal
	Periodic abstinence
Spermicial	Foam
	Cream
	Suppository
	Gel
	Film
Mechanical	Male Condom
	Vaginal Barriers
	Diaphragm
	Cervical Cap
	Vaginal Sponge
	Female Condom
Intrauterine Devices (IUD)	Copper IUD (ParaGuard®)
	Hormonal IUD
	Progesterone (Progestasert®)
	Levonorgestrel (Mirena®)

Hormonal Contraception

Combined Hormonal Contraception	Combined Oral Contraceptives
	Injectable (Lunelle®)
Progestin Only Contraception	Progestin-Only Pills
	Subdermal Implalnts (Norplant®)
	Injectable (Depo-Provera®)

(Table 2). It should be acknowledged to the patient that any contraceptive use represents a compromise, and that they need to understand the limitations of each method. In choosing a contraceptive method, important considerations include the degree of effectiveness, the spectrum of untoward effects, the presence of particular contraindications, the requirement for daily patient responsibility, as well as the necessity of interrupting sexual spontaneity. The selection of a contraceptive method for an adolescent patient with an endocrine disorder may even require additional considerations. Regardless of method, unmarried adolescents experience higher rates of contraceptive failure than older, married women, presumably from incorrect or inconsistent use (7) (Table 3).

In counseling patients, it should be emphasized that contraceptive use also confers health benefits unrelated to family planning. Hormonal contraceptive methods, in particular, have been used in management of dysfunctional uterine bleeding, pubertal disorders, acne, endometriosis, hirsutism, and osteoporosis. Hormonal contraceptives have also been shown to reduce the risk of endometrial cancers. The potential prevention of sexually transmitted disease (STD) may be an important consideration for young patients not in long-term, stable relationships. Unfortunately, spermicides and barriers are the most effective in preventing transmission of infections (8), but are the least effective methods of contraception, particularly in the adolescent population (7).

Table 2
Limitations of Current Contraceptive Methods

	Failure rate <10% (typical use)	Prevents STD	Daily patient responsibility	Interrupts spontaneity	Side effects
Ideal Method	Yes	Yes	No	No	No
Permanent Sterilization	Yes	No	No	No	No
Behavioral	No	No	Yes	Yes	No
Spermicide	No	Maybe	No	Yes	Yes
Barrier	No	Some types	No	Yes	Yes
IUD	Yes	No	No	No	Yes
Injectible Contraceptives	Yes	No	No	No	Yes
Oral Contraceptives	Yes	No	Yes	No	Yes

Both hormonal and non-hormonal contraceptive methods are available. In the adolescent population, hormonal methods are the most effective contraceptive methods, but because these methods are metabolically active, it is necessary to consider the possible interactions with the patient's disease or medical treatment. Non-hormonal contraceptive methods can be classified as behavioral, spermicidal, mechanical, and intrauterine. There are no medical contraindications to behavioral, spermicidal, and barrier contraceptive methods, but these methods are associated with high failure rates in adolescents (7).

NON-HORMONAL METHODS OF CONTRACEPTION

Behavioral

Behavioral methods include coitus interruptus and periodic abstinence. Coitus interruptus refers to withdrawal of the penis prior to ejaculation, so that sperm will not be deposited in the vagina. The withdrawal method, however, is associated with up to 38.3% failure rate in adolescents (7) and cannot be considered an adequate birth control method. Periodic abstinence involves abstaining from intercourse during the fertile time of the menstrual cycle when ovulation occurs. Perfect use of this method would require careful monitoring of menstrual cycles, assessments of cervical mucous quality, and daily measurements of basal body temperature. With avoidance of intercourse during the periovulatory period, the probability of pregnancy during the first year has been estimated at 3.1% (9). In theory, if intercourse were restricted to the 14-d luteal phase, after ovulation occurred, the failure rate would be zero (10). In practice, the failure rates associated with rhythm methods are as high as 86.4% (11) owing to imperfect identification of the periovulatory period or inability to abstain from intercourse during this time.

Spermicides

Vaginal spermicides are available, without a prescription, as foam, suppositories, gels, films, and cream, but probably do not represent an adequate birth control method

Table 3
Contraceptive Failure Rates During First Year Of Use

Method	Perfect use (percent)[1]	Routine use (percent)[2]	Age < 20 Unmarried not cohabiting (percent)[3]
Withdrawal	4	18.8	38.3
Periodic Abstinence	1	19.8	40.4
Spermicides	3	15.3	44.4
Male Condoms (alone)	2	8.7	22.5
Diphragm/Cervical Cap (with spermicide)	6	8.1	na
Intrauterine Device	<2	3.7	na
Combination Oral Contraceptive	0.1	6.9	12.1
Progestin-Only Pill	0.5	na	na
Subdermal Implant	0.04	2.3	2.3
Depo-Provera	0.3	3.2	4.2

[1] Adapted from Trussell et al 1990; [2] Adapted from Trussell and Vaughan 1999; [3] Adapted from ref. *(7)*.

for adolescents. If used correctly, vaginal spermicides have a 3% failure rate *(11)*, but perfect use is cumbersome. These agents are administered intravaginally and must be replenished prior to every act of intercourse. Ideally, foams, gels, and creams are inserted immediately prior to coitus, whereas suppositories and films are inserted several minutes prior. In practice, the failure has been estimated at 44.4% in adolescents *(7)*, so that spermicidal agents can be recommended only as an adjunctive measure, either to increase the efficacy of barrier methods or to provide protection from the transmission of sexually transmitted infections. Many of these spermicides are also effective anti-microbial agents *(12)*.

Barriers

Mechanical barriers to fertilization include male condoms and several vaginal barriers, including the female condom, diaphragm, vaginal sponge, and the cervical cap. Barrier methods not only prevent pregnancy, but also prevent the transmission of sexually transmitted infections *(8)*. It should be emphasized to adolescents that prevention of sexually transmitted infections is a critical step for the preservation of future fertility. Pelvic inflammatory disease (PID) usually results from ascending passage of bacteria from the lower reproductive tract into the tubal lumen *(13)*. It has been clearly demonstrated that the risk of infertility increases with the number of PID episodes. Infertility developed in 11.4% of women after one episode, in 23.1% of women after two episodes, and in 54.3% of women after three episodes *(14)*.

The male condom represents a mechanical barrier to fertilization and is the most frequently used method of contraception used at first intercourse *(15)*. Numerous different types of condoms are available over the counter and are similar in their ability to prevent pregnancy. With perfect use, condoms are an effective method of contraception with a failure rate of 2% *(11)*. Perfect use requires placing the condom prior to any genital contact and withdrawal of the penis prior to the loss of the erection. In adolescents, however, the failure rate with condom use is as high as 22.5% *(7)*, unacceptably high for adequate contraception. In the adolescent population, the primary role for the male condom may be to minimize the spread of sexually transmitted infections. The male condom provides the best available protection from STDs, providing protection from both bacterial and viral infections, including HIV *(8)*. It should be noted that natural condoms, made from sheep intestine, may not be as effective as latex and polyurethane in the prevention of STDs *(8)*.

The diaphragm, cervical cap, and contraceptive sponge prevent pregnancy by blocking the cervix, as well as holding spermicide around the cervix. These methods require the insertion of the device prior to intercourse and leaving it in place for several hours after intercourse. Although studies have not determined the optimal timing, clinical practice has been to insert the barrier no more than 6 h prior to intercourse and to leave it in place for at least 6 h afterwards *(16)*. It is recommended that the vaginal barriers be removed after 24 h due to concern about Toxic Shock Syndrome (TSS). The contraceptive sponge and diaphragm were found to significantly increase the risk of non-menstrual TSS in a case-control study *(17)*.

The diaphragm and cap are reusable latex barriers. They are available in several sizes and are fitted by trained personnel. The fit should be re-assessed annually or with changes in weight or after a pregnancy *(16)*. They should be used in conjunction with spermicides, and when used alone, are not as effective against pregnancy *(16)*. Additional spermicide is inserted prior to each act of coitus. With perfect use, the failure rate has been estimated at 6% (11), but with routine use, the failure rate has been reported to be three times as high (18%) during the first year of use *(11)*. There is no data available for specific failure rates in the adolescent population because female barriers were not widely used among the adolescents in the 1995 National Survey of Family Growth *(7)*.

There are several other drawbacks to the diaphragm and cervical cap. Oil-based lubricants cannot be used in conjunction with these barriers since oils destroy the integrity of the latex. Additionally, some women are allergic or sensitive to latex and will not be able to use these methods. Both the diaphragm and the cervical cap are associated with an increased risk of urinary tract infections *(16)*, presumably as a result of alterations in vaginal flora *(18,19)*.

The vaginal contraceptive sponge is disposable and is available over the counter. It is effective for multiple acts of coitus during a 24-h period. It appears to be slightly more effective in the nulliparous woman with a similar failure rate as the diaphragm and cervical cap *(11)*. In the women who have previously given birth, the annual failure rate is 9% for perfect users and 28% for typical users. The Today® sponge contains non-oxynol-9 as the spermicidal agent. It has been unavailable since 1995, but according to its website, it is expected to be available soon. The newer Protectaid® contraceptive sponge is available now, and is impregnated with 3 spermicidal agents, nonoxynyl-9, benzalkonoium chloride, and sodium cholate. These agents have anti-microbial, as well as spermicidal effects.

The Reality® female condom is a disposable method of contraception that was FDA approved for non-prescription sale in 1994. It consists of a polyurethane bag or sheath that fits into the vagina and is held in place by an internal vaginal ring. The open end of the sheath remains outside the vagina and covers part of the labia. It is pre-lubricated with a silicone-based lubricant and must be placed before coitus. It is disposable after one use.

According to the product literature, the annual failure rate is estimated at 5% with correct and consistent use and at 21% for typical use. This method may be overly cumbersome for the adolescent to use as a primary contraceptive method, but may have a role in STD prevention when the male partner will not wear a condom. In vitro studies indicate that polyurethane is an effective barrier to microorganisms, including HIV. Because part of the labia is also covered, this device may protect from transmission of human papilloma virus (HPV) by minimizing external genital contact. The female and male condom should not be used simultaneously because friction between the two could pull off the male condom or push in the female condom.

Intrauterine Devices

The intrauterine device (IUD) is a very effective, long-term contraceptive method that appears to work by producing an endometrial environment that is both spermicidal and unsuitable for implantation. IUDs require a prescription and are placed into the uterine cavity by trained personnel. The 3 IUDs, which are currently available in the US, provide differing lengths of contraceptive protection: 1 yr for Progestasert® (progesterone-releasing), 10 yr for ParaGuard® (Copper-releasing), and 5 yr for Mirena® (levonorgestrel-releasing). Because of the long period of effectiveness, the ParaGuard® IUD is the most cost-effective reversible contraceptive available to American women (20).

The IUD is generally thought to be inappropriate for use in the adolescent population. The ideal IUD candidate is a woman who is in a mutually monogamous relationship, who desires long-term contraception, and has had at least one child. The ParaGuard® IUD has a failure rate of less than 1% for perfect use and 3% for typical use. Perfect use requires checking for the IUD strings prior to each coital act to rule out expulsion of the IUD. The cumulative 5-yr expulsion rate has been approximated at 6%, and expulsions are even more common among young, nulliparous women (21). Because of the possible increased risk for PID in IUD users, IUDs are only appropriate for women in mutually monogamous relations with no risk of STDs. For this reason, IUDs are contraindicated in women with recent history of STD, and should be used cautiously when other conditions may increase susceptibility to infections, such as HIV infection, diabetes, valvular heart disease, or chronic steroid use.

HORMONAL METHODS OF CONTRACEPTION

Overview

Hormonal contraception, particularly long-acting methods, have proven to be the most effective contraceptive methods in the adolescent population (7). In the past, there had been concern that use of hormonal contraception in adolescents might adversely impact on the development of normal reproductive function and growth, but these fears have not been substantiated (22,23). After reviewing the literature in 1996, a consensus of 72 international experts concluded that healthy menstruating adolescents can take combined oral contraceptive therapy without any special assessment (22). In fact, hormonal contraception may be particularly safe in adolescents because contraindications to oral contraceptive therapy, such as risk factors for cardiovascular disease, are rarely seen in the adolescent population (23).

Hormonal contraceptive agents can be delivered as subdermal implants, intramuscular injections, and oral contraceptive pills (Table 1). Oral contraceptive pills (OCPs) are taken daily and are available as progestin-only "mini-pills"(POPs) or as combination oral contraceptive pills (COCs) containing both estrogen and progestin. Long-acting hormonal contraception is available with progestin only as a 3-mo depot intramuscular injection of medroxyprogesterone acetate (DMPA), sold under the brand name Depo-Provera® in the US. Subdermal implants that release levonorgestrel for a 5-yr period (Norplant®) are also available. Recently, the FDA has approved a monthly combination contraceptive injection containing estradiol cypionate and medroxyprogesterone acetate (Lunelle®).

Hormonal contraception prevents pregnancy via multiple mechanisms. At high circulating levels, progestins inhibit the mid-cycle surge of luteinizing hormone and block ovulation. Because ovulation occurs in approximately half of oral progestin users *(24)* and one third of Norplant® users *(25)*, suppression of ovulation in unlikely to be the primary contraceptive mechanism. Progestins inhibit sperm transport into the uterine cavity by producing a thick, but scant, cervical mucus that is not receptive to sperm penetration *(26)*. Progestins also produce an atrophic endometrium in which embryo implantation would be unlikely *(27)*. In combination contraceptive methods, estrogens augment the progestational effects so that lower progestin doses are necessary. Estrogens prevent follicular development by inhibiting pituitary gonadotropin production, and in combination with progestins, reliably inhibit ovulation *(24)*. It is also possible that exogenous hormones may impair fertilization and early embryo development by altering Fallopian tube secretion and peristalsis *(28)*.

The estrogenic component of the combined hormonal contraceptive methods also provides an important non-contraceptive benefit of predictable uterine withdrawal bleeding. With progestin-only contraceptive methods, endogenous estrogen is suppressed. The continuous presence of progestin without endogenous estrogen leads to atrophic endometrium that sheds unpredictably. Unpredictable irregular uterine bleeding is the major reason for discontinuation of both Depo-Provera® *(29)* and Norplant® *(30)*, particularly among adolescent women *(31)*.

Systemic Effects of Hormonal Contraception

Unlike the previously described contraceptive methods, which are metabolically inert, hormonal contraceptive methods have systemic metabolic effects. Studies performed in the 1960s and 1970s suggested that women using oral contraceptive pills were at increased risk for cardiovascular disease, but these data were derived from older pills containing higher steroid doses and different formulations compared to what is available today. Enovid, the first oral contraceptive released in the US contained 150 µg of mestranol (equivalent to approx 105 µg of ethinyl estradiol *[32]*), whereas today's low-dose combination oral contraceptive pill contains 20–35 µg of ethinyl estradiol *(33)*. Reduction in the steroid content of combination oral contraceptive pills has been accompanied by a decrease in adverse metabolic effects, such as stroke, myocardial infarction, and deep vein thrombosis, as well as reductions in side-effects, such as nausea and breast tenderness *(33)*.

Fear of complications, therefore, should not be a deterrent to the use of hormonal contraception by patients and clinicians. Prior to prescribing hormonal contraception, candidates need to be screened to identify any contraindications. The screening, however, does not need to be overly burdensome. In order to avoid unnecessary restriction of contraception use, the World Health Organization (WHO) held two meetings of experts in 1994 and 1995 to guide practitioners in a variety of health care settings around the world *(34)*. Using evidence-based criteria, these experts assessed the risk of pregnancy vs contraceptive use in setting of various medical conditions, and identified only a few medical conditions that precluded the use of hormonal contraception. Additionally, with the exception of blood pressure measurement, a physical exam was not a prerequisite to hormonal contraception. In 1996, another international consensus of 72 international experts concluded that the only two clinical assessments relevant to oral contraceptive use were blood pressure measurement and family and personal history, with particular attention to risk factors for thromboembolism and cardiovascular disease *(22)*.

Drug Interactions

Prior to initiating hormonal contraceptive therapy, a careful medication history should be obtained from patients, and patients should be counseled that the efficacy of hormonal contraception may be reduced by the concomitant use of certain medications *(35)*. Certain medications, through induction of liver enzymes, enhance the metabolism of estrogens and progestins. As a result, these medications may reduce the efficacy of COCs, POPs, and Norplant® *(36)*. In particular, WHO guidelines indicate that these contraceptive methods should not be used if certain anticonvulants (phenytoin, carbamezapine, barbituates, primadone) or antibiotics (griseofulvin, rifampin) are required *(34)*. WHO guidelines suggest that the Depo-Provera® may be used cautiously with these medications *(34)*. Contraceptive failure has not been reported in users of Depo-Provera® taking anticonvulsants, presumably due to the higher circulating levels of progestin *(36)*. Additionally, because estrogens and progestins are metabolized through the liver, WHO guidelines consider active liver disease contraindications for hormonal contraception *(34)*.

The use of hormonal contraception may also modulate the effects of other medications. Steroids weakly inhibit hepatic drug oxidation, but enhance glucuronosyltransferase activity *(35)*. For this reason, hormonal contraceptives may reduce the clearance (increase plasma levels) of certain medications and increase the clearance (lower plasma concentrations) of others. For example, increased serum levels of corticosteroids have been reported after high doses of estrogens *(35)*, so that corticosteroid doses may need to be adjusted with COC use. Post-menopausal women with hypothyroidism have an increased need for thyroxine during estrogen therapy, presumably from increases in thyroid binding globulin *(37)*. It seems reasonable to believe that COC users may similarly experience a need for increased thyroxine doses.

Thromboembolism

The most serious risk for adolescent users of combined hormonal contraception is venous thromboembolism (VTE), including pulmonary embolism. The increased risk appears to be related to estrogen, which increases hepatic production of coagulation factors in a dose-dependent manner *(38,39)*. Accordingly, the risk of VTE has decreased along with decreases in the estrogen content of the combination OCPs. Nevertheless, users of modern COCs, containing 30–35 µg of ethinyl estradiol, still have a three to four fold elevated relative risk of VTE compared with nonusers *(40)*. Although combination OCPs with 20 µg of ethinyl estradiol do not appear to have an effect on clotting factors *(39)*, there is no evidence that lowering the estrogen content below 30 µg further reduces the risk of VTE *(41–43)*. It is important to remember, however, that venous thromboembolic events occur less frequently in users of combination OCPs (10–40 cases per 100,000 woman per year) than during pregnancy (60 cases per 100,000 pregnancies) *(41)*.

In 1995–1996, several European studies suggested that the progestin component of combination OCPs may also contribute to the risk of VTE . These studies noted a small (1.5–2.6-fold) increase in the risk of VTE in users of COCs containing the newer progestins (gestodene and desogestrel) compared with users of COCs containing the older progestins *(21,45–49)*. Since then, newer studies have revealed biases in these studies *(44)*. Because women who develop VTE on COCs discontinue COC use, the increased risk of VTE in COC users decreases with duration of use *(50,51)*. Furthermore, because these new progestins were thought to be safer than older formulations, a high proportion of new COC starters were prescribed the new 3rd generation progestins, particularly if they were at increased risk for VTE *(52)*. More recent studies that controlled for preferential prescribing and duration of use have found the risk of VTE with the new progestins to be equivalent to other COCs *(50,51,53–55)*.

Due to the increased risk of thromboembolism, WHO guidelines recommend that individuals who are less than 3 wk postpartum or have a personal history of VTE do not use combination OCPs *(34)*. Because prolonged immobilization is also a risk factor for VTE, WHO guidelines recommend that COCs should be discontinued when major surgery with prolonged immobilization is anticipated *(34)*. If possible, COCs should be discontinued well in advance of the scheduled surgery date, since the hypercoaguable state associated with combination OCPs has been found to persist for 6 wk after OCPs were discontinued *(56)*. In the absence of other risk factors, however, COCs do not need to be discontinued pre-operatively on a routine basis *(34)*. WHO guidelines do not consider thromboembolic risk factors to be relevant for the prescription of progestin-only contraceptive methods, since no increased risk of thromboembolism has been identified in users of these contraceptive methods *(34)*.

Use of combination OCPs also increases the risk of VTE in women with thrombophilic disorders, such as the factor V Leiden mutation that occurs in approx 3–4% of the European population . Women heterozygous for the factor V Leiden mutation who use COCs have a 30-fold higher risk of VTE compared with a 6–8 fold risk for carriers who do not use COCs *(44)*. Laboratory screening may be indicated to identify thrombophilic disorders in women with a family history of VTE or thrombophilic disorder, but routine screening is not currently recommended *(22,44)*. The carrier frequencies of the factor V Leiden mutation in the US is lower than in Europe with the following ethnic distribution: 5.27% in Caucasian Americans, 2.21% in Hispanic Americans, 1.25% in Native Americans, 1.23% in African-Americans, and 0.45% in Asian Americans *(57)*. Even among women with factor V Leiden mutation, the vast majority will never get a VTE, and most VTE occur in women without a thrombophilic disorder *(22)*.

Cardiovascular Disease

With the decreasing estrogen content of combination OCPs over the past years, their cardiovascular safety has improved dramatically *(41,43)*. A review of the epidemiologic data found that in the absence of smoking, use of modern COCs, containing less than 50 µg of ethinyl estradiol, is not associated with any meaningful increase in the risk of myocardial infarction or stroke—regardless of age *(40)*. The increased risk for cardiovascular disease is concentrated in current users of COCs who are past their mid-thirties and who smoke cigarettes *(22)*. The WHO recommends that COCs be used cautiously in women over 35 yr of age who smoke *(34)*, whereas healthy, non-smokers can continue to use combination OCPs as long as they remain at risk for pregnancy *(22)*. In the adolescent population, cigarette smoking is not a contraindication for COC use, since they are at particularly low risk of cardiovascular disease.

Because the adolescent population is at extremely low risk for cardiovascular disease, screening may be of limited utility. Nevertheless, the initial assessment is to identify other risk factors for cardiovascular disease, such as cigarette use, hypertension, lipid disorders, diabetes mellitus, as well as family history of coronary artery disease or ischemic stroke *(22)*. The impact of these other cardiovascular risk factors will become more important as the patient ages, and sequelae of medical conditions, such as diabetes, may worsen over time. WHO guidelines consider pre-existing mild to moderate hypertension a relative contraindication to combination OCP use *(34)*.

The follow-up assessment should include blood pressure measurement after the first few months of OCP use, since there is evidence from older formulations that use of combination OCPs increases the risk of malignant hypertension *(58)*. Combination OCPs also appear to cause reversible blood pressure elevations in some women *(24,59)*. In the nurses health study, 41.5 per 10,000 person-years of OCP-related increases in blood pressure were identified *(59)*. The prevalence of hypertension, however, is age-related and it is unlikely that use of combination OCPs would cause hypertension in adolescents *(23)*. If blood pressure elevations are identified, another method of contraception should be considered.

Many of the progestin-only methods have the same package labeling as for combination OCPs despite the fact that the absence of the estrogen component in progesterone-only contraceptive methods appears to eliminate the cardiovascular risk. WHO guidelines do not consider cigarette smoking or age over 35 to be contraindications for progestin-only contraceptive methods *(34)*. A review of the epidemiologic data also concluded that women over age 35 who smoke can safely use progestin-only contraceptives *(40)*. Studies have not demonstrated significant changes in blood pressure with contraceptive methods containing only progestational agents *(34)*, so that progestin-only pills and Norplant® may be used without restriction in mild hypertension (up to 179/109), and DMPA may be used cautiously *(34)*.

Serum Lipids

Atherosclerotic heart disease and coronary artery disease are associated with increased triglycerides, increased LDL cholesterol, and decreased HDL cholesterol *(35,61)*. Some hormonal contraceptive agents have been shown to induce these types of changes in the serum lipid profile. Women taking combination OCPs were found to have higher fasting triglyceride levels compared with controls *(61)*. Levonorgestrel containing COCs and DMPA seem to depress HDL cholesterol *(35,61)*. Other COCs produced more favorable changes in the serum lipid profile. Preparations using desogestrel or low dose norethindrone depressed LDL cholesterol and increased HDL levels *(61)*. The progestin-only methods, Norplant® and DMPA appear to decrease triglyceride levels *(35)*. It is not clear, however, whether any of these changes in serum lipids increases the risk for cardiovascular disease, particularly in the adolescent.

Carbohydrate Metabolism

Insulin resistance, elevated insulin levels with poor glucose tolerance, is also associated with atherosclerotic heart disease and coronary artery disease. Hormonal contraception has been shown to induce these adverse changes in carbohydrate metabolism. Combination OCPs appear to impaired glucose tolerance and elevated insulin levels *(35,61,62)*. Both estrogen and progestins influence carbohydrate metabolism, but since the COCs contain the same estrogen component (ethinyl estradiol) at similar doses (20–35 µg), the differences in the carbohydrate metabolism between the various COC formulations have been attributed to the progestin component. In combination with estrogen, levonorgestrel appeared to have greater adverse effects on glucose tolerance and insulin resistance than those containing norethindrone or desogestrel. In contrast, progestin-only OCPs, containing either levonorgestrel or norethindrone alone, have minimal effects on carbohydrate metabolism. Deterioration of glucose tolerance has also been demonstrated in healthy users of DMPA *(63,64)*, and Norplant® *(65–67)*.

It is not clear whether these alterations in carbohydrate metabolism are clinically significant. The long-acting progestin methods did not produce clinically significant alterations in carbohydrate metabolism in normal women despite the changes in glucose tolerance. All of the changes in glucose tolerance remained within normal limits for Norplant® users over 30 mo *(65)* and for DMPA users after 12 mo *(63)*. In a study of 130 healthy women using triphasic COCs, statistically significant increases in plasma glucose and insulin levels were noted after initiating OCPs *(68)*. These changes, however, were not associated with impaired glucose tolerance and appear clinically unimportant. A large review found that use of the low dose COC is accompanied by a low risk of impaired glucose tolerance, even in previous gestational diabetics *(69)*.

Because a history of gestational diabetes increases risk of developing diabetes, gestational diabetics need close postpartum monitoring. The use of low dose COCs, however, does not appear to influence the risk of developing diabetes *(70)*, and WHO guidelines do not consider a history of gestational diabetes to be relevant for the prescription of hormonal contraception *(34)*. One study found that lactating women with recent gestational diabetes who used progestin-only pills had nearly a three-fold increase in the risk of diabetes *(70)*, suggesting that progestin-only pills should be prescribed cautiously in this group.

Although there are theoretical concerns about prescribing hormonal contraception for women with insulin-requiring diabetes, the current data suggests that modern COCs have little effect on glycemic control or the insulin requirements of diabetic women *(71)*. Furthermore, neither current, past, or duration of COC use was associated with current gycosylated hemoglobin or the development of diabetic sequelae, such as retinopathy, nephropathy, and hypertension *(72,73)*. There have been no studies specifically examining use of long-acting progestational contraceptives by diabetic women, so COCs or progestin-only OCPs may be preferable in this setting *(71)*. Given that an unplanned pregnancy in a diabetic woman may be associated with poor glycemic control and poor pregnancy outcomes, WHO guidelines indicate that the advantages of hormonal contraception generally outweigh the risks for diabetic women, unless there is nephropathy, retinopathy, neuropathy, or vascular disease *(34)*.

Weight Gain

It is widely believed that use of hormonal contraception may be associated with weight gain and may be a reason that adolescents are reluctant to initiate hormonal contraception. Adolescents appear to be particularly concerned about maintenance of their body weight. In a survey of women ages 13–21, 50% reported that they would not accept a contraceptive method if it were associated with a 5 lb weight gain *(74)*. In fact, 41% of adolescents listed weight gain as the primary reason for discontinuing contraception with long acting progestin *(31)*.

Theoretically, both the estrogenic and progestational components of the COCs can contribute to weight gain. Progestins are thought to directly stimulate hypothalamic center to increase appetite *(75)*. Progestins have also been shown to increase insulin levels, which can be associated with symptoms of hypoglycemia and increased appetite *(35)*. Estrogen can result in increased subcutaneous fat deposition *(35)*. Additionally, fluid retention has been associated with both the estrogen and progestin component of COCs *(35)*.

Despite the theoretical concerns about weight gain related to COC use, the existing data does not support this concern. Several prospective studies have demonstrated that OCP use was not associated with significant weight gain *(76–79)*. In another study, only 5% of women cited weight gain as a reason for discontinuing OCPs *(80)*. It appears that as many women lose weight as gain weight while taking COCs *(35)*.

In contrast to COCs, it appears that DMPA may be associated with significant weight gain. The FDA package labeling for DMPA states the method is associated with progressive weight gain, with an average weight gain of 5.4 lb after the first year, 8.1 lb after the second year, and 13.8 lb after the fourth year. These weight changes were identified in a large US study involving 3857 women *(81)*. Later studies, however, suggest that weight gain should not deter women from considering DMPA as a contraceptive method. Despite increases in weight by some women, many do lose weight while using DMPA. As many as 44–56% percent of DMPA users, including adolescents, were found to have lost or maintain their body weight in retrospective studies *(82,83)*. Another study had IUD users as controls and found that users of both types of contraception gained a similar amount of weight over the 120 mo study period: 10.9 kg for DMPA users and 11.2 kg for the IUD users *(84)*. This study suggests that weight gain is common in reproductive age women, so that weight changes should not be immediately attributed to contraceptive therapy.

Reproductive Cancer

Fear of breast and reproductive cancers is a major reason that women are reluctant to use hormonal contraception *(23)*, although strong epidemiologic data demonstrate a protective effect of combination OCPs against ovarian and endometrial cancers *(85,86)*. Furthermore, the benefit of combination OCPs are enhanced with duration of use and persist years after OCPs are discontinued *(22)*. In a review of the literature, ovarian cancer risk was found to decrease by 10% after 1 yr of using combination OCP and by approx 50% after 5 yr of use *(87)*. The cancer and steroid hormone (CASH) study demonstrated that the use of combination OCPs for as little as 3–6 mo reduces the risk of ovarian cancer, and the protective effect persists 15 yr after use ended *(88)*. The CASH study also found combination OCPs to be similarly protective against endometrial cancer *(89,90)*. Because endometrial cancer is common, it is estimated that combination OCP use prevents 2000 cases of endometrial cancer annually in the US *(89)*.

It is not yet clear whether combination OCPs containing less than 20 µg of ethinyl estradiol and progestin-only contraceptive methods offer the same protection against ovarian and endometrial cancer. Most of the COC users in the above studies were using formulations containing at least 30 µg of ethinyl estradiol. COCs are thought to reduce the risk of ovarian cancer by suppressing gonadotropin stimulation of the ovary and by preventing the trauma to the ovarian epithelium that occurs with ovulation *(91)*. Because ovulation occurs in users of progestin-only pills and Norplant®, these methods may not be as protective against the development of ovarian cancer. Daily exposure to progestins is thought to be the mechanism by which COCs protect the endometrium from endometrial cancer. Use of DMPA appears to reduce the risk of endometrial cancer at least as well as COCs *(92)*, and may even reduce the risk further *(93)*.

Despite numerous studies, it is not clear whether there is any association with combination OCP use and breast cancer *(22)*. Recently, a collaborative analysis examined data from 53,297 women with breast cancer and 100,239 controls obtained in 54 studies conducted in 26 different countries *(94,95)*. Regardless of duration of use, no increase in breast cancer risk was found in women who had not used OCPs in the past 10 yr. In this analysis, family history of breast cancer did not affect breast cancer risk associated with OCP use. Current OCP users were at a small increased risk of being diagnosed with breast cancer while they were using OCPs and for 10 yr after discontinuation *(95)*. Compared to non-users, cancers were diagnosed at an earlier stage in users—suggesting that the increased diagnosis of breast cancer may reflect a bias in cancer surveillance. Because OCP users are more likely to have contact with the health care system, cancer is detected more frequently, but at earlier stages *(23,96)*.

Approval for Depo-Provera® was delayed for over 20 yr over concerns about breast cancer. DMPA was approved for use in several countries in the 1970s, but did not receive FDA approval for contraceptive use in the US until 1992 *(29)*. A large case-control study by the World Health Organization, published in 1991, provided reassurance that long-term users of DMPA were not at increased risk of breast cancer *(92)*. The risk of breast cancer was not increased with increased duration of use, or for women who had initiated DMPA use more than 5 yr previously. The WHO study did detect a slightly increased risk of breast cancer in the first 4 yr of DMPA use, mainly in women <35-yr-old *(97)*. These results were interpreted to suggest that rather than cause new tumors, DMPA enhances growth of already existing tumors *(29)*.

There has also been concern that use of hormonal contraception during adolescence when the breast was developing would make the individual particularly at risk for breast cancer. A large study suggested that women aged 20–34 yr who had ever used OCPs had a slightly increased risk of being diagnosed with breast cancer compared to those who had never used OCPs *(98)*. The international collaborative breast cancer study, however, did not find an increased risk for breast cancer with long duration of use or use of OCPs at a young age *(95)*.

Studies have suggested an increased risk of cervical cancer in long-term users of combination oral contraception, compared with non-users, but is unclear whether OCP use is causal *(22)*. The major cause of squamous cervical neoplasia is infection with particular types of human papilloma virus (HPV), so there are many confounding factors that may contribute to the observed association between OCP use and cervical neoplasia.

Users of OCPs probably do not use barrier methods of contraception that protect against STDs such as HPV. Users of OCPs may have more sexual partners than nonusers. More recent studies that control for potential confounding factors are somewhat reassuring about the association between cervical neoplasia and OCP use. These well-controlled studies found that neither the risk of invasive cervical cancer nor the risk of cervical intraepithelial neoplasia (CIN) was increased in OCP users *(23,99–101)*.

OCP users also appear to have an increased risk for cervical adenocarcinoma *(99,102)*, unrelated to HPV infection and accounts for approx 10% of cervical cancers *(23)*. The risk of cervical adenocarcinoma in the adolescent population, however, is very low and has been estimated at approx 1 in 350,000 in women age 15–19 from 1992–1996 *(23)*. Current recommendations from the American College of Obstetricians and Gynecologists suggest that history of CIN is not a contraindication to OCP use, but regular cytology screening should be performed *(23)*.

Combined Oral Contraception

With perfect use, OCPs are an extremely effective method of contraception with a failure rate of less than 1% *(11)*. In actual use by adolescents, however, OCPs are associated with a much higher failure rate of 12.1% after a year, presumably due to inconsistent use *(7)*. Combination oral contraceptive pills contain both estrogenic as well as progestational agents. The pills differ in their total estrogen content, the progestational agent used, and the ratio of estrogen to progestin. In monophasic preparations, the dose of estrogen and progestin are constant throughout the pill pack. In biphasic and triphasic preparations, the dose of the progestin or estrogen component varies during the cycle to minimize the total amount of hormone required and to duplicate a normal menstrual cycle.

All combination OCPs contain either ethinyl estradiol or mestranol as their estrogenic component. The addition of an ethinyl group to estradiol makes the steroid orally active *(33)*. Mestranol, the methyl ether of ethinyl estradiol, is converted to ethinyl estradiol to exert its estrogenic effects *(33)*. Ethinyl estradiol, at doses of 20–35 µg, is the estrogenic component of all low dose combination OCPs available in the US. The metabolism of ethinyl estradiol varies between individuals so that the same dose can cause side effects in one woman and none in another *(32,103)*.

There are several different progestins used in the combination OCPs *(33)*. The first generation progestins were derived from testosterone and include norethindrone acetate, ethynodiol diacetate, and norethindrone. The addition of a methyl group to norethindrone increased its potency and created the second-generation progestins, norgestrel and levonorgestrel (the biologically active optical isomers of norgestrel). Norgestimate is metabolized to levonorgestrel and is classified as a second-generation progestin by some and as a third-generation by others *(44)*. The third-generation progestins, gestodene, desogestrel, and norgestimate, are derived from levonorgestrel, but have fewer androgenic effects. Gestodene containing products are not available in the US.

Drospirenone is a newer progestin that may have a pharmacologic profile more closely related to endogenous progesterone *(104)*. Drospirenone is an analog of Spironolactone, the aldosterone antagonist, and like progesterone, has mild anti-mineralocorticoid activity *(105)*. It may result in fewer side effects resulting from fluid retention (e.g., breast tenderness and weight gain) by counteracting the estrogen-induced stimulation of the renin-angiotensin-aldosterone system *(104)*. In contrast to the other progestins, drospirenone has no androgenic activity and, in fact, appears to have mild anti-androgenic activity like spironolactone *(104)*.

Combination OCPs are traditionally taken daily for 21 d. After 21 d, pills are stopped for 7 d to allow a hormone withdrawal bleed to occur. COCs are also packaged as 28-d packs with 7 placebo pills. The placebo pills contain no hormone, but keep the patient in the daily routine of pill taking. Because the synthetic steroids in COCs are not completely eliminated from the body within 24 h, there is a cumulative build-up over several days and maximal effectiveness is not achieved until after several days *(35)*. A back-up contraceptive method is usually recommended during the first combination OCP cycle, but immediate protection from pregnancy is thought to be present if COCs are started with the first day of the menstrual cycle. If COCs are started after the fifth day of the cycle, however, breakthrough ovulation may occur, and a back-up contraceptive method should be used *(35)*.

Many clinicians are using "Sunday starts" so that a patient will start her first pack of pills on the Sunday following the start of her menstrual cycle. If menses begin on Sunday, the patient will begin taking pills on that Sunday. Intuitively, it seemed that patients would be less likely to forget starting a new pill pack if the event were synchronized with the beginning of the week. The "Sunday start" also has the advantage of scheduling the hormonal withdrawal bleeding on Tuesday or Wednesday, so that bleeding on weekends is avoided. A drawback to the Sunday start is that a back-up contraceptive method will be necessary for at least 7 d if COCs are started after the fifth day cycle day.

Recently, the 21-d schedule and the necessity of a monthly withdrawal bleed have been questioned. During the placebo week, some COC users can experience hormonal withdrawal symptoms, such as pelvic pain and bleeding *(106)*. One strategy to reduce hormonal withdrawal symptoms is to decrease the hormone-free interval. Mircette® is packaged as 21 d of desogestrel (150 µg) and ethinyl estradiol (20 µg), followed by 2 d of inert tablets and 5 d of ethinyl estradiol (10 µg) only.

Alternatively, several groups have investigated increasing the duration of active pills to minimize these symptoms by reducing the frequency of hormone free intervals *(107–110)*. Although some women can take COCs continuously without any break, many experience breakthrough bleeding after prolonged continuous COC use *(111)*. It has been suggested that women may individualize their COC regimen and begin a 7-d pill free interval when they begin to have breakthrough bleeding or at whatever interval is convenient. Because irregular bleeding was more common in women who were initiating COC therapy, this continuous COC regimen should probably not be started until a woman has used COCs for several cycles *(109)*.

Patients occasionally forget to take a pill. It seems that patients are most likely to forget or skip pills during first cycles of use before pill-taking has become part of their daily routine *(35)*. Instructions for missed pills should be given to the patient when OCPs are initiated. If one pill is missed, the missed pill should be taken immediately and the next pill should be taken at the regular time. If 2 consecutive pills are missed during the first 2 wk, the standard recommendation is to take 2 pills daily for 2 d and to use back-up contraception for the remainder of the pack. If 2 or more pills are missed during the 3rd wk or if 3 or more pills are missed at any time, the standard recommendation is to start a new pack and use a back-up contraceptive method for at least 7 d. If the patient uses a Sunday start, she should take 1 pill daily until Sunday and then start a new pack on Sunday.

Table 4
Biological Activity of Selected Monophasic and Progestin-Only Oral Contraceptive Formulations[1]

Formulation EE (µg) + progestin (mg)	Endometrial activity	Estrogenic activity	Progestational activity	Androgenic activity
EE (30) Norgestrel (0.3)	9.6	25	0.8	0.46
EE (35) Norethindrone (0.4)	11.0	40	0.4	.15
EE (30) Desogestrel (0.15)	13.1	30	1.5	.17
EE (30) Levonorgestrel (0.15)	14.0	25	0.8	0.46
EE (35) Norgestimate (0.25)	14.3	35	0.3	0.18
EE (35) Norethindrone (1.0)	14.7	38	1	0.34
EE (35) Norethindrone (0.5)	24.6	42	0.5	0.17
EE (30) Norethindrone Acetate (1.5)	25.2	14	1.7	0.8
EE (20) Levonorgestrel (0.1)	26.5	17	0.5	0.31
EE (20) Norethindrone Acetate (1.0)	29.7	13	1.2	0.53
EE (35) Ethynodiol Diacetate (1.0)	37.4	19	1.4	0.21
EE (0) Norgestrel (0.075)	34.9	0	0.08	0.13
EE (0) Norethindrone (0.35)	42.3	1	0.12	0.13

[1]Adapted from Dickey 1998. Activities are defined as follows: endometrial is percent of users with irregular bleeding in third cycle or use, estrogenic refers to ethinyl estradiol (µg) equivalents per day, progestational refers to norethindrone (mg) equivalents per day, and androgenic refers to methyltestosterone (mg) equivalents per day.

It has been estimated that nearly one third to one half of women who start OCPs will discontinue them within a year due to side-effects. Proper counseling may be critical for compliance since discontinuation was found to be more likely in the first 2 mo of OCP use, particularly if side effects were unexpected *(80)*. The more common side effects (bleeding irregularities, nausea, weight gain, mood changes, breast engorgement, and headaches) should be reviewed with the patient, but it should be emphasized that breakthrough bleeding and nausea will usually resolve spontaneously with continued OCP use *(35)*. Since side-effects decrease with continued use, patients with irregular bleeding and nausea should be encouraged to try OCPs for three cycles prior to discontinuing.

It should also be emphasized to patients that there are many different formulations of COCs available today (Table 4). If a particular side effect is still troubling after 3 cycles, a different COC preparation can be tried. The choice of a different COC preparation can be tailored to alleviate her particular symptoms (Table 5). Although the progestins are

Table 5
Relation of Side Effects to Hormonal Biologic Activity[1]

Estrogen excess	Progestin excess	Androgen excess
Bloating	Appetite increase	Acne
Breast cystic changes	Bloating	Hirsutism
Breast engorgement	Depression	Libido increase
Cholasma	Fatigue	Oily skin
Fluid retention	Hypoglycemic symptoms	
Headache	Libido decrease	
Nausea	Menstrual flow decrease	
Menorrhagia/hypermenorrhea	Weight gain (noncyclic)	
Weight gain (cyclic)	Headache	
Estrogen deficiency	*Progestin deficiency*	*Androgen deficiency*
Amenorrhea		
Atrophic vaginitis	Irregular bleeding (d 10–21)	Libido decrease
Irregular bleeding (d 1–9)	Menorrhagia	
Irregular bleeding (continuous)	Withdrawal bleeding delayed	
Withdrawal bleeding decrease		

[1] Adapted from Dickey 1998.

used at such low doses that the differences in their biologic effects should be negligible, different combination OCPs may have slightly different side-effect profiles in a particular patient. The side-effect profile of a particular COC is due to differences in estrogen content, type of progestin, and ratio of progestin to estrogen. Side effects of COCs can be estrogenic, progestational, and androgenic (Table 5). The hormone content of the COCs can differentially effect the endometrium as well *(35)*.

The estrogenic effects of a particular COC formulation is caused by the dose of estrogen, the type of progestin used, and the ratio of estrogen to progestin. A small percentage of the first generation progestins is metabolized to ethinyl estradiol and therefore may contribute to the estrogenic effect of the combination OCP *(35)*. Progestins, however, also reduce the biological activity of estrogen by acting as estrogen antagonists *(35)*. So for the same dose of ethinyl estradiol, a patient may experience symptoms of estrogen excess (breast engorgement, fluid retention, nausea, hypermenorrhea, cholasma) or estrogen deficiency (vaginal dryness, loss of hormonal withdrawal bleeding) depending on the dose and type of progestin used. If a patient experiences symptoms or estrogen excess or deficiency, a COC preparation with different estrogenic activity can be tried (Table 4).

In tests of biological activity, the various progestational agents used in combination OCPs can exert androgenic, anti-mineralocorticoid, as well as progestational effects. In combination with estrogen, however, the specific differences between these progestins are less significant. For example, the number of progesterone receptors depends on the estrogen content *(35)*. OCP users, therefore, can experience symptoms of progesterone deficiency (breakthrough bleeding) or progesterone excess (decreased menstrual bleeding, increased appetite, depression) depending on the estrogen content and the estrogen to progesterone ratio.

With the exception of drospirenone, the synthetic progestins all have androgenic biological activity. These synthetic progestins can increase free androgen by depressing sex-hormone-binding globulin (SHBG) and also by displacing bound androgen from SHBG *(35)*. Nevertheless, all of the COCs exert an anti-androgenic effect. The estrogenic component increases SHBG to decrease free testosterone, and the progestational component suppresses the hypothalamic pituitary ovarian axis to decrease ovarian androgen production *(112)*. Some women may experience symptoms of androgen deficiency, such as decreased libido, due to these effects. In these women, a COC with lower estrogenic and progestational activity may have a less suppressive effect on ovarian androgen production *(35)*. On the other hand, if a patient has symptoms of androgen excess such as hirsutism or acne, a progestin with less androgenic activity may be worth trying. Norethindrone and desogestrel have a less depressive effect on SHBG than norgestrel *(35)*, and drospirenone appears to compete with androgen to exert an anti-androgenic effect *(104)*.

Endometrial activity is measured by the ability of the COC to prevent irregular bleeding while the active hormone pills are being taken *(35)*. Breakthrough bleeding results when the COC cannot stimulate endometrial growth, which can result from relative estrogen deficiency, or when the COC cannot adequately support the endometrium due to progesterone deficiency. Because irregular bleeding is so common after initiating OCPs, patients should be encouraged to make no changes for 3 cycles. If breakthrough bleeding or amenorrhea persists after the third cycle, a COC with greater endometrial activity may be helpful. Irregular bleeding during the first 9 pills is usually associated with estrogen deficiency while bleeding after the 10th d is usually a result of a deficiency in the progestational activity *(35)*. When a patient presents with new irregular bleeding after many cycles of COC use, other causes of bleeding per vagina, such as cervicitis, anatomic defects, or pregnancy should be investigated.

Combined Injectable Contraception

A monthly combination contraceptive injection containing 25 mg medroxyprogesterone acetate and 5 mg estradiol cypionate (Lunelle®) has recently become available. Like COCs, it is immediately effective if it is taken within the first 5 d of the menstrual cycle. Repeat injections are needed every 28 d with a ± 5 d grace period. In clinical trials, Lunelle® was found to be an extremely effective method of contraception with a failure rate of less than 1% *(29)*, but it has not yet been determined whether adolescents will return reliably for monthly injections. The current recommendation is to rule out pregnancy if a patient returns for injection after 33 d *(29)*, but there is data suggesting that after multiple injections, the return to ovulation does not occur until 63 d *(113)*.

As with COCs, the progestin component suppresses ovulation and the estrogen component provides predictable withdrawal bleeding. Irregular bleeding is common during the initial cycles, but with continued use, menses become more predictable occurring 10–20 d after injection *(29)*. Bleeding irregularities, including amenorrhea, occur more frequently than with OCPs, but seem to be tolerated by patients. In a US study, only 2.5% of women discontinued treatment due to spotting *(114)*.

Progestin-Only Contraception

Progestin-only contraception is useful for women who either cannot tolerate estrogenic side effects or have contraindications to estrogen use. These methods are available as progestin-only OCPs, a 3-mo depot intramuscular injection of medroxyprogesterone acetate (Depo-Provera®), or as subdermal implants that release levonorgestrel for a 5-yr period (Norplant®). In particular, these two long-acting progestin contraceptives have the lowest failure rate in actual use by adolescents *(7)*. Actual failure rates for Norplant® and Depo-Provera® are similar to those for perfect use, presumably because perfect use does not require daily pill taking, interrupting sexual activity, or frequent trips to the pharmacy.

Progestin-Only Pills

Progestin-only OCPs are available as norethindrone (0.35 mg) or norgestrel (0.3 mg) only preparations. Unlike COCs, they are packaged with 28 active tablets and are taken continuously. The progestin doses used in the POPs are lower than the doses used in COCs. At these low doses, ovulation is not reliably suppressed *(115)* and occurs in approximately half of oral progestin users *(24)*. With perfect use, the failure rate for POPs is 0.5%, but perfect use is difficult. Meticulous pill taking every 24 h appears critical for contraceptive efficacy, and a back-up contraceptive method is recommended if a pill is taken more than 3 h late *(36)*. For this reason, POPs are not usually used in the adolescent population.

Norplant® Subdermal Implants

The Norplant® system was approved by the FDA in 1990. The system consists of 6 Silastic capsules, each containing 36 mg of dry crystalline levonorgestrel (216 mg/6 capsules) *(35)*. The capsules are inserted under the skin of the upper arm, and insertion and removal of the capsules requires a minor surgical procedure under local anesthesia. Ideally, implants should be inserted within 7 d of the onset of menses to avoid the need for a backup contraceptive method *(35)*. Upon removal of the implants, the levonorgestrel is immediately cleared from the circulation so that the contraceptive effects of Norplant® are rapidly reversible. In adolescents, 81% of users resumed menstrual regularity within the first month after discontinuation *(31)*.

Because the method does not require daily (or even yearly) effort on the part of the user, the failure rates with routine use by adolescent is the same as in the general populations *(7)*. It is highly effective method of contraception with a failure rate of 0.04% after 1 yr of perfect use *(11)*, and 2.3 % with routine use *(116)*. Unfortunately, due to adverse publicity about side effects and painful removal, there has been a sharp decline in the sales of Norplant® from 800 sets/d to fewer than 100 sets/d in 1995 *(117)*. Perhaps, Norplant-2®, which consists of 2 capsules each containing 70 mg of levonorgestrel *(35)*, will be more successful.

Initially, Norplant® capsules release levonorgestrel at a rate of 85 µg/d. Over time, the release rate declines until 5 yr when the rate of release is approx 30 µg/d *(35)*. Although body weight does not affect the release rate of levonorgestrel, the circulating levels are inversely correlated with body weight, so that heavier women have lower levonorgestrel concentrations *(118)*. Accordingly, the rates of contraceptive failure over the 5-yr period was correlated with increased body weight *(30)*. In an American study of 511 women, no pregnancies occurred in women weighing less than 79 kg over the 5-yr study period *(119)*. Extrapolation of these data would suggest that in thinner women, Norplant® would remain effective for more than 5 yr, and prolonged effectiveness over 7 yr has been demonstrated *(120)*.

The circulating levonorgestrel levels are not high enough to reliably inhibit ovulation, and one third of Norplant® user experience cyclic luteal activity and regular withdrawal bleeding *(25)*. Progesterone levels, however, are lower than seen in normal ovulatory women, and this luteal phase deficiency may contribute to the contraceptive efficacy *(25)*, along with the effects of levonorgestrel on the cervical mucus *(26)*. The incidence of regular monthly cycles increases with continued use of Norplant®, with 50–60% of users having regular cycles after the first year of use *(121)*. The women with regular cyclic bleeding are at greatest risk of pregnancy, and these patients should be tested for pregnancy and monitored carefully if they suddenly cease to have regular menses *(121)*. One third of pregnancies occurring as a result of Norplant® failure are ectopic *(118)*.

The most common reason for discontinuation of Norplant® by adolescents is irregular bleeding . During the first year after Norplant® insertion, irregular bleeding, occurs in approximately two thirds of users *(119,121)*, with an average of 92.3 d of bleeding or spotting during the year *(118)*. The menstrual irregularity improves with continued Norplant® use, and by the fifth year after insertion, only 37.5% of users experienced irregular bleeding *(121)*, with an average of 70.2 d of bleeding during the year *(118)*. Despite the many days of irregular bleeding, the actual blood loss is probably less than with menstrual cycles. After three years of Norplant® use, the mean hemoglobin levels were found to increase *(118)*. Treatment with estrogen has been found to decrease the duration of bleeding episodes *(122)*, and may be considered if the patient finds the continued days of bleeding troublesome.

In addition to irregular bleeding, cited by 68% of adolescents as a reason for discontinuing Norplant®, adolescents also experienced other side effects, mostly related progestational excess, associated with fluid retention and fatigue *(35)*. The following side effects were also cited by adolescents as a reason for discontinuing Norplant®: weight gain (42%), mood changes (42%), increased headaches (35%), fatigue (29%), breast tenderness (19%), amenorrhea (16%), alopecia (10%) *(31)*, and acne (10%). Many adolescents, however, enjoy the convenience of Norplant and are satisfied with the method. In a small study, only 8% of adolescents discontinued Norplant® within the 6 mo study period.

Depo-Provera® Injectable Contraception

Depo-Provera® received FDA approval in 1992. It is given as an intramuscular shot of 150 mg DMPA in a crystalline suspension every 12 wk. After injection, crystalline deposits form in the tissue and are resorbed slowly *(35)*. As with other forms of hormonal contraception, the ideal time to initiate therapy is within the first 5 d of the menstrual cycle, so that the contraceptive effect is immediate *(35)*. The dose of progestin is high enough to block the LH surge and ovulation *(29)*. Although ovulation does not occur for 14 wk after injection, repeat injections are recommended every 12 wk, and the recommendation is to rule out pregnancy in women who come after 13 wk *(29)*.

Depo-Provera® is one of the most effective contraceptive methods for adolescents, with a failure rate of 0.3 % with perfect use *(11)*. With typical use, the failure rate after 12 mo is 3.2% for the general population *(116)* and 4.2% for adolescents *(7)*. Unlike Norplant®, increases in body weight and use of concomitant medications do not appear to reduce the efficacy of Depo-Provera®. The return to fertility can be unpredictable after the last injection, which can be advantageous for the adolescent who is not meticulous about returning every 12 wk. On the other hand, because the contraceptive effect is not immediately reversible, Depo-Provera® is not recommended for women who are planning pregnancies in the next 1–2 yr *(29)*. Although 50% of women will conceive within 10 mo of the last injection, some women will not conceive until after 18 mo *(29)*.

As for all progestin-only methods, the most prominent side effect of Depo-Provera® is irregular, unpredictable bleeding, and this is the most common reason for discontinuation of this method by adolescents *(31)*. In a multicenter US study, 46.0% of women reported amenorrhea, and 46.2% of women reported irregular bleeding after 3 mo of use *(124)*. With increased duration of use, menstrual bleeding decreased in frequency and duration, and in this multicenter study, 58.5% of users were amenorrheic after 9 mo *(124)*. In another study, 73% of users were found to be amenorrheic after 12 mo *(125)*. Many women, including adolescents, will view the amenorrhea as a benefit of DMPA therapy. Although supplemental estrogen has been shown to stop the irregular bleeding associated with of Depo-Provera®, estrogen treatment has not been shown to increase the continuation rate *(126)*. It appears that pre-treatment counseling may be the critical factor-if women are counseled about the menstrual changes prior to initiation of treatment, they are more likely to continue with subsequent injections *(127)*.

Because Depo-Provera® suppresses gonadotropin production and ovarian steroidogenesis, estradiol levels in users of DMPA (52.67 pg/mL) are lower than for a normal menstrual cycle *(84,128)*. This is in contrast to levonorgestrel implants that do not reliably suppress gonadotropin production, so that Norplant® users have levels of circulating estradiol levels (189.9 pg/mL) similar to ovulatory women using an IUD (147.51 pg/mL) *(128)*. In 1991, a cross-sectional study from New Zealand found that compared to pre-menopausal controls, women who had used DMPA for at least 5 yr had significantly reduced bone density *(129)*. This raised the concern that this relative hypoestrogenism decreases bone mineral density during reproductive life and puts DMPA users at increased risk for post-menopausal osteoporosis *(29)*. Since then, there have been numerous studies examining the relationship between DMPA use and bone mineral density with somewhat conflicting results *(29,130)*. Some of the discrepancies may be due to the anatomic sites where bone mineral density is measured with the forearm being less sensitive to hormonal changes.

Because adolescence is a critical time for increasing bone mineral density, the use of DMPA in adolescents was thought to be particularly concerning, and it does appear that use of DMPA may impair bone mineralization in adolescents. A small study of 48 women, ages 12–21, found that after 1 yr, bone mineral density decreased by 1.5% in DMPA users. In contrast, an increase in bone mineral density was found in adolescents who received no hormonal treatment (2.9%), users of Norplant® (2.5%), and users of OCPs (1.5%) *(131)*. Another study found the largest differences in bone mineral density between DMPA users and nonusers was in women 18–21 yr old *(132)*. A dose-response relationship between longer use of DMPA and decreased bone density was also found in this age group *(132)*.

The clinical significance of decreased bone mineral density in DMPA users has not been determined, but the data is reassuring. A large study of 2474 women found that despite reduction in bone mineral density, none of the DMPA users would be considered osteopenic *(130)*. The New Zealand investigators have continued their studies of DMPA use and found that the deficits in bone mineral density are reversible after discontinuation of DMPA *(133)*. Furthermore, the bone mineral density in post-menopausal former DMPA users was not found to be significantly different from never-users *(134)*. At this time, the theoretical risks of post-menopausal osteoporosis should be considered along with the need for reliable, effective contraception. Certainly, adolescents on DMPA should be counseled about appropriate intake of calcium (1200 mg/d), vitamin D, and weight bearing exercise, all of which have been shown to have positive effect on bone density *(135)*.

The side effects of DMPA are related to estrogen deficiency or progestational excess *(35)*. Irregular bleeding was the most common reason, cited by 60% of adolescents, for discontinuing DMPA. In addition, the following side effects were also cited by adolescents as a reason for discontinuing Depo-Provera®: weight gain (40%), increased headaches (26%), mood changes (20%), fatigue (20%), alopecia (20%), breast tenderness (14%), amenorrhea (14%), and acne (9%). The FDA package insert mentions depression as a side effect of DMPA *(35)*, but published studies indicate that DMPA does not cause depression *(29)*. A large prospective study evaluated 393 women before and after 12 mo of DMPA and found no increase in depressive symptoms, suggesting that use of DMPA would not exacerbate symptoms in women with pre-exisiting depression *(136)*.

NON-CONTRACEPTIVE BENEFITS OF HORMONAL CONTRACEPTION

Health Benefits of Hormonal Contraception

Aside from contraception, there are numerous health benefits associated with the use of hormonal contraception. The protection from ovarian and endometrial cancer is well established and has already been discussed. Hormonal contraceptive methods also offer protection from several benign conditions. COC users are less likely to suffer from benign breast disease, functional ovarian cysts, pelvic inflammatory disease, and ectopic pregnancy *(36,91)*. DMPA also seems to offer protection from pelvic inflammatory disease and ectopic pregnancy *(29)*. It is not clear whether Norplant® offers the same protection. Because it does not reliably suppress ovulation, it is not as protective against ectopic pregnancy *(119)*, and may increase the incidence of functional ovarian cysts *(118)*.

Although barrier methods of contraception offer the best protection against STDs, it appears that hormonal contraception may prevent the infection from entering the upper genital tract and are protective against salpingitis and the resulting tubal disease. One study demonstrated that COC users with chlamydial infections were less likely to suffer upper tract infections *(137)*. Another study demonstrated that OCP users with PID are more likely to have milder disease with less tubal damage *(138)*. The proposed mechanisms by which ascending infection is reduced appear to be related to the progestational effects of COCs *(36,91)*. Thickened cervical mucus may be less penetrable by bacteria. Endometrial atrophy with reduced menstrual blood flow may decrease the medium for bacterial proliferation. Decreased contractility of the Fallopian tube and decreased retrograde menstruation may reduce the intraperitoneal spread of bacteria.

Therapeutic Uses of Hormonal Contraception

Hormonal contraception also has therapeutic uses that are unrelated to contraception. All these methods will reduce the amount of menstrual blood flow and can be used to treat both iron-deficiency anemia associated with menorrhagia and dysmenorrhea *(35,36)*. Studies in OCP users demonstrated an improvement in dysmenorrhea *(139)* and reduction of menstrual flow *(140)*. OCP use has been associated with an increase in iron stores in some women *(140)*, and hemoglobin levels were found to rise in Norplant®

users *(118)*. Depo-Provera may be particularly appropriate for treatment of menstrual disorders, given its high rate of associated amenorrhea.

There is some evidence that OCP use protects against endometriosis, but the data is conflicting *(91)*. Hormonal methods, however, have been used to treat endometriosis by producing an environment that promotes endometrial atrophy *(141)*. Before gonadotropin-releasing hormone agonists were available, high dose COCs were used for the treatment of endometriosis *(35)*, and modern low dose COCs are still a staple of medical management *(141)*. Oral progestins can be used to treat endometriosis as well, but at much higher doses than in POPs *(91)*. Medroxyprogesterone (20–30 mg daily) or norethindrone (15 mg daily) are commonly used.

Hyperandrogenism can be associated with anovulation (sometimes called polycystic ovary syndrome), hirsutism, and acne. After serious illnesses, such as androgen-secreting tumor, Cushing's syndrome, and congenital adrenal hyperplasia are excluded, medical treatment can be initiated. COCs are the mainstay of medical therapy for hyperandrogenism *(112,142)*. In combination, estrogens and progestins are anti-androgenic. COCs decrease gonadotropin production, and as a result, suppress androgen production by the ovary. Estrogens increase the hepatic production of SHBG decreasing the bioavailability of the androgens. COCs have been also been shown to decrease adrenal androgen secretion *(143)*. Additionally, COCs restore cyclic endometrial shedding and protect against the endometrial hyperplasia associated with hyperandrogenic chronic anovulation *(112)*.

COCs can also be used for hormonal replacement therapy for women who undergo premature menopause or for girls who fail to develop secondary sexual characteristics as a result of Turner's syndrome or other causes of gonadal dysgenesis *(35)*. In patients with gonadal dysgenesis, estrogen therapy is usually required to induce and maintain the development of secondary sexual characteristics and achieve optimal bone density *(144)*. Hormonal treatment is initiated after adult height is achieved and is initiated with estrogen alone at low doses (0.3 mg conjugated estrogens, 0.5 mg of micronized estradiol, or 0.3 mg of esterified estrogens). The estrogen dose is doubled after 3–6 mo and then 2–3 mo later. Final doses are 1.25 mg conjugated estrogens, 2 mg of micronized estradiol, or 1.25 mg of esterified estrogens *(144)*. Cyclic progestin therapy is initiated after vaginal bleeding first occurs or after 12–24 mo of estrogen therapy. Alternatively, COCs can be initiated at this time *(144)*.

HORMONAL CONTRACEPTION: NEW DELIVERY METHODS

Recently, the FDA has approved two new methods of hormone delivery for contraception: a transdermal patch and a vaginal ring. Both methods contain ethinyl estradiol along with a progestin and appear to have a similar mechanism of action as COCs. Because these methods do not require daily dosing, compliance may be higher. Ortho Evra® is a transdermal patch that releases a daily dose of 20 µg ethinyl estradiol and 150 µg norelgestromin, the primary metabolite of norgestimate *(146)*. The patch is changed weekly for 3 wk, then is removed for one week to allow a withdrawal bleed. The NuvaRing® is a flexible vaginal ring that releases 15 µg of ethinyl estradiol and 120 µg of etonogestrel, the biologically active metabolite of desogestrel, daily *(147)*. The ring is inserted by the patient and left in place for 3 wk. It is removed for one week to allow for a withdrawal bleed.

CONCLUSIONS

For almost every contraceptive method, unmarried adolescents experience higher rates of contraceptive failure compared to older, married women . In the adolescent population, hormonal contraceptive methods appear to be more effective, than non-hormonal ones. Long-acting progestins, in particular, have similar failure rates for adolescents and adults, presumably because these methods do not interrupt spontaneity and do not require daily patient responsibility.

Each contraceptive method has its own set of limitations, and the limitations of hormonal contraception need to be considered. Hormonal contraceptive methods may have drug interactions that reduce contraceptive efficacy or alter require changes in medication doses. Disease processes, such as diabetes, may be altered by the use of hormonal contraception. Because hormonal contraceptive methods have systemic effects, untoward effects may occur in some individuals. The common side-effects should be discussed prior to treatment since compliance appears to improve with pre-treatment counseling. Additionally, hormonal contraception does not offer any protection against STDs, so a barrier method must also be recommended to individuals who are not in monogamous relationships.

In addition to providing reliable contraception, these hormonal methods also provide many non-contraceptive health benefits, including protection from certain cancer and benign medical conditions, such as PID, ectopic pregnancy, and benign breast disease. Because these health benefits have not received as much publicity as the health risks, adolescents may not be aware that there are secondary benefits to hormonal contraception. Hormonal contraception is associated with decreased menstrual flow and decreased menstrual cramps. Although menstrual regulation is a life-style benefit, it has also been shown to improve iron-deficiency anemia.

In summary, hormonal contraceptive methods appear to be particularly well-suited for the adolescent population. Adolescents generally are not at risk for cardiovascular disease and do not have contraindications to hormonal contraception. Hormonal contraceptive methods appear to be the most efficacious in this age group, providing reliable contraception with numerous non-contraceptive health benefits.

REFERENCES

1. Ventura SJ, Mosher WD, Curtin SC, Abma JC, Henshaw S. Trends in pregnancies and pregnancy rates by outcome: estimates for the United States, 1976–96. Vital Health Stat 21, 2000(56):1–47.
2. Mandel SJ, Larsen PR, Seely EW, Brent GA. Increased need for thyroxine during pregnancy in women with primary hypothyroidism. N Engl J Med 1990;323(2):91–96.
3. Davis LE, Leveno KJ, Cunningham FG. Hypothyroidism complicating pregnancy. Obstet Gynecol 1988;72(1):108–112.
4. Haddow JE, et al. Maternal thyroid deficiency during pregnancy and subsequent neuropsychological development of the child. N Engl J Med 1999;341(8):549–555.
5. Mills JL, et al. Incidence of spontaneous abortion among normal women and insulin-dependent diabetic women whose pregnancies were identified within 21 days of conception. N Engl J Med 1988;319(25):1617–1623.
6. Mills JL, et al. Lack of relation of increased malformation rates in infants of diabetic mothers to glycemic control during organogenesis. N Engl J Med 1988;318(11):671–676.
7. Fu H, Darroch JE, Haas T, Ranjit N. Contraceptive failure rates: new estimates from the 1995 National Survey of Family Growth. Fam Plann Perspect 1999;31(2):56–63.
8. Cates WJ. Sexually Transmitted Diseases, HIV, and Contraception. Infertility Reprod Med Clin N Am 2000;11(4):669–704.

9. Trussell J, Grummer-Strawn L. Contraceptive failure of the ovulation method of periodic abstinence. Fam Plann Perspect 1990;22(2):65–75.
10. Wilcox AJ, Weinberg CR, Baird DD. Timing of sexual intercourse in relation to ovulation. Effects on the probability of conception, survival of the pregnancy, and sex of the baby. N Engl J Med 1995;333(23):1517–1521.
11. Trussell J, Hatcher RA, Cates W, Stewart FH, Kost K. Contraceptive failure in the United States: an update. Stud Fam Plann 1990;21(1):51–54.
12. Mauck C, Doncel GF. Spermicides. Infertility Reprod Med Clin N Am 2000;11(4):657–667.
13. McCormack WM. Pelvic inflammatory disease. N Engl J Med 1994;330(2):115–119.
14. Westrom L. Incidence, prevalence, and trends of acute pelvic inflammatory disease and its consequences in industrialized countries. Am J Obstet Gynecol 1980;138(7 Pt 2):880–892.
15. Nelson AL. Barrier Methods of Contraception. Infertility Reprod Med Clin N Am 2000;11(4):669–685.
16. Gilliam ML, Derman RJ. Barrier methods of contraception. Obstet Gynecol Clin N Am 2000;27(4):841–858.
17. Schwartz B, Gaventa S, Broome CV, et al. Nonmenstrual toxic shock syndrome associated with barrier contraceptives: report of a case-control study. Rev Infect Dis 1989;11(Suppl 1):S43–48; discussion S48–49.
18. Fihn SD, Latham RH, Roberts P, Running K, Stamm WE. Association between diaphragm use and urinary tract infection. JAMA 1985;254(2):240–245.
19. Hooton TM, Hillier S, Johnson C, Roberts PL, Stamm WE. Escherichia coli bacteriuria and contraceptive method. JAMA 1991;265(1):64–69.
20. Trussell J, et al. The economic value of contraception: a comparison of 15 methods. Am J Public Health 1995;85(4):494–503.
21. Sivin I. Contraception and Therapy; Intrauterine Devices of the Twenty-first Century. Infertility Reprod Clin N Am 2000;11(4):597–608.
22. Hannaford PC, Webb AM. Evidence-guided prescribing of combined oral contraceptives: consensus statement. An International Workshop at Mottram Hall, Wilmslow, U.K., March, 1996. Contraception 1996;54(3):125–129.
23. American College of Obstetrics and Gynecology, Oral Contraceptives for Adolescents: Benefits and Safety, in American College of Obstetricians and Gynecologists (ACOG) Educational Bulletin. 1999, 1–8.
24. Baird DT, Glasier AF. Hormonal contraception. N Engl J Med 1993;328(21):1543–1549.
25. Shoupe D, Horenstein J, Mishell DR Jr, Lacarra M, Medearis A. Characteristics of ovarian follicular development in Norplant users. Fert Steril 1991;55(4):766–770.
26. Croxatto HB, Diaz S, Salvatierra AM, Morales P, Ebensperger C, Brandeis A. Treatment with Norplant subdermal implants inhibits sperm penetration through cervical mucus in vitro. Contraception 1987;36(2):193–201.
27. Johannisson E, Landgren BM, Diczfalusy E. Endometrial morphology and peripheral steroid levels in women with and without intermenstrual bleeding during contraception with the 300 microgram norethisterone (NET) minipill. Contraception 1982;25(1):13–30.
28. Kim HH, Fox JH. The Fallopian Tube and Ectopic Pregnancy. In: Kistner's Gynecology and Women's Health (Ryan KJ, et al., eds.) Mosby, St. Louis, MO, 1999, pp. 143–165.
29. Kaunitz AM. Injectable Contraception. Infertility Reprod Med Clin N Am 2000;11(4):609–643.
30. Gu SJ, Du MK, Zhang LD, Liu YL, Wang SH, Sivin I. A 5-year evaluation of NORPLANT contraceptive implants in China. Obstet Gynecol 1994;83(5 Pt 1):673–678.
31. Harel Z, Biro FM, Kollar LM, Rauh JL. Adolescents' reasons for and experience after discontinuation of the long-acting contraceptives Depo-Provera and Norplant. J Adolesc Health 1996;19(2):118–123.
32. Goldzieher JW, Brody SA. Pharmacokinetics of ethinyl estradiol and mestranol. Am J Obstet Gynecol 1990;163(6 Pt 2):2114–2119.
33. Thorneycroft IH. New Pills/New Progestins. Infertility Reprod Clin N Am 2000;11(4):515–529.
34. World Health Organization, Improving Access To Quality Care In Family Planning: Medical Eligibility Criteria For Contraceptive Use. 1996, Geneva: World Health Organization.
35. Dickey RP. Managing Contraceptive Pill Patients, Ninth Edition. 1998, Durant, OK: EMIS, Inc.
36. American College of Obstetrics and Gynecology, Hormonal Contraception. In: American College of Obstetricians and Gynecologists (ACOG) Educational Bulletin, 1994, pp. 1–12.

37. Arafah BM. Increased Need for Thyroxine in Women with Hypothyroidism During Estrogen Therapy. N Engl J Med 2001;344(23):1743–1749.
38. Westhoff CL. Oral contraceptives and thrombosis: an overview of study methods and recent results. Am J Obstet Gynecol 1998;179(3 Pt 2):S38–42.
39. Fruzzetti F, Ricci C, Fioretti P. Haemostasis profile in smoking and nonsmoking women taking low-dose oral contraceptives. Contraception 1994;49(6):579–592.
40. Carr BR, Ory H. Estrogen and progestin components of oral contraceptives: relationship to vascular disease. Contraception 1997;55(5):267–272.
41. Ory HW. Cardiovascular safety of oral contraceptives. What has changed in the last decade? Contraception 1998;58(3 Suppl):9S–13S; quiz 65S.
42. Shulman LP. Oral contraceptives. Risks. Obstet Gynecol Clin N Am 2000;27(4):695–704, v–vi.
43. Mishell DR Jr. Cardiovascular risks: perception versus reality. Contraception 1999;59(1 Suppl): 21S–24S.
44. Speroff L. Oral contraceptives and arterial and venous thrombosis: a clinician's formulation. Am J Obstet Gynecol 1998;179(1):S25–S36.
45. Spitzer WO, Lewis MA, Heinemann LA, Thorogood M, MacRae KD. Third generation oral contraceptives and risk of venous thromboembolic disorders: an international case-control study. Transnational Research Group on Oral Contraceptives and the Health of Young Women. BMJ 1996;312(7023):83–88.
46. Bloemenkamp KW, Rosendaal FR, Helmerhorst FM, Buller HR Vandenbroucke JP. Enhancement by factor V Leiden mutation of risk of deep-vein thrombosis associated with oral contraceptives containing a third-generation progestagen. Lancet 1995;346(8990):1593–1596.
47. Jick H, Jick SS, Gurewich V, Myers MW, Vasilakis C. Risk of idiopathic cardiovascular death and nonfatal venous thromboembolism in women using oral contraceptives with differing progestagen components. Lancet 1995;346(8990):1589–1593.
48. World Health Organization Collaborative Study of Cardiovascular Disease and Steroid Hormone Contraception, Venous thromboembolic disease and combined oral contraceptives: results of international multicentre case-control study. World Health Organization Collaborative Study of Cardiovascular Disease and Steroid Hormone Contraception. Lancet 1995;346(8990):1575–1582.
49. World Health Organization Collaborative Study of Cardiovascular Disease and Steroid Hormone Contraception, Effect of different progestagens in low oestrogen oral contraceptives on venous thromboembolic disease. World Health Organization Collaborative Study of Cardiovascular Disease and Steroid Hormone Contraception. Lancet 1995;346(8990):1582–1588.
50. Lidegaard O, Edstrom B, Kreiner S. Oral contraceptives and venous thromboembolism. A case-control study. Contraception 1998;57(5):291–301.
51. Lewis MA, Heinemann LA, MacRae KD, Bruppacher R, Spitzer WO. The increased risk of venous thromboembolism and the use of third generation progestagens: role of bias in observational research. The Transnational Research Group on Oral Contraceptives and the Health of Young Women. Contraception 1996;54(1):5–13.
52. Jamin C, de Mouzon J. Selective prescribing of third generation oral contraceptives (OCs). Contraception 1996;54(1):55–56.
53. Suissa S, Blais L, Spitzer WO, Cusson J, Lewis M, Heinemann L. First-time use of newer oral contraceptives and the risk of venous thromboembolism. Contraception 1997;56(3):141–146.
54. Farmer RD, Todd JC, Lewis MA, MacRae KD, Williams TJ. The risks of venous thromboembolic disease among German women using oral contraceptives: a database study. Contraception 1998;57(2):67–70.
55. Lewis MA, MacRae KD, Kuhl-Habichl D, Bruppacher R, Heinemann LA, Spitzer WO. The differential risk of oral contraceptives: the impact of full exposure history. Hum Reprod 1999;14(6):1493–1499.
56. Robinson GE, Burren T, Mackie IJ, Bounds W, Walshe K, Faint R, Guillebaud J, Machin SJ. Changes in haemostasis after stopping the combined contraceptive pill: implications for major surgery. BMJ 1991;302(6771):269–271.
57. Ridker PM, Miletich JP, Hennekens CH, Buring JE. Ethnic distribution of factor V Leiden in 4047 men and women. Implications for venous thromboembolism screening. JAMA 1997;277(16):1305–1307.
58. Petitti DB, Klatsky AL. Malignant hypertension in women aged 15 to 44 years and its relation to cigarette smoking and oral contraceptives. Am J Cardiol 1983;52(3):297–298.
59. Chasan-Taber L, Willett WC, Manson JE, et al. Prospective study of oral contraceptives and hypertension among women in the United States. Circulation, 1996;94(3):483–489.

60. Benson V, Marano MA. Current estimates from the National Health Interview Survey, 1995. Vital & Health Statistics - Series 10: Data From the National Health Survey 1998;(199):1–428.
61. Godsland IF, Crook D, Simpson R, et al. The effects of different formulations of oral contraceptive agents on lipid and carbohydrate metabolism. N Engl J Med 1990;323(20):1375–1381.
62. Wynn V, Godsland I. Effects of oral contraceptives on carbohydrate metabolism. J Reprod Med 1986;31(9 Suppl):892–897.
63. Fahmy K, Abdel-Razik M, Shaaraway M, et al. Effect of long-acting progestagen-only injectable contraceptives on carbohydrate metabolism and its hormonal profile. Contraception 1991;44(4):419–430.
64. Liew DF, Ng CS, Yong YM, Ratnam SS. Long-term effects of Depo-Provera on carbohydrate and lipid metabolism. Contraception 1985;31(1):51–64.
65. Konje JC, Otolorin EO, Ladipo OA. Changes in carbohydrate metabolism during 30 months on Norplant. Contraception 1991;44(2):163–172.
66. Konje JC, Odukoya OA, Otolorin EO, Ewings PD, Ladipo OA. Carbohydrate metabolism before and after Norplant removal. Contraception 1992;46(1):61–69.
67. Konje JC, Otolorin EO, Ladipo OA. The effect of continuous subdermal levonorgestrel (Norplant) on carbohydrate metabolism. Am J Obstet Gynecol 1992;166(1 Pt 1):15–19.
68. Bowes WA Jr, Katta LR, Droegemueller W, Bright TG. Triphasic Randomized Clinical Trial: Comparison of effects on carbohydrate metabolism. Am J Obstet Gynecol 1989;161(5):1402–1407.
69. Gaspard UJ, Lefebvre PJ. Clinical aspects of the relationship between oral contraceptives, abnormalities in carbohydrate metabolism, and the development of cardiovascular disease. Am J Obstet Gynecol 1990;163(1 Pt 2):334–343.
70. Kjos SL, Peters RK, Xiang A, Thomas D, Schaefer U, Buchanan TA. Contraception and the risk of type 2 diabetes mellitus in Latina women with prior gestational diabetes mellitus. JAMA 1998;280(6):533–538.
71. Kjos SL. Contraception in diabetic women. Obstet Gynecol Clin North Am 1996;23(1):243–258.
72. Garg SK, Chase HP, Marshall G, Hoops SL, Holmes DL, Jackson WE. Oral contraceptives and renal and retinal complications in young women with insulin-dependent diabetes mellitus. JAMA 1994;271(14):1099–1102.
73. Klein BE, Moss SE, Klein R. Oral contraceptives in women with diabetes. Diabetes Care 1990;13(8):895–898.
74. Gold MA, Coupey SM. Young women's attitudes toward injectable and implantable contraceptives. J Pediatr Adolesc Gynecol 1998;11(1):17–24.
75. Rees HD, Bonsall RW, Michael RP. Pre-optic and hypothalamic neurons accumulate [^{3}H]medroxyprogesterone acetate in male cynomolgus monkeys. Life Sci 1986;39(15):1353–1359.
76. Rosenberg M. Weight change with oral contraceptive use and during the menstrual cycle. Results of daily measurements. Contraception 1998;58(6):345–349.
77. Reubinoff BE, Grubstein A, Meirow D, Berry E, Schenker JG, Brzezinski A. Effects of low-dose estrogen oral contraceptives on weight, body composition, and fat distribution in young women. Fertil Steril 1995;63(3):516–521.
78. Redmond G, Godwin AJ, Olson W, Lippman JS. Use of placebo controls in an oral contraceptive trial: methodological issues and adverse event incidence. Contraception 1999;60(2):81–85.
79. Endrikat J, Muller U, Dusterberg B. A twelve-month comparative clinical investigation of two low-dose oral contraceptives containing 20 micrograms ethinylestradiol/75 micrograms gestodene and 30 micrograms ethinylestradiol/75 micrograms gestodene, with respect to efficacy, cycle control, and tolerance. Contraception 1997;55(3):131–137.
80. Rosenberg MJ, Waugh MS. Oral contraceptive discontinuation: a prospective evaluation of frequency and reasons. Am J Obstet Gynecol 1998;179(3 Pt 1):577–582.
81. Schwallie PC, Assenzo JR. Contraceptive use—efficacy study utilizing medroxyprogesterone acetate administered as an intramuscular injection once every 90 days. Fertil Steril 1973;24(5):331–339.
82. Risser WL, Gefter LR, Barratt MS, Risser JM. Weight change in adolescents who used hormonal contraception. J Adolesc Health 1999;24(6):433–436.
83. Polaneczky M, Guarnaccia M, Alon J, Wiley J. Early experience with the contraceptive use of depot medroxyprogesterone acetate in an inner-city clinic population. Fam Plann Perspect 1996;28(4):174–178.
84. Taneepanichskul S, Reinprayoon D, Khaosaad P. Comparative Study of Weight Change Between Long-term DMPA and IUD Acceptors. Contraception 1998;58:149–151.

85. Grimes DA. The safety of oral contraceptives: epidemiologic insights from the first 30 years. Am J Obstet Gynecol 1992;166(6 Pt 2):1950–1954.
86. Kaunitz AM. Oral contraceptive estrogen dose considerations. Contraception 1998;58(3 Suppl): 15S–21S; quiz 66S.
87. Hankinson SE, Colditz GA, Hunter DJ, Spencer TL, Rosner B, Stampfer MJ. A quantitative assessment of oral contraceptive use and risk of ovarian cancer. Obstet Gynecol 1992;80(4):708–714.
88. Cancer and Steroid Hormone Study Group, The reduction in risk of ovarian cancer associated with oral-contraceptive use. The Cancer and Steroid Hormone Study of the Centers for Disease Control and the National Institute of Child Health and Human Development. N Engl J Med 1987;316(11):650–655.
89. Cancer and Steroid Hormone Study Group, Oral contraceptive use and the risk of endometrial cancer. The Centers for Disease Control Cancer and Steroid Hormone Study. JAMA 1983;249(12): 1600–1604.
90. Cancer and Steroid Hormone Study Group, Combination oral contraceptive use and the risk of endometrial cancer. The Cancer and Steroid Hormone Study of the Centers for Disease Control and the National Institute of Child Health and Human Development. JAMA 1987;257(6):796–800.
91. Gutmann JN. Health Benefits of Contraceptives. Infertility Reprod Med Clin N Am 2000;11(4):755–777.
92. World Health Organization Collaborative Study of Neoplasia and Steroid Contraceptives, Depot-medroxyprogesterone acetate (DMPA) and risk of endometrial cancer. The WHO Collaborative Study of Neoplasia and Steroid Contraceptives. Int J Cancer 1991;49(2):186–190.
93. Kaunitz AM. Depot medroxyprogesterone acetate contraception and the risk of breast and gynecologic cancer. J Reprod Med 1996;41(5 Suppl):419–3427.
94. Collaborative Group on Hormonal Factors in Breast Cancer, Breast cancer and hormonal contraceptives: collaborative reanalysis of individual data on 53 297 women with breast cancer and 100 239 women without breast cancer from 54 epidemiological studies. Collaborative Group on Hormonal Factors in Breast Cancer. Lancet 1996;347(9017):1713–1727.
95. Collaborative Group on Hormonal Factors in Breast Cancer, Breast cancer and hormonal contraceptives: further results. Collaborative Group on Hormonal Factors in Breast Cancer. Contraception 1996;54(3 Suppl):1S–106S.
96. Westhoff CL. Breast cancer risk: perception versus reality. Contraception 1999;59(1 Suppl): 25S–28S.
97. World Health Organization Collaborative Study of Neoplasia and Steroid Contraceptives, Breast cancer and depot-medroxyprogesterone acetate: a multinational study. WHO Collaborative Study of Neoplasia and Steroid Contraceptives. Lancet 1991;338(8771):833–838.
98. Wingo PA, Lee NC, Ory HW, Beral V, Peterson HB, Rhodes P. Age-specific differences in the relationship between oral contraceptive use and breast cancer. Obstet Gynecol 1991;78(2):161–170.
99. Brinton LA, Reeves WC, Brenes MM, et al. Oral contraceptive use and risk of invasive cervical cancer. Int J Epidemiol 1990;19(1):4–11.
100. Kjaer SK, Engholm G, Dahl C, Bock JE, Lynge E, Jensen OM. Case-control study of risk factors for cervical squamous-cell neoplasia in Denmark. III. Role of oral contraceptive use. Cancer Causes Control 1993;4(6):513–519.
101. Coker AL, McCann MF, Hulka BS, Walton LA. Oral contraceptive use and cervical intraepithelial neoplasia. J Clin Epidemiol 1992;45(10):1111–1118.
102. Ursin G, Peters RK, Henderson BE, d'Ablaing G, 3rd, Monroe KR, Pike MC. Oral contraceptive use and adenocarcinoma of cervix. Lancet 1994;344(8934):1390–1394.
103. Goldzieher JW. Selected aspects of the pharmacokinetics and metabolism of ethinyl estrogens and their clinical implications. Am J Obstet Gynecol 1990;163(1 Pt 2):318–322.
104. Krattenmacher R. Drospirenone: pharmacology and pharmacokinetics of a unique progestogen. Contraception 2000;62(1):29–38.
105. Oelkers W. Drospirenone—a new progestogen with antimineralocorticoid activity, resembling natural progesterone. Eur J Contracept Reprod Health Care 2000;5(Suppl 3):17–24.
106. Sulak PJ, Scow RD, Preece C, Riggs MW, Kuehl TJ. Hormone withdrawal symptoms in oral contraceptive users. Obstet Gynecol 2000;95(2):261–266.
107. Kornaat H, Geerdink MH, Klitsie JW. The acceptance of a 7-week cycle with a modern low-dose oral contraceptive (Minulet). Contraception 1992;45(2):119–127.
108. de Voogd WS. Postponement of withdrawal bleeding with a monophasic oral contraceptive containing desogestrel and ethinylestradiol. Contraception 1991;44(2):107–112.
109. Cachrimanidou AC, Hellberg D, Nilsson S, Waldenstrom U, Olsson SE, Sikstrom B. Long-interval treatment regimen with a desogestrel-containing oral contraceptive. Contraception 1993;48(3):205–216.
110. Hamerlynck JV, Vollebregt JA, Doornebos CM, Muntendam P. Postponement of withdrawal bleeding in women using low-dose combined oral contraceptives. Contraception 1987;35(3):199–205.

111. Sulak PJ, Cressman BE, Waldrop E, Holleman S, Kuehl TJ. Extending the duration of active oral contraceptive pills to manage hormone withdrawal symptoms. Obstet Gynecol 1997;89(2):179–183.
112. American College of Obstetrics and Gynecology, Hyperandrogenic Chronic Anovulation. In: American College of Obstetricians and Gynecologists (ACOG) Educational Bulletin, 1995, pp. 1–7.
113. Rahimy MH, Ryan KK. Lunelle monthly contraceptive injection (medroxyprogesterone acetate and estradiol cypionate injectable suspension): assessment of return of ovulation after three monthly injections in surgically sterile women. Contraception 1999;60(4):189–200.
114. Kaunitz AM, Garceau RJ, Cromie MA. Comparative safety, efficacy, and cycle control of Lunelle monthly contraceptive injection (medroxyprogesterone acetate and estradiol cypionate injectable suspension) and Ortho-Novum 7/7/7 oral contraceptive (norethindrone/ethinyl estradiol triphasic). Lunelle Study Group. Contraception 1999;60(4):179–187.
115. McCann MF, Potter LS. Progestin-only oral contraception: a comprehensive review. Contraception 1994;50(6 Suppl 1):S1–195.
116. Trussell J, Vaughan B. Contraceptive failure, method-related discontinuation and resumption of use: results from the 1995 National Survey of Family Growth. Fam Plann Perspect 1999;31(2):64–72, 93.
117. Berenson AB, Wiemann CM, McCombs SL, Somma-Garcia A. The rise and fall of levonorgestrel implants: 1992–1996. Obstet Gynecol 1998;92(5):790–794.
118. Sivin I. International Experience with NORPLANT® and NORPLANT®-2 Contraceptives. Stud Fam Plann 1988;19(2):81–94.
119. Sivin I, Mishell DR Jr, Darney P, Wan L, Christ M. Levonorgestrel capsule implants in the United States: a 5-year study. Obstet Gynecol 1998;92(3):337–344.
120. Sivin I, et al. Prolonged effectiveness of Norplant® capsule implants: a 7-year study. Contraception 2000;61(3):187–194.
121. Shoupe D, Mishell DR Jr, Bopp BL, Fielding M. The significance of bleeding patterns in Norplant implant users. Obstet Gynecol 1991;77(2):256–260.
122. Diaz S, Croxatto HB, Pavez M, Belhadj H, Stern J, Sivin I. Clinical assessment of treatments for prolonged bleeding in users of Norplant implants. Contraception 1990;42(1):97–109.
123. Berenson AB, Wiemann CM. Patient Satisfaction and Side Effects With Levonorgestrel Implant (Norplant) Use in Adolescents 18 years of Age or Younger. Pediatrics 1993;92(2):257–260.
124. Sangi-Haghpeykar H, Poindexter AN, 3rd, Bateman L, Ditmore JR. Experiences of injectable contraceptive users in an urban setting. Obstet Gynecol 1996;88(2):227–233.
125. Mainwaring R, Hales HA, Stevenson K, et al. Metabolic parameter, bleeding, and weight changes in U.S. women using progestin only contraceptives. Contraception 1995;51(3):149–153.
126. Said S, et al. Clinical evaluation of the therapeutic effectiveness of ethinyl oestradiol and oestrone sulphate on prolonged bleeding in women using depot medroxyprogesterone acetate for contraception. World Health Organization, Special Programme of Research, Development and Research Training in Human Reproduction, Task Force on Long-acting Systemic Agents for Fertility Regulation. Hum Reprod 1996;11(Suppl 2):1–13.
127. Lei ZW, Wu SC, Garceau RJ, et al. Effect of pretreatment counseling on discontinuation rates in Chinese women given depo-medroxyprogesterone acetate for contraception. Contraception 1996;53(6):357–361.
128. Taneepanichskul S, Intaraprasert S, Theppisai U, Chaturachinda K. Bone mineral density in long-term depot medroxyprogesterone acetate acceptors. Contraception 1997;56(1):1–3.
129. Cundy T, Evans M, Roberts H, Wattie D, Ames R, Reid IR. Bone density in women receiving depot medroxyprogesterone acetate for contraception. BMJ 1991;303(6793):13–16.
130. Petitti DB, Piaggio G, Mehta S, Cravioto MC, Meirik O. Steroid hormone contraception and bone mineral density: a cross-sectional study in an international population. The WHO Study of Hormonal Contraception and Bone Health. Obstet Gynecol 2000;95(5):736–744.
131. Cromer BA, Blair JM, Mahan JD, Zibners L, Naumovski Z. A prospective comparison of bone density in adolescent girls receiving depot medroxyprogesterone acetate (Depo-Provera), levonorgestrel (Norplant), or oral contraceptives. J Pediatr 1996;129(5):671–676.
132. Scholes D, Lacroix AZ, Ott SM, Ichikawa LE, Barlow WE. Bone mineral density in women using depot medroxyprogesterone acetate for contraception. Obstet Gynecol 1999;93(2):233–238.
133. Cundy T, Cornish J, Evans MC, Roberts H, Reid IR. Recovery of bone density in women who stop using medroxyprogesterone acetate. BMJ 1994;308(6923):247–248.
134. Orr-Walker BJ, Evans MC, Ames RW, Clearwater JM, Cundy T, Reid IR. The effect of past use of the injectable contraceptive depot medroxyprogesterone acetate on bone mineral density in normal post-menopausal women. Clin Endocrinol 1998;49:615–618.

135. Cromer B, Harel Z. Adolescents: at increased risk for osteoporosis? Clin Pediatr (Phila) 2000;39(10):565–574.
136. Westhoff C, Truman C, Kalmuss D, et al. Depressive Symptoms and Depo-Provera. Contraception 1998;57:237–240.
137. Wolner-Hanssen P, Eschenbach DA, Paavonen J, et al. Decreased risk of symptomatic chlamydial pelvic inflammatory disease associated with oral contraceptive use. JAMA 1990;263(1):54–59.
138. Svensson L, Westrom L, Mardh PA. Contraceptives and acute salpingitis. JAMA1984;251(19): 2553–2555.
139. Milsom I, Sundell G, Andersch B. The influence of different combined oral contraceptives on the prevalence and severity of dysmenorrhea. Contraception 42(5):497–506.
140. Larsson G, Milsom I, Lindstedt G, Rybo G. The influence of a low-dose combined oral contraceptive on menstrual blood loss and iron status. Contraception 46(4):327–334.
141. Olive DL, Pritts EA. Treatment of endometriosis. N Engl J Med 345(4):266–275.
142. American College of Obstetrics and Gynecology, Evaluation and Treatment of Hirsute Women, in American College of Obstetricians and Gynecologists (ACOG) Educational Bulletin, 1995, pp. 1–6.
143. Klove KL, Roy S, Lobo RA. The effect of different contraceptive treatments on the serum concentration of dehydroepiandrosterone sulfate. Contraception 1984;29(4):319–324.
144. Saenger P. Management of Turner syndrome (gonadal dysgenesis). Endocrinology Up To Date® On Line 9.3, 2001. pp. 1–5.
145. Saenger P, et al. Recommendations for the diagnosis and management of Turner syndrome. J Clin Endocrinol Metab 2001;86(7):3061–3069.
146. Dittrich R, Parker L, Rosen JB, Shangold G, Creasy GW, and Fisher AC. Transdermal contraception: Evaluation of three transdermal norelgestromin/ethinyl estradiol doses in a randomized multicenter, dose-response study. Am J Obstet Gynecol 2002;186(1): 15–20.
147. Mulders, TMT, Dieben TOM, Coelingh Bennink HJT. Ovarian function with a novel combined contraceptive vaginal ring. Human Reproduction 2002;17(10):2595–2599.

VII Metabolic Disorders

27 Hypoglycemia

Charles A. Stanley, MD

CONTENTS

INTRODUCTION
DEFINITION OF HYPOGLYCEMIA
THE FASTING SYSTEMS APPROACH
REFERENCES

INTRODUCTINON

Hypoglycemia is a medical emergency that may result in seizures, permanent brain damage, or even sudden death. Because hypoglycemia can result from a long list of causes, it is necessary to have a comprehensive strategy for diagnosis and therapy that includes not only hormonal disorders, but also metabolic defects, as well as drugs and toxins. This chapter presents an approach to disorders of hypoglycemia based on the metabolic and endocrine systems involved in successful adaptation to fasting. This "Fasting Systems" approach takes advantage of the fact that all of the hypoglycemia problems in infants and children involve fasting. Since the integrity of these various systems is reflected in plasma levels of critical fuels and hormones at the time of hypoglycemia, the most important specimens for diagnosis are the ones obtained at the point of hypoglycemia. These specimens of plasma and urine are known as the "Critical Samples" or the "Didja Tubes" and should be routinely obtained immediately prior to beginning treatment of the hypoglycemia.

DEFINITION OF HYPOGLYCEMIA

With regard to the "When is it hypoglycemia?" question, the plasma glucose thresholds for older infants, children, and adults include the following: normal levels = 70–100 mg/dL; detectable neurophysiologic signs of hypoglycemia = 50–70 mg/dL; usual definition of severe hypoglycemia = <40 mg/dL; therapeutic goal = >60 mg/dL.

Lower limits for defining hypoglycemia have traditionally been applied in neonates (e.g., as low as 20 mg/dL for "lowbirthweight" neonates). However, it must be remembered that these values reflect only a statistical definition of hypoglycemia based on infants fasted for what would now be considered exceptionally long times of 12 h or more immediately after delivery on the first day of life. Such "statistically normal" values

From: *Contemporary Endocrinology: Pediatric Endocrinology: A Practical Clinical Guide*
Edited by: S. Radovick and M. H. MacGillivray © Humana Press Inc., Totowa, NJ

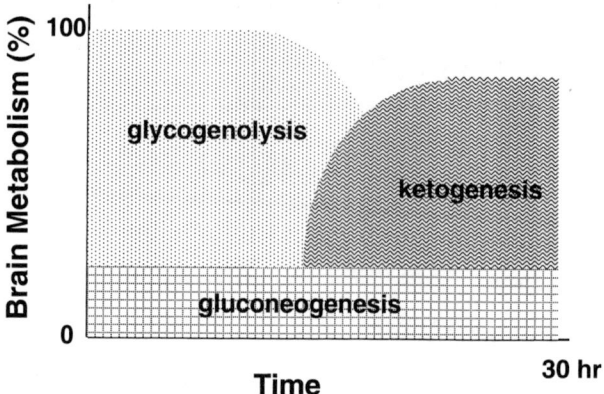

Fig. 1. Contribution of major fasting systems to brain metabolism over time in a typical normal infant. Note that glycogen stores are depleted by 8–12 h and that ketogenesis becomes the major source of brain substrate by 24–36 h.

merely represent blood glucose levels that were common under the circumstances in nurseries 40–50 yr ago and clearly do not represent what is physiologically normal. There is no good evidence that the brain is more resistant to effects of hypoglycemia in neonates than in older children. In the absence of such evidence, this author recommends using the same thresholds noted above for neonates as older children and adults *(1)*. The better question about neonates is, "Why is there hypoglycemia?" As indicated below, major advances have been made in answering this question during the past 5 yr.

THE FASTING SYSTEMS APPROACH

In older infants and children, hypoglycemia (almost) always means fasting hypoglycemia. The physiology of normal successful fasting adaptation provides a useful framework that encompasses the diagnosis and treatment of all the potential hypoglycemia disorders. This "Fasting Systems Approach" was originally developed at the Children's Hospital of Philadelphia by Dr. Lester Baker *(2)*.

The Fasting Systems

Three metabolic systems ([1] hepatic glycogenolysis, [2] hepatic gluconeogenesis, [3] hepatic ketogenesis) are coordinated by the *(4)* endocrine system, consisting of insulin (which suppresses all 3 metabolic systems) balanced by a relatively redundant set of counter-regulatory hormones that activate one or more of the 3 metabolic systems: cortisol (gluconeogenesis), glucagon (glycogenolysis), epinephrine (glycogenolysis, gluconeogenesis, ketogenesis & suppression of insulin), growth hormone (ketogenesis via increased lipolysis) (*see* Figs. 1 and 2).

The essential function of fasting adaptation is to maintain fuel supply to the brain, since the brain has no fuel stores of its own. As shown in Fig. 1, early in fasting, glucose is the primary brain fuel and accounts for over 90% of total body oxygen consumption. Glucose is provided chiefly from hepatic glycogenolysis, supplemented by hepatic gluconeogenesis utilizing amino acids released by muscle protein turnover. After 12–16 h in normal infants (24–36 h in adults), glucose production declines, since the supply of liver glycogen is limited and the rate of gluconeogenesis from amino acids remains

	Glycogenolysis	Gluconeo-genesis	Lipolysis	Ketogenesis
Insulin	−	−	−	−
Glucagon	+	+		
Epinephrine	+		+	+
Cortisol		+		
Growth Hormone		+		

Fig. 2. Hormonal regulation of fasting metabolic systems.

constant. At this time, a transition to fat as the major fuel for the body begins with accelerated adipose tissue lipolysis and increased fatty acid oxidation in muscle and ketogenesis in liver. The brain cannot utilize fatty acids directly, therefore, ketones provide an alternative fat-derived fuel for the brain and permit a reduction of brain glucose consumption and the drain on essential muscle proteins. In late stages of fasting adaptation, fatty acid oxidation and ketone utilization account for 90% of total oxygen consumption.

The Critical Samples (Didja Tubes)

The circulating levels of certain key fuels and hormones at the time of fasting hypoglycemia reflect the integrity of the metabolic and hormonal systems of fasting. As shown in Fig. 3, in a normal infant fasted until hypoglycemia approaches at 24–30 h, i.e., at a plasma glucose of 50 mg/dL: 1) glycogen stores are exhausted (no glycemic response to glucagon) *(3)*, 2) gluconeogenic substrate levels have declined modestly compared to the fed state (lactate <1.5 mM), 3) free fatty acids have tripled (1.5–2.0 mM) and β–hydroxybutyrate, the major ketone, has risen 50–100 fold (2–5 mM), 4) insulin has declined to essentially undetectable levels (<2 μU/mL). A comparison of these normal expected values to the values from a patient obtained at the "critical" time when fasting adaptation fails and the plasma glucose falls below 50 mg/dL provides the information "critical" to diagnosing the underlying cause. These "critical" samples can be obtained during a formal fasting study, but are also extremely useful when obtained during a spontaneous attack. Pediatricians and residents should be trained to get these "Didja Tubes" whenever a child is treated for hypoglycemia (i.e., "Didja" remember to order a __ test?).

Categories of Hypoglycemia Based on the Critical Samples

Since it is easily obtained, we begin with the serum bicarbonate at the time of hypoglycemia to segregate the hypoglycemia disorders into 4 groups (Fig. 4), with and without acidemia (HCO_3 <15–17 vs >16–18 mEq/L). Additional tests can then be selected within each of the groups to distinguish specific defects.

1) Acidemia due to lactate typifies defects in hepatic gluconeogenesis: glucose-6- phosphatase deficiency (type 1 GSD), fructose-1,6-diphosphatase deficiency, normal neonates on d 1 of life, and ethanol ingestion (lactate and glucose responses to glucagon, galactose, fructose stimulation, enzyme assay, mutation identification, and the like).

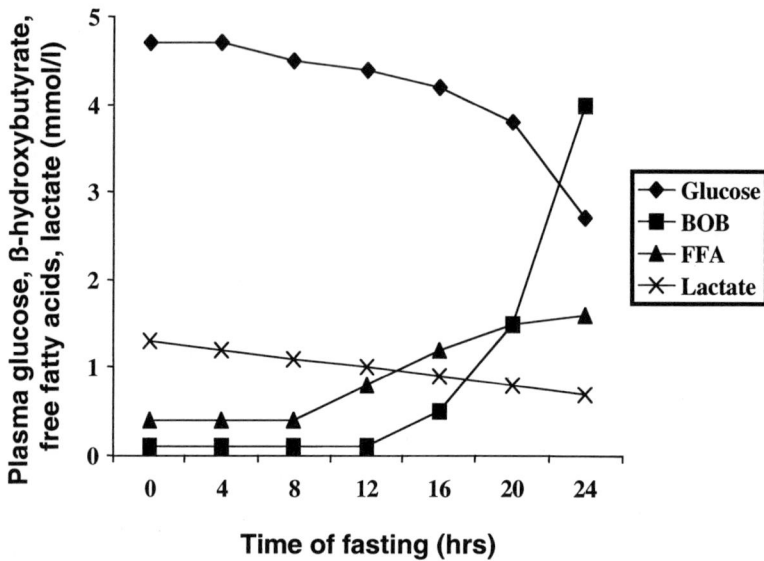

Fig. 3. Changes in plasma concentrations of major substrates during the course of fasting in a normal child.

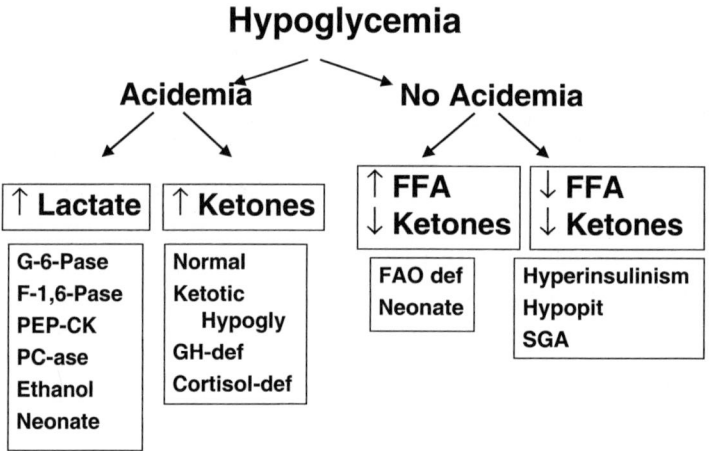

Fig. 4. Algorithm for diagnosis of hypoglycemia based on specimens obtained at time of fasting hypoglycemia.

2) Acidemia due to ketones typifies normal children, ketotic hypoglycemia (probably also normal, but with low fasting tolerance), defects in glycogenolysis (types 3, 6, 9 GSD) growth hormone and/or cortisol deficiencies. (GH & cortisol assay, liver biopsy for enzyme assay, mutation identification, and the like).

3) No acidemia with ketones and free fatty acids both suppressed: congenital hyperinsulinism, IDM, insulin Rx, oral hypoglycemics, SGA and birth asphyxia, neonatal hypopituitarism. (insulin, C-peptide, mutation identification, and the like).

4) No acidemia with suppressed ketones, but elevated free fatty acids: genetic defects in fatty acid oxidation and ketogenesis. (serum acylcarnitine profile, urinary organic acids, assays in cultured cells, mutation identification, and the like).

Specific Disorders

ACIDEMIA OWING TO LACTATE

1) Examples include, glucose-6-phosphatase deficiency. (Type 1a and Type 1b Glycogen Storage Disease), fructose- 1,6-diphosphatase deficiency (*see* Fig. 5). These often do not present with symptoms in the newborn period, since the elevated levels of lactate provide an alternative fuel for the brain when glucose is low.
2) Normal neonates. Gluconeogenesis and ketogenesis are both poorly developed at birth, probably accounting for the high risk of hypoglycemia in the first 12–24 h of life in all groups of newborns. Both of these systems appear to mature quickly, perhaps accelerated by feeding, by 12–24 h of age.
3) Ethanol intoxication. Ethanol metabolism shifts the $NADH/NAD^+$ redox potential to a more reduced state and blocks gluconeogenesis by diverting pyruvate to lactate. Hypoglycemia ensues if liver glycogen stores have been depleted.

ACIDEMIA DUE TO KETONES

1) Examples include, debrancher, liver phosphorylase, or phosphorylase kinase deficiencies (Type 3, 6, 9 Glycogen Storage Disease) (*see* Fig. 5); growth hormone and cortisol deficiency (e.g., hypopituitarism, adrenal insufficiency).
   N.B. neonatal presentation of hypopituitarism may mimic hyperinsulinism.
2) Ketotic hypoglycemia. These are children, usually 1–4 yr of age, with episodes of symptomatic fasting hypoglycemia but without any identifiable metabolic or endocrine defect. In some cases, this can be thought of as merely a quantitative, rather than a specific qualitative abnormality of fasting adaptation. These children can be thought of as representing the low end of the normal distribution of fasting tolerance. Note however, that the features of abbreviated, but otherwise normal fasting response are shared by the milder glycogenoses, and a few cases have been shown to have deficiency of hepatic glycogen synthase (GSD type 0).

NO ACIDEMIA WITH KETONES AND FREE FATTY ACIDS BOTH SUPPRESSED

1) Congenital hyperinsulinism (HI) *(4–6)*. Fasting tolerance: nil to 12+ h (depends on severity), low lactate, ↓ FFA, ↓ BOB, glucagon stimulation (++glucose) *(3)*. N.B. hyperinsulinemia can often be difficult to document, because available insulin assays are too insensitive (>3–5 µU/mL): thus, it is often necessary to make the diagnosis based on evidence of excessive insulin effects on the 3 fasting metabolic systems. Clinical features and treatment depend on the specific type (*see* Fig. 6):
   a) Recessive mutations of KATP-channel genes (SUR1, sulfonylurea receptor; Kir6.2, ion pore) *(7–11)*. Severe neonatal onset, LGA birthweight, diazoxide unresponsive, ↑↑↑↑glucose requirement (up to 20–30 mg/kg/min). Therapy: diazoxide is unlikely to work (because it acts by binding to SUR1): octreotide is effective acutely, but tachyphylaxis may make it inadequate for long-term therapy; 95% subtotal pancreatectomy; glucagon via continuous infusion. (identical phenotype in focal disease).
   b) Dominant mutations of glutamate dehydrogenase (GLUDI): Hyperinsulinism/ Hyperammonemia (HI/HA) Syndrome *(12–16)*. Milder, later onset, diazoxide responsive, protein/leucine sensitive hypoglycemia. Associated with persistent mild hyperammonemia (plasma ammonium, 50–200 µM). Mutations cause a gain of GDH enzyme function with excessive enzyme activity in liver, in addition to β-cells.
   c) Dominant mutations of glucokinase (GK) *(17)*. Also milder, later onset, diazoxide responsive. Due to mutations that lower the K_m for glucose of GK and reduce the glucose threshold for insulin release. Loss of function mutations of GK occur in MODY2 (maturity onset type diabetes of the young type 2).

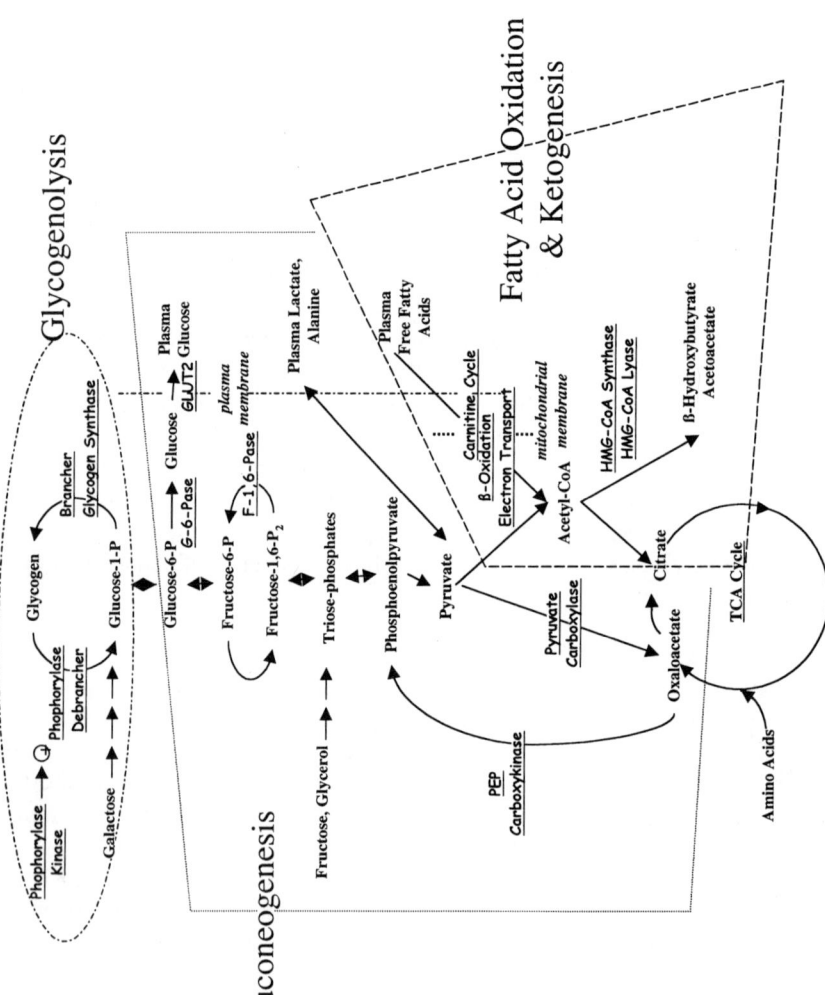

Fig. 5. Metabolic pathways of fasting adaptation. Sites of genetic defects are underlined.

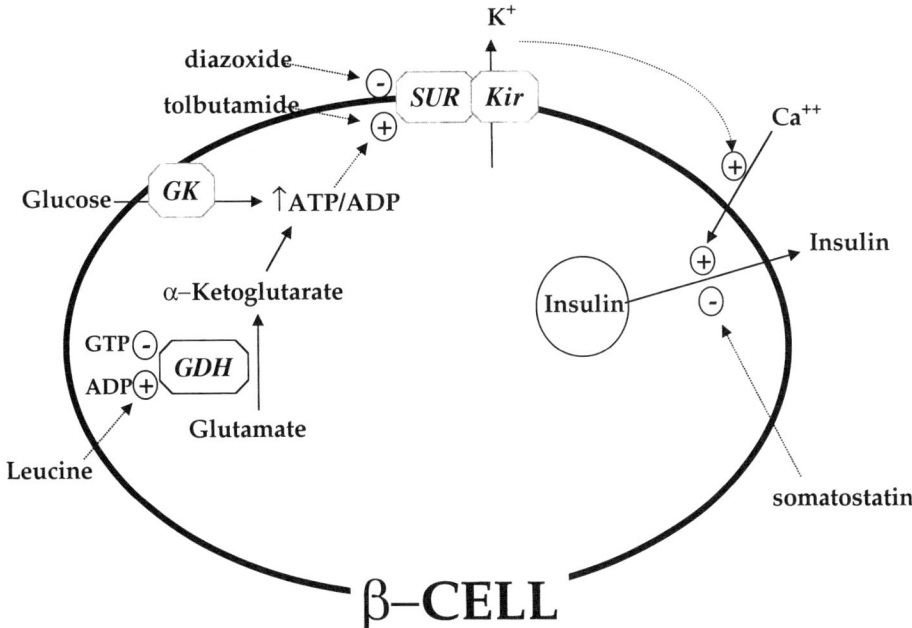

Fig. 6. Pathways pancreatic beta-cell insulin secretion. Glucose stimulates insulin secretion via an increase in ATP/ADP ratio which leads to inhibition of plasma membrane ATP-dependent potassium channel, membrane depolarization, and activation of a voltage-gated calcium channel with subsequent influx of calcium to trigger insulin exocytosis. Note that leucine stimulates insulin secretion by allosteric activation of glutamate oxidation via glutamate dehydrogenase. Drugs may stimulate or inhibit insulin secretion by activation or inhibition of the plasma membrane ATP-sensitive potassium channel (e.g., diazoxide or tolbutamide) or by downstream inhibition of insulin release (e.g., octreotide).

    d) Dominant mutations of SUR1 *(18)*. One family from Finland has been described in which a missense mutation of SUR1 caused hyperinsulinism, presumably by acting as a dominant negative. Unlike the severe disease often associated with recessive mutations of SUR1, hypoglycemia in this family appeared to be mild and was responsive to treatment with diazoxide.

    e) Focal hyperinsulinism *(19,20)*. Associated with focal loss of heterozygosity for maternal 11p and expression of paternally-transmitted K-channel mutation (either SUR1 or Kir6.2). Phenotype identical to recessive K-channel disease. May account for 40–60% of cases of severe, neonatal onset diazoxide unresponsive, hyperinsulinism.

2) Transient Neonatal Hyperinsulinism

    a) Infant of diabetic mother (IDM). Fetal hyperinsulinism secondary to maternal hyperglycemia. Features include LGA birthweight. Usually resolves in 1–2 d. Rx: early feeds, iv dextrose.

    b) Perinatal stress-induced hyperinsulinism *(21,22)*. Mechanism unknown. Associated with SGA birthweight, birth asphyxia, maternal toxemia; may persist for 1–2 mo after birth; ↑↑↑↑ glucose requirement (up to 20–30 mg/kg/min). Rx: diazoxide, glucagon, continuous iv dextrose.

3) Neonatal hypopituitarism. Features may mimic hyperinsulinism, including high glucose requirement, low FFA & BOB, glycemic response to glucagon. Suspect especially with midline malformations of face, microphthalmia, micropenis. May be associated with

	Hours	Lactate	BOB	FFA	Response to glucagon
G-6-Pase	2-4	↑	±↑	↑	-
Debrancher	4-8	↓	↑	↑	-
F-1,6-Pase	8-12	↑	↓	↑	-
MCAD	12-16	N	↓	↑	-
Hyperinsulinism	0-?	N	↓	↓	↑
Hypopit	12-16	N	±↑	±↑	-
Neonate	0-8	↑	↓	↑	-

Fig. 7. Differential diagnosis of hypoglycemia disorders based on critical specimens obtained at time of fasting hypoglycmia.

laboratory features of cholestatic liver disease. Rx: replacement therapy for deficient hormones.

NO ACIDEMIA WITH SUPPRESSED KETONES, BUT ELEVATED FREE FATTY ACIDS

1) Examples presenting usually beyond the newborn period include, genetic fatty acid oxidation and ketogenesis defects (medium-chain acyl-CoA dehydrogenase deficiency, MCAD, is the most common of these) (see Fig. 5) (23–27). These infants present with acute life-threatening episodes of illness which are provoked by fasting stress beyond 8–14 h. Hypoketotic hypoglycemia, often with elevated liver transaminases, uric acid, or ammonia, but nearly normal levels of bicarbonate are typical. The presentation mimicks Reye syndrome. Cardiac and skeletal muscle involvement occur in the more complete defects. Most (but not all) can be diagnosed from plasma acyl-carnitine profiles by tandem mass spectrometry (28).
2) Normal Neonates. Gluconeogenesis and ketogenesis are poorly developed at birth, accounting, in part for the high risk of hypoglycemia in the first 12–24 h of life in all groups of newborns. The defect in ketogenesis has recently been shown to involve developmental delays in both CPT-1 and HMG-CoA synthase for the first 12 h of life: first feedings containing fat may aid in CPT-1 development through induction of transcription by long-chain free fatty acids (29,30).

Therapeutic Goals for Managing Hypoglycemia

In order to minimize the risk of brain damage, aim to maintain plasma glucose >60 mg/dL (1). Delays in development of fasting systems make low glucose common in the first day of life. However, as noted above, the therapeutic targets for blood glucose should not be set lower in neonates than in older children. Ideally, treatment should maintain normoglycemia on a normal feeding schedule for age. Neonates who are suspected to have hypoglycemia persisting beyond the first day after birth should be tested for ability to fast >10–12 h: older infants for >16–20 h. It is advisable to periodically re-assess efficacy of treatment of any form of hypoglycemia by a formal fasting study on treatment.

Rare Post-Prandial Hypoglycemia Disorders in Pediatrics

The following are the sole exceptions to the rule that all of hypoglycemia is fasting:

1) Post-Nissen Dumping Hypoglycemia. This occurs in some infants following surgery for reflux and may be severe enough to cause seizures and brain damage. The mechanism involves rapid stomach emptying with an excessive rise of plasma glucose, followed by an overshoot of insulin secretion and rapid fall of glucose to hypoglycemic levels 1–2 h following a carbohydrate load. This is the sole circumstance in pediatrics that warrants an oral glucose tolerance test to demonstrate the exaggerated glucose swings. Rx: frequent feedings, reduced free sugar, inhibitors of gastric motility; a newly-introduced drug for type 2 diabetics, acarbose, may be useful as a means to delay digestion and absorption of complex carbohydrates *(32)*.

Selected Drugs for Hypoglycemic Disorders

- Dextrose (emergency Rx): iv 0.2 g/kg bolus (2 cc/kg of D10), followed by D10 continuous.
- Glucagon (emergency Rx only in case of insulin-induced hypoglycemia): 1 mg sq or iv (may use 0.5 mg in neonates).
- Diazoxide. 5–15 mg/kg/d divided into 2 or 3 doses. Start with maximum dose, 15 mg/kg to test efficacy (1–2 d sufficient), then lower as possible. Responders usually require 10 mg/kg or less.
- Octreotide: starting at 2–10 μg/kg/d; may increase to >50 μg/kg/d: sq divided q 6–8 h. or continuous iv or sq. Tachyphylaxis is commonly encountered, unfortunately *(31)*.

Formal Fasting Study Protocol

Requirements: experienced nurses and physicians, blood-drawing iv, rapid and accurate plasma glucose monitoring (N.B. Standard bedside glucose meters not accurate enough). Fast usually begins with 8 PM bedtime snack, but may be adjusted later if very short fasting tolerance suspected (consider monitoring for 24 h on usual diet before starting fasting study to assess glucose stability). From beginning of fast, monitor plasma glucose closely (e.g., q 4 h until <80, q 2 h until <70, q 1 h until <60, then q 30 min to end at 50 mg/dL): obtain additional "critical" specimens for key fuels and hormones q 4–6 h and especially, at end of fast. End study at plasma glucose 50 mg/dL or 36 h (24 h if <1-yr-old) or any worrisome symptoms (can end early if urinary ketones = "large"). If considering hyperinsulinism, may end with glucagon stimulation test, 1 mg iv, to test glycogen reserve (at plasma glucose <50 mg/dL, appropriate glycemic response <30 mg/dL within 15–30 min after glucagon; glycemic response above 30 mg/dL is consistent with hyperinsulinism) *(3)*. Critical specimen assays should include lactate, FFA, BOB, insulin. Include additional blood or urine tests depending on suspected diagnosis, e.g., serum HCO_3; plasma GH & cortisol: plasma NH_3: plasma acyl-carnitine profile: plasma total and free carnitine; urinary organic acid profile. *CAUTION*: fasting studies are provocative tests that, like water deprivation tests, must be closely monitored for patient safety; sudden deaths during fasting tests have been reported in patients with fatty acid oxidation defects. The latter patients may develop life-threatening symptoms before plasma glucose levels fall below 60–65 mg/dL, including progressive lethargy, nausea, vomiting, or unexplained tachycardia; fasts should be terminated in these cases without waiting for plasma glucose to reach 50 mg/dL.

Other Tests

1. Plasma acyl-carnitine profile. This test using tandem mass spectrometry measures the different fatty acids bound to carnitine to detect many of the genetic defects in fatty acid oxidation. The method is now employed in many state newborn screening programs using filter paper blood spots to screen for 20 or more inborn errors of metabolism. Medium-chain acyl-CoA dehydrogenase (MCAD) deficiency is particularly common (1/5000) and easily detected by this method *(28)*.
2. Genetic testing. Mutation screening is useful for glucose-6-phosphatase deficiency, since 80% of patients have 1 of 5 common mutations. 90% of MCAD patients have the common A985G mutation.
3. Cultured cells. Lymphoblasts or fibroblasts are useful for diagnosis of some inborn errors of metabolism (such as fatty acid oxidation disorders) and as sources of DNA for mutation analysis for other genetic defects.

REFERENCES

1. Stanley CA, Baker L. The causes of neonatal hypoglycemia [editorial; comment]. N Engl J Med 1999;340(15):1200–1201.
2. Stanley CA, Baker L. Hypoglycemia. In: Kaye R, Oski FA, Barness LA, eds. Core Textbook of Pediatrics. Lippincott, Philadelphia, 1978, pp. 280–305.
3. Finegold DN, Stanley CA, Baker L. Glycemic response to glucagon during fasting hypoglycemia: an aid in the diagnosis of hyperinsulinism. J Pediatr 1980;96(2):257–259.
4. Stanley CA, Baker L. Hyperinsulinism in infants and children: diagnosis and therapy. Adv Pediatr 1976;23:315–355.
5. Stanley CA. Hyperinsulinism in infants and children. Pediatr Clin North Am 1997;44(2):363–374.
6. Aynsley-Green A, Hussain K, Hall J, et al. Practical management of hyperinsulinism in infancy. Arch Dis Child Fetal Neonatal Ed 2000;82(2):F98–F107.
7. Baker L, Thornton PS, Stanley CA. Management of hyperinsulinism in infants. J Pediatr 1991;119(5):755–757.
8. Nestorowicz A, Wilson BA, Schoor KP, et al. Mutations in the sulonylurea receptor gene are associated with familial hyperinsulinism in Ashkenazi Jews. Hum Mol Genet 1996;5(11):1813–1822.
9. Nestorowicz A, Inagaki N, Gonoi T, et al. A nonsense mutation in the inward rectifier potassium channel gene, Kir6.2, is associated with familial hyperinsulinism. Diabetes 1997;46(11):1743–1748.
10. Thomas P, Ye YY, Lightner E. Mutations of the pancreatic islet inward rectifier Kir6.2 also leads to familial persistent hyperinsulinemic hypoglycemia of infancy. Hum Mol Genet 1996;5:1809–1812.
11. Thomas PM, Cote GJ, Wohllk N, et al. Mutations in the sulfonylurea receptor gene in familial persistent hyperinsulinemic hypoglycemia of infancy. Science 1995;268:426–429.
12. Weinzimer SA, Stanley CA, Berry GT, Yudkoff M, Tuchman M, Thornton PS. A syndrome of congenital hyperinsulinism and hyperammonemia. J Pediatr 1997;130(4):661–664.
13. Stanley CA, Lieu YK, Hsu BY, et al. Hyperinsulinism and hyperammonemia in infants with regulatory mutations of the glutamate dehydrogenase gene. N Engl J Med 1998;338(19):1352–1357.
14. Hsu BY, Kelly A, Thornton PS, Greenberg CR, Dilling LA, Stanley CA. Protein-sensitive and fasting hypoglycemia in children with the hyperinsulinism/hyperammonemia syndrome. J Pediatr 2001;138(3):383–389.
15. Kelly A, Ng D, Ferry RJ, Jr., et al. Acute insulin responses to leucine in children with the hyperinsulinism/hyperammonemia syndrome. J Clin Endocrinol Metab 2001;86(8):3724–3728.
16. MacMullen C, Fang J, Hsu BYL, et al. Hyperinsulinism/hyperammonemia syndrome in children with regulatory mutations in the inhibitory GTP binding domain of glutamate dehydrogenase. J Clin Endocrinol Metab 2001;86:1782–1787.
17. Glaser B, Kesavan P, Heyman M, et al. Familial hyperinsulinism caused by an activating glucokinase mutation. N Engl J Med 1998;338(4):226–230.
18. Huopio H, Reimann F, Ashfield R, et al. Dominantly inherited hyperinsulinism caused by a mutation in the sulfonylurea receptor type 1. J Clin Invest 2000;106(7):897–906.
19. de Lonlay-Debeney P, Poggi-Travert F, Fournet JC, et al. Clinical features of 52 neonates with hyperinsulinism. N Engl J Med 1999;340:1169–1175.

20. Glaser B, Furth J, Stanley CA, et al. Intragenic single nucleotide polymorphism haplotype analysis of SUR1 mutations in familial hyperinsulinism. Hum Mutat 1999;14(1):23–29.
21. Collins JE, Leonard JV. Hyperinsulinsim in asphyxiated and small-for-dates infants with hypoglycaemia. Lancet 1984;2:311–313.
22. Collins JE, Leonard JV, Teale D, et al. Hyperinsulinaemic hypoglycaemia in small for dates babies. Arch Dis Childhood 1990;65:1118–1120.
23. Stanley CA, Coates PM. Inherited defects of fatty acid oxidation which resemble Reye's Syndrome. In: Pollack JD, ed. Reye's Syndrome IV. NRSF, Bryan, OH, 1985.
24. Stanley CA. Disorders of fatty acid metabolism. In: Behrman RE, ed. Nelson Textbook of Pediatics. 14th ed. W. B. Saunders, Philadelphia, 1992, pp. 328–338.
25. Roe CR, Coates PM. Mitochondrial fatty acid oxidation disorders. In: Scriver CR, Beaudet AL, Sly WS, Valle D, ed. The Metabolic and Molecular Bases of Inherited Disease. VI ed. New York: McGraw Hill; 1995. p. 1501–1534.
26. Stanley CA. Dissecting the spectrum of fatty acid oxidation disorders. J Pediatr 1998;132:384–386.
27. Saudubray JM, Martin D, DeLonlay P. Recognition and management of fatty acid oxidation defects: a series of 107 patients. J Inher Met D 1999;22:488–502.
28. Ziadeh R, Hoffman EP, Finegold DM, et al. Medium chain acyl-CoA dehydrogenase deficiency in Pennsylvania: neonatal screening shows high incidence and unexpected mutation frequencies. Pediatr Res 1995;37:675–678.
29. Girard J, Pegorier JP. An overview of early post-partum nutrition and metabolism. Biochem Soc Trans 1998;26(2):69–74.
30. Pegorier JP, Chatelain F, Thumelin S, Girard J. Role of long-chain fatty acids in the postnatal induction of genes coding for liver mitochondrial beta-oxidative enzymes. Biochem Soc Trans 1998;26(2): 113–120.
31. Thornton PS, Alter CA, Katz LE, Baker L, Stanley CA. Short- and long-term use of octreotide in the treatment of congenital hyperinsulinism. J Pediatr 1993;123(4):637–643.
32. Ng D, Ferry RJ, Weinzimer SA, Stanley CA, Levitt Katz LE. Acarbose treatment of postprandial hypoglycemia in children after Nissen fundoplication. J Pediatr 2002;139:877–879.

28 Diabetes Mellitus in Children and Adolescents

William V. Tamborlane, MD
and JoAnn Ahern, MSN, APRN, CDE

CONTENTS

INTRODUCTION
CLASSIFICATION
TREATMENT OF T1DM
TREATMENT OF TYPE 2 DIABETES
REFERENCES

INTRODUCTION

Diabetes mellitus is a chronic disorder characterized by impaired metabolism of glucose and other energy-yielding fuels, as well as the late development of vascular and neuropathic complications. Diabetes mellitus consists of a group of disorders involving distinct pathogenic mechanisms in which hyperglycemia is the common denominator. Regardless of the cause, the disease is associated with insulin deficiency that in children with Type 1 diabetes is usually total, and in adults and adolescents with type 2 diabetes partial or relative when viewed in the context of coexisting insulin resistance. Lack of insulin plays a primary role in the metabolic derangements linked to diabetes, and hyperglycemia, in turn, plays a key role in the complications of the disease.

CLASSIFICATION

Diabetes mellitus is a heterogeneous group of disorders that can be divided into at least three subclasses: type 1 or insulin-dependent diabetes mellitus (T1DM): type 2, or non-insulin-dependent diabetes mellitus (T2DM); and secondary diabetes linked to another identifiable condition or syndrome. The majority of children with diabetes have T1DM, but the prevalence of T2DM is increasing dramatically especially in obese adolescents of African-American, Native American, and Hispanic origin.

Patients with T1DM have little or no insulin secretory capacity and are dependent on exogenous insulin to prevent metabolic decompensation (e.g., ketoacidosis) and death.

From: *Contemporary Endocrinology: Pediatric Endocrinology: A Practical Clinical Guide*
Edited by: S. Radovick and M. H. MacGillivray © Humana Press Inc., Totowa, NJ

Commonly, T1DM appears abruptly over days or weeks in previously healthy nonobese children or young adults. At the time of intial presentation, the patient appears ill; has symptoms of polyuria, polydipsia, polyphagia, and weight loss; and may demonstrate ketoacidosis. T1DM actually has a long asymptomatic preclinical stage often lasting years, during which pancreatic β-cells are gradually destroyed by an autoimmune attack.

Patients with T2DM retain some endogenous insulin secretory capacity, but insulin levels are low relative to the magnitude of insulin resistance and ambient glucose levels. It is not uncommon, however, for adolescents with T2DM to present with marked hyperglycemia and even ketosis, especially in the context of a stressful intercurrent illness. Impairments in insulin sensitivity induced by obesity, ethnicity, and puberty, as well as genetic defects in insulin secretory capacity, contribute to the pathogenesis of this condition. The presence of acanthosis nigricans is a characteristic finding on physical examination.

TREATMENT OF T1DM

T1DM in childhood and adolescence presents special challenges to pediatric health care providers. The combination of severe insulin deficiency and the physical and psychosocial changes that accompany normal growth and development make day-to-day management of pediatric patients especially difficult. Moreover, the results of the Diabetes Control and Complicaiton Trial (DCCT) have raised the bar considerably higher with respect to goals of treatment, since intensive treatment significantly reduced the risk of progression of retinopathy and the development of microalbuminuria *(1–3)*. Current recommendations mandate that youth with type 1 diabetes should aim to achieve metabolic control as close to normal as possible and as early in the course of the disease as possible. Remarkably, a much greater proportion of young patients are meeting strict standards of care than ever imagined possible only a few years ago. Our approach to treatment of children and adolescents with T1DM is discussed below.

Goals of Treatment

The traditional goals of treatment of children and adolescents with diabetes were to use insulin, diet, and exercise to minimize symptoms of hypoglycemia and hyperglycemia and promote normal growth and development. Intensive education and psychosocial support are used to maximize independence and self-efficacy in order to reduce the adverse psychosocial effects of this chronic disease. Since the results of the DCCT were published, additional primary aims of therapy are to lower blood glucose and glycosylated hemoglobin values to as close to normal as possible. In pediatric patients, achievement of such stringent treatment goals is best accomplished with a multidisciplinary team of clinicians to provide ongoing education and support of aggressive self-management efforts on the part of parents and patients. Matching the treatment to the patient (rather than vice versa) by taking a flexible and varied approach to insulin replacement, diet, and exercise are critically important.

It is recognized that intensive treatment places extra burdens on patients and families and that practical considerations such as acceptability of and compliance to the treatment regimens must be balanced appropriately in order to obtain all of these aims of therapy. Nevertheless, recent data suggest that an intensive approach to diabetes education and aggressive self-management by patients and families may reduce rather than increase the adverse psychosocial effects of this chronic illness *(4)*.

Table 1
Insulin Injection Regimens

Doses	Breakfast[a]	Lunch/afternoon snack	Dinner[a]	Bedtime[a]
Two	R + I		R + I	
	R + I + L		R + I + L	
	I + L		I + L	
Three	R + I		R	R + I or L
	R + I	R	R + I + L	
Four	R	R	R	I or L

[a]Types of insulin: R = rapid acting (regular, lispro, aspart) insulin.
                I = intermediate acting (NPH, lente) insulin.
                L = long acting (ultra lente, glargine[b]).
[b]Cannot be mixed with other and must be given as a separate injection.

Insulin Regimens

Initiation of insulin treatment can be accomplished either in the inpatient or outpatient setting. Many youngsters require hospital admission due to vomiting, dehydration, and/or moderate to severe ketoacidosis. In patients who are not ill at presentation, admission to the hospital may also provide the child and parent with a safe and supportive environment in which to adjust to the shock of the diagnosis. Outpatient management in a comprehensive day treatment program staffed by individuals knowledgeable in the care of children with diabetes can also provide a supportive environment to initiate therapy *(5)*, and such programs are becoming more widely available.

Once so simple, the choice of types of insulin and insulin regimens has become much more complicated. To the standard human regular, NPH, lente, and ultralente insulins have been added new insulin analogs. Lispro and aspart insulin are produced by amino acid substitutions near the C-terminal end of the β-chain. These substitutions do not affect the biologic actions of insulin but result in more rapid absorption than regular insulin following subcutaneous injection. The sharper peak and shorter duration of these insulins vs regular insulin may be of particular advantage in teenagers who require large premeal bolus doses of rapid action insulin. There are fixed mixtures of both human insulin (i.e., regular and NPH) and human insulin analogs (i.e., lispro and NPL) and inhaled insulin preparations are currently under study *(6)*. A sampling of the variety of conventional and unconventional insulin regimens that can be employed is given in Table 1.

Although many clinicians start insulin treatment with three or more daily injections, we begin most newly diagnosed patients on two injections of insulin per day using mixtures of human lente and lispro insulins. Each dose is given as two-thirds lente and one third lispro insulin. The rationale for using two rather than three or more injections at onset of diabetes is that with aggressive control of blood levels, most children enter a "honeymoon" or partial remission period after a few weeks of therapy. This remission period is a result of increased insulin secretion by residual β-cells and improved insulin sensitivity with normalization of blood glucose levels *(7)*. To achieve these effects, patients are started on a total daily dose of at least one unit per kilogram body weight per day. Even more important, each component of the insulin regimen is adjusted on the basis of finger stick blood glucose levels measured at least four times a day. The goal is to obtain premeal blood glucose values within the normal range and this is achieved via daily telephone contracts with the family for at least the first three weeks of treatment. The DCCT data indicate that strict control of diabetes also serves to prolong the period of residual β-cell function in patients with T1DM *(8)*.

During the "honeymoon", insulin requirements rapidly decrease. Commonly, the doses of rapid acting insulin are sharply reduced or discontinued during this time; many children are well managed with two injections of intermediate-acting insulin, and some may not even require an evening injection. A major reason why the two daily injections regimen is effective during the honeymoon phase is that endogenous insulin secretion provides much of the overnight basal insulin requirements, leading to normal fasting blood glucose values. Conversely, increased and more labile pre-breakfast glucose levels often herald the loss of the relatively small amount of residual endogenous insulin secretion that is required for overnight glucose control. When residual β-cell function wanes, problems with the two-injection regimen become apparent. One problem is that the peak of the pre-dinner intermediate-acting insulin may coincide with the time of minimal insulin requirements (i.e., midnight to 4 AM). Subsequently, insulin levels fall off when basal requirements are increasing (i.e., 4–8 AM). Increasing the pre-supper dose of intermediate-acting insulin to lower fasting glucose values often leads to hypoglycemia in the middle of the night without correcting hyperglycemia before breakfast. Adolescents using relatively large doses of regular insulin before supper may also have elevations in plasma insulin levels after midnight *(9)*. Patients are especially vulnerable to hypoglycemia in the middle of the night because the normal plasma epinephrine response to low blood glucose levels is markedly blunted during deep sleep *(10)*. Another problem with the conventional two-injection regimen is high pre-supper glucose levels, despite normal or low pre-lunch and mid-afternoon values. This is owing, in part, to eating an afternoon snack when the effects of the pre-breakfast dose of intermediate acting insulin is waning.

One way to deal with these problems without increasing the number of injections is to add ultralente insulin to the pre-breakfast and pre-supper mixtures of lispro and lente. With this combination in the morning, lispro covers breakfast, lente covers lunch, and ultralente the late afternoon period. With the pre-supper dose, lispro covers supper, lente covers the bedtime snack and part of the overnight period, and ultralente helps limit the pre-breakfast rise in plasma glucose. However, when strict control cannot be achieved with two daily injections, we do not hesitate to switch to a regimen involving three or more daily injections. A common approach to the problem in the overnight period is to use a three injection regimen, lispro and lente at breakfast, lispro only at dinner and lente at bedtime. In youngsters who go to bed early, we recommend that the parents give the third shot at their bedtime (i.e., 10:00–11:00 PM). Lispro can also be added to the bedtime dose, especially if glucose levels are elevated. For patients with elevated pre-supper glucose levels, a pre-lunch dose of regular or a pre-afternoon snack dose of lispro can be added. Such extra doses of insulin can be facilitated by the use of insulin pens, which are small, light, and easy to use. Only a small number of our patients are using a four or more injection regimen of rapid acting insulin before meals and intermediate insulin at bedtime.

Over the past few years, there has been a rediscovery of the effectiveness of insulin pump therapy in the management of young patients with diabetes *(11)*. Indeed, we are much more likely to turn to this method of insulin replacement rather than more frequent injections in patients who are coming out of their honeymoon phase of diabetes.

With insulin pump treatment, small amounts of rapid-acting insulin are infused as a basal rate and larger bolus doses are given at each meal or snack. Although not yet labeled by the FDA for use in pumps, lispro insulin appears to have advantages over regular insulin in pump therapy *(12)*. The pumps are battery powered and about the size of a beeper. The "basal" rate can be programmed to change every half hour, but it is unusual to need more than five or six basal rates. Varying the basal rate can be particularly helpful in regulating overnight blood glucose levels, since it can be lowered for the early part of the night to prevent hypoglycemia and increased in the hours before dawn to keep glucose from rising. However, younger children seem to need a higher basal rate during the earlier part of the night perhaps due to earlier nocturnal peaks of growth hormone in this age group. Bolus doses are given before meals based on glucose level, carbohydrate content of the meal, and anticipated exercise after the meal. Pump treatment can be especially useful in infants and toddlers who are picky eaters. In this setting, part of the usual premeal bolus can be given prior to the meal and the rest given at the end of the meal depending on the actual amount of carbohydrate intake. Indeed, most children and parents are encouraged to use carbohydrate counting as a means to adjust premeal bolus doses. Pump therapy also enhances flexibility in children with variable exercise and meal routines.

The pump employs a reservoir (syringe) to hold the insulin and the infusion set, which consists of tubing with a small plastic catheter at the end. The insertion site can be the abdomen or hip area, except in the young child in whom there may not be sufficient subcutaneous tissue in the abdomen. Our patients are encouraged to change their catheters every 2–3 d. Because only rapid acting insulin is used in this pump, the child and parent must understand that the insulin infusion should not be discontinued for more than 4 h at a time.

New Insulin Preparations

Intermediate and long acting preparations of human insulin suffer from a number of pharmacologic problems, not the least of which is the failure to uniformly mix these suspensions prior to injection. Human NPH insulin is a particularly poor choice for basal insulin replacement, since there is a substantial peak in insulin levels and insulin action 2–6 h after subcutaneous injection. Even human ultralente has a significant peak action 8–12 h after injection, and the dose-to-dose variability in absorption of all human insulin suspensions is substantial.

Glargine insulin (Aventis Pharmaceuticals) is an analog of human insulin with C-terminal elongation of the β-chain by two arginines and replacement of asparagine in position A21 by glycine. This molecule is soluble in the acidic solution in which it is packaged, but relatively insoluble in the physiologic pH of the extracellular fluid. Consequently, microprecipitates of glargine insulin are formed following subcutaneous injection, which markedly delays its absorption into the systemic circulation. Pharamacokinetic and pharmacodynamic studies have demonstrated that the insulin analog has a very flat and prolonged time-action profile *(13)*. Results of a 6-mo study of the efficacy and safety of glargine in adolescents and children with diabetes showed modestly lower fasting blood glucose levels and reduced risk for hypoglycemia with glargine vs human NPH insulin. Additional studies and more clinical experience need to be accumulated regarding use of this analog in youth with type 1 diabetes. Because glargine cannot be mixed with other insulins, it has to be given by separate injection, which might affect its acceptability by some youngsters.

Although there have been many failed attempts at finding alternatives to insulin injections *(14)*, use of aerosolized preparations for inhaled insulin delivery is currently under active investigation. Preliminary studies in adults have been promising enough *(6)* that Phase III studies are already underway in pre-adolescents as well as adolescents with type 1 diabetes. As with pump therapy, inhaled insulin allows the patients to take premeal boluses of insulin with each meal and snack without having to take extra insulin injections. However, one or more injections of intermediate or long-acting insulin are still needed for basal insulin replacement.

Adjusting Insulin Doses

Insulin replacement in children is a special challenge because insulin requirements increase as weight and calorie intake increase and as residual endogenous secretion declines. Regular self-monitoring of blood glucose (SMBG) allows the family and clinicians to keep up with the child's steadily increasing insulin needs. We request that blood glucose levels be checked at least four times per day (before each meal and at bedtime). The most important component of SMBG is the interpretation of the results. The parent or child must be taught what the target value is and what the relationship is between diet, exercise, and insulin. If the parent and/or child grasp these concepts, they will make accurate adjustments aimed at achieving target goals. If they are unable to make accurate adjustments, they should be given guidelines of when to call the diabetes service for help. Day to day adjustments in the doses of rapid-acting insulin can be made based on the premeal blood glucose value, amount of carbohydrate in the meal, and the amount of anticipated exercise. In addition, patients and parents should be taught to look for repetitive patterns of hypo- or hyperglycemia, in order to make ongoing changes in their usual insulin doses. To facilitate identification of trends, families are encouraged to maintain either a handwritten or computer generated record of each glucose value in a spread sheet format.

Self-monitoring of blood glucose is subject to a variety of problems, especially making up false numbers *(15)*. These issues must be addressed with the child and family. They must understand the reason for the tests and that they are only used to make proper adjustments to keep them healthy. Elevated glucose levels are not an indication of worsening of diabetes or that they have been cheating on their diet. Instead, we emphasize that the tests are being done primarily to determine when they have outgrown their current dose of insulin.

Even when performed correctly, four blood tests daily gives only a limited glimpse of wide fluctuations in blood glucose that occur during a 24-h period in children with diabetes. Consequently, the recent introduction of continuous glucose monitoring systems has the potential to be the most important advance in assessing diabetes control in the past 20 y. In intensively-treated children and adolescents with type 1 diabetes, preliminary results in a relatively small number of children suggest that continuous glucose monitoring will provide a wealth of data regarding post-prandial glycemic excursions and asymptomatic nocturnal hypoglycemia that were unavailable from capillary blood glucose measurements *(16)*. We anticipate that these technological breakthroughs will have a great impact on diabetes management over the next few years. Continuous monitoring of nocturnal glucose levels is likely to be particularly useful in programming overnight basal rates in pump-treated patients.

Measurements of glycosyolated hemoglobin (HbA$_{1c}$) provide the gold standard by which to judge the adequacy of the insulin regimen. A variety of methods are available for assaying glycosylated hemoglobin. A simple method that can be performed in the office in 6 mins (Bayer DCA 2000) offers the opportunity to make immediate changes in the insulin regimen, while the patient is being seen. The goal of treatment is to achieve HbA$_{1c}$ levels as close to normal as possible. Based on DCCT results *(2)*, our general goal of therapy is to try to keep all patients under 8.0%. HbA$_{1c}$ levels are determined at least every 3 mo.

Matching Insulin to Food Intake

Dietary guidance for children with diabetes is provided best by a nutritionist who is an integral part of the treatment team and is comfortable working with children. In addition to helping achieve optimal glucose levels and normal growth and development, nutritional management of diabetes is aimed at reducing the risk for other diseases such as obesity, high blood cholesterol, or high blood pressure. Underlying all of these is the establishment of sound eating patterns that include balanced, nutritious foods and consistent timing of food intake *(17)*.

The American Diabetes Association dietary guidelines are used for dietary counseling. In addition to incorporating sound nutritional principles concerning the fat, fiber, and carbohydrate content, the importance of consistency in meal size and regularity in the timing of meals is emphasized. The prohibition of simple sugar in the diet has been de-emphasized, but it should still comprise no more than 10% of total carbohydrate intake. The success of the nutritional program may ultimately depend on the degree to which the meal planning is individualized and tailored to well-established eating patterns in the family. Moreover, flexibility can be enhanced if blood glucose-monitoring results are used to evaluate the impact of change in dietary intake. As with other aspects of the treatment regimen, we preach consistency and teach how to adjust for deviations from the prescribed diet.

Carbohydrate counting is an increasingly popular way to increase flexibility in food intake that is commonly used by patients using insulin pumps or multiple daily injections. The amount of insulin that is needed for each gram or serving of carbohydrate is used to calculate the amount of regular or lispro to be taken depending on the amount of carbohydrate in the meal. With instructions on how to use nutritional labels on food packages, even relatively young children can become expert at counting carbohydrates. An even simpler method is to vary the dose of regular or lispro by one or two units if it is a small, regular, or large meal. Some foods, like pizza, that cause a prolonged increase in blood glucose levels may require an increase in the amount of intermediate-acting insulin or a temporary change in overnight basal rates in pump-treated patients.

Exercise

Regular exercise and active participation in organized sports have positive implications concerning the psychosocial and physical well being of our patients. Parents and patients should be advised that different types of exercise might have different effects on blood glucose levels. For example, sports that involve short bursts of intensive exercise may increase rather than decrease blood glucose levels *(18)*. On the other hand, long-distance running and other prolonged activities are more likely to lower blood glucose levels. Parents also need to be warned that a long bout of exercise during the day may lead to hypoglycemia while the child is sleeping during the night, which may require a reduction in the dose of intermediate or long-acting insulin.

Outpatient Care

Children and adolescents with T1DM should be routinely cared for by a diabetes center that uses a multidisciplinary team knowledgeable about and experienced in the management of young patients. This team should ideally consist of pediatric diabetologists, diabetes nurse specialists, nutritionists, and social workers or psychologists.

In newly diagnosed patients, the first few weeks are critically important in the process of teaching self-management skills to the parent and child. Glucose levels, adjustment to diabetes, diet, and exercise are reviewed. The timing of the phone calls should be prearranged and ideally made to the same clinician. Usually within 3 wk the parents or patients are feeling more confident and many are ready to attempt to make their own adjustments.

Once stabilized, regular follow-up visits on a 2- to 3-monthly basis are recommended for most patients *(19)*. The main purpose of these visits is to ensure that the patient is achieving primary treatment goals. In addition to serial measurements of height and weight, particular attention should be paid to monitoring of blood pressure and examinations of the optic fundus, thyroid, and subcutaneous injection sites. Routine outpatient visits provide an opportunity to review glucose monitoring, to adjust the treatment regimen and to assess child and family adjustment. Follow-up advice and support are given by the nutritionist, diabetes nurse specialist, and psychologist or social worker. Use of the telephone, fax, or email should be encouraged for adjustments in the treatment regimen between office visits.

Hypoglycemia

Severe hypoglycemia is a common problem in patients striving for strict glycemic control with intensive treatment regimens. In the DCCT, the risk of severe hypoglycemia was three-fold higher in intensively treated than in conventionally treated patients, and adolescence was an independent risk factor for a severe hypoglycemic event *(2)*. The majority of severe hypoglycemic events occur overnight owing, in part, to sleep-induced defects in counterregulatory hormone responses to hypoglycemia *(10)*.

Monitoring glucose is critical in order to detect asymptomatic hypoglycemia especially in the young child with diabetes. The older child is usually aware of symptoms such as weakness, shakiness, hunger, or a headache and is encouraged to treat these symptoms as soon as they occur. The older child who can accurately recognize symptoms is taught to immediately treat with 15 g of carbohydrate (e.g., 3–4 glucose tablets, 4 oz of juice or 15 g of a glucose gel) without waiting to check a glucose level. Each episode should be assessed in order to make proper adjustments if a cause can be identified. Every family should have a glucagon emergency kit at home in order to treat severe hypoglycemia.

Sick Day Rules

Children with intercurrent illnesses, such as infections or vomiting, should be closely monitored for elevations in blood glucose levels and ketonuria. On sick days, blood glucose levels should be checked every 2 h and the urine should be checked for ketones with every void. Supplemental doses of short-acting insulin (0.13–0.3 U/k) should be given every 2–4 h for elevations in glucose and ketones. Because of its more rapid absorption, lispro will lower plasma glucose faster than regular insulin. If the morning dose has not been given and the child has a modestly elevated glucose level (150–250 mg/dL), small doses of NPH can be given to avoid a too rapid fall in plasma glucose levels. This works especially well in young children whose glucose levels fall quickly with rapid acting insulin. Adequate fluid intake is essential to prevent dehydration. Fluids such as flat soda, clear soups, popsicles, and gelatin water are recommended to provide some electrolyte and carbohydrate replacement. If vomiting is persistent and ketones remain moderate or large after several supplemental insulin doses, arrangements should be made for parenteral hydration and evaluation in the emergency department.

Children receiving ultralente insulin seem to be prone to the development of hypoglycemia and ketonuria during episodes of gastroenteritis. If the child is unable to retain oral carbohydrate, then small doses of glucagon (i.e., 0.1–0.2 mg), given subcutaneously every 2–4 h, can be used to maintain normal blood glucose levels.

TREATMENT OF TYPE 2 DIABETES

Except for some special considerations, our approach to T2DM is very similar to that in T2DM, especially with respect to goals of treatment, monitoring of glycemic control, and follow-up care. Since obesity-induced insulin resistance is hallmark of most cases of T2DM in children and adolescents, a comprehensive program of behavior modification, dietary counseling, and physical fitness should be an integral part of all treatment regimes. The choice of drug therapy will vary depending on the clinical presentation. Patients who have marked hyperglycemia with or without ketosis at diagnosis require insulin in order to correct metabolic abnormalities and limit glucotoxic effects of hyperglycemia on β-cell function. While continuing treatment with insulin might be considered to be more burdensome than treatment with oral agents, long-term compliance with insulin therapy may, paradoxically, be better. Most pediatric diabetes treatment centers have well-established and intensive education and support programs for youngsters starting on insulin. In contrast, both clinicians and families may take a more relaxed attitude toward patients whose diabetes is "sufficiently mild" to require "only" oral agents. Consequently, the urgency to achieve strict metabolic control and to comply with therapy may also be reduced.

Oral hypoglycemic agents are being used with increasing frequency in youth, either as initial monotherapy in youngsters who are not ill on presentation or as an adjunct to treatment in patients who are started on insulin. Although sulfonylureas continue to be used, metformin is currently the drug most commonly prescribed for young patients with T2DM because of its ability to enhance hepatic sensitivity to insulin, its tendency to promote weight loss (or at least reduce weight gain), and its relatively favorable safety profile. However, gastrointestinal tolerance to metformin is a relatively common problem. To minimize this problem, we initiate treatment with a relatively low dose (i.e., 500 mg daily) and gradually increase dose in 500 mg steps to a maximum dose of 1000 mg twice daily.

Although the new peripheral sensitizers (e.g., pioglitazone) and short acting insulin secretagogs (e.g., repaglinide) have been extensively used in adults, much less experience has been obtained with these agents in pediatric patients. A multi-center group is being assembled by the National Institutes of Health to better define optimal treatment of T2DM in children and adolescents.

REFERENCES

1. DCCT Research Group. The effects of intensive diabetes treatment on the development and progression of long-term complications in insulin-dependent diabetes mellitus. The Diabetes Control and Complications Trial. N Engl J Med 1993;329:977–986.
2. The DCCT Research Group. The effect of intensive diabetes treatment on the development and progression of long-term complications in adolescents with insulin-dependent diabetes mellitus: the Diabetes Control and Complications Trial. J Pediatr 1994;125:177–188.
3. DCCT Research Group. Prolonged effect of intensive therapy on the risk of advanced complications in the Epidemiology of Diabetes Intervention and Complications (EDIC) follow-up of the DCCT cohort. N Engl J Med 2000;342:381–389.
4. Grey M, Boland EA, Davidson M, Li J, Tamborlane W. Coping skills training for youth on intensive therapy has long lasting effects on metabolic control and quality of life. J Pediatr 2000;137:107–114.
5. Dougherty G, Schiffrin A, White D, Soderstrom I, Sufrategui M. Home-based management can achieve intensification cost-effectively in type I diabetes. Pediatrics 1999;103:122–128.
6. Patton JW, Bukar J, Nagarajan S. Inhaled insulin. Adv Drug Deliv Rev 1999;36:235–247.
7. Yki-Jarvinen H, Koivisto VA. Natural course of insulin resistance in type I diabetes. N Engl J Med 1986;315:224–230.
8. The DCCT Research Group. The effect of intensive diabetes treatment in the DCCT on residual insulin secretion in IDDM. Ann Int Med 1998;128:517–523.
9. Mohn A, Matyka K, Harris D, Ross K, Edge J, Dunger DB. Lispro or regular insulin for multiple injection therapy in adolescents: differences in the insulin and glucose levels overnight. Diabetes Care 1999;23:27–32.
10. Jones TW, Porter P, David EA, et al. Suppressed epinephrine responses during sleep: a contributing factor to the risk of nocturnal hypoglycemia in insulin-dependent diabetes. N Engl J Med 1999;338:1657–1662
11. Boland EA, Grey M, Fredrickson L, Tamborlane WV. CSII: a "new" way to achieve strict metabolic control, decrease severe hypoglycemia and enhance coping in adolescents with type I diabetes. Diabetes Care 1999;22:1779–1894.
12. Zinman B, Tildesley H, Chiasson TJ, Tsue E, Strack T. Insulin lispro in CSII: results of a double-blind crossover study [published erratum appears in Diabetes 1997, July 46:1239]. Diabetes 1997;46: 440–443.
13. Moses AC, Gordon GS, Carey MC, Flier JS. Insulin administration intranasally as an insulin-bile salt aerosol. Effectiveness and reproducibility in normal and diabetic subjects. Diabetes 1983;32: 1040–1047.
14. Mazze RS, Shamoon H, Pasmantier R, et al. Reliability of blood glucose monitoring by patients with diabetes mellitus. Am J Med 1984;77:211–217.
15. Boland EA, DeLucia M, Brandt C, Grey MJ, Tamborlane WV. Limitations of conventional methods of self blood glucose monitoring: lessons learned from three days of continuous glucose monitoring in pediatric patients with type I diabetes. Diabetes 2000:49(Suppl 1):A98.
16. Tamborlane WV, Held N. Diabetes. In: Yale Guide to Children's Nutrition. (Tamborlane WV, ed.) Yale University Press, New Haven, CT, 1997, pp. 161–169.
17. Mitchell TH, Abraham G, Schiffrin A, Leiter LA, Marls EB. Hyperglycemia after intensive exercise in IDDM subjects during continuous subcutaneous insulin infusion. Diabetes Care 1988;11:311–317.
18. American Diabetes Association: Clinical Practice Recommendations, 1992–1993. Diabetes Care 1993;16(Suppl 2):1–113.

VIII MEN

29 Multiple Endocrine Neoplasia Syndromes

Michael S. Racine, MD
and Pamela Thomas, MD

CONTENTS

OVERVIEW
MULTIPLE ENDOCRINE NEOPLASIA TYPE 1
PRIMARY HYPERPARATHYROIDISM
PANCREATIC NEUROENDOCRINE TUMORS
TUMORS OF THE ANTERIOR PITUITARY
GENETICS OF MEN 1
SCREENING OF CHILDREN AND ADOLESCENTS AT RISK
   OF DEVELOPING MEN 1
MULTIPLE ENDOCRINE NEOPLASIA TYPE 2
MEDULLARY THYROID CARCINOMA
PHEOCHROMOCYTOMA
PRIMARY HYPERPARATHYROIDISM
DIAGNOSTIC GUIDELINES: SCREENING FOR THE PRESENCE OF MEN 2
CONCLUSION
REFERENCES

OVERVIEW

The multiple endocrine neoplasia (MEN) syndromes form a heterogeneous set of familial neoplastic disorders featuring, as a common denominator, groupings of tumors of diverse endocrine glands. They are made up of MEN types 1, 2A, and 2B, and the related familial medullary thyroid carcinoma (FMTC). All variants of MEN are caused by mutations of discrete genetic loci and are transmitted in an autosomal dominant pattern. MEN 1 is caused by a loss-of-function mutation in the tumor-suppressor gene *menin*, while MEN 2A, 2B, and FMTC are caused by inherited gain-of-function mutations in the *RET* proto-oncogene. Prior to the localization and detailed characterization of the causative genes (MEN 2 in 1993 and MEN 1 in 1997), all children of affected parents were

From: *Contemporary Endocrinology: Pediatric Endocrinology: A Practical Clinical Guide*
Edited by: S. Radovick and M. H. MacGillivray © Humana Press Inc., Totowa, NJ

deemed at-risk and were subjected to annual biochemical screening. Genetic testing has obviated this need for routine biochemical screening in all such children, as it has made possible the positive identification of carriers of the causative genetic mutation.

Other neoplastic syndromes featuring endocrine gland oncogenesis (Von Hippel-Lindau disease, Carney complex, Peutz-Jeghers syndrome, and Cowden syndrome) are beyond the scope of this review. We limit our discussion here to the presentation, diagnosis, genetic basis, and treatment of the different MEN syndromes as they pertain to children.

MULTIPLE ENDOCRINE NEOPLASIA TYPE 1

Introduction

Approximately twenty individuals afflicted with multiple adenomas of varied endocrine glands had previously been described in Europe and the US when Dr. Paul Wermer's paper entitled "Genetic Aspects of Adenomatosis of Endocrine Glands" appeared in 1954 *(1)*. In it, Dr. Wermer described the presentation of various collections of endocrine gland tumors in a man and four of his nine adult offspring. Though the possibility that this was a familial disorder had occurred to previous investigators, Dr. Wermer was the first to propose that it was the result of a single genetic defect with autosomal dominant transmission and a high degree of penetrance. In the half-century since the appearance of his paper, Wermer's syndrome (now known as multiple endocrine neoplasia type 1) has proven to fulfill perfectly the assertions made by Dr. Wermer in 1954.

With an estimated prevalence of between 1/10,000 and 1/25,000 in the general population *(2)*, MEN 1 is a rare autosomal dominant, familial syndrome of neoplastic transformation of variable combinations of endocrine glands. Primary hyperparathyroidism, tumors of the pancreatic islet cells, and adenomas of the anterior pituitary are the most common manifestations of the disorder *(1,3)*, with other findings such as carcinoid tumors, tumors of the adrenal cortex, lipomas, facial angiofibromas, and skin collagenomas, occasionally present *(4,5)*. The specific constellation of glandular involvement varies between kindreds, and even between individuals within a family. Each of the three principal components of MEN 1 may be the presenting manifestation. MEN 1 is caused by mutations of a gene located on chromosome 11. The gene has been cloned, and multiple pathogenic mutations have been documented *(6)*.

PRIMARY HYPERPARATHYROIDISM

Overview

Primary hyperparathyroidism eventually develops in nearly all patients (85–95%) with MEN 1, and features the highest penetrance of the MEN 1 tumors *(2,7–9)*. It is characterized by hypercalcemia with inappropriately normal or elevated concentrations of serum parathyroid hormone, with asymmetric hyperplasia of all four parathyroid glands *(10)*, a feature that differentiates it from the solitary parathyroid adenoma of sporadic primary hyperparathyroidism.

Clinical Presentation

The average age at clinical detection of MEN 1-related primary hyperparathyroidism is 25 yr, but MEN 1-related asymptomatic hypercalcemia has been reported in a child as young as 5 yr of age *(11)*. Primary hyperparathyroidism is often, though not always, the first disorder of MEN 1 to present clinically. With careful biochemical screening of adolescents at risk (*see* Screening), the mean age of detection of primary hyperparathyroidism may be lowered to 19 yr, as shown by Skogseid et al. *(12)*. The hypercalcemia of MEN 1-related hyperparathyroidism is usually mild *(13)*, and classic symptoms of hypercalcemia such as polyuria, constipation, muscle aches, and abdominal pain are frequently absent.

Diagnosis

In a child known to be at risk for MEN 1, primary hyperparathyroidism is suggested by a serum calcium concentration above 10.4 mg/dL. The finding of an inappropriately normal or elevated concentration of serum parathyroid hormone (by an amino-terminal or intact PTH assay) is necessary for confirmation.

Therapy

Primary hyperparathyroidism is amenable to surgery, and sure indications for surgery include a serum calcium concentration higher than 12 mg/dL, nephrolithiasis, or evidence of bone loss *(5)*. It is agreed that surgery is the primary mode of treatment, however the best approach is a matter of debate, and two strategies have their proponents *(14,15)*. The total parathyroidectomy approach involves excision of all four parathyroid glands, with transfer of parathyroid tissue to the non-dominant forearm. In contrast, subtotal parathyroidectomy features the excision of 31/2 glands, leaving residual parathyroid tissue in the neck with its existing vascular supply. Thymectomy is included in both approaches. With subtotal parathyroidectomy, persistent postoperative hypocalcemia can be avoided when as little as 50 mg of parathyroid tissue is left intact *(15)*, however recurrent hyperplasia of residual parathyroid tissue commonly leads to a reappearance of hypercalcemia. The rate of recurrent hypercalcemia following both surgical strategies exceeds that seen following excision of a primary sporadic parathyroid adenoma, with rates at 10 yr averaging 50% in long term follow-up series *(14,16)*.

PANCREATIC NEUROENDOCRINE TUMORS

Overview

Neoplastic transformation of pancreatic islet cells is the second most common manifestation of MEN 1, occurring in 30–80% of patients with MEN 1. Because of their potential for malignant transformation and metastasis, occuring in one-third to one-half of patients, pancreatic neuroendocrine tumors (PNTs) represent the most pressing threat to life associated with MEN 1 *(9)*. Pancreatic neuroendocrine tumors are characteristically multifocal. They are classified according to the hormone(s) they secrete and on the clinical syndrome produced by their hormones. Tumors secreting pancreatic polypeptide are the most common, but are clinically silent unless they reach a size large enough to cause mass effects. Among PNTs that secrete clinically relevant hormones, gastrinomas are most common, followed by insulinomas. Tumors that produce somatostatin, vasoactive intestinal polypeptide, glucagon, and adrenocorticotropic hormone (ACTH) are far less common.

Clinical Presentation

Involvement of the endocrine pancreas may present before hyperparathyroidism in some patients with MEN 1. In a 10-yr, prospective screening study involving 80 individuals from 4 Swedish kindreds with MEN 1, Skogseid et al. *(12)* prospectively identified 7 new cases of MEN 1. Of those seven, primary hyperparathyroidism (HPT) was the sole initial presenting tumor in only two. HPT was identified simultaneously with pancreatic neuroendocrine tumors in another two subjects, and PNTs were the solitary presenting manifestation in three of seven patients. The mean age of patients prospectively diagnosed with a PNT in this series was 25 yr; the youngest was 16. This contrasts with previously published series' in which the average age of presentation of PNT was 44 yr, and demonstrates that carefully conducted regular screening of adolescents at risk for MEN 1 may lead to earlier diagnosis of these potentially malignant tumors. Screening strategies to secure early identification of PNTs in children at risk have been proposed and are recommended *(5,17)*, as detailed later in this discussion.

Gastrinoma with Zollinger-Ellison syndrome (ZES) eventually develops in up to 30% of adults with MEN 1 *(18)*. These tumors may be as small as 1–2 mm and often arise within the duodenal wall, whereas other PNTs are found mostly in the body or the tail of the pancreas. ZES in MEN 1 occurs at a younger age than in sporadic cases. In a recent large NIH review of ZES *(19)*, age of onset of symptomatic gastrinoma was 43.5 yr in sporadic cases, and 33.2 yr in MEN 1-associated cases; the youngest patient with MEN 1-associated gastrinoma was 12 yr old. In the NIH review, the most consistent presenting complaints were diarrhea, epigastric pain, and heartburn (in 76, 66, and 52% of cases, respectively) *(19)*. ZES leading to duodenal or gastric ulceration and perforation with massive bleeding has historically been the commonest cause of death related to MEN 1. The incidence of this complication has been greatly reduced by medical management of gastrinomas with proton pump inhibitors and histamine-2 receptor blockers. Insulin-secreting PNTs present with recurrent, often severe postabsorptive and fasting hypoglycemia.

Diagnosis

The diagnosis of a pancreatic neuroendocrine tumor hinges upon measurement of the hormone fitting the clinical syndrome. Biochemical findings suggestive of abnormal gastrin secretion include an elevated fasting plasma gastrin (>200 pg/mL), with a concurrent fasting gastric pH <2.5. Provocative testing with intravenous secretin or calcium infusion produces further elevation of serum gastrin concentration, >200 pg/mL in adults with gastrinoma *(20)*. The standardized meal test, with measurement of basal and meal-stimulated pancreatic polypeptide and gastrin, may be useful in detecting early pancreatic involvement in MEN 1 *(21)*. In a child at risk for MEN 1, insulinoma is strongly suggested when plasma insulin and C-peptide concentrations above 6 (μU/mL, and 0.6 ng/mL, respectively, accompany hypoglycemia (plasma glucose <45 mg/dL) *(22)*. Measurement of other pancreatic neuroendocrine hormones may be indicated as necessary. T1-weighted magnetic resonance imaging (MRI) of the pancreas is used to assess tumor location and size.

Therapy

Once the presence of a pancreatic neuroendocrine tumor is recognized, the best approach to management must be determined by a number of factors, and may not be entirely clear. The motivation to remove tumors with an inherent risk of malignancy as high as 50% (as in the case of gastrinomas) is counterbalanced by the potential morbidity of iatrogenic insulin-dependant diabetes mellitus and exocrine pancreas dysfunction.

More conservative surgical management aimed at identifying and enucleating all pancreatic tumors while leaving the gland intact appears to be a more promising approach, and is facilitated by intraoperative pancreatic ultrasound *(18,23)*. Pharmacologic gastrectomy has revolutionized the treatment of hypergastrinemia and can be effected with proton-pump inhibition (e.g., omeprazole), or H2 blockade (e.g., ranitidine). Still, surgery may yet be necessary to diminish the risk of malignant transformation of larger gastrin-secreting PNTs. No satisfactory medical management of insulinomas is currently available, and surgical removal provides the best management of these tumors.

TUMORS OF THE ANTERIOR PITUITARY

Overview

Tumors of the anterior pituitary gland, whether associated with a hereditary endocrine syndrome or not, are characteristically benign adenomas whose major morbidity results from hormone over-secretion, mass effect, or both. The overall rate of occurrence in MEN 1 is 10–65%. Prolactin-secreting tumors are the most common pituitary adenoma in MEN 1 and account for the third most prevalent manifestation of the disorder. Lactotroph adenomas are followed in frequency by somatotroph and corticotroph adenomas.

Clinical Presentation

Clinical features of pituitary adenomas are dependent on the hormone being secreted (if any), and on the presence of mass-effects. Common presenting signs in children and adolescents, regardless of cell type, include delayed puberty, headache, primary or secondary amenorrhea, central diabetes insipidus, and visual field defects *(24)*. Prolactinomas may be heralded by galactorrhea and growth deceleration, whereas growth hormone-secreting tumors produce gigantism, or acromegaly, if fusion of epiphyseal growth plates is complete. A child with an ACTH-secreting adenoma will present with Cushingoid features, accelerated weight gain, and decelerated growth *(24,25)*. MEN 1-associated pituitary tumors are frequently multicentric, and may be large. The appearance of a prolactinoma associated with MEN 1 has been reported in a patient as young as 16 yr of age *(17)*, however pituitary involvement in children or adolescents with MEN 1 is uncommon.

Diagnosis

In a child with presenting features suggestive of a prolactinoma, serum prolactin concentration greater than 200 ng/mL is diagnostic, while lower levels may be seen early in the course of a microadenoma *(24)*. Serum for insulin-like growth factor 1 (IGF-1) should be sent to a reference lab capable of providing age-adjusted normative data (e.g., Esoterix Inc., Calabasas Hills, California) when a somatotroph adenoma is suspected. An elevated serum IGF-1 is suggestive, but the conclusive test for diagnosis of a growth hormone-secreting tumor remains the oral glucose challenge, in which growth hormone will fail to suppress to less than 1 µg/L after 75 g of glucose are administered orally *(26)*. Measurement of serum cortisol and 24-h-urine free cortisol may be useful, as clinically indicated to screen for MEN 1-related Cushing's disease. Magnetic resonance imaging of the pituitary gland before and after gadolinium enhancement is the best radiological modality for a suspected pituitary adenoma. Normally the posterior pituitary is hyperintense (the pituitary "bright spot") and the anterior pituitary is isointense, as compared with the rest of the brain *(27)*. With gadolinium enhancement, adenomas of the anterior pituitary appear hypointense, as they are slow to take up contrast, in comparison with the normal part of the gland.

Therapy

As in sporadic prolactinomas, reduction of hyperprolactinemia with dopamine agonists such as bromocriptine or pergolide is nearly always the best method of treatment and can reduce tumor size markedly. Bromocriptine has been used most in children, and should be started at a low dose (1.25 mg po qd), to minimize its side effects of nausea and hypotension. Daily doses of 2.5–20 mg are usually successful in inducing normal prolactin levels *(24)*. Transsphenoidal surgery is reserved for the treatment of somatotroph adenomas, corticotroph adenomas, enlarging nonsecretory adenomas, and prolactinomas that present an immediate threat to eyesight because of their size or those that are unyielding to medical management *(25,27)*.

GENETICS OF MEN 1

The *MEN 1* gene was isolated in 1997 by positional cloning, a technique in which the size of the candidate gene interval on the chromosome is progressively narrowed, and many or all genes within that interval are found and tested *(6)*. The *MEN 1* gene is located in the 13th band of the long arm of chromosome 11 (11q13) and codes for a novel protein called menin. The structure of menin is similar to no previously known protein. However, molecular investigations suggest that menin functions within the nucleus as a repressor of gene transcription through interaction with the AP1 transcription factor JunD *(28,29)*. The loss of heterozygosity of many tumors associated with MEN 1 is suggestive of the role of the *MEN 1* gene as a tumor suppressor as well *(6)*. Individuals with MEN 1 inherit a defective copy of the gene from their affected parent. Tumorigenesis is then triggered when the remaining functional copy of the gene is inactivated by an acquired mutation (the "two-hit" theory of loss of tumor suppression). A recent review notes more than 70 mutations of the menin gene have been identified across the 9 coding exons. No apparent correlation exists between genotype and phenotype *(17)*.

Genetic screening has significantly facilitated the evaluation of families with MEN 1, and is extremely useful in identifying children at risk. The specific causative mutation of the menin gene should be sought in all patients affected by MEN 1*. When it has been identified, the children of adult patients should be screened for the mutation also. Children lacking the mutation present in their affected parent are non-carriers and can be spared years of needless biochemical and radiological screening. On the other hand, the child of an affected patient whose mutation cannot be positively identified should be screened annually as if she or he was known to be a carrier of a mutation of the MEN 1 gene.

SCREENING OF CHILDREN AND ADOLESCENTS AT RISK OF DEVELOPING MEN 1

A protocol of annual biochemical screening and periodic radiographic imaging (*see* Table 1) in children has recently been proposed by Johnston et al. *(17)*. The best age at which to begin routine biochemical screening is not firmly established, but the very low risk of tumorigenesis before the second decade and the considerable volume of blood

Table 1
Proposed MEN-1 Screening Protocol in Children

	Biochemical	Radiology	Age to start	Frequency
Parathyroid	Serum calcium (intact PTH)		10–15 yr	Annual
Pancreas	Pancreatic polypeptide Gastrin	US pancreas	10–15 yr	Annual
		MRI pancreas	10–15 yr	3 yearly
Pituitary	Prolactin IGF-1		10–15 yr	Annual
		MRI pituitary	10–15 yr	5 yearly

PTH = parathyroid hormone; US = ultrasound; MRI = magnetic resonance imaging; IGF-1 = insulin-like growth factor 1.
Reproduced from (17) with permission.

required suggest the discretion of waiting until the child has reached 10 yr of age. The goal of vigilant screening is to detect biochemical evidence of tumors before they become symptomatic or malignant. Screening for primary hyperparathyroidism with annual measurement of plasma total calcium is suggested. The intact-parathyrod hormone (PTH) concentration should be measured if the calcium concentration is elevated. Imaging for primary hyperparathyroidism is not indicated as a screening tool. Pancreatic neuroendocrine tumors should be screened for with yearly measurement of plasma gastrin and pancreatic polypeptide concentrations, accompanied by annual transabdominal pancreatic ultrasound. T1-weighted contrast-enhanced MRI of the pancreas every 3 yr has been suggested (9,17). Screening for pituitary involvement with annual measurement of serum prolactin and IGF-1 is suggested, and IGF-1 should be measured at a lab with age-adjusted norms, bearing in mind that IGF-1 concentrations in adolescents during the accelerated height growth of puberty are above the normal range for adults. Pituitary MRI every 5 yr is recommended.

MULTIPLE ENDOCRINE NEOPLASIA TYPE 2

Introduction

Since the initial description of the MEN 2 syndromes 40 yr ago (30), a gradual advance in understanding of these syndromes of endocrine gland tumorigenesis has revolutionized clinical practice. Recognition of the clinical components and inheritance patterns comprised the most basic level of understanding, and was followed by the development of methods for screening for the syndrome before overt symptoms became apparent (31). The final step in this course to date has been the delineation of activating point mutations of the *RET* proto-oncogene as the initiating molecular defect for both the MEN 2 syndrome and the familial medullary thyroid carcinoma (FMTC) variant (32,33). This has allowed predictive DNA testing of at-risk family members to be performed with great accuracy.

The MEN 2 syndromes are composed of the following distinct categories: MEN 2A, MEN 2B, and FMTC. MEN 2A is the most common form, and includes medullary thyroid carcinoma (MTC) in association with pheochromocytoma and parathyroid

Table 2
Incidence of Clinical Features in the MEN-2 Syndromes

	MEN 2A	MEN 2B	FMTC
MTC	>90%	>90%	100%
Parathyroid hyperplasia	20%	~0%	0%
Pheochromocytoma	≤ 50%	50%	0%
Mucosal ganglioneuromatosis	0%	~100%	0%

hyperplasia *(34)*. The additional feature of a pruritic skin rash caused by the deposition of keratin-like peptides in the dermal-epidermal junction characterizes the variant of MEN 2A known as cutaneous lichen amyloidosis (CLA) *(35,36)*. MEN 2B accounts for about 5% of all MEN 2 cases. The findings are similar to those of MEN 2A, with the additional unique features of both a Marfanoid habitus (without the lens, palate, or cardiac anomalies associated with true Marfan's syndrome), and diffuse ganglioneuromatosis of the alimentary tract and ocular system *(37, reviewed in 38)*. The unique features of MEN 2B, owing to the unsubtle presence of diffuse ganglioneuromatosis, may result in a characteristic appearance identifiable early in childhood. Parathyroid hyperplasia is almost universally absent in MEN 2B *(34)*. FMTC is a distinct entity, which occurs without associated endocrinopathy *(39)*. The incidence of the clinical manifestations associated with each of these variants is summarized in Table 2.

MEDULLARY THYROID CARCINOMA

Although only 20% of all cases of medullary thyroid carcinoma (MTC) are associated with MEN 2, more than 90% of those affected with the MEN 2 syndrome will develop MTC, often as the initial manifestation of disease *(40)*. MTC of the MEN 2 syndrome is a bilateral, multifocal process most likely to be present in the upper and middle thirds of the lateral thyroid lobes. Hyperplastic change of the C-cell has been demonstrated to be the precursor of MTC *(41)*. The time course for the progression from C-cell hyperplasia to microscopic carcinoma, metastasis, or both remains unclear, but may take years (reviewed in *38,42*). However, in those with MEN 2A, C-cell hyperplasia has been demonstrated as early as 20 mo of age *(43)*, MTC as early as 3 yr of age *(44)*, and metastatic disease as early as 6 yr of age *(45)*. In general, the MTC of MEN 2B is more aggressive, with an earlier clinical presentation of neoplasia *(46)*, and C-cell hyperplasia has been demonstrated at birth in patients with this form of endocrinopathy *(43)*. Because of the capacity of MEN 2-related MTC to present so early, prophylactic thyroidectomy is recommended by the age of 3 yr in children known to harbor the genetic mutation.

PHEOCHROMOCYTOMA

MEN 2-related pheochromocytoma usually presents later than MTC. Less than 20% of patients with this tumor present earlier than 20 yr of age, and it is rarely detected before the onset of MTC *(42)*. As with MTC, the pheochromocytomas of MEN 2 are usually multicentric and are found in the context of diffuse adrenomedullary hyperplasia *(36)*. About half of pheochromocytomas are bilateral in the MEN 2 syndromes *(47)*. Malignant pheochromocytoma is a rare feature of the MEN 2 syndrome, with an incidence in the range of 0–8% *(47,48)*.

The classic history of facial flushing, episodic hypertension, and headache is not reliably present in MEN 2-related pheochromocytoma. Clinical manifestations are usually subtle, and more than half of individuals are asymptomatic and normotensive. Early clinical signs and symptoms of adrenal medullary hyperplasia or of pheochromocytoma in MEN 2 include palpitations, nervousness, and jitteriness. Initial biochemical findings include elevated plasma epinephrine concentrations, with an increase in the ratio of epinephrine to norepinephrine in timed urine collections (reviewed in *49*).

PRIMARY HYPERPARATHYROIDISM

Approximately 20% of MEN 2A patients develop hyperparathyroidism as a later manifestation of the syndrome *(27)*. The usual pathologic findings are those of chief cell hyperplasia involving multiple glands *(36)*. Pheochromocytoma is a rare cause of hypercalcemia, but should be ruled out prior to parathyroid exploration in those with MEN 2 *(42)*.

DIAGNOSTIC GUIDELINES: SCREENING FOR THE PRESENCE OF MEN 2

Genetics of MEN 2 Syndromes

All current discussions of screening paradigms for the presence of MEN 2 must be prefaced by an understanding of the molecular genetics of the disorder, since current standards of care are predicated on methods of DNA-testing. The MEN 2 syndromes are either inherited as autosomal-dominant disorders or occur as new mutations in the absence of a family history for the syndrome. In 1987, the gene locus for *MEN 2* was linked to the centromeric region of chromosome 10 *(49,50)*. Subsequently, single activating point mutations within the *RET* proto-oncogene were found to be associated with the range of clinical phenotypes of the MEN 2 syndrome (reviewed in *51*). The *RET* gene, which maps to chromosome 10q11.2, encodes a transmembrane protein of the receptor tyrosine kinase family and is expressed in derivatives and tumors of neural crest origin (reviewed in *38* and *51*). The activating mutations that cause MEN 2 are located in either the first cysteine-rich extracellular domain (codons 609, 611, 618, 620, 630, 634) or in an intracellular region affecting codons 768, 790, 791, 804, 891, and 918 (reviewed in *38*). Codon 634 mutations are found to be present in about 80% of individuals affected with the classic MEN 2A syndrome, although a small percentage of families harboring this mutation have FMTC only. MEN 2B is most commonly associated with a germline codon 918 mutation. Codon 883 mutations may also occur in those affected with MEN 2B (reviewed in *52*).

Prior to the era of a molecular genetic screening approach for the MEN 2 syndrome, the preferred screening method for MTC was provocative stimulation of calcitonin release using pentagastrin stimulation *(42)*. The test is administered by giving 0.5 µg/kg of pentagastrin as an intravenous bolus over 5–10 s and calcitonin measurements are made at 2 and 5 min. Commonly experienced side effects that usually resolve within 2–3 min, include nausea, flushing, and substernal tightness.

There are clear advantages to the use of DNA-testing in at-risk family members as opposed to screening by pentagastrin stimulation testing and measurement of calcitonin levels. First, DNA testing allows the possibility of detection of the presence of the MEN 2 syndrome prior to the development of C-cell abnormalities. Second, it eliminates the need for repeated pentagastrin testing, which is unpleasant at best and therefore may make compliance with annual testing an issue. Finally, DNA testing eliminates the false-positive rate of the pentagastrin test, estimated at 3–5%, and the variable reported specificity *(52)*. Screening for RET germ-line mutations can be performed at any age, but children at risk should be screened by 3 yr of age, when possible. To avoid the possibility of potential sample misclassification or test error, many centers recommend testing of two samples drawn on different occasions prior to referral for surgical intervention *(53)*. In addition to those with established MEN 2, 6–8% of those with MTC and no apparent family history for the disorder nonetheless harbor germ-line RET mutations and, therefore, would have the risk of familial transmission. Because of this, it has been thought prudent to also offer *RET* gene screening to those with apparent sporadic MTC *(54)*. Multiple centers now offer screening of genomic DNA obtained from peripheral blood samples for mutations of the RET locus. Perhaps the greatest difficulty occurs in the rare situation where germ-line transmission of MTC is proven, but no *RET* gene mutations are identified. It becomes necessary in this case to identify a research laboratory that will analyze regions of the RET gene outside the most commonly mutated regions *(55)*.

Screening: Pheochromocytoma and Hyperparathyroidism

Annual screening for pheochromocytoma should be performed beginning at around age 6 yr and is accomplished by a thorough review of relevant signs and symptoms and measurement of urine or plasma catecholamine levels *(56)*. Hypertensive encephalopathy secondary to a pheochromocytoma in MEN 2A has been described in a 13-yr-old child *(57)*. The presence of pheochromocytoma must be ruled out prior to any operative procedure.

It is currently recommended that screening for hyperparathyroidism in patients with MEN 2A consist of a measurement of serum calcium every other year after the age of 10 yr. An elevated level should be followed up with parathyroid hormone measurements. Treatment is as discussed above for MEN 1-related primary hyperparathyroidism.

Management of MEN 2 Kindreds: Incorporating Genetic Data

The availability of the highly sensitive and specific DNA-based screening for identification of the MEN 2 syndromes spares half of patients at risk–those without a demonstrable genetic mutation–from further specialized medical follow-up. Because pheochromocytoma is rarely malignant in the MEN 2 syndromes, genetic identification of a RET mutation does not dictate prophylactic surgical therapy. Hyperparathyroidism occurs in the minority of patients and also does not have malignant potential. Therefore, recommendations for screening for these components of the syndrome remain unchanged by the recent genetic advances, with the exception that only those with mutations demonstrated by DNA-based testing need to undergo recurrent screening.

Most influenced by the advent of DNA-based diagnostic testing is the management of MTC. The opportunity to improve the outcome for those with MTC lies in the performance of a safe and comprehensive initial surgical procedure *(52,53)*. Multiple studies have demonstrated that stage of disease at diagnosis most accurately predicts the length of patient survival (reviewed in *52*). Current recommendations are for prophylactic thyroidectomy to occur in the early preschool yr for those with positive DNA-based testing, typically before 5 yr of age, and with some centers pursuing intervention at 3 yr of age. For those with MEN 2B, the more aggressive form, prophylactic thyroidectomy is recommended as early as possible *(52)*.

CONCLUSION

When not recognized and treated definitively, the multiple endocrine neoplasia syndromes are capable of producing significant morbidity and mortality. The past reliance upon biochemical screening of all children from families with a history of MEN has given way to molecular genetic analysis and conclusive identification of children at risk. This has allowed screening efforts to focus upon those individuals known to be genetically at-risk, and relieves those *not* at-risk, of needless, costly, and often difficult surveillance. At the same time, better experience with screening at-risk children has yielded further benefit in improved biochemical and radiographic screening protocols, and has significantly enhanced the odds of prospective diagnosis of the presence of disease. Still, the management of some MEN-related tumors remains challenging. Further advancement in medical and surgical treatment is expected, and looked for with anticipation.

REFERENCES

1. Wermer P. Genetic aspects of adenomatosis of endocrine glands. Am J Med 1954;16:363–367.
2. Waterlot C, Porchett N, Bauters C, et al. Type 1 multiple endocrine neoplasia (MEN1): contribution of genetic analysis to the screening and follow-up of a large French kindred. Clin Endocrinol 1991;51:101–107.
3. Trump D, Farren B, Wooding C, et.al.: Clinical studies of multiple endocrine neoplasia type 1 (MEN1). Q J Med 1996;89:653–669.
4. Veldhuis JD, Norton JA, Wells SA, Vinik AI, Perry RR. Therapeutic Controversy: Surgical versus Medical Management of Multiple Endocrine Neoplasia (MEN) Type 1. J Clin Endocrin Metab 1997;82:357–364.
5. Hoff AO, Gagel RF. Multiple endocrine neoplasia types 1 and 2: phenotype, genotype, diagnosis, and therapeutic plan with special reference to children and adolescents. Curr Opin Endocrin Diab 1997;4:91–99.
6. Chandrasekharappa SC, Guru SC, Manickam P, et al. Positional cloning of the gene for multiple endocrine neoplasia-type 1. Science 1997;276:404–407.
7. Benson L, Ljunghall S, Åkerström G, Öberg K. Hyperparathyroidism presenting as the first lesion in multiple endocrine neoplasia type 1. Am J Med 1987;82:731–737
8. Marx S, Spiegel AM, Skarulis MC, Doppman JL, Collins FS, Liotta LA. Multiple Endocrine Neoplasia Type 1: Clinical and Genetic Topics. Ann Int Med 1988;129(6):484–494.
9. Chanson P, Cadiot G, Murat A. Management of Patients and Subjects at Risk for Multiple Endocrine Neoplasia Type 1: MEN 1. Horm Res 47:211–220, 1997.
10. Block MA. Familial hyperparathyroidism and hyperparathyroidism associated with multiple endocrine neoplasia syndrome. In: Cady B, Rossi RL, eds. Surgery of the Thyroid and Parathyroid Glands, 3rd ed. W.B. Saunders, Philadelphia, 1991.
11. Ballard HS, Frame B, Hartsock RJ, Familial multiple endocrine adenoma-peptic ulcer complex. Medicine 1964;43:481–516.
12. Skogseid B, Eriksson B, Lundqvist G, et al. Multiple Endocrine Neoplasia Type 1: A 10-Year Prospective Screening Study in Four Kindreds. J Clin Endocrinol Metab 1991;73:281–287.
13. Eberle F, Grum R. Multiple endocrine neoplasia type 1 (MEN-I). Ergberg Inn Med Kinderheilkd 1981;46:76–149.
14. Malmaeus J, Benson L, Johansson H, et.al.: Parathyroid surgery in the multiple endocrine neoplasia type 1 syndrome: Choice of surgical procedure. World J Surg 1986;10:668–672.
15. Thompson NW. The techniques of initial parathyroid explorative and reoperative parathyroidectomy. In: Thompson NW, Vinik AI, eds. Endocrine Surgery Update. Grune and Stratton, New York, NY, 1983, pp. 365–383.
16. Rizzoli R, Green J III, Marx SJ. Primary hyperparathyroidism in familial multiple endocrine neoplasia type 1: Long term follow-up of serum calcium levels after parathyroidectomy. Am J Med 1985;78: 467–474.
17. Johnston LB, Chew SL, Trainer PJ, et al. Screening children at risk of developing inherited endocrine neoplasia syndromes. Clin Endocrinol 2000;52:127–136.

18. Thompson NW. The surgical management of hyperparathyroidism and endocrine disease of the pancreas in the multiple endocrine neoplasia type 1 patient. J Intern Med 1995;238:269–280.
19. Roy PK, Venzon DJ, Shojamanesh H, et al. Zollinger-Ellison Syndrome. Medicine 2000;79:46–49.
20. Gagel RF. Multiple endocrine neoplasia. In: Wilson JD, Foster DW, Kronenberg HM, Larsen PR, eds. Williams Textbook of Endocrinology, 9th ed. Saunders, Philadelphia, 1998, pp.1630–1631.
21. Skogseid, B, Öberg K, Benson L, et al. A standardized meal stimulation test of the endocrine pancreas for early detection of pancreatic endocrine tumors in MEN type 1 syndrome: five yr experience. J Clin Endocrinol Metab 1987;64:1233–1240.
22. Cryer PE, Polonsky KS. Glucose homeostasis and hypoglycemia. In: Wilson JD, Foster DW, Kronenberg HM, Larsen PR, eds. Williams Textbook of Endocrinology, 9th ed. Saunders, Philadelphia, 1998, p. 959.
23. Skogseid B, Grama D, Rastad J, et al. Operative tumour yield obviates preoperative pancreatic tumour localization in multiple endocrine neoplasia type 1. J Intern Med 1995;238:281–288.
24. Colao A, Loche S, Cappabianca P, de Divitiis E, Lombardi G. Pituitary adenomas in children and adolescents. Clinical presentation, diagnosis, and therapeutic strategies. The Endocrinologist 2000;10:314–327.
25. Mindermann T, Wilson CB. Pediatric pituitary adenomas. Neurosurgery 1995; 36:259–269.
26. Thorner MO, Vance ML, Laws ER, Horvath E, Kovacs K. In: Wilson JD, Foster DW, Kronenberg HM, Larsen PR, eds. Williams Textbook of Endocrinology, 9th ed. Saunders, Philadelphia, 1998, pp. 300–301.
27. Lafferty AR, Chrousos GP. Pituitary tumors in children and adolescence. J Clin Endocrinol Metab 1999;84;4317–4323.
28. Agarwal SK, Guru SC, Heppner C, et al. Menin interacts with the AP1 transcription factor JunD and represses JunD-activated transcription. Cell 1999;96:143–152.
29. Huang SC, Zhuang Z, Weil RJ, et al. Nuclear/cytoplasmic localisation of the multiple endocrine neoplasia type 1 gene product, menin. Lab Invest.1999;79:301–310.
30. Sipple JH. The association of pheochromocytoma with carcinoma of the thyroid gland. Am J Med 1961;31:163–166.
31. Tashjian AH Jr, Howland BG, Melin KEW, Hill CS Jr. Immunoassay of human calcitonin: clinical measurement, relation to serum calcium and studies in patients with medullary carcinoma. N Engl J Med 1970;283:90–95.
32. Mulligan LM, Kwok JBJ, Healey CS, et al. Germ-line mutations of the RET proto-oncogene in multiple endocrine neoplasia type 2A. Nature 1993;363:458–461.
33. Donis-Keller H, Dou S, Chi D, et al. Mutations in the RET proto-oncogene are associated with MEN 2A and FMTC. Hum Mol Genet 1993;2:851–856.
34. Saad MF, Ordonez NG, Rashid RK, et al. Medullary carcinoma of the thyroid: a study of the clinical features and prognostic factors in 161 patients. Medicine 1984;63:319–442.
35. Nunziata V, Giannattosio R, di Giovanni G, D'Armiento MR, Mancini M. Hereditary localized pruritus in affected members of a kindred with multiple endocrine neoplasia type 2A (Sipple's syndrome). Clin Endocrinol 1989;30:57–63.
36. Gagel RF, Levy ML, Donovan DT, Alford BR, Wheeler T, Tschen JA. Multiple endocrine neoplasia type 2a associated with cutaneous lichen amyloidosis. Ann Inter Med 1989;111:802–806.
37. Williams ED, Pollock DJ. Multiple mucosa neuromata with endocrine tumours. A syndrome allied to von Recklinghausen's disease. J Pathol Bacteriol 1966;91:71–80.
38. Eng C. RET proto-oncogene in the development of human cancer. J Clin Oncol 1999;17:380–393.
39. Farndon JR, Leight GS, Dilley WG, et al. Familial medullary thyroid carcinoma without associated endocrinopathies: a distinct clinical entity. Br J Surg 1986;73:2278–2281.
40. Padberg BC, Holl K, Schroder S. Pathology of multiple endocrine neoplasia 2A and 2B: a review. Horm Res 1992;38 (Suppl 2):24–30.
41. Wolfe HJ, Melvin KE, Cervi-Skinner SJ, et al. C-cell hyperplasia preceding medullary thyroid carcinoma. N Engl J Med 1973;289:437–441.
42. Gagel RF, Tashjian AH Jr, Cummings T, et al. The clinical outcome of prospective screening for multiple endocrine neoplasia type 2a: an 18-year experience. N Engl J Med 1988;318:478–484.
43. Gagel RF, Jackson CE, Block MA, et al. Age-related probability of development of hereditary medullary thyroid carcinoma. J Pediatr 1982;101:941–946.
44. Telander RL, Zimmerman D, van Heerden JA, Sizemore GW. Results of early thyroidectomy for medullary thyroid carcinoma in children with multiple endocrine neoplasia type 2. J Pediatr Surg 1986;21:1190–1194.

45. Graham SM, Genel M, Touloukian RJ, Barwick KW, Gertner JM, Torony C. Provocative testing for occult medullary carcinoma of the thyroid: findings in seven children with MEN type IIa. J Pediatr Surg 1987;22:501–503.
46. Norton JA, Froome LC, Farrell RE, Wells SA Jr. MEN 2b. The most aggressive form of medullary thyroid carcinoma. Surg Clin North Am 1979;59:109–118.
47. Scott HW, Halter SA. Oncologic aspects of pheochromocytoma: the importance of follow-up. Surgery 1984;96:1061–1066.
48. Stenstrom G, Ernest I, Tisell LE. Long-term results in 64 patients operated upon for pheochromocytoma. Acta Med Scand 1988;223:345–352.
49. Mathew CG, Chin KS, Easton DF, et al. A linked genetic marker for multiple endocrine neoplasia type 2A on chromosome 10. Nature 1987;328:527–528.
50. Simpson NE, Kidd KK, Goodfellow PJ, et al. Assignment of multiple endocrine neoplasia type 2A on chromosome 10 by linkage. Nature 1987;328:528–530.
51. Ponder BAJ. The phenotypes associated with RET mutations in the multiple endocrine neoplasia type 2 syndrome. Cancer Res Suppl. 59 1999;59:1736s–1742s.
52. Evans DR, Fleming JB, Lee JE, Cote G, Gagel RF. The surgical treatment of medullary thyroid carcinoma. Sem Surg Oncol 1999;16:50–63.
53. Kebebew E, Tresler PA, Siperstein AE, Duh QY, Clark OH. Normal thyroid pathology in patients undergoing thyroidectomy for finding a RET gene germline mutation: a report of three cases and review of the literature. Thyroid 1999;9:127–131.
54. Stratakis CA, Ball DW. A concise genetic and clinical guide to multiple endocrine neoplasia and related syndromes. J Pediatr Endocrinol Metab. 2000;13:457–465.
55. Gagel RF. Multiple Endocrine Neoplasia type 2 - Impact of genetic screening on management. In: Arnold, A, ed. Endocrine Neoplasms, Kluwer Academic, 1997, pp. 421–441.
56. Gagel RF. Multiple endocrine neoplasia type 2. In: Degroot LJ, Jameson JL, eds. Endocrinology, 4th ed., WB Saunders, Philadelphia, 2001, pp. 2424–2425.
57. Jadoul M, Leo JR, Berends MJ, et al. Pheochromocytoma-induced hypertensive encephalopathy revealing MEN 2A syndrome in a 13-year old boy: implications for screening procedures and surgery. Horm Metab Res Suppl 1989;21:46–49.

IX ENDOCRINE AND CRITICAL ILLNESS

30 The Endocrine Response to Critical Illness

Michael S. D. Agus, MD

CONTENTS

> PARADIGM OF ENDOCRINE RESPONSE TO ACUTE VERSUS CHRONIC CRITICAL ILLNESS
> ADRENAL AXIS
> THYROID AXIS
> GROWTH HORMONE AXIS
> GONADAL AXIS
> POTENTIAL FOR THERAPEUTIC HORMONAL INTERVENTIONS TO TREAT THE PROTEIN CATABOLISM OF CRITICAL ILLNESS
> REFERENCES

PARADIGM OF ENDOCRINE RESPONSE TO ACUTE VERSUS CHRONIC CRITICAL ILLNESS

The traditional view of the hormonal response to critical illness, including severe infection, trauma, and hemodynamic collapse, has described a singular set of changes. Over recent years, however, clinical research has uncovered two unique sets of responses to severe illness: one to the acute onset, and a chronic response stimulated by the continuation of extreme stress (Fig. 1).

The acute response is considered fully adaptive, and involves changes in every hormonal axis. It involves stimulation of the hypothalamic-pituitary-adrenal (HPA) axis, peripheral inactivation of the hypothalamic-pituitary-thyroid (HPT) and hypothalamic-pituitary-gonadal (HPG) axes, induction of insulin resistance, and upregulated secretion of growth hormone (GH) and prolactin (PRL).

The chronic response, on the other hand, involves central suppression of the HPT, HPG and GH axes as well as decreased production of PRL. These changes are associated with continued insulin resistance and the onset of a profound protein catabolic state, which has, to date, not been reversible and is associated with significant morbidity and mortality. With the advent of modern critical care, humans may survive prolonged catastrophic illness that would have been universally fatal prior to the development of artificial life support technologies. It can be argued, therefore, that the hormonal response

From: *Contemporary Endocrinology: Pediatric Endocrinology: A Practical Clinical Guide*
Edited by: S. Radovick and M. H. MacGillivray © Humana Press Inc., Totowa, NJ

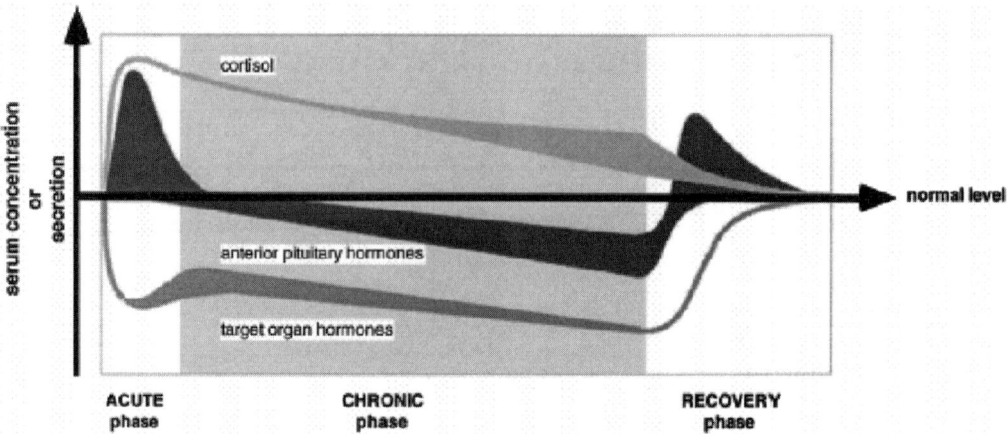

Fig. 1. Endocrine changes in critical illness. At the onset of illness, anterior pituitary hormones surge with an associated peripheral inactivation of target organ hormones. Once the chronic response has been engaged, the sensitivity to pituitary hormones is restored, but both remain low due to failure of the pituitary to resume normal secretory activity. (Reproduced with permission from Van den Berghe, G., de Zegher, F. & Bouillon, R. Clinical review 95: Acute and prolonged critical illness as different neuroendocrine paradigms. J Clin Endocrinol Metab 1998;83:1828.)

to this unnatural scenario may not be adaptive, as any response would have been inadequate to yield a meaningful evolutionary survival advantage. In fact, a close examination of these hormonal responses demonstrates what can be reasonably considered quite maladaptive changes.

ADRENAL AXIS

The adrenocortical response to critical illness is arguably the single most important hormonal response. Lacking it, patients may quickly succumb to their illness, as documented by Brown-Sequard in 1856 *(1)*. The initial response is characterized by high serum adrenocorticotropic hormone (ACTH) and cortisol concentrations. A high level of cortisol, up to six times normal, produces profound insulin resistance that accelerates glycogenolysis and mobilizes precursors for gluconeogenesis via increased protein catabolism and lipolysis—creating a relative shunt of energy resources away from peripheral organs and towards brain and heart. It also promotes intravascular fluid retention, enhances the inotropic and vasopressor response to catecholamines and angiotensin II, and suppresses the immune response. This suppression is thought to be important in preventing an overexuberant, and potentially destructive, immune response *(2)*.

Once the patient enters the chronic phase of critical illness, ACTH levels decrease, while cortisol concentrations remain elevated. Potential suppressors of ACTH and stimulators of cortisol production include atrial natriuretic peptide, substance P, and endothelin. Production of other adrenal steroids, including mineralocorticoids and androgens are relatively suppressed during the chronic phase. This appears to constitute an overall shift by the adrenal towards prioritizing cortisol production.

The potential disadvantages of this hormonal constellation include increased protein catabolism leading to impaired wound healing and myopathy, as well as continued immune suppression at a time when the patient becomes increasingly susceptible to

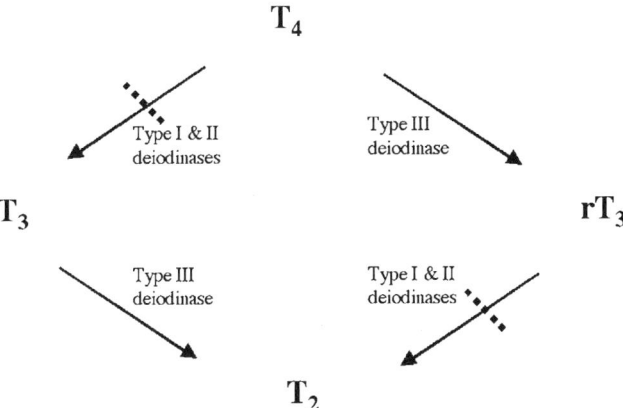

Fig. 2. Thyroid hormone metabolism. --- indicates downregulation of Type I and II deiodinases in critical illness leading to a decreased T_3, increased rT_3, and having no direct effect on T_4.

infectious complications. Potential benefits may relate to the hemodynamic effects, both direct and indirect, mediated through the adrenal medulla. Epinephrine is produced via methylation of norepinephrine by phenylethanolamine-N-methyltransferase (PNMT), whose mRNA expression and enzymatic activity are induced by high intra-adrenal concentrations of cortisol (estimated at 50 times above circulating concentrations). These high intra-adrenal concentrations are only achievable if normal cortisol synthesis continues in the adrenal cortex *(3,4)*.

Diagnosis

The diagnosis and therapy of adrenal insufficiency are discussed in a different chapter.

THYROID AXIS

Assessing thyroid function in healthy as well as critically ill patients is a non-exact science. Ultimately, a clinician is concerned about quantifying the systemic metabolic actions of circulating thyroid hormones, then determining whether that level of activity is appropriate to the given clinical scenario. As there is currently no available measure of peripheral thyroid function, we generally depend on each patient's own thyroid stimulating hormone (TSH) serum concentration to give us an index of whether the brain is satisfied with the total production of thyroxine (T_4) and triiodothyronine (T_3). In the critically ill patient, however, this is no longer relevant, as the TSH level may remain in the normal range despite a low T_3 concentration, and possibly a low T_4 as well. This constellation of thyroid function tests has been named the "sick euthyroid syndrome" as well as the "low T_3 syndrome" and hypothyroxinemia of "non-thyroidal illness" (NTI).

The two most significant components of NTI are the drop in T_3 and the concomitant failure of TSH to rise in response. Within hours of the onset of acute illness or trauma, circulating T_3 concentrations decline significantly due both to decreased conversion of T_4 to T_3 by the outer-ring monodeiodinases (Types I and II; *see* Fig. 2) *(5)* and to increased turnover of thyroid hormones *(6)*. T_4 uptake by the liver is also suppressed, reducing the available substrate for conversion to T_3 *(7)*. The magnitude of this drop in T_3 within the first 24 h reflects the severity of illness *(8)*.

Under normal conditions, 35–40% of the T_4 produced by the thyroid is eventually monodeiodinated to T_3, accounting for almost all (80–90%) of circulating T_3 *(9)*. The thyroid directly produces the remaining percentage. As type I and II monodeiodinases are suppressed, excess T_4 is converted by type III monodeiodinases into the biologically inactive reverse T_3 (rT_3), and circulating T_3 is degraded into T_2. This peripheral inactivation of thyroid hormones characterizes the acute phase of critical illness. It is adaptive for the patient in that it produces decreased overall metabolic rate, allowing available resources to remain available for critical functions: brain, heart, and immune system.

In the chronic phase, TSH concentrations begin to decline into the lower third of the normal range, despite low circulating T_3 and possibly T_4. In addition to absolute levels being depressed, TSH pulsatility is diminished, hypothalamic thyrotropin releasing hormone (TRH) is suppressed, and both correlate with low serum T_3 *(10,11)*. These argue for a hypothalamic etiology of the euthyroid sick syndrome in the chronic phase of critical illness. Supporting this is the ability of TRH infusion to re-establish normal TSH pulsatility and increased T_3 and T_4 concentrations *(12)*. In prolonged critical illness, these changes may become maladaptive, as normal levels of T_3 are required for protein synthesis, lipolysis, fuel utilization by muscle, and GH secretion and responsiveness.

Diagnosis

The clinical effects of low serum concentrations of T_4 and T_3 may be difficult to discern in the critically ill patient, and the indications for therapy are therefore difficult to define. Physiologic effects of a deficiency in thyroid hormones include elevated systemic vascular resistance by up to 50%, decreased cardiac output, hyponatremia, hypoglycemia, hypercholesterolemia, induction of a hypocoagulable state, hypothermia, and decreased metabolic rate *(13)*. Additionally, in children, pulmonary function and the ventilatory response to hypoxia are diminished in this setting *(9)*. Though individual responses vary, these factors are rarely significant enough to warrant thyroid hormone therapy, in the absence of true hypothyroidism.

Necessary information prior to instituting therapy includes a full panel of thyroid function tests (TFTs), including TSH, total T_4, total T_3 and an index of unbound thyroid binding globulin (TBG) *(1)*. Depending on the complexity of the clinical scenario, an rT_3 level may be helpful, as well, although it is generally not available in a timely fashion. Given the variability of techniques and accuracy of the various measurements of free T_4 and T_3, they are not recommended as part of standard thyroid function testing at this time.

The most likely laboratory value to be abnormal in children with hypothyroxinemia of NTI is the total T_3. Free T_3, however, when measured by equilibrium dialysis and radioimmunoassay, was found to be normal in 21 of 25 (84%) adults with NTI *(14)*. Thus, the laboratory difference may, in fact, be caused by alterations in binding rather than absolute drops in hormonal concentrations.

rT_3 measurement in NTI may be helpful early on in the course, as excess T_4 is converted to rT_3, instead of T_3. After the syndrome has been established for several days, however, and T_4 production is decreased, less substrate may be available for conversion to rT_3, and the serum concentration may be misleadingly low. Unfortunately, while these laboratory value changes are common, they are not absolute and not diagnostic *(15)*. Furthermore, rT_3 may be decreased in patients with renal failure, AIDS, and occasionally elevated in patients with mild hypothyroidism.

Measurement of TSH must be accomplished using a third-generation assay, and ought to be interpreted in the context of the patient's overall clinical condition. During the acute phase of illness TSH may be slightly elevated. During the chronic phase, it is usually normal or slightly low. During a period of clinical recovery, however, TSH is generally elevated above the normal range, driving a resurgence of T_4 output from the thyroid. The most reliable way to identify the etiology for a high TSH level is to obtain a repeat set of TFTs 5–7 d later: if the abnormalities are associated with clinical recovery, T_4, T_3, and TSH will each have migrated closer to normal range, while in primary hypothyroidism, the TSH will remain elevated.

A final helpful measurement in NTI is an index of free T_4 or T_3 (e.g., thyroid binding globulin index [TBGI], thyroid hormone binding resin [THBR], T_3 resin uptake [T3RU]). An elevated index, indicating a paucity of available TBG binding sites, has been consistently associated with NTI, and not primary hypothyroidism.

Another significant consideration prior to instituting therapy is concomitant medications. Many of those commonly used in the intensive care unit (ICU) setting have profound effects on various aspects of the HPT axis, and are listed in Table 1 *(16)*.

Treatment

NON-THYROIDAL ILLNESS

Direct supplementation with thyroid hormone in the setting of NTI currently does not appear to be beneficial in non-cardiac adult patients, as demonstrated in two PRCTs *(17,18)*. It cannot, therefore, be recommended as standard therapy for NTI in non-cardiac pediatric critically ill patients. If, however, T_3 is extremely low and important clinical sequelae of hypothyroxinemia are apparent, including severely elevated SVR, severe hyponatremia, and/or uncontrolled coagulopathy, therapy may be justified, although no data are currently available regarding this issue.

POST-OPERATIVE CARDIAC PATIENTS

T_3 may have beneficial inotropic and chronotropic effects on the myocardium, as demonstrated by clinical data obtained from T_3 infusions in brain dead organ donors *(19)*. This data prompted two prospective, randomized, controlled trials (PRCTs) in post-operative cardiac adults and one in children. In adults, no benefit was demonstrated with an intravenous load of 0.8 µg/kg, followed by an infusion of 0.11–0.12 µg/kg/h *(20,21)*. A recent PRCT in neonates after cardiac surgery, however, did show promising benefits, as post-operative myocardial function was improved and the need for postoperative intensive care was reduced using an intravenous loading dose 2 µg/kg, followed on subsequent days with 1 µg/kg/d *(22)*.

CHOICE OF THERAPEUTIC AGENT AND DOSE

Levothyroxine is the mainstay of thyroid hormone replacement strategies, although with replacement in the setting of critical illness, rT_3 may rise without any increase in T_3 *(18)*. For patients with diagnosed hypothyroidism, which is not associated with NTI, their T_4 therapy should be continued at their usual dose while in the ICU. Based on incomplete absorption of enteral T_4, 75% of the enteral dose should be given intravenously to those patients who cannot continue to take the medication enterally *(23)*.

A continuous intravenous infusion of T_3, in the unique situation of severe hypothyroidism, on the other hand, may theoretically be titrated to the desired T_3 concentration and effect. The danger of a T_3 infusion is that overdosage may result in a fatal arrhythmia, and a prolonged infusion would be expected to fully suppress TSH, creating an iatrogenic risk of myxedema coma upon cessation of therapy. General recommendations

Table 1
Drugs That Influence Thyroid Function (Data adapted with permission
from Surks MI, Sievert R. Drugs and thyroid function. N Engl J Med 1995;333, 1691.)

Drugs that decrease TSH secretion
Dopamine
Glucocorticoids
Octreotide
Drugs that alter thyroid hormone secretion
Decreased thyroid hormone secretion
Lithium
Iodide
Amiodarone
Aminoglutethimide
Increased thyroid hormone secretion
Iodide
Amiodarone

Drugs that decrease T4 absorption
Colestipol
Cholestyramine
Aluminum hydroxide
Ferrous sulfate
Sucralfate

Drugs that alter T4 and T3 transport in serum
Increased serum TBG concentration
Estrogens
Tamoxifen
Heroin
Methadone
Mitotane
Fluorouracil
Decreased serum TBG concentration
Androgens
Anabolic steroids (e.g., danazol)
Slow-release nicotinic acid
Glucocorticoids
Displacement from protein-binding sites
Furosemide
Fenclofenac
Mefenamic acid
Salicylates

Drugs that alter T4 and T3 metabolism
Increased hepatic metabolism
Phenobarbital
Rifampin
Phenytoin
Carbamazepine
Decreased T4 5'-monodeiodinase activity
Propylthiouracil
Amiodarone
Beta-adrenergic-antagonist drugs
Glucocorticoids

Cytokines
Interferon alfa
Interleukin-2

even for the treatment of myxedema coma do not recommend sole therapy with T_3, rather a combination of T_3 and T_4 *(24)*.

Continuous infusion of TRH is a theoretical treatment that has been demonstrated, in the chronic phase of critical illness, to be effective in restoring normal TSH pulsatility and increasing T_4 and T_3 concentrations *(12)*. It is a safer option than direct end hormone replacement, as the negative feedback exerted by thyroid hormones on the thyrotropes is maintained, thus precluding overstimulation of the thyroid axis. No clinical outcome data has yet been reported.

GROWTH HORMONE AXIS

The response of the GH axis to stress also follows a bi-phasic response to critical illness: acute and chronic. In the acute phase, GH increases by a factor of three to five above baseline, initially associated with a concomitant rise in insulin-like growth factor (IGF-I). After several days of critical illness, GH continues to have an elevated baseline level, with pulsatile secretion at a rate similar to healthy controls, but with a lower pulse amplitude. During this latter period, a single GH/IGF-1 ratio may be elevated well above normal, indicating what has been described as a state of GH insensitivity *(25)*. The integrated production of GH over time, however, is decreased, and IGF-I is known to be much more responsive to pulsatile GH production *(26)*. Furthermore, unlike the acute phase of critical illness, during the chronic phase normal GH pulsatility and normal concentrations of IGF-I can be restored by continuous infusion of GH secretagogues *(27)*. These data suggest a primary hypothalamic origin for the alterations in the GH axis during chronic critical illness, and not GH insensitivity.

Important non-hypothalamic regulators of GH secretion in the ICU setting include thyroid hormone, glucocorticoids, and dopamine. In the setting of true hypothyroidism or the hypothyroxinemia of non-thyroidal illness, GH has markedly decreased pulsatility. This is predominantly a pituitary effect, as thyroid hormones are needed for GH gene transcription, translation, and GH secretion, but there are documented hypothalamic and peripheral effects as well *(28,29)*.

Glucocorticoids acutely stimulate GH secretion, but beyond 12 h lead to a prolonged suppression of GH concentrations. Glucocorticoids also raise IGF-I concentrations, but inhibit its biological activity. Glucocorticoid deficiency, on the other hand, impairs the GH response to growth hormone releasing hormone (GHRH) *(30–33)*.

Dopamine infusions suppress GH production at the level of the pituitary, with doses as low as 5 µg/kg/min. Rebound elevations in GH concentrations occur within 20 min of discontinuation of dopamine, however, and persist for at least an additional day *(34,35)*.

Diagnosis

The diagnosis of true GH insufficiency during critical illness is extremely difficult to make, owing to the relative dissociation of IGF-I levels from GH secretion, and to the lack of predictability of random GH levels. Stimulation testing is often impractical and may be uninformative, given the already stressed state of the individual. Documentation of an elevated concentration, however, will reliably rule out GH insufficiency.

Treatment

Initiation of GH therapy is appropriate in the setting of the Neonatal Intensive Care Unit (NICU) at the time of a new diagnosis of GH insufficiency. The usual replacement dose for a neonate is 0.18 mg/kg/wk divided into daily subcutaneous doses. The use of

GH in any other setting in critically ill patients is contraindicated (including in non-neonates who have previously been on replacement therapy), as the only large prospective, randomized, controlled trial demonstrated significantly increased mortality in adult ICU patients treated with daily GH *(36)*. This will be discussed further in the final section of this chapter.

GONADAL AXIS

Hypogonadotropic hypogonadism has been demonstrated in virtually all studies of sex hormones in critically ill adults. There are currently no available data for children. In adults who are responding to a variety of severe stresses (e.g., sepsis, trauma, burns, starvation) there is an initial surge in LH in the acute phase, while FSH and inhibin remain in the normal range, and serum testosterone and estradiol concentrations abruptly decrease *(37,38)*. As the patient enters the chronic phase of critical illness, she or he becomes hypogonadotropic, and the low sex steroid levels continue *(39,40)*. This likely represents the common pattern of peripheral hormonal suppression and pituitary activation in the acute phase of illness, followed by hypothalamic-based pituitary and peripheral suppression in the chronic phase. This has not yet been confirmed experimentally with a gonadotropin releasing hormone (GnRH) pulsatile infusion.

Diagnosis

Laboratory evaluation of hypogonadism should be approached skeptically in the setting of critical illness. High or "normal" concentrations of gonadotropins may be encountered early on in the clinical course and do not necessarily indicate gonadal failure. Likewise, suppressed concentrations are uninformative even in the acute phase, as prolactin may be elevated, dopamine may be infusing, or the patient may have a variably paced progression into the chronic phase of critical illness.

Treatment

Several hormonal replacement trials have been attempted, largely in the context of attempting to treat the catabolic state of critical illness. These will be addressed in the final section of this chapter.

For those on hormonal replacement therapy prior to critical illness, we recommend discontinuing it for the duration of the ICU stay, or until the child has begun to show signs of significant clinical recovery.

POTENTIAL FOR THERAPEUTIC HORMONAL INTERVENTIONS TO TREAT THE PROTEIN CATABOLISM OF CRITICAL ILLNESS

Critically ill infants and children are under severe catabolic stress. Protein loss is the hallmark of the metabolic stress response, and its extent is determined by the severity of illness *(41,42)*. If protein loss persists, it is associated with increased morbidity and mortality *(43)*. Limiting protein degradation and maximizing protein accretion is of particular importance in critically ill children because of their restricted protein reserves and their requirement for growth and development. Infants on extracorporeal life support (ECLS, also known as ECMO), for example, who are among the most profoundly ill children in pediatric critical care, quantitatively demonstrate the highest rates of protein loss ever reported *(44)*. Children who have suffered severe burns have also been studied extensively in this regard, and have recently been shown to remain catabolic for at least 9 mo after their injury (45).

The hormonal changes detailed earlier in the chapter, in particular, suppressed GH, elevated cortisol, and insulin resistance, contribute to this state of catabolism. This produces a scenario of protein catabolism, carbohydrate intolerance, and paradoxical fat sparing. Hormonal anabolic therapies been administered in the past in an effort to counteract these maladaptive changes have included GH, IGF-I, insulin, and androgens.

GH was first used in an animal model of traumatic injury in 1941 to improve nitrogen retention and reduce weight loss, in the form of injected human pituitary extracts (46). Its recombinant formulation has been investigated since then in a variety of small clinical trials over a period of approx 25 yr. Improvements in various indices of protein turnover and clinical outcome were documented in a wide variety of ICU adult patients, using a wide variety of dosages of GH, largely in the context of small, prospective, randomized, controlled trials (PRCTs) (47–50). One moderate-sized pediatric study ($n = 72$) demonstrated decreased protein catabolism in burned children treated from ICU discharge until 1 yr from burn (51). The adult studies prompted a large scale PRCT in two European adult ICUs using a daily dose 0.1 mg/kg, in which the relative risk of mortality was raised to 1.9–2.4 (36). Interestingly, there was a dose dependent increase in mortality over time in the population whose dose was slowly increased over the course of the study. No clear rationale for the increased mortality has yet been demonstrated, although hyperglycemia and associated immune compromise are suspected mediators. The FDA has since warned against any use of GH in patients suffering from acute critical illness, and all related clinical trials have effectively ceased (52).

Other attempts to augment the suppressed somatotrope axis have focused on the delivery of IGF-I, with or without GH. In normal adult subjects, IGF-I therapy has multiple effects that might be desirable in critically ill patients, including: 1) increasing glucose uptake 3-fold; 2) reducing hepatic glucose output by 60–70%; 3) lowering blood glucose acutely (iv, not sq); 4) lowering insulin, c-peptide, glucagon, free fatty acids, ketones; and 5) decreasing proteolysis and thereby decreasing plasma amino acid concentrations (53). These effects persist in the fed state with glucocorticoid-induced catabolism (54), and were confirmed in a non-randomized fashion in stable, post-burn adults (55). Unfortunately, three PRCTs failed to demonstrate significant effect in ill, post-operative adult patients (56–58). In stable, post-burn children, one PRCT demonstrated significant effects in mitigating the extent of protein catabolism using IGF-I in combination with insulin-like growth factor binding protein 3 (IGF-BP3) (59). IGF-I has been shown to be safe in a Phase I clinical trial in critically ill adults (60)—further clinical data are imminent.

Anabolic steroid therapy in the critically ill adult with burns or trauma has produced several reports of positive results in adults (61–63), and one in burned children (51). In fact, the pediatric data demonstrated a doubling of the fractional synthetic rate of protein, and a substantial improvement in net protein balance. Oxandrolone, a non-aromatizable androgen, has been the therapeutic agent of choice due its decreased virilizing potency and hepatotoxicity as compared to testosterone. Further studies designed as large PRCTs are needed to draw definitive conclusions, based on these promising data.

Insulin therapy has been studied in a wide variety of clinical situations in order to reduce protein breakdown, and to stimulate protein synthesis and growth. In small numbers of healthy volunteers, insulin has suppressed proteolysis by 59–91%, in a dose-dependent manner *(64–67)*. In burned adults, protein synthesis was stimulated, and wound healing was accelerated *(68–70)*. A single study in children demonstrated an 80% suppression of proteolysis in four stable, premature neonates, but noted a significant rise plasma lactate during the insulin infusion *(71)*. Two large PRCTs have recently demonstrated that tight glucose control, using an intravenous insulin infusion, produces remarkable and significant reductions in mortality of 29% in adult diabetics after myocardial infarction, and 34% in adult post-operative surgical ICU patients *(72,73)*. Based upon these data, the standard of care of adult, and ultimately pediatric, critically ill patients will soon likely include insulin infusion aimed at strict maintenance of euglycemia, despite the logistical challenges that insulin infusions present.

A final approach to hormonal therapies in critical illness is replacement of hypothalamic peptides by continuous infusion, in order to re-activate normal pulsatile production of pituitary hormones. The primary advantage of this approach is that it maintains the negative feedback on the pituitary, preventing overproduction of end hormones with their own untoward side effects at excessive concentrations. Although GH has been deemed unsafe for use in this population, infusion of GH secretagogs (e.g., GHRH, Ghrelin), for example, as has been shown by Van den Berghe, would normalize GH and IGF-I concentrations in a physiologic, pulsatile manner *(27)*.

Co-administration of GH secretagogues, TRH, and potentially pulsatile GnRH, makes theoretical sense during the chronic state of critical illness. This is a state that, but for modern critical care, human beings would not have survived to reach, and would not have been designed to endure. It is during this phase of critical illness that the hypothalamus continues to be suppressed, despite normal responsiveness of the remainder of the components of each hormonal axis. Further research aimed at clinical outcomes using infusions of hypothalamic peptides is required to definitively address this issue.

REFERENCES

1. Brown-Sequard CE. Recherches experimentales sur la physiologie et la pathologie des capsules surrenales. C R Acad Sci [D] Paris 1956;43:422–425.
2. Munck A, Guyre PM, Holbrook NJ. Physiological functions of glucocorticoids in stress and their relation to pharmacological actions. Endocr Rev 1984;5:25–44.
3. Wurtman RJ, Axelrod J. Adrenaline synthesis: control by the pituitary gland and adrenal glucocorticoids. Science 1965;150:1464–1465.
4. Wong DL, Lesage A, Siddall B, Funder JW. Glucocorticoid regulation of phenylethanolamine N-methyltransferase in vivo. FASEB J 1992;6:3310–3315.
5. Chopra IJ, Huang TS, Beredo A, Solomon DH, Chua Teco GN, Mead JF. Evidence for an inhibitor of extrathyroidal conversion of thyroxine to 3,5,3'-triiodothyronine in sera of patients with nonthyroidal illnesses. J Clin Endocrinol Metab 1985;60:666–672.
6. Kaptein EM, Grieb DA, Spencer CA, Wheeler WS, Nicoloff JT. Thyroxine metabolism in the low thyroxine state of critical nonthyroidal illnesses. J Clin Endocrinol Metab 1981;53:764–771.
7. Vos RA, De Jong M, Bernard BF, Docter R, Krenning EP, Hennemann G. Impaired thyroxine and 3,5,3'-triiodothyronine handling by rat hepatocytes in the presence of serum of patients with nonthyroidal illness. J Clin Endocrinol Metab 1995;80:2364–2370.
8. Rothwell PM, Lawler PG. Prediction of outcome in intensive care patients using endocrine parameters. Crit Care Med 1995;23:78–83.
9. Engler D, Burger AG. The deiodination of the iodothyronines and of their derivatives in man. Endocr Rev 1984;5:151–184.
10. Bacci V, Schussler GC, Kaplan TB. The relationship between serum triiodothyronine and thyrotropin during systemic illness. J Clin Endocrinol Metab 1982;54:1229–1235.

11. Van den Berghe G, de Zegher F, Veldhuis JD, et al. Thyrotrophin and prolactin release in prolonged critical illness: dynamics of spontaneous secretion and effects of growth hormone- secretagogues. Clin Endocrinol (Oxf) 1997;47:599–612.
12. Van den Berghe G, de Zegher F, Baxter RC, et al. Neuroendocrinology of prolonged critical illness: effects of exogenous thyrotropin-releasing hormone and its combination with growth hormone secretagogues. J Clin Endocrinol Metab 1998;83:309–319.
13. Murkin JM. Anesthesia and hypothyroidism: a review of thyroxine physiology, pharmacology, and anesthetic implications. Anesth Analg 1982;61:371–383.
14. Chopra IJ. Simultaneous measurement of free thyroxine and free 3,5,3'- triiodothyronine in undiluted serum by direct equilibrium dialysis/radioimmunoassay: evidence that free triiodothyronine and free thyroxine are normal in many patients with the low triiodothyronine syndrome. Thyroid 1998;8: 249–257.
15. Burmeister LA. Reverse T3 does not reliably differentiate hypothyroid sick syndrome from euthyroid sick syndrome. Thyroid 1995;5:435–441.
16. Surks MI, Sievert R. Drugs and thyroid function. N Engl J Med 1995;333:1688–1694.
17. Becker RA, Vaughan GM, Ziegler MG, et al. Hypermetabolic low triiodothyronine syndrome of burn injury. Crit Care Med 1982;10:870–875 (1982).
18. Brent GA, Hershman JM. Thyroxine therapy in patients with severe nonthyroidal illnesses and low serum thyroxine concentration. J Clin Endocrinol Metab 1986;63:1–8.
19. Novitzky D. Heart transplantation, euthyroid sick syndrome, and triiodothyronine replacement. J Heart Lung Transplant 1992;11:S196–S198.
20. Bennett-Guerrero E, Jimenez JL, White WD, D'Amico EB, Baldwin BI, Schwinn DA. Cardiovascular effects of intravenous triiodothyronine in patients undergoing coronary artery bypass graft surgery. A randomized, double- blind, placebo- controlled trial. Duke T_3 study group. JAMA 1996;275:687–692.
21. Klemperer JD, Klein I, Gomez M, et al. Thyroid hormone treatment after coronary-artery bypass surgery. N Engl J Med 1995;333:1522–1527.
22. Bettendorf M, Schmidt KG, Grulich-Henn J, Ulmer HE, Heinrich UE. Tri-iodothyronine treatment in children after cardiac surgery: a double- blind, randomised, placebo-controlled study. Lancet 2000;356:529–534.
23. Hays MT, Nielsen KR. Human thyroxine absorption: age effects and methodological analyses. Thyroid 1994;4:55–64. (1994).
24. Wartofsky L. In: The Thyroid: A Fundamental and Clinical Text (Braverman LE, Utiger RD, eds.) Lippincott-Raven, Philadelphia, 1995, pp. 871–877.
25. Ross R, Miell J, Freeman E, et al. Critically ill patients have high basal growth hormone levels with attenuated oscillatory activity associated with low levels of insulin- like growth factor-I. Clin Endocrinol (Oxf) 1991;35:47–54.
26. Maiter D, Walker JL, Adam E, et al. Differential regulation by growth hormone (GH) of insulin-like growth factor I and GH receptor/binding protein gene expression in rat liver. Endocrinology 1992;130:3257–3264.
27. Van den Berghe G, de Zegher F, Veldhuis JD, et al. The somatotropic axis in critical illness: effect of continuous growth hormone (GH)-releasing hormone and GH-releasing peptide-2 infusion. J Clin Endocrinol Metab 1997;82:590–599.
28. Giustina A, Wehrenberg WB. Influence of thyroid hormones on the regulation of growth hormone secretion. Eur J Endocrinol 1995;133:646-53.
29. Valcavi R, Zini M, Portioli I. Thyroid hormones and growth hormone secretion. J Endocrinol Invest 1992;15:313–330.
30. Wajchenberg BL, Liberman B, Giannella Neto D, et al. Growth hormone axis in cushing's syndrome. Horm Res 1996;45:99–107.
31. Dieguez C, Mallo F, Senaris R, et al. Role of glucocorticoids in the neuroregulation of growth hormone secretion. J Pediatr Endocrinol Metab 1996;9(Suppl 3):255–260.
32. Casanueva FF. Physiology of growth hormone secretion and action. Endocrinol Metab Clin North Am 1992;21:483–517.
33. Strobl JS, Thomas MJ. Human growth hormone. Pharmacol Rev 1994;46:1–34.
34. Van den Berghe G, de Zegher F, Lauwers P. Dopamine suppresses pituitary function in infants and children. Crit Care Med 1994;22:1747–1753.
35. Van den Berghe G, de Zegher F. Anterior pituitary function during critical illness and dopamine treatment. Crit Care Med 1996;24:1580–1590.

36. Takala J, Ruokonen E, Webster NR, et al. Increased mortality associated with growth hormone treatment in critically ill adults. N Engl J Med 1999;341:785–792.
37. van Steenbergen W, Naert J, Lambrecht S, Scheys I, Lesaffre E, Pelemans W. Suppression of gonadotropin secretion in the hospitalized postmenopausal female as an effect of acute critical illness. Neuroendocrinology 1994;60:165–172.
38. Spratt DI, Cox P, Orav J, Moloney J, Bigos T. Reproductive axis suppression in acute illness is related to disease severity. J Clin Endocrinol Metab 1993;76:1548–1554.
39. Woolf PD, Hamill RW, McDonald JV, Lee LA, Kelly M. Transient hypogonadotropic hypogonadism caused by critical illness. J Clin Endocrinol Metab 1985;60:444–450.
40. Vogel AV, Peake GT, Rada RT. Pituitary-testicular axis dysfunction in burned men. J Clin Endocrinol Metab 1985;60:658–665.
41. Jaksic T, Wagner DA, Burke JF, Young VR. Proline metabolism in adult male burned patients and healthy control subjects. Am J Clin Nutr 1991;54:408–413.
42. Cuthbertson DP. Further observations on the disturbance of metabolism caused by injury, with particular reference to the dietary requirements of fracture cases. Br J Surg 1936;23:505–520.
43. Moyer E, Cerra F, Chenier R, et al. Multiple systems organ failure: VI. Death predictors in the trauma-septic state—the most critical determinants. J Trauma 1981;21:862–869.
44. Shew SB, Keshen TH, Jahoor F, Jaksic T. The determinants of protein catabolism in neonates on extracorporeal membrane oxygenation. J Pediatr Surg 1999;34:1086–1090.
45. Hart DW, Wolf SE, Mlcak R, et al. Persistence of muscle catabolism after severe burn. Surgery 2000;128:312–319.
46. Cuthbertson DP, Shaw GB, Young FG. The anterior pituitary gland and protein metabolism: the nitrogen retaining action of anterior lobe extracts. J Clin Endocrinol Metab 1941;2:459–467.
47. Voerman BJ, Strack van Schijndel RJ, Groeneveld AB, de Boer H, Nauta J. P, Thijs LG. Effects of human growth hormone in critically ill nonseptic patients: results from a prospective, randomized, placebo-controlled trial. Crit Care Med 1995;23:665–673.
48. Petersen SR, Holaday NJ, Jeevanandam M. Enhancement of protein synthesis efficiency in parenterally fed trauma victims by adjuvant recombinant human growth hormone. J Trauma 1994;36:726–733.
49. Dahn MS, Lange MP. Systemic and splanchnic metabolic response to exogenous human growth hormone. Surgery 1998;123:528–538.
50. Gamrin L, Essen P, Hultman E, McNurlan MA, Garlick PJ, Wernerman J. Protein-sparing effect in skeletal muscle of growth hormone treatment in critically ill patients. Ann Surg 2000;231:577–586.
51. Hart DW, Herndon DN, Klein G, et al. Attenuation of posttraumatic muscle catabolism and osteopenia by long-term growth hormone therapy. Ann Surg 2001;233:827–834.
52. Genentech Nutropin AQ package insert, 1999.
53. Turkalj I, Keller U, Ninnis R, Vosmeer S, Stauffacher W. Effect of increasing doses of recombinant human insulin-like growth factor-I on glucose, lipid, and leucine metabolism in man. J Clin Endocrinol Metab 1992;75:1186–1191.
54. Berneis K, Ninnis R, Girard J, Frey BM Keller U. Effects of insulin-like growth factor I combined with growth hormone on glucocorticoid-induced whole-body protein catabolism in man. J Clin Endocrinol Metab 1997;82:2528–2534.
55. Cioffi WG, Gore DC, Rue LW, 3rd, et al. Insulin-like growth factor-1 lowers protein oxidation in patients with thermal injury. Ann Surg 1994;220:310–316; discussion 316–319.
56. Leinskold T, Permert J, Olaison G, Larsson J. Effect of postoperative insulin-like growth factor I supplementation on protein metabolism in humans. Br J Surg 1995;82:921–925.
57. Sandstrom R, Svanberg E, Hyltander A, et al. The effect of recombinant human IGF-I on protein metabolism in post-operative patients without nutrition compared to effects in experimental animals. Eur J Clin Invest 1995;25:784–792.
58. Goeters C, Mertes N, Tacke J, et al. Repeated administration of recombinant human insulin-like growth factor-I in patients after gastric surgery. Effect on metabolic and hormonal patterns. Ann Surg 1995;222:646–653.
59. Herndon DN, Ramzy PI, DebRoy MA, et al. Muscle protein catabolism after severe burn: effects of IGF-1/IGFBP-3 treatment. Ann Surg 1999;229:713–720; discussion 720–722.
60. Yarwood GD, Ross RJ, Medbak S, Coakley J, Hinds CJ. Administration of human recombinant insulin-like growth factor-I in critically ill patients. Crit Care Med 1997;25:1352–1361.
61. Hausmann DF, Nutz V, Rommelsheim K, Caspari R, Mosebach KO. Anabolic steroids in polytrauma patients. Influence on renal nitrogen and amino acid losses: a double-blind study. JPEN J Parenter Enteral Nutr 1990;14:111–114.

62. Gervasio JM, Dickerson RN, Swearingen J, et al. Oxandrolone in trauma patients. Pharmacotherapy 2000;20:1328–1334.
63. Demling RH, Orgill DP. The anticatabolic and wound healing effects of the testosterone analog oxandrolone after severe burn injury. J Crit Care 2000;15:12–17. (2000).
64. Denne SC, Liechty EA, Liu YM, Brechtel G, Baron AD. Proteolysis in skeletal muscle and whole body in response to euglycemic hyperinsulinemia in normal adults. Am J Physiol 1991;261:E809–E814.
65. Fukagawa NK, Minaker KL, Rowe JW, et al. Insulin-mediated reduction of whole body protein breakdown. Dose- response effects on leucine metabolism in postabsorptive men. J Clin Invest 1985;76:2306–2311.
66. Heslin MJ, Newman E, Wolf RF, Pisters PW, Brennan MF. Effect of hyperinsulinemia on whole body and skeletal muscle leucine carbon kinetics in humans [published erratum appears in Am J Physiol 1993;265(1 Pt 1):section E following table of contents]. Am J Physiol 1992;262:E911–E918.
67. Tessari P, Trevisan R, Inchiostro S, et al. Dose-response curves of effects of insulin on leucine kinetics in humans. Am J Physiol 1986;251:E334–E342.
68. Ferrando AA, Chinkes DL, Wolf SE, Matin S, Herndon DN, Wolfe RR. A submaximal dose of insulin promotes net skeletal muscle protein synthesis in patients with severe burns [see comments]. Ann Surg 1999;229:11–18.
69. Pierre EJ, Barrow RE, Hawkins HK, Nguyen TT, Sakurai Y, Desai M, Wolfe RR, Herndon DN. Effects of insulin on wound healing. J Trauma 1998;44:342–345.
70. Sakurai Y, Aarsland A, Herndon DN, Chinkes DL, Pierre E, Nguyen TT, Patterson BW, Wolfe RR. Stimulation of muscle protein synthesis by long-term insulin infusion in severely burned patients. Ann Surg 1995;222:283–294; 294–297.
71. Poindexter BB, Karn CA, Denne SC. Exogenous insulin reduces proteolysis and protein synthesis in extremely low birth weight infants. J Pediatr 1998;132:948–953.
72. van den Berghe G, Wouters P, Weekers F, et al. Intensive insulin therapy in the surgical intensive care unit. N Engl J Med 2001;345:1359–1367.
73. Malmberg K, Ryden L, Efendic S, et al. Randomized trial of insulin-glucose infusion followed by subcutaneous insulin treatment in diabetic patients with acute myocardial infarction (DIGAMI study): effects on mortality at 1 year. J Am Coll Cardiol 1995;26;57–65.

Index

A

Ablation
  thyroid cancer, 333
Acanthosis nigricans, 253f
Acidemia
  ketones, 515
  lactate, 515
Acquired gonadotropin deficiency, 454–455
Acquired nephrogenic diabetes insipidus
  causes, 159–160
ACTH, 190, 229
  overproduction, 251
Acute hypocalcemia
  management, 354
Acute lymphoblastic leukemia (ALL), 8–9
Addison's disease. *See* Primary adrenal insufficiency
ADHD, 309
Adrenal axis, 552–553
Adrenalectomy
  CAH, 239
Adrenal failure
  clinical presentation, 212–213
  therapy, 216, 218
Adrenal hyperandrogenism
  functional
    causes, 459–460
Adrenal hypoplasia congenita (AHC), 386
  X-linked, 209
Adrenal insufficiency, 203–220
  age of onset, 349
  causes, 208t
  clinical presentation, 212–213
  diagnosis, 213–216
  etiology, 206–212
  evaluation and treatment, 182–183
  psychosocial quality of life, 219–220
  therapy, 216–219, 216t
Adrenal insufficiency test, 214–215
Adrenal neoplasms
  precocious puberty, 418
Adrenal steroidogenesis, 227–243, 228f
  biosynthetic pathway, 410f
  enzymes and genes, 229t
Adrenocortical neoplasms, 251
Adrenocorticotropic hormone (ACTH), 190, 229
  overproduction, 251
Adrenoleukodystrophy
  psychosocial quality of life, 220
Adult growth hormone deficiency
  etiology, 140t
  persistence, 140–143
  therapy, 139–149
Adult height
  prediction, 20
African American infants
  rickets, 372–373
AHC, 386
  X-linked, 209
Aldosterone
  ion flow, 263f
  production, 262f
  synthetase, 265f
ALL, 8–9
Ambiguous genitalia, 429–447
  care, 437–439
  diagnostic tests, 440–444
  differential diagnosis, 442f
  history, 439
  medical management, 439–447
  physical examination, 439–440

f: figure
t: table

AME, 268
Amenorrhea
 defined, 451
 differential diagnosis, 462f–463f,
  464f–465f
Amiloride (Midamor)
 nephrogenic diabetes insipidus, 169
Aminoglutethimide
 Cushing syndrome, 257
Aminoglutethimide-induced adrenal
  insufficiency, 211
Anabolic steroids
 critical illness, 559
 safety, 130
Androgen
 deficiency
  anorexia nervosa, 193f
 insensitivity, 390
Aneuploidy, 118
Anorexia nervosa
 bone loss
  etiology, 193f
 dietary history, 194
 DSM-IV criteria, 190t
 endocrinologic sequelae, 189–196
 GH abnormalities, 191
 hospitalization indications, 194
 HPA, 190
 hypothalamic-pituitary-ovarian abnormalities, 192
 insulin abnormalities, 191
 leptin abnormalities, 191
 management, 194–195
 osteopenia, 193
 osteoporosis, 194–195
 patient evaluation, 194–195
 physical examination, 194
 prolactin, 192
 TH abnormalities, 191
 vasopressin, 192
Anovulatory tract disorders
 differential diagnosis, 466f–467f
 menstrual disorders, 452–455
Anterior pituitary
 development, 10f
 formation, 3
 tumors, 539–540

Antiandrogens
 hirsutism, 474
Antibiotics
 hormonal contraceptive interaction, 486
Anticonvulsants
 hormonal contraceptive interaction, 486
Antidiuretic hormone deficiency. *See*
  Diabetes insipidus
APECED, 207
Apparent mineralocorticoid excess
  (AME), 268
Arginine, 16
Asherman's syndrome, 452
Astrocytomas, 8
Attention-deficit hyperactivity disorder
  (ADHD), 309
Autoimmune disorders
 with Turner syndrome, 122–123
 therapy, 131
Autoimmune hypophysitis, 148
Autoimmune polyendocrinopathy
  candidiasis ectodermal dystrophy
  (APECED), 207
Autoimmune thyroid disease, 291–304
 Graves' disease, 296–304
Autoimmune thyroiditis, 291–296
 classification, 292t
 clinical presentation, 293
 diagnosis, 293–294
 pathophysiology, 292
 terminology, 291–292
 therapy, 294–296

B

Barbiturate-induced adrenal
  insufficiency, 211
Barriers, 482–484
Baseline hormone measurements
 adrenal insufficiency, 213–214
Behavioral control
 contraception, 481
Benign intracranial hypertension
 following GH therapy, 24
Benign premature pubertal development,
  405–411
Bilateral total adrenalectomy
 Cushing syndrome, 257

Bioinactive growth hormone, 13
Bipotential external genitalia, 435–436
Bipotential gonad, 431–435
Blastomycosis, 211
Body fat percentage
  GHD, 146t
Bone
  age
    evaluation, 19
  loss
    anorexia nervosa, 193f
Brain tumor treatment
  endocrine dysfunction, 173–185
Breast cancer
  hormonal contraceptives, 490–491
Breast development
  Tanner stages, 403f
Bromocriptine
  anterior pituitary tumors, 540

C

CAH. *See* Congenital adrenal hyperplasia
Calciopenic rickets, 366
  heritable forms, 370
  therapy
    complications, 374
Calcitonin
  hypercalcemia, 361
  serum calcium, 345–346
Calcitriol
  chronic hypocalcemia, 354
  serum calcium, 345–346
Calcium
  acute hypocalcemia, 354
  serum hormonal regulation, 344–347
Calcium deficiency rickets
  treatment, 373
Calcium homeostasis abnormalities, 343–362
  hypercalcemia, 356–362
  hypocalcemia, 347–356
Carbamazepine
  diabetes insipidus, 168
Carbohydrate metabolism
  hormonal contraceptives, 488
Cardiovascular abnormalities
  with Turner syndrome, 119–120
    therapy, 126

CDGP, 67, 384
Central adrenal failure
  therapy, 218
Central adrenal insufficiency
  psychosocial quality of life, 219–220
Central diabetes insipidus
  non-traumatic, 157
  vasopressin therapy, 166t
Central nervous system tumors recurrence
  following GH therapy, 23
Central precocious puberty (CPP), 411–414
Central resistance to thyroid hormone (CRTH), 309
Cerebral salt-wasting, 184
Cervical caps, 482, 483
Chemotherapy
  endocrine system, 175–176
Chlorpropamide
  diabetes insipidus, 168
Cholecalciferol
  serum calcium, 345–346
Chronic autoimmune thyroiditis, 291–296
  clinical presentation, 293
  diagnosis, 293–294
  pathophysiology, 292
  terminology, 291–292
  therapy, 294–296
Chronic hypocalcemia
  management, 354–355
Chronic lymphocytic thyroiditis. *See* Chronic autoimmune thyroiditis
Chronic systemic disease
  delayed puberty, 384
Clofibrate
  diabetes insipidus, 168
Clonidine, 16
Coccidomycosis, 211
COCs, 485, 492–496
Coitus interruptus, 481
Combination oral contraceptive pills (COCs), 485, 492–496
Combined dexamethasone-corticotropin-releasing hormone (CRH) test, 255
Combined injectable contraception, 496
Combined pituitary hormone deficiency (CPHD), 9–10

Computed tomography (CT)
  adrenal insufficiency, 215
  Cushing syndrome, 256
Condoms
  female, 482
  male, 482
Congenial lipoid adrenal hyperplasia, 209
Congenital adrenal hyperplasia (CAH), 209, 227–242, 417
  3beta hydroxysteroid/delta 4,5-isomerase deficiency, 233
  11beta-hydroxylase deficiency, 236–237
  12-hydroxylase deficiency, 234–236
  17-hydroxylase/17,20 lyase deficiency, 234
  clinical and hormonal data, 230t–232t
  lipoid adrenal hyperplasia, 228–229
  newborn screening, 243
  prenatal diagnosis and treatment, 240–241
  prenatal therapy
    maternal complications, 242
    protocol, 242–243
  psychosocial quality of life, 220
  therapy, 237–240
    monitoring, 239–240
    outcome, 240
  virilizing forms
    therapy, 218–219
Congenital anorchia, 388
Congenital hypothyroidism, 275–287
  cause, 277t
  clinical presentation, 278–280
  diagnosis, 280–284
  mechanism, 276–278
  treatment, 284–286
Congenital Leydig cell aplasia, 389
Conjugated estrogen, 181
Constitutional delay of growth and puberty (CDGP), 67, 384
Contraception, 479–502
  failure rates, 482t
  hormonal methods, 484–500
    cardiovascular disease, 487–488
    drug interactions, 486
    new delivery methods, 501
    non-contraceptive benefits, 500–501
    systemic effects, 485–486
    thromboembolism, 486–487
  limitations, 481t
  methods, 480t
  non-hormonal methods, 481–484
Contraceptive sponge, 483
Corticotropin-releasing hormone (CRH), 190, 249–250
  adrenal insufficiency test, 214–215
  ovine
    stimulation test, 255
Cortisol, 204
  biosynthetic pathway, 210f
  CAH virilizing forms, 218–219
  secretion, 250f
Cosyntropin stimulation test
  adrenal insufficiency, 214
CPHD, 9–10
CPP, 411–414
Craniopharyngiomas, 8, 147
CRH. See Corticotropin-releasing hormone
CRH test, 255
Critical illness
  endocrine response, 551–560
  protein catabolism
    therapeutic hormonal intervention, 558–560
Critical samples, 513–514
CRTH, 309
Cryptococcus, 211
CT
  adrenal insufficiency, 215
  Cushing syndrome, 256
Cushing's disease, 251
Cushing syndrome, 249–258
  clinical presentation, 252, 252t
  diagnostic algorithm, 254f
  diagnostic guidelines, 253–256
  epidemiology, 250–251
  food-dependent, 251
  glucocorticoid replacement, 258
  striae, 253f
  treatment, 256–257
CYP11B2 gene, 263
Cypionate (Lunelle), 485, 496
Cyproterone acetate, 474

D

dDAVP, 165, 184
Dehydroepiandrosteredione (DHEA)
   anorexia nervosa, 193f
Delayed puberty, 383–395, 455
   classification, 383–395
   etiology, 385t
   evaluation, 391–395
   history, 391
   physical examination, 391
   treatment, 393–395
Deoxycorticosterone (DOC), 262
Depo-Provera, 485, 497, 498–500
   breast cancer, 491
   drug interactions, 486
Desmopressin, 166t
Desogestrel, 473
Development. *See* Growth
      and development
DEXA bone density
   GHD, 146t
Dexamethasone
   CAH, 241
   primary aldosteronism, 270
Dexamethasone-resistant forms
      of hyperandrogenism, 459–460
Dextrose
   hypoglycemic disorders, 519
DHEA
   anorexia nervosa, 193f
Diabetes
   gestational
      hormonal contraceptives, 488
Diabetes insipidus, 8, 155–171, 183–184
   causes, 158–160, 158t
   clinical presentation, 156–157
   diagnosis, 160–165
      tests, 162t
   familial
      causes, 158
   growth and development, 157
   idiopathic central
      causes, 159
   nephrogenic, 157–160
   non-traumatic, 157
   perioperative management, 166–167
   postoperative management, 168
   treatment, 165–170
   vasopressin therapy, 166t
Diabetes mellitus, 523–532
   classification, 523–524
   insulin-dependent. *See* Type 1 diabetes
      mellitus.
   noninsulin-dependent. *See* Type 2
      diabetes mellitus.
Diaphragms, 482, 483
Diazoxide
   hypoglycemic disorders, 519
Didja tubes, 513–514
Dietary history
   anorexia nervosa, 194
Diuretics
   nephrogenic diabetes insipidus, 169
DMPA. *See* Medroxyprogesterone acetate
DOC, 262
Drospirenone, 492
Drug-induced adrenal insufficiency, 211
Drug-induced nephrogenic diabetes
      insipidus, 169
Dysfunctional uterine bleeding
   defined, 451
Dysgenic gonad
   defined, 437
Dysmorphic features
   with Turner syndrome, 119
      therapy, 126

E

ECLS, 558
Endocrine disorders
   evaluation and treatment, 177–184
Endocrinopathies
   delayed puberty, 384
Endometrial cancer
   hormonal contraceptives, 491
Estrogen
   delayed puberty, 394–395
   menstrual disorders, 471
Ethics
   GH therapy
      normal short stature variants, 72
Ethynyl estradiol, 181, 472
Etidronate
   hypercalcemia, 361

Etomidate-induced adrenal
    insufficiency, 211
Euthyroid hyperthyroxinemia, 315
    causes, 315t
Exercise
    T1DM, 529–530
    test, 17
Exogenous sex steroid exposure, 414
External beam radiotherapy
    thyroid cancer, 336
External sex
    defined, 437
Extracorporeal life support (ECLS), 558
Eye problems
    with Turner syndrome, 122
        therapy, 131

F
Familial diabetes insipidus
    causes, 158
Familial dysalbuminemic
    hyperthyroxinemia (FDH), 316
Familial glucocorticoid deficiency, 210
Familial hypocalciuric hypercalcemia, 358
Familial male precocious puberty
    (FMPP), 416–417
Familial medullary thyroid carcinoma
    (FMTC), 535
Family history
    RTH, 317
Fanconi syndrome, 371
Fasting adaptation
    metabolic pathways, 516f
Fasting metabolic systems
    hormonal regulation, 513f
FDH, 316
Female athlete triad, 194
Female breast and pubic hair development
    Tanner stages, 403f
Female condoms, 482
Female external genitalia, 436
Female hormone replacement, 181
Female pseudohermaphroditism, 443
Fetus
    calcium homeostasis, 346
    growth retardation
        causes, 81t
Fine needle aspiration biopsy (FNAB), 331

Fludrocortisone
    mineralocorticoid deficiency, 266
Flutamide
    CAH, 219
FMPP, 416–417
FMTC, 535
FNAB, 331
Focal hyperinsulinism, 517
Food-dependent Cushing syndrome, 251
Formal fasting study protocol, 519
46, XY testicular dysgenesis, 441
    causes, 435t
Free fatty acids, 515–518
Functional adrenal hyperandrogenism
    causes, 459–460
Functional ovarian hyperandrogenism
    causes, 459
Fungal disease, 211
Furosemide
    hypercalcemia, 361

G
Gastrointestinal disorders
    with Turner syndrome, 122
        therapy, 131
Gender identity
    defined, 437
Gender role
    defined, 437
Generalized resistance to thyroid hormone
    (GRTH), 309
Genetic sex
    defined, 436
Genetic testing
    hypoglycemia, 520
Genital and pubic hair development
    male
        Tanner stages, 402f
Genitalia
    ambiguous. See Ambiguous genitalia.
    bipotential external, 435–436
    female external, 436
    male external, 436
    surgery
        CAH, 238–239
Genital tract disorders
    menstrual disorders, 452
Germ-cell tumors, 8

Gestational diabetes
    hormonal contraceptives, 488
GH. *See* Growth hormone
GH-1
    gene, 4
        point mutations, 14f
GHD
    adult
        etiology, 140t
    cranial irradiation, 174
    evaluation and treatment, 177–180
GHF-1, 11
GHIS. *See* Growth hormone insensitivity syndrome
GH-R
    gene, 41
        mutations, 41–42, 75
    mutations, 13–14
GHRD. *See* Growth hormone receptor deficiency
GHRH, 4–5
    receptor mutations, 9, 16–17, 74
GHRP, 5
GHS, 5, 74, 178
GHS-R, 5, 6f
Glargine insulin, 527
Glucagon, 16
    hypoglycemic disorders, 519
Glucagon stimulation test
    adrenal insufficiency, 215
Glucocorticoids
    CAH, 237–238
    deficiency
        familial, 210
    growth suppression, 93–101
        treatment, 98–101
    replacement therapy
        NCAH, 411
Glucose homeostasis
    with Turner syndrome, 123
        therapy, 131–132
GnRH, 192
    delayed puberty, 394–395
    stimulation test, 412
Gonad
    bipotential, 431–435
    cranial irradiation, 175

Gonadal axis, 558
Gonadal dysgenesis, 389
Gonadal failure
    acquired causes, 390–391
    with Turner syndrome, 123–124
        therapy, 132–133
Gonadal sex
    defined, 436
Gonadotropin
    deficiency, 8
Gonadotropin deficiency, 455
    acquired, 454–455
Gonadotropin-dependent precocious puberty
    differential diagnosis, 406t
Gonadotropin releasing hormone (GnRH), 192
    delayed puberty, 394–395
    stimulation test, 412
Gonadotropin therapy
    delayed puberty, 394–395
Graves' disease, 296–304
    antithyroid medications, 300–301
    clinical presentation, 297
    definitive therapy, 301–303
    diagnosis, 298–300
    monitoring, 303
    neonatal, 303–304
    pathophysiology, 296–297
Greulich and Pyle method, 19
Growth and development
    chemotherapy, 175–176
    diabetes insipidus, 157
    skeletal tissue irradiation, 175
    spinal irradiation, 175
Growth failure
    evaluation and treatment, 177–180
    idiopathic, 67
Growth hormone (GH), 3
    action, 6–8
    adult deficiency
        diagnosis, 25
    axis, 557–558
    bioinactive, 13
    body proportion, 128
    bone mineral density, 128
    conditions characterized by
        unresponsiveness to, 38t

continuance
  contraindications for, 144–146
  examples, 145–146
craniofacial development, 128–129
critical illness, 559
deficiency, 7–15, 8t
  diagnosis, 15–21
  MRI, 20
dosage, 22
following intrauterine growth failure, 79–90
follow-up, 22–23
gene activation, 5f
gene mutation, 12–13, 74–75
GHR signal transduction abnormality, 43
IGF-I axis, 39–40, 39f
linear growth, 127–128
molecular basis, 41–43
monitoring therapy, 148–149
neurosecretory dysfunction, 67
physiology, 4–5
psychosocial function, 129
replacement, 24–25
safety, 129–130
secretion, 4–5
  physiologic assessment, 17–19
side effects, 23–24
stimulation tests, 18t
therapy, 21–24
  adverse effects, 73
  CAH, 239
tumor recurrence, 180
X-linked hypophosphatemic rickets, 376
Growth hormone-1 (GH-1)
  gene, 4
    point mutations, 14f
Growth hormone deficiency (GHD)
  adult
    etiology, 140t
  cranial irradiation, 174
  evaluation and treatment, 177–180
Growth hormone factor-1 (GHF-1), 11
Growth hormone insensitivity syndrome (GHIS), 37–61
  biochemical features, 50–52
    growth hormone, 50

growth hormone binding protein, 51
IGF binding proteins, 52
insulin-like growth factors, 51
classification, 37–39
defined, 37–39
diagnosis, 52–54
IGF-1
  long-term treatment, 55–59
Growth hormone receptor (GH-R)
  gene, 41
    mutations, 41–42, 75
  mutations, 13–14
Growth hormone receptor deficiency (GHRD)
  clinical findings, 44–52
  craniofacial characteristics, 47
  E180 splice mutation, 48f, 49f
  epidemiology, 43–44
  ethnic origin, 43
  growth, 44–50
  growth velocities, 45f
  IGF-1, 57f
  intellectual and social development, 49–50
  morbidity and mortality, 44
  musculoskeletal and body composition, 47
  reproduction, 49
  treatment, 54–59
    IGF-1, 54–55
Growth hormone releasing hormone (GHRH), 4–5
  receptor mutations, 9, 16–17, 74
Growth hormone releasing peptides (GHRP), 5
Growth hormone secretagogues (GHS), 5, 74, 178
Growth hormone secretagogues receptor (GHS-R), 5, 6f
Growth hormone stimulation tests, 15–16
Growth regulatory genes
  childhood growth, 73–74
Growth retardation
  fetal
    causes, 81t
GRTH, 309
Gynecomastia
  precocious puberty, 419–422

H

Hair development
  female
    Tanner stages, 403f
Hamartoma
  hypothalamic, 411
HCG, 182f, 229
HCG-producing tumors
  precocious puberty, 418–419
Head trauma, 7–8
Hearing loss
  with Turner syndrome, 121
    therapy, 130–131
Height. *See also* Short stature
  adult
    prediction, 20
Hemochromatosis, 8
Hereditary hypophosphatemic rickets with hypercalciuria (HHRH), 371, 377
Hereditary vitamin D resistance, 370
Hereditary vitamin D rickets
  treatment, 373–374
Hermaphroditism
  true, 443
Hesx1 gene, 9
HHRH, 371, 377
High dose dexamethasone suppression test, 255
Hirsutism
  defined, 461
  differential diagnosis, 468t–470t
  Ferriman and Gallwey scoring, 409f
Hormone replacement
  female, 181
  male, 181
HPA axis. *See* Hypothalamic-pituitary adrenal axis
HPG, 551
HPT, 551
Human chorionic gonadotropin (HCG), 229
Hydrochlorothiazide
  nephrogenic diabetes insipidus, 169
Hydrocortisone, 183
  CAH, 219, 237–238
Hydroxylase, 390
  deficiency, 370
    treatment, 373
Hydroxylase deficiency
  CAH, 236–237
Hydroxysteroid deficiency
  CAH, 233
Hydroxysteroid dehydrogenase deficiency, 390
Hyperandrogenism, 455, 456–460
  causes, 456t, 460
  differential diagnosis, 468t–470t
Hypercalcemia, 356–362
  calciotropic hormones, 356–358
  diagnosis and evaluation, 359–360
  differential diagnosis, 357t
  management, 360–362
Hypercortisolism, 253
Hypergonadotropic hypogonadism, 181, 388–391, 454
Hyperinsulinism
  focal, 517
  transient neonatal, 517
Hypernatremia, 157
Hyperparathyroidism, 536–537, 543
  hypercalcemia, 356–358
  screening, 544
Hyperprolactinemia, 455, 473
Hypertension
  benign intracranial
    following GH therapy, 24
Hyperthyroidism
  signs, 298t
  symptoms, 316
Hyperthyroxinemia
  euthyroid, 315
Hypertrichosis, 253f
Hypocalcemia, 347–356
  acute
    management, 354
  calciotropic hormone alterations, 347–350
  diagnosis, 351–354
  differential diagnosis, 348t
  management, 354–356
    goals, 518–519

neonates
    causes, 351t
    classification, 350–351
    management, 355–356
Hypocalciuric hypercalcemia
    familial, 358
Hypoestrogenism, 454, 471
    oral contraceptive pills, 472
Hypoglycemia, 511–520
    defined, 511–512
    fasting systems, 512–520
    insulin-induced
        adrenal insufficiency, 214
    post-Nissen dumping, 519
    T1DM, 530
Hypoglycemia disorders
    differential diagnosis, 518f
Hypogonadism
    true, 181
Hypogonadotropic hypogonadism, 181
    acquired causes, 387–388
    delayed puberty, 385
    idiopathic
        delayed puberty, 386–388
Hypoparathyroidism
    age of onset, 349
    hypocalcemia, 347–348
Hypophosphatasia, 372
Hypophysitis
    autoimmune, 148
    lymphocytic, 8
Hypopituitarism, 3, 8
    acquired forms, 7–8
    congenital forms, 9–15
Hypospadius, 441
Hypothalamic-chiasmatic glioma
    (HCG), 182f
Hypothalamic hamartoma, 411
Hypothalamic peptides
    replacement, 560
Hypothalamic-pituitary adrenal (HPA)
    axis, 399–401, 551
    anorexia nervosa, 190
    normal, 249–250
    regulation, 205, 206f
Hypothalamic-pituitary-gonadal
    (HPG), 551

Hypothalamic-pituitary-thyroid
    (HPT), 551
Hypothyroidism
    cranial irradiation, 174
    evaluation and treatment, 181–182
    precocious puberty, 419, 419f
    signs, 293t
    with Turner syndrome, 122–123
        therapy, 131

I

I-131
    Graves' disease, 302
ICS
    adverse effects, 96
    growth, 95–98
Idiopathic central diabetes insipidus
    causes, 159
Idiopathic growth failure, 67
Idiopathic hypogonadotropic
        hypogonadism
    delayed puberty, 386–388
Idiopathic short stature (ISS), 67
    defined, 68–69
    GH therapy
        height outcomes, 69–72
IGF, 19
IGF-1. See Insulin-like growth factor-I
IGFBP, 19
IGFBP-3, 178, 179f
    reference values, 53t
Immunometric assays, 15
Immunoradiometric assay (IRMA), 344
Indomethacin
    nephrogenic diabetes insipidus, 169
Infants
    African American
        rickets, 372–373
    diabetes insipidus
        management, 168
Inhaled corticosteroids (ICS)
    adverse effects, 96
    growth, 95–98
Insulin
    abnormalities, 191
        anorexia nervosa, 191
    adjusting doses, 528–529
    critical illness, 559–560

injection regimens, 525t
  matching to food intake, 529
  T1DM, 525–527
Insulin-dependent diabetes mellitus. *See*
    Type 1 diabetes mellitus
Insulin-induced hypoglycemia
  adrenal insufficiency, 214
Insulin-like growth factor (IGF), 19
Insulin-like growth factor binding
    protein (IGFBP), 19
Insulin-like growth factor binding
    protein-3 (IGFBP-3), 178, 179f
  reference values, 53t
Insulin-like growth factor-I (IGF-I),
    178, 179f
  critical illness, 559
  deficiency
    clinical features, 46f
    gene deletion, 75
    mutations, 14–15
  reference values, 53t
Insulin pump therapy, 526–527
Insulin tolerance test (ITT), 16
  for GHD, 146f
Internal sex
  defined, 437
Intersex Society of North America
    (ISNA), 444
Intrauterine devices, 484
Intrauterine growth retardation (IUGR)
  clinical presentation, 82
  diagnosis, 82–84
  growth hormone, 79–90
    future, 89–90
    somatic growth, 84–89
  mechanisms, 80–82
Iodine-131 (I-131)
  Graves' disease, 302
IRMA, 344
ISNA, 444
Isomerase deficiency
  CAH, 233
ISS, 67
  defined, 68–69
  GH therapy
    height outcomes, 69–72
  ITT, 16
    for GHD, 146f
IUGR. *See* Intrauterine growth retardation

K

Kallman syndrome, 386
Kaposi's sarcoma, 211
Keloids
  with Turner syndrome, 122
  therapy, 131
Ketoconazole
  FMPP, 417
  hypercalcemia, 361
Ketoconazole-induced adrenal
    insufficiency, 211
  Cushing syndrome, 257
Ketones, 515–518
Klinefelter's syndrome, 388

L

Langerhans cell histiocytosis, 8
Laron syndrome
  discovery, 41
Laurence-Moon-Beidl syndrome, 387
Learning disabilities
  with Turner syndrome, 124–125
  therapy, 133
Length standard deviation, 45f
Leptin abnormalities
  anorexia nervosa, 191
Leukemia
  cranial irradiation, 147
  following GH therapy, 23
Levodopa, 16
Levothyroxine, 182, 555
  chronic autoimmune thyroiditis, 295
  conditions altering, 297t
  congenital hypothyroidism, 285
  replacement doses, 296t
LHRH agonists
  CAH, 239
Lhx3, 11
Liddle's syndrome, 270
Liddle's test, 255
Lipids
  with Turner syndrome, 123
  therapy, 131–132
Lithium-induced nephrogenic diabetes
    insipidus, 169
Low-dose dexamethasone suppression
    test, 254
Lunelle, 485, 496

Lupron Depot-Pet
  CAH, 239
  CPP, 413
Luteinizing hormone releasing hormone (LHRH) agonists
  CAH, 239
Lymphedema
  with Turner syndrome, 119
    therapy, 125
Lymphocytic hypophysitis, 8

M
Macrobiotic diet, 367
Magnetic resonance imaging (MRI)
  adrenal insufficiency, 215
  Cushing syndrome, 255–256
  RTH, 317
Male condoms, 482
Male external genitalia, 436
Male genital and pubic hair development
  Tanner stages, 402f
Male hormone replacement, 181
Male pseudohermaphroditism, 442
Malignancy
  hypercalcemia, 358
Massive macronodular adrenal hyperplasia (MMAD), 251
McCune-Albright syndrome, 371, 415–416
Medroxyprogesterone acetate, 485
  CPP, 413
  FMPP, 417
  menstrual disorders, 472
Medullary thyroid carcinoma, 542
Medulloblastoma, 175–176, 176f
Meiosis
  abnormal pairing, 118
Melanocyte-stimulating hormone (MSH), 212
MEN. See Multiple endocrine neoplasia
Menorrhagia, 473
Menstrual cycle
  lengths, 452f
Menstrual disorders, 451–475
  causes, 453t
  differential diagnosis, 460–461
  etiology, 452–461
  management, 461–475
Metabolic disorders, 8

Metformin
  T2DM, 531–532
Metyrapone-induced adrenal insufficiency, 211
Metyrapone test
  adrenal insufficiency, 215
  Cushing syndrome, 257
Micropenis, 441
Midamor
  nephrogenic diabetes insipidus, 169
Mineralocorticoid
  CAH, 238
  mineralocorticoid excess, 267–270
Mineralocorticoid deficiency, 263–269
  clinical presentation, 265
  diagnosis, 266
  isolated, 264t
  molecular mechanisms, 264–265
  treatment, 266–267
Mineralocorticoid disorders, 261–270
Mineralocorticoid excess
  clinical presentation, 269
  diagnosis, 269–270
  molecular mechanisms, 268
  treatment, 270
Mirena, 484
Mixed gonadal dysgenesis, 443
MMAD, 251
MRI
  adrenal insufficiency, 215
  Cushing syndrome, 255–256
  RTH, 317
MSH, 212
Mucocutaneous candidiases
  age of onset, 349
Mullerian ducts, 435
Multiple endocrine neoplasia (MEN)
  syndromes, 535–545
  type 1, 536
    gastrinoma with Zollinger-Ellison syndrome, 538
    genetics, 540
    screening, 540–541, 541t
  type 2, 541–542
    clinical features, 542t
    genetic data, 544
    screening, 543–544
  type 2B, 359–360
Murine gene deletions
  growth, 81
Mycobacterium avium-intracellulare, 211

N

NCAH, 410–411
Neisseria meningitides, 211
Neonatal hypopituitarism, 517–518
Neonates
   calcium homeostasis, 346
   hypocalcemia
      causes, 351t
      classification, 350–351
      management, 355–356
   RTH, 318
   screening
      congenital hypothyroidism, 280–282
Nephrocalcinosis, 376
Nephrogenic diabetes insipidus, 157
   acquired
      causes, 159–160
   causes, 160t
   treatment, 169
Nervous system tumors recurrence following GH therapy, 23
Neurofibromatosis, 371
Nevi
   with Turner syndrome, 122
Newborn screening
   congenital hypothyroidism, 280–282
Nonclassical congenital adrenal hyperplasia (NCAH), 410–411
Non-GH deficient short stature, 68
Noninsulin-dependent diabetes mellitus. *See* Type 2 diabetes mellitus
Non-traumatic central diabetes insipidus, 157
Noonan's syndrome, 389
Norgestimate, 473
Normal variant short stature (NVSS), 67
Norplant, 485, 497–498
Nutritional deficiency rickets, 367, 369–370
NVSS, 67

O

Obesity
   with Turner syndrome, 123
      therapy, 131–132
OCPs, 484–485
   combination, 485
   menstrual disorders, 461, 472–473
oCRH
   stimulation test, 255
Octreotide hypoglycemic disorders, 519
Oligomenorrhea
   defined, 451
Oral contraceptive pills (OCPs), 484–485
   combination, 485
   menstrual disorders, 461, 472–473
Orthodontic problems
   with Turner syndrome, 121
      therapy, 130
Osteomalacia, 365
Osteopenia, 365
   anorexia nervosa, 193
Osteoporosis, 365
   anorexia nervosa, 194–195
Outpatient care
   T1DM, 530
Ovarian cysts, 415
Ovarian differentiation, 432–435
Ovarian hyperandrogenism
   functional
      causes, 459
Ovarian tumors
   precocious puberty, 417–418
Ovine corticotropin-releasing hormone (oCRH)
   stimulation test, 255

P

Paired internal ducts, 435
Pamidronate
   hypercalcemia, 361
Pancreatic beta-cell insulin secretion pathways, 517f
Pancreatic neuroendocrine tumors, 537–539
ParaGuard, 484
Parathyroid hormone (PTH)
   serum calcium, 344–345
Parathyroid hormone related protein (PTHrP), 344
Pars distalis, 3
Pars intermedia, 3
Pars tuberalis, 3
Partial growth hormone (GH) resistance, 53–54

PCOS, 456–458, 473
   manifestations, 457f
Pelvic inflammatory disease (PID), 482
Peptides, 3
Pergolide
   anterior pituitary tumors, 540
Periodic abstinence, 481
Peripheral precocious puberty, 414–422
Phenytoin-induced adrenal insufficiency, 211
Pheochromocytoma, 542–543
   screening, 544
Phosphopenic rickets, 366, 374–377
   heritable forms, 370–372
   nutritional phosphate deprivation, 374–375
   psychosocial considerations, 377–378
   X-linked hypophosphatemic, 375–376
PID, 482
Pioglitazone
   T2DM, 531–532
Pit-1, 11, 12f, 74
Pitressin Tannate, 165
Pituitary gland
   formation, 3
Pituitary transcription factor mutations, 9–10
Plasma acyl-carnitine profile, 520
Plasma renin activity (PRA), 229
Plasma vasopressin
   diabetes insipidus, 162
Polycystic ovary syndrome (PCOS), 456–458, 473
   manifestations, 457f
Polydipsia, 156
Polyglandular autoimmune disease I, 207
Polyglandular autoimmune disease III, 206–207
Polyglandular autoimmune syndromes
   psychosocial quality of life, 219
POPs, 485
Post-Nissen dumping hypoglycemia, 519
Postprandial hypoglycemia disorders, 519
PPNAD, 251
PRA, 229
Prader-Willi syndrome, 387
   body composition, 107–108

growth hormone therapy, 105–114
   body composition, 109–111
   linear growth, 108
   muscle strength and agility, 109–112
   safety, 112–114
linear growth, 106
Precocious puberty, 399–422
   brain tumors, 181
   defined, 404–405
   diagnosis, 420t–421t
   gonadotropin-dependent
      differential diagnosis, 406t
   gonadotropin-independent
      differential diagnosis, 407t
   hypothyroidism, 419, 419f
   peripheral, 414–422
Premature pubarche, 408–411
Premature pubertal development
   benign, 405–411
Premature thelarche, 405–408
Primary adrenal failure
   clinical presentation, 212–213
   therapy, 216
Primary adrenal insufficiency, 204
   etiology, 206–211
Primary amenorrhea
   defined, 451, 460
   differential diagnosis, 462f–463f
Primary hyperparathyroidism, 536–537, 543
Primary hypothyroidism
   cranial irradiation, 174
Primary pigmented adrenocortical nodular disease (PPNAD), 251
Primary polydipsia, 156
PRL, 3
Progestasert, 484
Progestin-only contraception, 496–497
Progestin only mini-pills (POPs), 485
Prolactin
   anorexia nervosa, 192
Prolactin (PRL), 3
Prop-1, 11, 74
Propylthiouracil
   Graves' disease, 300
Protectaid contraceptive sponge, 483

Pseudohermaphroditism
   female, 443
   male, 442
Pseudohypoaldosteronism, 266
Pseudohypoparathyroidism, 349
PTH
   serum calcium, 344–345
PTHrP, 344
Ptx2, 10
Pubertal development
   normal, 401–404
Pubertal disorders
   evaluation and treatment, 180–181
Puberty
   delayed. See Delayed puberty.
   precocious. See Precocious puberty.
Pubic hair development
   Tanner stages
      female, 403f
      male, 402f

R
Rachitic bone deformities, 367
Radioactive iodide uptake (RAIU), 299
Radioimmunoassays (RIAs), 15
Radioiodine therapy
   thyroid cancer, 333
Radiological tests
   adrenal insufficiency, 214–215
Radiotherapy
   endocrine system, 173–177
RAIU, 299
Reality female condom, 483
Recombinant human growth hormone
      targets, 21
Reductase deficiency, 390
Renal abnormalities
   with Turner syndrome, 122
      therapy, 131
Replacement growth hormone therapy, 179
Reproductive cancer
   hormonal contraceptives, 490–492
Resistance to thyroid hormone (RTH), 309–319
   clinical presentation, 313–314, 313t
   diagnostic considerations, 315–318
   mechanisms, 310–313
   therapy, 318–319

RIAs, 15
Rickets, 365–378. See also specific types
   biochemical abnormalities, 368–369
   causes, 366t
   history/physical exam, 367–372
   radiographic abnormalities, 368
   treatment, 372–378
Rickets-like disorders, 372
RIEG, 10
Rifampicin-induced adrenal
      insufficiency, 211
Ringworm, 253f
Rokitansky-Kustner-Hauser syndrome, 452
Rpx gene, 9
RTH. See Resistance to thyroid hormone

S
Saline infusion test, 163–164
Salt
   CAH, 238
Salt-wasting
   cerebral, 184
Salt-wasting crisis
   treatment, 266
Sandwich immunoradiometric assay, 344
Sarcoidosis, 8
SCFE
   following GH therapy, 24
Secondary adrenal failure
   clinical presentation, 213
Secondary adrenal insufficiency, 211–212
Secondary amenorrhea
   defined, 451
   differential diagnosis, 464f–465f
Self-monitoring of blood glucose
      (SMBG), 528
Serum calcium
   set point, 346
Serum lipids
   hormonal contraceptives, 488
Sex assignment decisions, 430
Sex determining genes, 434t
Sex-hormone-binding globulin
      (SHBG), 496
Sex of assignment
   defined, 437

Sex steroids
  CAH, 238
  exposure
    exogenous, 414
  priming, 17
Sex terminology, 436–437
Sexual differentiation, 431–436
  pathway, 433f
Sexual dimorphism, 446–447
Sexual orientation
  defined, 437
SHBG, 496
Short non-growth hormone (GH)
    deficient children, 21
Short stature
  psychosocial considerations, 72–73
  with Turner syndrome, 120–121
    therapy, 126–127
SHOX gene (Short Stature HOmeoboX-
    containing gene), 75
SIADH, 183–184
Sick day rules
  T1DM, 530–531
Skeletal abnormalities
  with Turner syndrome, 120–121
Skeletal age
  evaluation, 19
Skin cancer
  following GH therapy, 24
Skin disorders
  with Turner syndrome, 122
    therapy, 131
Slipped capital femoral epiphysis
    (SCFE)
  following GH therapy, 24
SMBG, 528
Smith-Lemli-Opitz syndrome, 209
Sodium iodide symporter, 277
Somatostatin (sst), 4–5
Somatotropin, 3
Somatotropin release-inhibiting factor
    (SRIF), 4–5
Spermicides, 481–482
Spironolactone
  AME, 270
  FMPP, 417
Sponge
  contraceptive, 482–483

Spontaneous growth hormone secretion
  overnight test, 17–18
Spot plasma ACTH, 255
SRIF, 4–5
SRY gene, 431–432
sst, 4–5
StAR, 209
Stature
  menstrual disorders, 471
  short. See Short stature.
Steroidogenic acute regulatory protein
    deficiency (StAR), 209
Steroids
  critical illness, 559
  safety, 130
Strabismus
  with Turner syndrome, 122
    therapy, 131
Stress replacement
  adrenal insufficiency, 216–218
Struma lymphomatosa, 291
Subclinical hyperthyroidism, 299
Sulfonylurea
  T2DM, 531–532
Surgery
  endocrine system, 176–177
  menstrual disorders, 471
  thyroid cancer, 332–333
Surgical resection
  Cushing syndrome, 257
Systemic disease
  delayed puberty, 384

T
T1DM, 523–524
  following GH therapy, 23
  treatment, 524–531
T2DM, 523–524
  treatment, 531–532
T3, 553
  postoperative cardiac patients, 555
T4, 553
Tanner-Whitehouse 2 (TW2) method, 19
Technetium (Tc99m) scan
  congenital hypothyroidism, 283
Tertiary adrenal insufficiency, 211–212
Testicular differentiation, 431–432
Testicular dysgenesis, 441
  causes, 435t

Testicular tumors
  precocious puberty, 418
Testolactone
  CAH, 219
  FMPP, 417
Testosterone, 177
  biosynthesis defects, 389–390
  delayed puberty, 394
Testosterone patches
  transdermal, 181
Testotoxicosis, 416–417
Thalassemia major, 8
Thiazide diuretics
  adverse effects, 169
Thromboembolism
  hormonal contraceptives, 486–487
Thymectomy
  primary hyperparathyroidism, 537
Thyroglobulin
  congenital hypothyroidism, 283
Thyroid
  newborn screening
    congenital hypothyroidism, 281–282
Thyroid axis, 553–557
  diagnosis, 554–555
  treatment, 555–556
Thyroid cancer, 327–337
  clinical presentation, 329–330
  diagnostic guidelines, 330–331
  follow-up, 336–337
  incidence, 328
  pathogenesis, 329
  patient characteristics, 328
  predisposing factors, 328–329
  recurrence, 332
  therapy, 331–336
Thyroid disease
  autoimmune, 291–304
Thyroid function
  drugs influencing, 556t
Thyroid hormone
  abnormalities
    anorexia nervosa, 191
  metabolism, 553f
  suppression
    thyroid cancer, 336
Thyroiditis
  autoimmune
    classification, 292t
    defined, 291
Thyroid releasing hormone (TRH)
  stimulation testing
    congenital hypothyroidism, 283
    RTH, 317
Thyroid scan-iodine (I-123) scan
  congenital hypothyroidism, 283
Thyroid-stimulating hormone (TSH), 3
  receptor mutations, 319–322
Thyrotoxicosis
  differential diagnosis, 299t
Thyrotropin, 3
Thyrotropin-receptor antibodies (TRAb)
  assays, 299
Thyrotropin receptor mutations, 319–322
  diagnostic considerations and therapy, 321–322
  mechanism, 320–321
Thyroxine (T4), 553
Today sponge, 483
Total adrenalectomy
  bilateral
    Cushing syndrome, 257
Total parathyroidectomy
  primary hyperparathyroidism, 537
Toxic Shock Syndrome (TSS), 483
TRAb assays, 299
Transdermal testosterone patches, 181
Transient neonatal hyperinsulinism, 517
Transsphenoidal surgery
  Cushing syndrome, 256
Trapazole
  Graves' disease, 300
TRH
  stimulation testing
    congenital hypothyroidism, 283
    RTH, 317
Triac, 319
Triiodothyronine (T3), 553
  postoperative cardiac patients, 555
Trilostane test
  Cushing syndrome, 257
True hermaphroditism, 443
True hypogonadism, 181

TSH, 3
  receptor mutations, 319–322
TSS, 483
Tumors
  precocious puberty, 417–419
Turner syndrome, 117–133, 388
  autoimmune disorders, 122–123
    therapy, 131
  clinical presentation, 119–125
  diagnosis, 125
  pathogenesis, 117–119
  therapy, 125–126
TW2 method, 19
24 hours urinary free cortisol excretion, 253
Type 1 diabetes mellitus (T1DM), 523–524
  following GH therapy, 23
  treatment, 524–531
Type 2 diabetes mellitus (T2DM), 523–524
  treatment, 531–532

U

Ultrasound
  Cushing syndrome, 256
Urinary free cortisol (UFC) excretion, 253
Urinary growth hormone, 18
Uterine aplasia, 452

V

Vaginal sponges, 482
Vanishing testes syndrome, 388
Vasopressin, 155–156, 162, 166t
  anorexia nervosa, 192
  central diabetes insipidus, 166t
  deficiency, 158
  plasma
    diabetes insipidus, 162
Vasopressin analog desmopressin, 165, 184
Vegetarian diet, 367
Virilizing tumors, 411
Vitamin D
  chronic hypocalcemia, 354
  deficiency
    hypocalcemia, 350
    treatment, 373
  excess, 358
  resistance
    hereditary, 370
  rickets
    hereditary treatment, 373–374
  serum calcium, 345
Vitamin D3 (cholecalciferol)
  serum calcium, 345–346

W

Water balance
  disorders, 183–184
  normal physiology, 155–156
Water deprivation test, 161–163
  endpoints, 163
Waterhouse-Friderichsen syndrome, 211
Weight gain
  hormonal contraceptives, 490
Williams syndrome
  hypercalcemia, 359
Wolffian ducts, 435
Wolman's disease, 210

X

XAHC, 209
X-ALD, 209
X chromosome gene
  haploinsufficiency, 117–118
XLH, 368, 370–371, 375–376
  therapy
    complications, 376
XLHN, 371
X-linked adrenal hypoplasia congenita (XAHC), 209
X-linked adrenoleukodystrophy (X-ALD), 209
X-linked hypercalciuric nephrolithiasis (XLHN), 371
X-linked hypophosphatemic rickets (XLH), 368, 370–371, 375–376
  therapy
    complications, 376
X-linked leukodystrophy, 219
XY testicular dysgenesis, 441
  causes, 435t